AF333836

AILMENTS OF AGING

FROM SYMPTOM TO TREATMENT

AILMENTS OF AGING

FROM SYMPTOM TO TREATMENT

Manuel M. Villaverde, M.D.
C. Wright MacMillan, M.D.

VAN NOSTRAND REINHOLD COMPANY
NEW YORK   CINCINNATI   ATLANTA   DALLAS   SAN FRANCISCO
LONDON   TORONTO   MELBOURNE

Van Nostrand Reinhold Company Regional Offices:
New York   Cincinnati   Atlanta   Dallas   San Francisco

Van Nostrand Reinhold Company International Offices:
London   Toronto   Melbourne

Copyright © 1980 by Litton Educational Publishing, Inc.

Library of Congress Catalog Card Number: 79-18553
ISBN: 0-442-25108-4

Manufactured in the United States of America

Published by Van Nostrand Reinhold Company
135 West 50th Street, New York, N.Y. 10020

Published simultaneously in Canada by Van Nostrand Reinhold Ltd.

15 14 13 12 11 10 9 8 7 6 5 4 3 2 1

Library of Congress Cataloging in Publication Data

Villaverde, Manuel Maria, 1905-
     Ailments of aging.

     Includes index.
     1. Geriatrics. 2. Aging. I. MacMillan, Charles
Wright, 1895-   joint author. II. Title. [DNLM:
1. Geriatrics.   WT100.3 V727a]
RC952.V45   618.9'7   79-18553
ISBN: 0-442-25108-4

Introduction

Aging is not felt, but suffered. For elderly persons, as a rule, boast of feeling young while complaining of pains here and there, tiredness, shortness of breath, and many other minor or major ailments. Certainly, aging begins at the time of conception, but the ravages of aging occur only after years of wear and tear—a variable time lapse, differing with each particular individual. Consequently, geriatrics, the medical specialty dealing with old age, should be considered as starting at a different time for each person. Geriatricians want to set a starting point that coincides with the climacterium, plus or minus five years: that is, from 40 to 50 years of age. This could have been true early in this century, when the life span was about 50 years. At the present time, when the life span averages a little over 70 years (somewhat more for women), the concept of when old age begins has to be changed. Of course, the climacterium (when the balance of endocrine functions changes, mainly gonadal and pituitary) will indicate the time of late maturity. Senescence and senility, synonyms meaning old age, are used by geriatricians to name the true start of old age—senescence—and the beginning of deterioration by age—senility, the latter at times also called involution.

Both senescence and involution vary considerably for each individual, and, at times, for different organic segments of the same individual. As a help in estimation of these conditions, the following figures may be useful:

Vital phase	*Starting age*
Climacterium	40 to 50 years
Senescence	50 to 60 years
Senility or involution	60 to 80 years

From the legal(?) point of view, old age begins at 65, the usual time for retirement. According to this view, 10% of the American population are elderly persons. Nevertheless, a large number of these persons are still capable of active and productive work because of their excellent physical condition. This time of life offers some actual advantages. In the first place, people enjoy better judgment and ability to interrelate facts. Studies * of I.Q. values at different stages of life showed that figures obtained in the early twenties were always inferior to those obtained 30 years later for the same individual, and equal or inferior after a 40-year interval only when some sort of organic decay had already taken place. Also noted was an improvement in interpretation of visual fields and better comprehension in analysis and criticism. The Bible supports this evaluation.

Among elderly persons many diseases show milder symptomatology, are chronic, and are frequently multiple. These persons may suffer any of the diseases common to man, some of which are very rare at this time, such as the eruptive fevers usually occurring in childhood, while others show a higher incidence or some peculiarities in their clinical course. Usually, the major geriatric problems are:

1. Circulatory disorders, mainly related to atherosclerosis, including hypertension, kidney diseases, and lesions affecting the brain, the coronary arteries, the retina, and the general circulation.
2. Metabolic disorders, presenting anemia, diabetes, gonadal disorders, and pituitary and other glandular diseases.
3. Arthritis.
4. Neoplasms.
5. Neurofunctional disorders.
6. Other diseases, such as prostatic, skin, gastrointestinal, and respiratory disorders.

To summarize: ailments of aging may start at any age; an attempt to predict a typical life chronology would be futile. Senescence and involution are individual patterns.

Consistent with the purposes of our program "From Symptom to Treatment," as presented in our previous books on *Pain* and *Fever,* the objective of this book is to evaluate symptoms and then to move to the next category—namely, treatment of ailments occurring during this late stage of life. As usual, the first part of the book deals with the pharmacology of drugs used. Since the ailments of aging will require almost any known medication, this part of our subject could include a complete treatise on pharmacology. However, since good books on pharmacology are available for the purpose, only the most frequently mentioned or needed drugs will be considered here. The second part will deal with diseases usually diagnosed during ailing aging, arranged according to the following categories: pain, unconsciousness,

---

* Studies made by Carl Eisdorfer and Wm. Owens, among others. See *A Good Age* by Dr. Alex Comfort or *Tests and Measurements* by Dr. Leona E. Tyler.

mental changes, neurological derangements, cough with or without expecto-ration and hoarseness, dyspnea, fever, hyper- and hypotension, ar-rhythmias, edema and changes of skin color, weight changes, tumors, ul-cers, other skin symptoms, and surgery for the elderly.

Manuel M. Villaverde
C. Wright MacMillan

Contents

AILMENTS OF AGING

FROM SYMPTOM TO TREATMENT

Part One

Pharmacology of Drugs Used in Gerontology

I. GENERAL INFORMATION

Drugs used for the treatment of elderly persons are the same as those used for the treatment of any other persons. Since we are dealing here with diseases that occur in the indefinite upper limits of life, almost any disease may be present, and all drugs used in pharmacology should be dealt with here. Of course, such a long list will not be considered, but only the most frequently prescribed, which will be presented in a very concise way: the essentials of indications, side effects, dosage and market presentation, all summarized, giving particular emphasis to use among older people.

Nevertheless, there are a few considerations that may help toward a better drug evaluation in these cases, and they are discussed in the following lines.

Personal Traits of the Individual Patient. There are some people whose age changes their susceptibility to drugs and who should be spared stress from unusual reactions.

Personal traits are important for accurate evaluation of changes and tolerances, both mental and physical. Dependability of character, such as reliability in following schedules and directions, and cheerful or pessimistic attitudes must be considered. Physical differences are also to be noted in the metabolism of drugs: weight and temperament affect the circulation and absorption of drugs; reactions of the nervous system to neurotropic drugs are varied. Previous signs of allergy should be carefully noted and prepared for.

Absorption of Drugs.   In the elderly, the absorption of drugs, particularly if given by mouth, is frankly slower. When a rapid response is needed, it is better to give the medication by the intravenous or subcutaneous route.

Elimination of Drugs.   Usually elimination is slower. This is a very important point: should a drug stay in the organism for a longer period, dosage and frequency of administration must be changed accordingly—namely, smaller dosage and less frequent intake.

Response.   Individual response to drugs is frequently changed by age and must be re-evaluated as to strength of drug action. There is a tendency, for instance, to increased action from cardiotonics, barbiturates, tranquilizers, bromides, and potassium cyanates and less effect from the opiates, histamines, and insulin.

Side Effects.   As the above statements would indicate, side effects are often exaggerated; but in regarding these symptoms do not rely entirely on the patient's complaints, but actively watch and check for any possible undesirable effects, particularly those of a serious nature. A case in point is that of a much feared gastrointestinal irritation, which not rarely will be followed by ulceration and bleeding after the use of acetylsalicylic acid, corticoids, reserpine, indomethacin, phenylbutazone, and others. Antacids may induce constipation (aluminum, calcium) or diarrhea (magnesium); laxatives may result in electrolyte depletion, or abnormal bowel motility. Also, hypotension is to be watched for when sedatives or tranquilizers are given, and urinary retention or glaucoma when anticholinergics are used. Agranulocytosis may result from amidopyrin, phenylbutazone, or chlorpromazine.

Dosage.   Since there is usually a reduction in elimination and possibly an individual reduced tolerance, dosage will always be established at the lower levels for all elderly persons, with particular attention paid to the small, the frail, and the ailing. Of course, as noted above, special care will be observed if there is renal insufficiency or any other chronic depleting condition.

Poly-pharmacy.   At the time of scheduling a treatment, most physicians will prescribe a number of drugs, very frequently more than two. The simultaneous use of two or more medicaments among the elderly has to be especially watched for intolerance and side effects. For this reason, it is better to keep the number of different medications to a workable minimum in all instances. The harmful interaction of drugs is more marked in these patients.

Aims of Geriatric Therapeutics.   As with any other patient, the principal aim has to be (1) to cure, but if this is not feasible—as so frequently it is not—at least (2) to improve, or (3) to encourage! In any instance, the very important considerations are the following:

Do not rely on self-administration of drugs when the patient may be forgetful or stubborn. Usually, when age starts to deteriorate the patient, forgetfulness is a necessary consequence; and those with even a moderate arteriosclerosis will actually skip more than one dose, if left alone.

Keep a careful watch at all times for any sort of side effects, or true toxic effects. Many of the aged will not give adequate information when it is needed. Their symptoms are not marked enough, or their sensitivity could be blurred so as to mask them.

Avoid continuing patients on bed rest, particularly when they are receiving sedatives, tranquilizers, or any other psychotropic drug, because depressions are very easily caused by these drugs as well as occurring spontaneously.

Carefully regulate all dosages, as suggested above.

Finally, it is necessary to be on the alert for the interaction of drugs, particularly when one of them may potentiate dangerous reactions of others, such as hypnotics showing greater power if given concomitantly with phenothiazines.

II. SULFONAMIDES

Sulfanilamides are derivatives of paraaminobenzenesulfonamide (sulfanilamid), usually white or white-yellowish crystalline powders, easily made soluble when changed to the corresponding sodium salts. They are bacteriostatic agents; and at high concentration in the urine may become bactericidal. Sensitive agents become resistant very frequently. Reciprocally, there are substances that can help to antagonize sulfonamide resistance activity. The *absorption* of most sulfonamides given orally or parenterally is rapid, with the exception of those used for gastrointestinal problems, which are poorly absorbed or not absorbed at all in the intestinal tract. Also, they are rapidly absorbed when injected subcutaneously. They *diffuse* throughout all fluids, tissues, and organs, including the cerebrospinal fluid.

Adverse Reactions. One of the adverse reactions to sulfa drugs is the production of crystalluria and renal stones. Drinking large quantities of water helps to solve the problem. Sensitivity reactions of the allergic type, including severe or deadly anaphylactic shock, do not occur frequently. Fever, purpura, pallor, and jaundice will warn of blood dyscrasias, as agranulocytosis and aplastic anemia. Blood disturbances are not rare complications, so blood counts should be done frequently during this therapy. Watch out also for thrombocytopenia, leukopenia, hypoprothrombinemia, hemolytic anemia, rashes, erythema multiforme (of the Stevens-Johnson type), serum sickness, exfoliative dermatitis, edema (mainly periorbital), eye inflammation, arthralgia, stomatitis, thyroid reactions, pancreatitis, hepatitis, gastrointestinal complaints, headache, neuritis, depression, or toxic nephrosis. When treating elderly persons, be extremely cautious.

Selection of a Sulfa Drug.   Response to sulfa therapy is expected for certain infections. Cultures and sensitivity tests should be performed, but the clinician cannot always rely on them because of lack of time. They can be repeatedly performed, but must be correlated with clinical results. It will be noted that resistant strains develop with relative ease, particularly when treating chronic or recurrent infections. Selection is based on absorption, distribution, excretion, and particular efficiency of each sulfa for a given disease.

In general, sulfa drugs are used for the treatment of urinary infections, meningitis, and otitis media, as follows: urinary tract infections due to *E. coli, Streptococcus* (mainly group A), *Staphylococcus aureus, Klebsiella,* and *Proteus;* meningeal infections due to any of the above, plus *H. influenzae;* and other infections due to *P. falciparum* (or resistant to chloroquine), malaria in general, chancroid, nocardiosis, toxoplasmosis (together with pyrimethamine), trachoma, inclusion conjunctivitis, and lymphogranulomatosis.

A more complete sulfa antibacterial spectrum follows:

Pneumococci
E. coli (some strains)
Streptococcus (mainly group A)
Staphylococcus aureus
Klebsiella
Proteus
B. anthracis (some strains)
H. influenzae
H. ducreyi
Brucella
C. diphtheriae
V. comma
P. pestis
Shigella (not all strains)
Actinomyces
Nocardia
D. granulomatosis
N. gonorrhoeae (many resistant strains)
A. aerogenes
P. aeruginosa
Agents causing trachoma, inclusion conjunctivitis and lymphogranuloma
   venereum

Classification of Sulfonamides.   There are three main groups:

1. *Poorly absorbed sulfas* (for gastrointestinal use: succinylsulfathiazole, phthalylsulfathiazole, sulfasalazine.
2. *Rapidly absorbed sulfas:* rapidly excreted—sulfadiazine, sulfamer-

azine, sulfamethazine, sulfamethizole, sulfisoxazole, sulfachlorpyridazine, sulfacyctine, sulfa mixtures; slowly excreted—sulfamethoxazole, sulfaethiodole.

3. *Long-acting sulfonamides:* sulfamethoxypyridazine, sulfadimethoxine.

GASTROINTESTINAL USE (POOR ABSORPTION)

Succinylsulfathiazole

Brand name: Sulfasuxidine. This is a sulfa derivative employed in gastrointestinal infections. Because of its delayed absorption, high concentrations are obtained in the intestinal lumen, especially the colon. Succinylsulfathiazole may be indicated as a prophylactic in surgery of the colon, and in bacillary dysentery, particularly in cases of *Shigella flexneri* or *Shigella sonnei.*

Dosage: 250 mg per kilo of body weight, the whole amount given as a starting dose, and then one sixth of the total given every 4 hours. Sulfadiazine, however, is considered a superior alternative.

Succinylsulfathiazole, tablets, 300 or 500 mg each.

Phthalylsulfathiazole

Brand name: Sulfathalidine. This drug is used only in intestinal infections with ulcerative lesions, or for prophylaxis in colon surgery. It is not recommended for shigellosis.

Dosage: 125 mg for each kilo of body weight, in divided doses.

Phthalylsulfathiazole, 500 mg tablets

Sulfasalazine (Salicylazosulfapyridine)

This drug is recommended as an adjunct therapy for ulcerative colitis. Other qualities correspond to what is generally known about sulfas.

Dosage: from 4000 to 8000 mg (if needed, 12,000 mg can be given) in 24 hours, in divided doses, every 3 to 6 hours. Larger doses may be given in severe cases. Following acute attacks, maintenance dosage may be 500 mg every 6 hours. Results will determine further dosage.

Sulfasalazine, 500 mg tablets (Brand name: S.A.S. 500)

RAPIDLY ABSORBED AND EXCRETED SULFAS

These short-acting sulfas are preferred for the treatment of systemic or urinary infections.

Sulfadiazine

This is the most widely used sulfa, rapidly absorbed, widely diffused, and promptly excreted.

Dosage: oral administration is preferred, at all times, and as soon as possible after the parenteral route is first used, 4000 mg to start, and thereafter 1000 mg every 4 hours; in urinary infections, 1000 mg every 6 hours, with no need of a "loading dose"; but when therapy may extend for months, use only 1000 mg every 24 hours. Parenteral administration: better by intravenous injection (never intrathecally!) in concentrations up to 5 %, administered very slowly (at least 10 minutes), and at a dosage of no more than 5000 mg (100 mg for each kilo of body weight) to start, followed by individual doses of 0.03 to 0.05% per kilo of body weight every 6 or 8 hours; change to oral therapy as soon as possible (in about 24 hours).

Sulfadiazine, 300 or 500 mg tablets.

Sulfadiazine, oral suspension, 500 mg per 5 ml.

Sodium sulfadiazine injection, ampoules of 10 ml, each ml containing 250 mg.

Sulfisoxazole

Brand names: Gantrisin, SK-Soxazole, Soxomide. Sulfisoxazole is used to treat infections usually responsive to sulfas.

Dosage: start the oral route with 2000 to 4000 mg, at once, and thereafter every 4 to 6 hours to reach 4000 to 8000 mg in 24 hours. If acetyl sulfisoxazole forms with delayed absorption are used, give 4000 to 5000 mg every 12 hours. Subcutaneous injections: dilute to 5% the 40% solution (combine a 5-ml ampoule with 35 ml of sterile water—or a 10-ml one with 70 ml of water) and give 100 mg per kilo of body weight in 24 hours; start with half the daily dose, and follow with one third of the dose every 8 hours. Intramuscular injection: undiluted ampoules will be used, but no more than 5 ml are to be injected in one site, the total daily dose is divided into two or three installments. Intravenous injection: same dosage as for subcutaneous administration, but the injection is to be given very slowly or, preferably, by infusion.

Sulfisoxazole, 500 mg tablets.

Sulfisoxazole, syrup containing 500 mg in each 5 ml (long-acting acetyl form).

Sulfisoxazole, 1000 mg in each 5 ml of injectable suspension (long-acting acetyl form).

Sulfisoxazole, 200 mg in 5-ml or 4000 mg in 10-ml ampoules (400 mg in each ml).

Sulfamethizole

Brand names: Thiosulfil, Thiosulfil Forte. This drug is used for the treatment of susceptible infections of the gastrointestinal tract, usually due to the following microorganisms: *E. coli, Staphylococcus* (mainly *S. aureus*), *Proteus* (not all strains), *Klebsiella,* and *Aerobacter.*

The diseases of the urinary tract that may respond to sulfamethizole are pyelonephritis, pyelitis, and cystitis.

Dosage: 500 to 1000 mg every 6 to 8 hours.

Sulfamethizole, tablets with 250 or 500 mg each.

Sulfachlorpyridazine

Brand name: Sonilyn. This drug is indicated in urinary tract infections, as above. Also, it is used for the treatment of other diseases responsive to sulfas.

Dosage: 2000 to 4000 mg to start, followed by the same amount every 24 hours, in divided doses.

Sulfachlorpyridazine, 500 mg tablets.

Sulfacytine

Brand name: Renoquid. This drug is mainly indicated for the treatment of pyelonephritis, pyelitis, and cystitis due to *E. coli, Proteus, Staphylococcus aureus,* and *Klebsiella.* Side effects are as with other sulfas (watch for crystalluria and blood dyscrasias).

Dosage: 500 mg to start, followed by 250 mg every 6 hours for about 10 days.

Sulfacytine, 250 mg tablets.

Sulfa Mixtures

Sulfa mixtures are frequently used, in order to reach the same results with lower amounts of each individual sulfa. This will protect against precipitation of crystals or growth of stones in the urinary tract. Usually, three different sulfas are mixed; occasionally, two. Sulfadiazine is present in practically all these mixtures. Sulfamerazine or sulfacetamide is generally the second drug. When a third drug is added, sulfamethazine is the usual selection.

Dosage: an initial total dose of 3000 to 4000 mg, followed by 1000 mg every 6 hours.

Sulfadiazine and sulfamerazine tablets.

Sulfadiazine, sulfamerazine, and sulfamethazine tablets.

Sulfadiazine, sulfamerazine, and sulfacetamide tablets.

There are mixtures of a sulfa (sulfamethoxazole) and a pyrimidine (trimethoprim), q.v. in the section on urinary antiseptics, with good activity as anti-infective agents.

RAPIDLY ABSORBED AND SLOWLY EXCRETED SULFAS

These sulfas have the advantage of maintaining high blood levels with only one or two doses a day, but the long-lasting high blood levels are an obstacle to treatment in the case of a severe reaction against the drug. They are of value for prophylactic or prolonged administration.

Sulfamethoxazole

Brand name: Gantanol. Administration will start with 2000 mg and will be followed by 1000 mg every 12 hours, for urinary and systemic infections. In no instance should a daily intake exceed 3000 mg. Uses are the same as for sulfisoxazole, q.v.

Sulfamethoxazole, 500 mg tablets.

Sulfamethoxazole, oral suspension containing 500 mg in each 5 ml.

LONG-ACTING SULFAS

Most sulfas with a slow excretion rate could be considered long-acting sulfas. Nevertheless, true long-acting sulfas have a half-life of 30 to 40 hours and are administered only once a day. The risk of reactions, which is thus maintained because of the long time the medication is in the blood, seriously curtails their use.

Sulfamethoxypyridazine

Brand names: Kynex, Midicol. This sulfa is advisable for prophylaxis and for prolonged therapy, provided low doses are always given, particularly in urinary infections. Specially sensitive to sulfamethoxypyridazine are *E. coli, B. proteus, Staphylococcus aureus,* gonococci, and dysenteric bacteria. Of course, special care in watching for complications will be observed.

Dosage: for prophylaxis give 500 mg, once a day; for treatment, 2000 mg to start, followed by 1000 mg once a day for no more than 1 week; then discontinue, or follow with 500 mg a day.

> Sulfamethoxypyridazine, 500 mg tablets.
> Sulfamethoxypyridazine, oral suspension containing 250 mg in each 5 ml.

Sulfadimethoxine

Brand name: Madribon. This sulfa presents similar properties to those of sulfamethoxypyridazine (q.v. above) and is particularly useful in infections due to pneumococci, *H. influenzae, Salmonella, Shigella,* staphylococci, and the usual gram-negative bacteria. Nevertheless, it will not be used when a safer sulfa is available for the individual patient.

Dosage: 100 mg, to be followed by 500 mg once a day. A double amount might be needed in severe infections.

> Sulfadimethoxine, 500 mg tablets.

> Sulfadimethoxine, oral suspension containing 250 mg in each 5 ml.

Sulfaethiodole

This is not a long-acting sulfa, but is suspended in a sustained-action formulation for slower release. The dosage is 4000 mg to start, followed by 2000 mg every 12 hours.

III. ANTIBIOTICS

Differing from disinfectants and similar substances, antibiotics act in very small amounts by interfering with the physiology of the bacterial cell wall and the general metabolism of disease-causing organisms, while they do little or no harm to cells and tissues of the host, except for those adverse reactions induced in some instances by allergy.

Classification of Antibiotics. For clinical purposes the best approach is to consider bactericidal and bacteriostatic antibiotics.

Bactericidal antibiotics interfere with chemical processes essential to the life of the bacterial cell, thus destroying the basic bacterial organism. The bacterial antibiotics are:

> Penicillin (penicillin G, penicillin V, ampicillin, amoxacillin, oxacillin, methicillin, napcillin, cloxacillin, carbenicillin, and also dicloxacillin and phenethicillin).

> Aminoglycosides (streptomycin, dihydrostreptomycin, gentamycin, kanamycin, neomycin, paromomycin, amikacin).

Polypeptides (bacitracin, colistin, polymyxin B, viomycin).

Cephalosporins (cephalothin, cephaloridine, cephalexin, cephaloglycin).

Vancomycin.

Cycloserine.

Bacteriostatic antibiotics interfere with metabolic cell reactions, making growth impossible. The bacteriostatic antibiotics are:

Tetracyclines (tetracycline, oxytetracycline, chlortetracycline, doxycycline).

Macrolides (erythromycin, oleandomycin, troleandomycin).

Chloramphenicol.

Rifampin.

Lincomycin.

Clindamycin.

Novobiocin.

Selection of an Antibiotic.   After the diagnosis of an infectious disease is established, all efforts should be made to find the antibiotics to which that germ is *sensitive*. Most frequently, it will be good practice to give antibiotherapy at once in adequate *dosage* with the drug most carefully selected at that time, until reports are received pointing out the preferred one; but use this therapy only for those cases which really *need* it, to avoid the growth of *resistant* strains. The *side-effects* will be very carefully watched, particularly for those well-known dangerous antibiotics, and always weighed against "to give or not to give." It is well established that at times a *combination* of at least two antibiotics is more efficient for best results.

The table giving "Susceptibility of Germs to Antibiotics" will help in selection of an adequate antibiotic for initial therapy before the specific one is known. When there is reasonable doubt, *broad-spectrum antibiotics* will be administered, such as the tetracyclines and chloramphenicol.

With respect to established clinical entities, the next table, on "Selecting Antibiotherapy in Cases of Diseases," will also be a very good help.

Use and Misuse of Antibiotics.   When the decision to use an antibiotic has been made, its administration will start immediately, using the right dosage and the appropriate route: in mild to moderate infections, the average dosage, and in severe ones, an appropriately higher dosage. These high dosages require a return to average medication when symptoms abate. Any dosage will be maintained until about 2 days after the clinical picture subsides, unless it is known that prolonged therapy is needed. Oral medication will not be given to those who have nausea, and avoid injections in persons with bleeding tendencies. Above all, avoid giving antibiotics that will cause an allergic reaction. Also, stop antibiotics as soon as they provoke any sort of untoward reaction, and use combined antibiotics whenever advisable.

It is generally useless to treat viral infections with antibiotics, but psittacosis, a typical viral pneumonia (mycoplasma), lymphogranuloma venereum, and trachoma usually respond to broad-spectrum antibiotics. It is

Susceptibility of Germs to Antibiotics

Germ	Antibiotic
Actinomyces	Penicillin—Tetracycline
Bacillus anthracis	Penicillin—Erythromycin
Bacteroides	Clindamycin—Chloramphenicol
Borrelia	Tetracycline—Penicillin
Brucella	Tetracycline plus streptomycin
Chlamydia	Tetracycline—Sulfa
Clostridium	Penicillin—Tetracycline
Corynebacterium	Erythromycin—Penicillin
Enterobacter	Kanamycin—Gentamycin
Enterococcus	Ampicillin plus aminoglycoside
Escherichia coli	Kanamycin—Sulfa
Gonococcus	Penicillin—Ampicillin
Hemophilus	Ampicillin—Chloramphenicol
Klebsiella	A cephalosporin—Kanamycin
Leptospira	Penicillin—Tetracycline
Listeria	Ampicillin plus aminoglycoside
Meningococcus	Penicillin—Chloramphenicol
Mima-Herellea	Cephalosporin—Kanamycin
Mycobacterium leprae	Sulfone drugs
Mycobacterium tuberculosis	Antitubercular combination
Mycoplasma	Tetracycline—Erythromycin
Nocardia	Sulfa—Tetracycline
Pasteurella	Streptomycin plus tetracycline
Pneumococcus	Penicillin—Erythromycin
Proteus mirabilis	Penicillin—Ampicillin
Proteus vulgaris, etc.	Kanamycin—Carbenicillin
Pseudomonas aeruginosa	Polymixin B—Gentamycin
Pseudomonas pseudomallei	Tetracycline plus sulfa
Pseudomonas mallei	Streptomycin plus tetracycline
Rickettsia	Tetracycline—Chloramphenicol
Salmonella	Chloramphenicol—Ampicillin
Serratia	Gentamycin—Kanamycin
Shigella	Ampicillin—Chloramphenicol
Spirochete (Treponema)	Penicillin—Erythromycin
Staphylococcus	Penicillin—Penicillase-resistant penicillin
Streptococcus	Penicillin—Erythromycin-Cephalosporin

Selecting Antibiotherapy in Cases of Disease

Disease/agent	First Choice	Alternate
Gram-positive agents:		
Pneumonia	Penicillin	Erythromycin
Streptococcal infections	Penicillin	Erythromycin or a cephalosporin
Staphylococcal infections	Oxacillin	A cephalosporin, vancomycin, or lincomycin
Actinomycosis	Penicillin	A tetracycline
Anthrax	Penicillin	Erthromycin
Diphtheria	Erythromycin or penicillin	A cephalosporin (always use antitoxin!)
Tetanus	Penicillin	A tetracycline
Gas gangrene	Penicillin	A tetracycline (always use antitoxin!)
Listeriosis	Ampicillin plus aminoglycoside	A tetracycline
Enterococcal infections	Ampicillin plus aminoglycoside	Penicillin plus gantamycin
Tuberculosis	INH plus rifampin or ethambutol	Three of the anti-tubercular drugs
Glanders (farcy)	Streptomycin plus a tetracycline	Chloramphenicol, sulfa
Leprosy	A sulfone	Other sulfone
Gram-negative agents:		
Gonorrhea	Penicillin or ampicillin	A tetracycline
Meningitis	Penicillin	Chloramphenicol
Salmonellosis	Chloramphenicol or ampicillin	
Shigellosis	Ampicillin	A tetracycline, chloramphenicol
Cholera	A tetracycline	Chloramphenicol
Brucellosis	A tetracycline, with or without streptomycin	Chloramphenicol
Gastrointestinal infections	Kanamycin or gentamycin	Chloramphenicol or ampicillin
Genitourinary infections	Trimethoprim (sulfa)	Ampicillin
Chancroid	A tetracycline	Streptomycin or a sulfa
Whooping cough	Erythromycin	Ampicillin
Hemophilus influenzae	Ampicillin	Chloramphenicol

Selecting Antibiotherapy in Cases of Disease (*Continued*)

Disease/Agent	First Choice	Alternate
Plague	Streptomycin plus a tetracycline	A sulfa
Tularemia	Streptomycin plus a tetracycline	A sulfa
Granuloma inguinale	Chloramphenicol or a tetracycline	Streptomycin
Spirochetes and others:		
Syphilis	Penicillin	Erythromycin or tetracycline
Pinta, yaws, bejel	Penicillin	Erythromycin or tetracycline
Relapsing fever	A tetracycline	Penicillin
Leptospirosis	Penicillin	A tetracycline
Nocardiosis	A sulfa	A tetracycline
Rickettsial	A tetracycline	Erythromycin
Psittacosis, trachoma	A tetracycline or a sulfa	Erythromycin
Lymphogranulomatosis	A tetracycline or a sulfa	Erythromycin
Mycoplasma	A tetracycline	Erythromycin

dangerous, without close monitoring, to use most antibiotics on patients with impaired renal function, particularly in elderly persons, as that condition will increase the concentration of the drug in the blood. Finally, either large or small amounts are equally wrong; the recognized adequate dosage should always be given, keeping in mind the dangers of overdosage, underdosage, and length of administration.

THE PENICILLIN GROUP

All penicillins act by preventing the formation of a rigid cell wall, thus making impossible the life of susceptible germs; but penicillinase-producing organisms will become resistant because the antibiotic is destroyed by the enzyme.

All the penicillin injected is rapidly absorbed, widely distributed in the body, and rapidly excreted in the urine. Kidney diseases, most frequently among the elderly, may impair excretion and keep large amounts of penicillin in the blood. When it is given by the oral route, the absorption of penicillin is notably decreased, but special forms have been developed for better gastrointestinal absorption.

Dosages vary for the different penicillins and for different diseases: low ranges in mild or moderate infections, higher ones for severe diseases, but, in all instances, adequate doses. Kidney insufficiency requires a reduction in dosage, since the drug is stored in the blood for a longer period, particularly in the older patient.

Adverse reactions to penicillin are mainly allergic. Anaphylactic shock may occur, even with oral penicillin; it should not be used when there is a history of previous reactions, nor should it be given to asthmatic patients. Other reactions are nausea, vomiting, diarrhea, black tongue, dermic reactions (particularly urticaria), and, the most serious, laryngeal edema. Hemolytic anemia, thrombocytopenia, and mental reactions may also occur. Treatment will be carried out with antihistaminics, corticosteroids, or epinephrine. *Penicillinase* should be tried in anaphylactic reactions because this enzyme can decrease blood levels of active penicillin, but it will be given only after epinephrine and other measures against shock are put into use. It is not entirely reliable.

> Penicillinase, 800,000-unit vials (to prepare 2 ml solution), repeat, if needed, after 3 days.

Germs and Diseases Sensitive to Penicillin.   The following lists present: (1) microorganisms usually sensitive to penicillin, (2) diseases provoked by such microorganisms, and (3) those responsive only to high intravenous doses:

1. Streptococci, mainly groups A, C, G, H, L, and M
   Staphylococci, except penicillinase-producing staphylococci
   Pneumococci
   Treponema pallidum, usually very sensitive to penicillin
   Other treponemas, pinta, yaws, bejel
   Neisseria gonorrhoeae
   Corynebacterium diphtheriae
   Leptospira
   Bacillus anthracis
   Clostridia
   Listeria monocytogenes
   Actinomyces bovis
   Streptobacillus moniliformis
   Fusobacterium fusiforme and *Borrelia vincentii* found together in Vincent's angina)
2. Infections of the upper respiratory tract
   Pneumonia
   Scarlet fever
   Erysipelas
   Vincent's angina (try to avoid using antibiotics!)
   Skin infections
   Prophylactic for rheumatic fever

Prophylactic for bacterial endocarditis
Prophylactic for surgical patients
Syphilis
Pinta, yaws, bejel
Rat-bite fever
Anthrax
Actinomycosis
Diphtheria
Tetanus
Gas gangrene
Gonorrhea
Meningitis
Leptospirosis

3. Salmonellae
Shigellae
Escherichia coli
Proteus mirabilis
Aerobacter aerogenes
Alcaligenes faecalis

Penicillin G

Brand names: Pentids, Pfizerpen G, QID pen G. This drug is rapidly absorbed from the duodenum and from injections. Large intravenous doses are to be injected very slowly, and better given by infusion. Topical applications are not recommended. If given by mouth (preferably the buffered tablets), it should be taken about 1 hour before or 3 hours after meals. This route is reserved only for minor infections. The injectables are diluted with sodium chloride solution, and can be given by any route, including intrathecally.

Crystalline penicillin G, tablets, with 200,000, 250,000, 400,000, or 500,000 units each.

Crystalline penicillin G, powder for oral suspension, 200,000, 250,000, or 400,000 units in each 5 ml, in vials to contain 60 ml, 80 ml, or 150 ml, respectively; to reconstitute immediately before use.

Crystalline penicillin G, aqueous suspension, 300,000 units in each ml, 10-ml vial, for injection.

Crystalline penicillin G, vials containing 200,000, 500,000, 1 million, 5 million, 10 million, or 20 million each, for injection.

Buffered potassium penicillin G, tablets with 200,000, 250,000, or 400,000 units each.

Buffered potassium penicillin G, powder, to provide 200,000 or 400,000 units in each 5 ml of prepared liquid.

Potassium penicillin G, powder, to provide 1,5, 10, or 20 million units for each vial, to give by infusion or intramuscularly (the 10 or 20 million units dose, only by infusion).

Repository Preparations of Penicillin G

Brand names: for procaine penicillin—Duracillin AS, Crysticillin 300 AS, Crysticillin 600 AS, Wycillin; for benzathine penicillin—Bicillin.

Procaine penicillin is slowly absorbed, and is to be given solely by intramuscular injection. In general, two injections of 600,000 units a day will suffice for infections of moderate severity. *Benzathine* penicillin has a very low water solubility, and its activity is longer-lasting than that of procaine penicillin, of which an injection of 600,000 units is usually given once a day. With benzathine penicillin, injections of 1.2 to 2.4 million units can be given. Used for prophylactic purposes, these dosages need not be repeated more often than every 3 or 4 weeks. Adverse reactions are the same as with other penicillins.

Dosage: for penicillin G administration, when given by injection (only intramuscularly for procaine or benzathine penicillin G suspensions):

Streptococcal infections: 600,000 to 1.2 million units a day, for at least 10 days.

Staphylococcal infections: same as above.

Pneumococcal pneumonia: same doses as above, to continue 2 days after all symptoms have subsided.

Treponema infections: 600,000 units a day, for a total of 8 days; up to 15 days in cases of tertiary or neurological syphilis.

Gonorrhea: inject 2.4 million units into each buttock (a total of 4.8 million). It is advised that 1 g probenecid be given half an hour before penicillin.

Diphtheria: 300,000 to 600,000 units a day until the disease clears up; to be given together with antitoxin.

Leptospirosis: up to 6 to 12 million units a day, starting before the fourth day of the disease, by intramuscular or intravenous injection.

Anthrax: as for pneumococcal pneumonia, above.

Tetanus: as for pneumococcal pneumonia, above; but always given together with antitoxin (prefer human tetanus immune globulin).

Rat-bite fever: as for pneumococcal pneumonia, above.

Vincent's angina: as for pneumococcal pneumonia, above, whenever penicillin is advisable.

Preparations include:

Procaine penicillin G, 300,000 units in 1 ml, in 10-ml vials or 1-ml ampoules.

Procaine penicillin G, 600,000 units in 1.2 ml, in 12-ml vials, or 1-ml ampoules or 1.2-ml ampoules.

Procaine penicillin G, 1.2 million units in 2 ml or 2.4 million units in 4 ml.

Benzathine penicillin G, 300,000 or 600,000 units for each ml, in 1- or 2-ml ampoules; also in individual dosages of 1.2 million or 2.4 million units.

Buffered sodium penicillin G, 5 million units in each vial, for intravenous or intramuscular injection.

Penicillin V (Phenoxymethyl Penicillin)

Brand names: Betapen VK, Compocillin VK, Ledercillin VK, Penapar VK, Pfizerpen VK, Pen Veek, QID pen VK, Robicillin VK, SK penicillin VK™, Uticillin VK, V-cellin F, Veetids. Penicillin V can be given orally in cases of infections due to susceptible streptococci, staphylococci, pneumococci, *Neisseria gonorrhoeae, Treponema pallidum, Leptospira, Corynebacterium diphtheriae, Bacillus anthracis, Actinomyces bovis, clostridia,* and *Listeria monocytogenes.* It should be given, preferably on an empty stomach, only to patients with mild infections; and in no instance to patients during the acute stage of pneumonia, bacteremia, meningitis, empyema, or pericarditis. Also it can be used when prolonged or prophylactic therapy is indicated.

Adverse reactions are of the same type as for any other penicillin, from mildly allergic to very serious anaphylactic shock.

Dosage: varies from 125 mg every 8 hours to 250 mg every 6 hours, usually for 10-day periods; different dosages can also be used.

Streptococcal infections: 125 to 250 mg every 6 to 8 hours, for at least 10 days.

Staphylococcal infections: as above.

Pneumococcal pneumonia: 250 mg every 6 to 8 hours, until 2 days after subsidence of all symptoms.

Treponema infections: give injections.

Gonorrhea: give injections.

Diphtheria: give injections.

Leptospirosis: give injections.

Anthrax: give injections.

Tetanus: give injections.

Rat-bite fever: give injections.

Vincent's angina: 250 mg every 6 to 8 hours, until 2 days after all symptoms subside.

Preparations include:

Penicillin V, 250 or 500 mg tablets.

Penicillin V, powder, to prepare solutions containing 125 or 250 mg in each 5 ml (each bottle will contain 100, 150, or 200 ml of liqsid).

Ampicillin

Brand names: Alpen, Omnipen, Omnipen N, Pen A, Penbritin, Principen, Principen N, QID amp, Totacillin. Ampicillin is active against some germs that do not respond to regular penicillin, or respond mildly. This list contains the following microorganisms: *Salmonella, Shigella, Escherichia coli, Proteus mirabilis, enterococcus,* and *Hemophylus influenzae,* which may cause infections of the gastrointestinal, the genitourinary, or the respiratory tracts. The drug may be given by mouth, but in severe cases, treatment should start by injection (either intramuscular, intravenous, or by continuous drip). It is best to resort to the oral route as soon as possible.

Dosage: Orally—500 mg every 6 hours, for most diseases. Respiratory diseases may respond to half the dosage. For gonorrhea, a single 3500-mg dose together with 1000 mg probenecid. Parenterally—50 mg every 6 hours; respiratory infections require 250 to 500 mg every 6 hours; in cases of gonorrhea, two injections of 500 mg 12 hours apart (intramuscularly).

Ampicillin, 250 or 500 mg capsules.

Ampicillin, 125 or 250 mg for each 5 ml of the oral suspension (bottles furnished to contain 80, 100, or 200 ml after reconstitution).

Ampicillin, 125, 250, 500, or 1000 mg vials for injection (also 2000 mg for infusions).

Amoxicillin

Brand names: Larotid (formerly Larocin), Amoxil, Polymox. Amoxicillin is an analog of ampicillin, also active against many gram-positive and gram-negative microorganisms, and resistant to gastric juices. It is not active against penicillinase-producing staphylococci, and is not indicated for the treatment of shigellosis, as ampicillin is. It is a good alternate for infections due to *H. influenzae, E. coli, N. gonorrhoeae, P. mirabilis, D. pneumoniae,* and streptococci.

Dosage: from 250 mg (milder cases) to 500 mg (more severe cases) every 8 hours, though in *N. gonorrhoeae* infections, a single dose of 3000 mg should be given.

Amoxycillin, 250 mg capsules.

Amoxycillin, powder for suspensions, 125 or 250 mg for each 5 ml.

Oxacillin

Brand names: Prostaphlin, Bactocill. The absorption and the distribution in tissues and organs are excellent. Previous lists of responsive organisms can be enlarged to include beta-hemolytic streptococci, and penicillinase-producing staphylococci.

Oxacillin is considered a good choice for the treatment of infections caused by pneumococci; beta-hemolytic streptococci, group A; and staphylococci. It is active either by mouth or injection; but the oral route is not advisable for any serious infection. Nevertheless, these penicillinase-resistant penicillins may increase the number of resistant strains, for which reason they should be used with extreme caution and only in selected cases, as indicated by sensitivity tests.

Dosage: for mild or moderate infections, 500 mg every 4 to 6 days, for no less than 5 days, preferring in these instances the oral route. For more serious infections use the parenteral route; doses as above, either intramuscularly, intravenously, or by slow infusion. For severe infections, doses can be increased to 1000 mg or even to 4000 mg every 4 to 6 hours for about 10 days.

Oxacyllin, 250 or 500 mg capsules.

Oxacyllin, powder for oral solution, to provide 250 mg in each ml.

Oxacyllin, for injection, 250, 500, 1000, 2000, or 4000 mg in each ampoule; the amount of liquid for reconstitution increases with the dose and the route for injection in muscle (sterile water) or vein (normal saline or 5% glucose).

Methicillin

Brand names: Staphcillin, Celbenin. Methicillin is indicated for the same situation, in general, as oxacillin.

Dosage: 1000 mg every 4 to 6 hours by deep intramuscular injection. Same dosage for intravenous injections (use isotonic sodium chloride or 5% glucose solutions). Dosage to be increased in severe infections; resort to oral administration as soon as possible, continuing for 2 days after symptoms subside.

Methicillin, 1000, 4000, or 6000 mg vials.

Nafcillin

Brand name: Unipen. Nafcillin activity is similar to that of oxacillin.

Dosage and indications are as for oxacillin.

Cloxacillin

Brand name: Tegopen. The uses are the same as for other penicillinase-resistant penicillins, particularly for the treatment of infections due to penicillinase-producing germs, pneumococci, and group A beta-hemolytic streptococci.

Dosages: 250 to 500 mg every 6 hours in mild to moderate cases; 500 mg or more every 6 hours for more serious cases, but not for the most severe ones.

Cloxacillin, 250 or 500 mg capsules.

Cloxacillin, powder, with 125 mg in each 5 ml when reconstituted.

Carbenicillin

Brand name: Bactocill. This drug is especially active against *Pseudomonas, Proteus,* and *Enterobacter* infections, but also active against other penicillin-responsive organisms, except for the penicillinase-producing cocci. Use is suggested for urinary infections due to *Pseudomonas* (some develop resistance), *Proteus, Enterobacter, Escherichia coli, enterococcus, Streptococcus,* and *Staphylococcus* (non-penicillinase-producing).

Dosage: one or two tablets every 6 hours; injectable, for urinary infections, 200 mg for each kilo of body weight in 24 hours, intravenously; injectable, for severe infections, 20,000 to 40,000 mg a day, in divided doses or continuous infusion; for infections, 500 mg per kilo of body weight in 24 hours, in divided doses; intramuscularly, 1000 to 2000 mg every six hours.

Carbenicillin, 382 mg tablets.

Carbenicillin, 1000, 2000, and 5000 mg vials, to prepare injectables.

Carbenicillin for intravenous use, vials containing 2000, 5000, or 10,000 mg.

Dicloxacillin

Brand name: Pathocil. A penicillin with the double advantage of resistance to acids and to penicillinase, used for mild to moderate infections.

Dosage: 125 mg every 6 hours in mild cases; to 250 mg or more every 6 hours, in moderate infections.

Dicloxacillin, 250 mg capsules.

Dicloxacillin, powder, 62.5 g per vial for solution.

Phenethicillin

This drug is resistant to the acid gastric contents and its uses are the same as for penicillin V, q.v. Of course, it should not be used for severe infections.

AMINOGLYCOSIDES (THE STREPTOMYCIN GROUP)

The streptomycin group is of help in cases of tuberculosis, *Staphylococcus* infections, and infections due to gram-negative bacteria, particularly when a severe disease occurs, though their use is drastically curtailed by the very serious side effects they provoke. Damage to the 8th cranial nerve may result in irreversible deafness, mainly when the drug is given in high dosages for more than one week. It is advisable to perform audiometric tests twice a week and frequent urine tests for kidney injury. Damage should be detected at the first sign, and special attention will be given to patients over 60 years of age.

Streptomycin

Streptomycin sulfate U.S.P. is the preparation usually prescribed. It is used for the treatment of the following diseases:

Tuberculosis
Bacterial endocarditis (if needed to help another antibiotic)
Brucellosis (with a tetracycline)
Tularemia (with a tetracycline)
Plague (with a tetracycline)
Meningitis due to *H. influenzae, K. pneumoniae,* or *E. coli*
Urinary infections due to *Proteus, K. pneumoniae, E. coli, S. fecalis,* or
   A. aerogenes
Peritonitis (particularly due to perforation)

Respiratory infections due to *K. pneumoniae* or *H. influenzae*
Chancroid (if a tetracycline fails)
Granuloma inguinale (if a tetracycline fails)

Dosage: 1000 to 2000 mg, given at a rate of 500 to 1000 mg every 12 hours. For subcutaneous injections it should be diluted about 100 mg for each ml; for intramuscular, 200 mg for each ml; and for intravenous drip, 1000 to 2000 mg in each liter of solution, using physiologic saline or 5% dextrose solution. Streptomycin may be given intrathecally; but not by mouth, except for local infections or as a prophylactic for surgery. Topical use is to be totally discouraged.

Streptomycin, powder, 1000 or 5000 mg vials.

Streptomycin, 500 mg in each ml, in vials containing 10 ml.

Streptomycin, 1000 mg in 2-, 2.5-, or 5-ml vials.

Streptomycin, 5000 mg in 12.5- or 30-ml vials.

With streptomycin, it is important to note that there are mutants in bacterial strains which, after they emerge after a few days of treatment, provoke infections unresponsive to the drug. Under these circumstances, an additional drug should be combined or the treatment switched to another antibiotic if response is not immediate.

Gentamycin

Brand name: Garamycin. Gentamycin is prescribed for local application or parenteral injection, particularly active against: streptococci, staphylococci (most varieties), gram-negative bacteria, *P. Aeruginosa, A. aerogenes, E. coli, K. pneumoniae, Proteus* species, and *Serratia.*

Similar to other aminoglycosides, it is oto- and nephrotoxic, and should be used only when other less toxic antibiotics fail to help, particularly when dealing with elderly persons.

Garamycin, 0.1% cream, for dermatologic use.

Garamycin, 0.1% ointment, as above.

Garamycin ophthalmic solution, to instill one or two drops, every 8 hours.

Garamycin, ophthalmic ointment.

Garamycin, 40 mg in each ml, 2-ml ampoule vials (80 mg); give 80 mg every 8 hours for individuals over 60 kg of body weight (about 130 lb); or 60 mg for smaller persons, assuming there is a normal kidney function (less frequent dosage in kidney impairment).

Kanamycin

Brand name: Kantrex. Kanamycin is particularly active against *E. coli, K. pneumoniae, A. aerogenes, S. marcescens, Mima-Herellea,* and the *Proteus* species. The drug may be administered either orally or by injection, but should not be given for prolonged periods of time owing to nephrotoxicity.

Oral administration is advised for suppression of intestinal bacteria and hepatic coma (for more prolonged administration). Parenteral administration is recommended for infections caused by susceptible germs and selected staphylococcal infections. Other routes may be intravenous, intraperitoneal, direct injection into abscesses, or by aerosol.

Kanamycin, 500 mg capsules, 1000 mg every 8 to 12 hours (hepatic coma), or larger doses for 2 or 3 days.

Kanamycin, 500 mg in 2 ml or 1000 mg in 3 ml per vial, for intramuscular injection.

Neomycin

Brand names: Mycipradin, Neobitic. Neomycin and kanamycin are very closely related, though neomycin is more toxic. Topical applications easily induce allergic reactions.

The drug may be administered: topically, particularly for skin, eyes, and ears; orally, for pre-surgery prophylaxis, hepatic coma, and *E. coli* diarrhea; and intramuscularly, for urinary infections with *P. aeruginosa, K. pneumoniae, E. coli,* when no other effective antibiotic is available.

Neomycin, 500 mg tablets.

Neomycin, oral solution, 125 mg in each 5 ml.

Neomycin, 500 mg per vial for intramuscular injection.

Paromomycin

Brand name: Humatin. The drug is used mainly for intestinal (*not* systemic) amebiasis, and as adjunct therapy in hepatic coma, when there are no ulcerative intestinal lesions.

Dosage: 30 mg for each kilo of body weight (25 mg in milder or 35 mg in very acute cases) in 24 hours, divided into three installments, preferably with meals, and for only 5 or 6 days. Patients in hepatic coma may receive 1000 mg every 6 hours (or lower doses at more frequent intervals, to reach 4000 mg a day).

Paromomycin, 250 mg capsules.

Paromomycin syrup, 125 mg in each 5 ml.

Amikacin

Brand name: Amikin. Amikacin is a derivative of kanamycin which shows minimal or no oto- or nephrotoxicity, when given at conservative dosage. After injection, it spreads to most of the body fluids and tissues, including the meninges, pleurae, and peritoneal fluids. Amikacin is reported to be active against gram-positive and particularly gram-negative bacteria, and is prescribed for *Proteus* species, *Providencia, Serratia,* and *Pseudomonas.*

Nevertheless, patients treated with amikacin, and particularly the elderly, have to be watched for evidence of damage to the 8th cranial nerve and the kidney. The dosage is to be decreased or suspended when urinary excretion is impaired.

Dosage: 15 mg for each kilo of body weight in 24 hours, not to exceed 1500 mg in 24 hours, divided into two or three installments, and discontinued before 10 days. When the condition of the patient is stable, dosage interval may be calculated as nine times the serum creatinine expressed in hours (creatinine $1.7 \times 9 = 15.3$, that is, injections can be given every 15 hours 18 minutes). Intravenously it should be administered at the same dosage and intervals, properly diluted.

Amikacin, 100 or 500 mg in 2-ml ampoules.

Amikacin, 1000 mg in 4-ml ampoules.

CHLORAMPHENICOL

Brand name: Chloromycetin. Because of the variety of germs under its action, chloramphenicol is considered a "broad-spectrum" antibiotic, with the advantage of very good diffusion into tissues and organs, including the spinal fluid. Unfortunately, it has been incriminated as the cause of severe bone marrow depression, leading to serious and fatal blood dyscrasias. For this reason, it should be used only when less dangerous agents are not suitable for treatment, and never for minor ailments. The oral route will be preferred in most instances, always checking blood counts every two days, and to stop administration as soon as any minor evidence of bone marrow depression is noted. Diseases treated by this antibiotic are typhoid fever and other salmonelloses, granuloma inguinale, *H. influenzae* meningitis, gram-negative meningitis, bacteremia or similar severe infections, and rickettsial diseases.

Dosage: For ophthalmic use, 1% ointment, to apply a small amount on the affected eye, repeating every 3 hours, day and night, for 2 days; then decrease frequency and continue treatment for 2 days after disappearance of symptoms. For otic use, 0.5% solution; instill 2 or 3 drops into the ear canal, every 8 hours. Cream, 1%, to apply locally every 6 or 8 hours. Capsules, to give 50 mg for each kilo of body weight in 24 hours, in divided doses every 6 hours; average dosage is one 250-mg capsule for each 4.5 kg (10 1b) of body weight; double dosage (100 mg) is given in unusually resistant cases, but the dosage has to be decreased as soon as possible; for infants use 25 mg for each kg. For intravenous injections the dosage is the same as for capsules.

Chloramphenicol, 50, 100, or 250 mg capsules.

Chloramphenicol, oral suspension containing 150 mg in each 5 ml.

Chloramphenicol, powder, 100 mg in each ml when reconstituted in 10-ml vials.

Chloramphenicol, 1% cream.

Chloramphenicol. 1% ophthalmic ointment.

Chloramphenicol, 0.5% otic solution.

THE TETRACYCLINE GROUP

Tetracyclines attack a wide variety of noxious germs, for which reason, like chloramphenicol, they are called broad-spectrum antibiotics. Also, tetracyclines offer the advantage of being tolerated better than many other antibiotics. They are advantageously used to treat:

Gram-positive infections
Gram-negative infections
Gonorrhea
Brucellosis (plus streptomycin)
Rickettsial diseases
    Typhus
    Rocky Mountain spotted fever
    Q fever
    Trench fever
    Rickettsialpox
Mycoplasma infections (pneumonia)
Chlamydiae infections
    Psittacosis
    Pneumonia
Lymphogranuloma venereum
Borrelia (relapsing fever)
Granuloma inguinale
Pasteurella (plus streptomycin, in many instances)
    Plague
    Tularemia
    Meningitis
    Bacteremia

Abscesses
Pseudomonas pseudomallei (plus sulfa)
Listeria
 Meningitis
 Bacteremia
 Endocarditis
Fusobacterium (Vincent's angina)
Spirillum (treponemas)
 Syphilis
 Pinta
 Yaws
 Bejel
H. ducreyi (chancroid)
Bacteroides (bacteremia)
Amebiasis
V. comma (cholera)
Acne (used as adjunct therapy).

The tetracyclines may provoke sensitivity reactions heralded by rashes, edema, anaphylaxis, itching, gastrointestinal upsets, or thrombopenic purpura; they may injure the liver, and care should be taken to avoid tetracyclines that have become chemically changed by aging or poor storage, which may give rise to a form of poisoning, the Fanconi syndrome, with polydypsia, polyuria, glycosuria, and aminoaciduria. This syndrome usually subsides about one month after cessation of therapy.

Tetracycline

Brand names: Achromycin, Achromycin V, QIDtet. Indications correspond fairly well with the information given on the above section on the tetracyclines, but it will be kept in mind that there are frequent resistant strains of *H. ducreyi, Pasteurella, Bacteroides, Brucella,* and *V. comma;* thus sensitivity tests will be carried out, whenever needed. If a patient is not doing well with tetracycline, an alternate antibiotic should be tried. The following diseases will be treated with tetracycline only in case penicillin cannot be used: gonorrhea, syphilis, pinta, yaws, Listeriosis, tetanus, gas gangrene, anthrax, actinomycoses, and Vincent's angina.

Oral administration: The dose is given about 1 hour before or 3 hours after meals. Avoid milk and antacids. For streptococcal infections maintain therapy for 10 days. Dosage: 500 mg every 6 hours. For syphilis use total of 30,000 or 40,000 mg in a period of 15 days; for gonorrhea, give 1500 mg to start, followed by 500 mg every 6 hours for 4 days (9000 mg total).

Intramuscular administration: 250 mg every 24 hours; alternate dosage,

100 mg every 8 hours, or 150 mg every 12 hours. When tetracycline is given by injection, resume the oral route as soon as possible.

Intravenous administration: slow injection, not to exceed 500 mg every 6 hours.

Tetracycline, 100, 250, or 500 capsules.

Tetracycline, syrup, 125 mg in each 5 ml.

Tetracycline, oral suspension, 250 mg in each 5 ml, after reconstitution.

Tetracycline, 100, 250, or 500 mg vials for intravenous injection, to be reconstituted.

Oxytetracycline

Brand name: Terramycin. Clinical indications are as for tetracycline, q.v. above. The dosage to be used when given by mouth or by intramuscular injection is the same. Intravenous injection is not used.

Oxytetracycline, 125 or 250 mg capsules.

Oxytetracycline, syrup, 125 mg in each 5 ml.

Oxytetracycline vials for deep intramuscular injection, containing 50 mg in 1 ml, or 100 or 250 mg in 2 ml.

Chlortetracycline

Brand name: Aureomycin. The foregoing indications (q.v.) are valid for chlortetracycline.

Chlortetracycline, 250 mg capsules.

Chlortetracycline, 3% dermatologic ointment.

Chlortetracycline, 1% ophthalmic ointment.

Chlortetracycline, 500 mg in each vial, for intravenous injection.

Demethylchlortetracycline

Brand name: Declomycin. In all senses demethylchlortetracycline is similar to the above-described tetracyclines, with the only difference being that it is excreted at a slower pace, thus maintaining prolonged high blood levels. All indications given above are valid here; except for dosage:

Dosage: 600 mg a day in divided doses every 6 to 12 hours. For gonorrhea, the initial dose will be 600 mg and thereafter 300 mg every 12 hours for 4 days (3000 mg total).

Demethylchlortetracycline, 75, 150, or 300 mg tablets.

Demethylchlortetracycline, syrup, containing 75 mg in each 5 ml.

Doxycycline

Brand name: Vibramycin. This antibiotic claims all properties and indications given by other tetracyclines; but there are a few important differences. It is almost completely absorbed with little interference from foods or antacids, and the dosage is considerably lower than for other tetracyclines.

Oral usage: 100 mg every 12 hours the first day; and once a day thereafter. In severe infections, it may be increased to 100 mg twice a day. It is advisable to give the drug together with food.

Intravenous usage: after diluting the powder in adequate solutions (0.9% saline, 5% glucose), prepare no more than 1 mg for each ml. Infusions are to be given *very* slowly. The dosage is 200 mg the first day, in one or two installments, followed by a daily dosage of 100 to 200 mg in one or two infusions. Oral administration will be given as soon as possible. Do not use doxycycline intramuscularly.

Dosage for gonorrhea: start with 200 mg, and give 100 mg after 12 hours; thereafter 100 mg every 12 hours for 3 days.

Dosage for syphilis: 300 mg every day in divided doses for a total of 10 days. This dosage may be given either by mouth or by intravenous injection.

Doxycycline, 50 or 100 mg capsules.

Doxycycline, syrup, containing 50 mg in each 5 ml.

Doxycycline, powder for oral suspension, giving 25 mg in each 5 ml after reconstituting.

Doxycycline, powder, for intravenous injection, vials containing 100 or 200 mg, to be reconstituted to give 0.1 to 1 mg in each ml of the infusion made with saline, 5% dextrose, Ringer's solution, lactated Ringer's injection, or 10% invert sugar.

OTHER ANTIBIOTICS

Erythromycin

Brand names: Erythrocin, Ibotycin, Kesso-mycin, Pediamycin, Pediamycin 400, Robimycin, Bristamycin, Ethril 250, Ethril 500, Pfizer E. QID mycin, SK erythromycin. Erythromycin belongs to the group of the macrolides. It is affected by gastric contents, but the pharmacologic preparations protect its stability and facilitate absorption. It is the drug of choice in infections caused by *Corynebacterium* and pertussis; and is a good alternate in *Mycoplasma, B. anthracis,* pneumococcal, spirochetal, and streptococcal infections. Responsive germs are:

Corynebacterium (diphtheriae)⎱ antibiotic of choice
Pertussis (whooping cough)   ⎰
Mycoplasma pneumoniae
B. anthracis (anthrax)
Pneumococcus (pneumonia, etc.)
Spirochetal (syphilis, etc.)
Rickettsial
Psittacosis
Trachoma
Lymphogranulomatosis
Streptococcal infections
Staphylococcal infections
Entoameba listolytica (only intestinal infection)
Listeriosis

It may be also tried, if needed, in gonorrhea and infections due to *H. influenzae.*

Dosage: 1000 mg a day, by mouth, in 250-mg installments every 6 hours or 500 mg every 12 hours. In severe infections it can be raised to 4000 mg a day (in no less than four daily installments). When injected intramuscularly, 100 mg will be given deep in the muscle every 4 or 8 hours. Intravenous injections: regular dosage about 1000 to 1500 mg a day, and up to 4000 mg in very severe infections, always administered *very slowly* in 1- to 4-hour drips.

For gonorrhea: 500 mg every 6 hours for 5 days. For syphilis: 30,000 to 40,000 mg in divided doses in a period of 10 to 15 days; that is, about 3000 mg a day, in divided doses. For amebic dysentery: 250 mg every 6 hours, for 10 to 14 days.

Erythromycin 125, 250, or 500 mg tablets.

Erythromycin, 125 or 250 mg capsules.

Erythromycin, oral suspension, to yield 200 or 400 mg in each 5 ml.

Erythromycin, drops, 200 mg in 5 ml (about 2 mg a drop).

Erythromycin, chewable tablets, 125, 200, or 250 mg each.

Erythromycin, suppositories, 125 mg each.

Erythromycin, ophthalmic ointment, 5 mg in each 1000 mg.

Erythromycin, intravenous injection, 500 and 1000 mg vials.

Erythromycin, intramuscular injection, 100 mg in 2 ml, or 250 and 500 mg vials.

Polymyxin B

Brand name: Aerosporin. Polymyxin B is active against most gram-negative organisms except *Proteus,* because it causes increased bacterial cell membrane permeability. The principal indication is in the treatment of *Pseudomonas aeruginosa* infections. It should be used in all severe cases of the following:

Pseudomonas aeruginosa infections
H. influenzae meningitis (intrathecal)
A. aerogenes bacteremia
K. pneumoniae bacteremia
E. coli urinary infections

This is not a safe drug, particularly for the elderly, since nephrotoxic reactions may occur, and should be carefully watched for. Dosage can be stated by weight or by units (1 unit equals $0.1 \mu g$, 1 mg equals 10,000 units); but regular dosages should be reduced as soon as possible.

Ophthalmic solution: dissolve 50 mg (500,000 units) in 50 or 20 ml of distilled water (0.1% or 0.25%); administer one to three drops every hour. Solutions in sterile saline may be used for subconjunctival injection of 1 mg (10,000) units) a day.

Intramuscular injections: cause severe pain and should be given in 1% procaine solution, 50 mg (500,000 units) in 2 ml of the solution; 25,000 to 30,000 units for each kilo of body weight in 24 hours in four to six injections.

Intravenous injection: dissolve 50 mg (500,000 units) in 300 to 500 ml of 5% dextrose, for infusion, 15,000 to 25,000 units for each kilo of body weight in 24 hours, in two installments.

Intrathecal injection: for meningitis caused by *Pseudomonas* or *H. influenzae;* the 50 mg (500,000 units) will be dissolved in 10 ml of sterile saline, to give 1 ml (50,000 units) every 24 hours the first 3 or 4 days, and thereafter every other day.

Polymyxin B, 50 mg (500,000 units) vials.

Bacitracin

Bacitracin is an antibiotic principally designed for topical use for the treatment of gram-negative superficial infections and used generally in combination with other agents.

Bacitracin, 10,000 or 50,000 units in vials, for intramuscular injection (to be dissolved in 2% procaine solution, to reach a concentration of no less than 5000, no more than 10,000 in each ml).

Bacitracin, ointment (usually 500 units per gram).

Bacitracin, ophthalmic (same as above).

Novobiocin

Brand names: Albamycin, Cathomycin. Novobiocin is active against pneumococci, *Staphylococcus aureus* (very sensitive), streptococci (less sensitive) enterococci, *H. influenzae, H. pertussis, N. meningitidis, C. diphtheriae,* and *Proteus* (some strains).

Novobiocin is recommended *only* if penicillin, a tetracycline, or erythromycin cannot be given because of reactions, which include skin rashes, Stevens-Johnson syndrome, diarrhea, anuria, leukopenia, agranulocytosis, and superinfections.

Dosage: 500 mg every 6 hours; 1000 mg in severe infections.

Novobiocin, 250 mg capsules.

Novobiocin, oral suspension containing 125 mg in each 5 ml.

Novobiocin, 500 mg powder, for injection

Oleandomycin

Brand name: Matromycin. Oleandomycin is a macrolide which shows similar properties to those of erythromycin, q.v. above. Specially sensitive are streptococci, pneumococci, *Neisseria, Hemophilus,* clostridia, *C. diphtheriae, Brucella,* and *Listeria.* Reactions include diarrhea, esophagitis and other gastrointestinal disturbances. Uses are the same as for erythromycin.

Dosage: 250 to 500 mg every 6 hours, never exceeding a daily amount of 3000 mg.

Oleandomycin, 250 mg capsules.

Oleandomycin, 500 mg powder, in ampoules, to be dissolved in 5% dextrose solution 2 mg or less per ml, for use intravenously.

Colistin

Brand names: Coly-mycin oral suspension, Coly-mycin M. Parenteral. This polypeptide antibiotic is used for oral administration and, in the form of colistimethate sodium, for parenteral injection. Given by mouth, it is indicated for diarrhea due to *E. coli* or *Shigella;* by injection, intramuscularly or intravenously, for infections due to *E. coli, Enterobacter, K. pneumoniae,* and *P. aeruginosa.* After prolonged use, there may be kidney damage and overgrowth of germs, particularly Proteus. Other side effects are due to neurological disturbances, as dizziness, vertigo, or impaired speech. It should not be used together with streptomycin, kanamycin, neomycin, or polymyxin; or with ether, curare, decamethonium, or sodium citrate.

Dosage: for oral administration give 5 to 15 mg for each kilo of body weight in 24 hours, divided into three installments. For parenteral administration, give 5 mg for each kilo of body weight (less with renal impairment), in two or more divided doses intramuscularly; every 12 hours or by infusion intravenously.

> Colistin, oral suspension, after reconstitution will contain 25 mg in each 5 ml.

> Colistimethate sodium, in vials containing 20 mg (reconstitute with 2.2 ml sterile water) or 150 mg (reconstitute with 2 ml sterile water for injection U.S.P.).

Rifampin and Cycloserine

Since these antibiotics are mainly used for the treatment of tuberculosis, they are discussed under the heading "Antituberculosis Drugs," q.v.

Vancomycin

Brand name: Vancocin. Vancocin is bactericidal against gram-positive bacteria, particularly streptococci and staphylococci. It is poorly absorbed by mouth, for which reason when so given it will be *only* for staphylococcal enterocolitis; parenteral use is preferred. Vancomycin given intravenously is recommended for extremely severe infections not responding to other drugs, or when those drugs cannot be given for individual reasons. Included are infections due to staphylococci, such as pneumonia, osteomyelitis, bacteremia, or local infections, and infections occurring with surgery. Vancomycin is nephrotoxic and ototoxic, and will not be given concurrently with other antibiotics similarly toxic. Injections must be given intravenously, since it causes necrosis of tissues.

Dosage: 500 mg every 6 hours or 1000 mg every 12 hours, either by mouth or by injection.

> Vancomycin, powder to be reconstituted for oral use as solution with 115 ml of distilled water (each 6 ml will contain 500 mg).

> Vancomycin, ampoules for parenteral use, containing 500 mg in each 10-ml ampoule, to be reconstituted (100 to 200 ml saline or 5% glucose for injections; or larger amounts for infusion).

Lincomycin

Brand name: Lincocin. Lincomycin is another of the toxic antibiotics, reserved for severe infections when there is no option to use other, less toxic drugs. It is active against streptococci (several varieties), pneumococci, staphylococci (mainly *S. aureus*), clostridia, and *C. diphtheriae*. It is not active against *S. fecalis, N. gonorrhoeae, N. meningitidis, H. influenzae,* and many gram-negative microorganisms.

Lincomycin may cause a severe, possibly fatal, pseudomembranous colitis (watch always for diarrhea together with abdominal cramps), which can occur not only during active treatment but also after several weeks of discontinuance of therapy. Other side effects may be gastrointestinal; hematopoietic, as agranulocytosis and aplastic anemia; dermatological, as rashes and exfoliative dermatitis; hepatic; or cardiovascular.

Dosage: for oral administration give 500 mg every 8 hours (every 6 hours in more severe cases); for intramuscular administration give 600 mg every 24 hours (every 12 hours or more often in severe cases); for intravenous administration, infusions should last no less than 1 hour, to give 600 mg or more every 8 to 12 hours.

Lincomycin, 250 or 500 mg capsules.

Lincomycin, ampoules, containing 300, 1000, or 2000 mg.

Clindamycin

Brand name: Cleocin. Clindamycin is derived from lincomycin. Large doses have been well tolerated experimentally, but the possible incidence of side effects similar to those caused by lincomycin limits its use. It is active against *Staphylococcus aureus,* streptococci (not *s. fecalis*), pneumococci, *Bacteroides, Pseudobacterium, Propionibacterium, Eubacterium Actinomyces, Peptococcus, Peptostreptococcus,* and *C. perfringens* (not other clostridia).

Dosage: for oral administration give 150 to 300 mg (300 to 450 mg in severe infections), every 6 hours, but in the case of pharyngitis there is no need for more than two doses a day. For parenteral administration give 600 mg a day, in two doses of 300 mg; more severe infections will require from 600 to 1200 mg daily, in 300-mg doses in three, four, or six installments; but in very serious cases, doses to 1200 or 2700 mg, also in three, four, or six installments.

Clindamycin, 150 mg capsules.

Clindamycin, for oral suspension, in bottles to be reconstituted, yielding 75 mg in each ml.

Clindamycin, ampoules: 2-ml ampoules, 300 mg; 4-ml ampoules, 600 mg; and 6-ml ampoules, 900 mg.

IV. ANTITUBERCULOSIS DRUGS

Mycobacteria causing tuberculosis and leprosy pose a special challenge to physicians because of their metabolic characteristics and their ability to become resistant to drugs. The lack of good antimycobacterial activity in most drugs and the tendency of some to cause serious side effects put streptomycin, rifampin, and ethambutol in a preferred position. Associate at least two of them in all instances. Among the ancillary drugs, paraaminosalicylic acid ranks first.

Streptomycin

For the treatment of tuberculosis, streptomycin was the first truly effective drug, regardless of its serious disadvantages, such as neural toxicity (8th cranial nerves) and the tendency of mycobacteria to develop resistance to it. A second important step in the treatment of tuberculosis was taken when the use of a second or third drug was advised, isoniazid with streptomycin being one of the active combinations. Streptomycin is given to patients sensitized to other agents.

Dosage: in tuberculosis, streptomycin is given only by injection, 500 to 1000 mg intramuscularly every 12 hours (or subcutaneously, if given more diluted). Intravenous infusions will provide 1 or 2 g in each liter of saline.

Streptomycin, vials containing 1 or 5 g of the drug, to be diluted, to a concentration of 500 mg in each ml, as a general rule.

For more details, see the section above devoted to streptomycin.

Isoniazid (INH)

Brand names: Isonicotinic acid, INH tablets, Nydrazid, Hydrazide, Nicozide, Niconyl. Toxicity is manifested by pyridoxine (vitamin B_6) deficiency (peripheral neuropathy), hepatitis, aplastic anemia, thrombocytopenia, or agranulocytosis. Overdosage produces immediate reactions (nausea, vomiting, blurring of vision, slurring of speech, dizziness, hallucinations); and with higher doses there will be stupor progressing to coma, respiratory distress, and signs of central nervous system depression. Optic neuritis may occur, which makes it necessary to perform frequent ophthalmologic examinations, particularly if any symptom associated with vision occurs, especially among elderly persons. Gastrointestinal distress is frequent but not always serious. The important concern is to detect liver damage early with signs of hepatitis, such as elevation of SGOT, SGPT, and bilirubin (with or without jaundice). Nevertheless, transient elevation of transaminase may occur during the first months of treatment, more rarely at later stages; if such elevations are mild and no other evidence of hepatic injury is noted, treatment should be continued and complete restoration expected, provided adequate care is strictly observed. Other reactions may be allergy, vasculitis, fever, hyperglycemia, metabolic acidosis, pellagra, gynecomastia, convulsions, a syndrome similar to lupus erythematosus, memory impairment, or encephalopathy.

IHN is among the two or three basic drugs prescribed for tuberculosis, as are streptomycin, rifampin, and ethambutol. It is also used as a preventive drug for contacts, recent converters, tuberculin reactors under 20 years of age, and tuberculosis patents who were not well treated previously. INH will be prescribed for tuberculin reactors who need to be treated with corticoids or immunosuppressive agents. Do not use it if the bacilli prove nonresponsive or the patient develops severe reactions. When treatment is effective, it must be continued for long periods of time, to avoid relapses. A good help is the administration of pyridoxine (vitamin B_6), at a dosage of 20 to 30 mg in 24 hours.

Dosage for adults: 300 mg a day, in one dose; those under 60 kg (about 130 lb) will take 5 mg for each kilo of body weight in 24 hours. Preventive therapy consists of 300 mg a day, in one dose.

Isoniazid, 50, 100, or 300 mg tablets.

Ethambutol

Brand name: Myambutol. Reactions are: decreased visual acuity, possibly related to degenerative central nervous system changes; reactions of an allergic nature—rashes, itching, articular pain, fever; or gastrointestinal upsets. Neurological and psychiatric symptoms, malaise, headache, increased uricemia capable of precipitating gout attacks, and impaired liver function have been reported.

Optic *neuritis* appears to be related to dose and time, and about 6% of all patients receiving ethambutol are affected. Visual changes are reversible if the drug is discontinued in time, for which reason patients should be instructed to watch for visual changes and report them promptly. The physician will check the eyes at least once a month, particularly in older patients and those receiving more than 15 mg for each kilo of body weight in 24 hours.

Ethambutol inhibits multiplication of mycobacteria, but some may develop resistance if the drug is given alone for a long time. If ethambutol is given together with isoniazid, the development of bacterial resistance against the germ is decreased. It is indicated in the treatment of tuberculosis, but only if given concurrently with isoniazid and streptomycin. If there is resistance to isoniazid (because of a previous treatment), rifampin and/or streptomycin, and ethambutol, will be given together with one of the secondary drugs not yet used for that particular patient, as paraaminosalicylic acid, viomycin, cycloserine, or ethionamide.

Dosage: for a primary treatment, 15 mg for each kilo of body weight, once a day. For a re-treatment, the dosage must be increased to 25 mg for each kilo of body weight, once a day; but after 2 months of treatment the dose should be decreased to 15 mg for each kilo.

Ethambutol, 100 mg tablets.

Ethambutol, 400 mg film-coated tablets.

Rifampin

Brand names: Rimactane, Rifamate. Rifampin is a derivative of rifamycin B with its metabolism taking place in the liver, which is often damaged by the drug. Blood changes, nausea, vomiting, cramps, or diarrhea may occur, as well as headache, visual disturbances, weakness, dizziness, confusion, rashes, itching, and soreness of the mouth. Most of these adverse effects take place after resumption of rifampin therapy following intermissions in treatment. Tests for sensitivity must always be done when persistent positive cultures are found. The drug is indicated in the treatment of tuberculosis and of asymptomatic *Neisseria meningitidis* carriers (not for the treatment of the meningeal infection) when the risk of meningitis is high.

Toxicity due to rifampin is diagnosed when reactive symptoms occur as indicated above, with possible hepatomegalia and, even, jaundice. This situation is treated by emptying the stomach, provoking active diuresis, and resorting to hemodialysis if it is deemed necessary.

Dosage: 600 mg in one dose in 24 hours, either 1 hour before or 2 hours after a meal. Therapy for tuberculosis is to continue until clinical improvement and bacterial elimination take place. To treat *Neisseria* carriers, give the medication for only 4 days.

Rifampin, 300 mg capsules.

Paraaminosalicylic Acid (PAS)

Brand names: Pas C (Pascorbic), Panrisyl, Parasal, Razipas, Parapas. Aminosalicylic acid, also paraaminosalicylic acid, PAS, is capable of inhibiting the development of resistance of the mycobacteria to streptomycin and isoniazid, and will always be given with those or other adjunctive agents.

The most frequently compained-of side effects are nausea, vomiting, abdominal pain, diarrhea, goiter, hypersensitivity reactions, and other serious problems mainly posed by blood dyscrasias, principally agranulocytosis.

Dosage for adults: 6000 to 8000 mg a day, in one or two installments, after meals.

PAS, 500 mg tablets (expiration date is given because the drug is relatively unstable).

Pyrazinamide

Brand names: Aldinamide, Tebrazid. Reactions include liver damage, leading in some cases to jaundice or even hepatic necrosis, and, less important, articular pain, anorexia, nausea, dysuria, fever, and an elevation of uric acid (gout), or of carbohydrates, causing difficult control of preexisting diabetes.

Pyrazinamide is recommended in cases of lung surgery with mycobacteria resistant to the first-line drugs, and for *hospitalized* patients. Treatment will start 7 to 14 days before and will continue for 4 to 6 weeks after the operation.

Dosage: 20 to 35 mg for each kilo of body weight in 24 hours divided into three or four equal doses; never exceeding 3000 mg a day.

Pyrazinamide, 500 mg tablets.

Cycloserine

Brand names: Seromycin, Oxamycin. Cycloserine was mentioned above because it is active against a number of microorganisms, particularly *E. coli* and *Enterobacter* when they cause infections of the urinary tract (pyelonephritis, pyelitis, and cystitis). It may be used in the treatment of tuberculosis, including tuberculosis of the urinary system, as one of the second-line drugs for this disease, and has to be given together with other antituberculosis drugs.

Reactions relate principally to the nervous system, usually when high dosages are used (500 mg or more): convulsions, headache, dysarthria, confusion, psychoses, paresis, and coma. Anticonvulsants may help, but cycloserine blood levels should be checked once a week.

Dosage: for the treatment of tuberculosis start with 250 mg every 12 hours, and increase gradually to 500 or 1000 mg a day, in divided doses.

Cycloserine, 250 mg capsules.

Ethionamide

Brand name: Trecator. Its side effects are similar to those of pyrazinamide (q.v. above), gastric irritation not allowing the intake of doses over 500 mg; it is recommended only as a secondary alternative to be used with other antituberculosis drugs. Otherwise, resistance develops rapidly.

Dosage: 250 mg every 12 hours, to be increased in amounts of 125 mg a day, every 5 days, until a dosage of 500 mg every 12 hours is reached, which should not be exceeded; preferably it is given after meals.

Ethionamide, 125 or 250 mg tablets.

Ethionamide, 125 or 250 mg enteric coated tablets (irregular absorption).

Viomycin

Brand names: Viocin sulfate, Vinactan sulfate. Resistance may develop; there is no cross resistance with streptomycin or isoniazid. To minimize resistance, it is better combined with other antitubercular drugs. Renal function may be impaired, and periodic urine examinations must be carried out frequently when this drug is used on elderly persons. Vestibular damage can also occur.

Dosage: 1000 mg every 12 hours by deep muscular injection only, twice a week for at least 4 to 6 months. Daily injections depend on urgency of need and tolerance. In all instances, it is better to give viomycin together with paraaminosalicylic acid (PAS), 12 g every day, by mouth.

Viomycin, 1 or 5 g vials.

Capreomycin

Brand name: Caqastat sulfate. Cross resistance is possible with viomycin, and to a variable extent with kanamycin and neomycin, but there is no cross resistance with other antibiotics used against tuberculosis. It is used only when isoniazid, streptomycin, ethambutol, or PAS has failed or is not tolerated, since it may cause oto- or renal toxicity.

Dosage: for the treatment of tuberculosis give 1000 mg in one daily dose (not to exceed 20 mg for each kilo of body weight in 24 hours) for 2 to 4 months; thereafter, same dosage two or three times a week, for a total of 18 to 24 months.

Capreomycin, 1000 mg in 5-ml ampoules.

V. ANTIVIRAL DRUGS

Idoxuridine (IDU)

Brand names: Stoxil, Herplex, Dendrid. Keratoconjunctivitis due to herpes simplex virus is the main indication for the use of topical idoxuridine. The drug should be stopped if there is no improvement after 1 week of treatment.

Dosage: the ophthalmic solution will be applied continuously, one drop every hour during the day and every 2 hours during sleep time; as soon as improvement is evident, give medication at intervals of 2 and 4 hours, and continue for 3 to 5 days after total recovery. If the ointment is used, apply five times a day, about every 4 hours, the last application when retiring. Do not use the drug for more than 3 weeks.

Idoxuridine, 0.1% ophthalmic solution.

Idoxuridine, 0.125% ophthalmic ointment.

Cytosine Arabinoside (Cytarabine)

Brand name: Cytosar. This drug is mainly recommended for cancer therapy, because of its powerful inhibition of deoxyribonucleic acid; it also inhibits DNA viruses and is used when idoxuridine fails to control keratoconjunctivitis due to herpes simplex virus. It may be tried in generalized herpes simplex and in varicella, but results have not been encouraging.

Dosage: 0.3 to 2 mg for each kilo of body weight in 24 hours, only administered once a day for 5 days, strictly intravenously.

Cytosine arabinoside, 100 or 500 mg vials, to be reconstituted to provide 20 or 50 mg, respectively, in each ml.

Amantadine Hydrochloride

Brand name: Symmetral. Amantadine is principally recommended for the treatment of Parkinson's disease, and also for influenza due to A_2 (Asian) virus. The main purpose is prophylaxis, but possibly it may also reduce the incidence and severity of complications of the disease. Adverse reactions are: congestive heart failure, hypotension, psychotic reactions, urinary retention, blood dyscrasias, and increased symptomatology in patients with epilepsy or heart disease. The medication will be given carefully to patients with diseases of the liver or the kidney, in the presence of rashes, or to patients with psychoses.

Dosage: 100 mg twice a day for as many days as will be needed, even to 90 days.

Amantadine hydrochloride, 100 mg capsules.

Amantadine hydrochloride, syrup containing 5 mg in each 5 ml.

Methisazone (Marboran)

This drug is recommended as a prophylactic against smallpox, to be given less than 2 days after exposure, at an oral dosage of 2000 to 4000 mg in 24 hours; it is also used for vaccinia complications.

VI. ANTIFUNGALS

Nystatin

Brand name: Mycostatin. Nystatin is very poorly absorbed from the gastrointestinal tract, for which reason it is indicated for the treatment of intestinal moniliasis. Topically, it is used for skin and vaginal infections caused by *Candida* species.

Topical application can be made two or three times a day to skin or vagina. Oral administration: 500,000 to 1 million units every 8 hours during the disease and for 2 or 3 days thereafter.

Nystatin, 500,000 units tablets.

Nystatin, 100,000 units in each g of cream.

Nystatin, 100,000 units in each g of ointment.

Nystatin, powder, 100,000 units in each g.

Griseofulvin

Griseofulvin is active against *Microsporon* (several varieties), *Trichophyton* (several varieties), and *Epidermophyton* (almost all varieties). It is not effective in moniliasis, tinea versicolor, actinomycosis, histoplasmosis, sporotrichosis, coccidioidomycosis, or torulosis. Since it is a penicillin, cross sensitivity with penicillin can occur. Before using griseofulvin, it is advised that an accurate diagnosis of the infecting microorganism be made.

Dosage: for tinea capitis give 500 mg every 24 hours, in four, two, or one dose(s); only severe cases will require 750 mg to start; reduce as soon as possible; continue 4 to 6 weeks. For tinea corporis, give same dosage as above, but only for 2 to 4 weeks. For ungueal infections, give same dosage as above, but for 4 months in fingernails and 6 months in toenails.

Griseofulvin, 125 or 250 mg capsules.

Griseofulvin, 125, 250, or 500 mg tablets.

Griseofulvin, suspension, with 250 mg in each 5 ml.

Amphotericin B

Brand name: Fungizone. This is a fungistatic antibiotic used, either topically or intravenously, against *Candida* (moniliasis), *Cryptococcus immitis* (torulosis), *Blastomyces* (blastomycosis), *Mucor mucedo* (mucormycosis), *Aspergillus fumigatus* (aspergillosis), *Histoplasma capsulatum* (histoplasmosis), *Sporotrichum schenkii* (sporotrichosis), *Rhizopus* (mucormycosis), and *Absidia* (mucormycosis).

The topical drug is mainly used for cutaneous moniliasis. By injection, it is used against severe infections caused by the above-mentioned fungi; but since it is a potent and dangerous drug, it will be used only when strictly needed, always watching for nephrotoxicity, blood dyscrasias, or neurotoxicity. Topical applications can be made liberally.

Dosage: for very slow infusions, use concentrations of 0.1 mg in each ml, to give 0.25 mg for each kilo of body weight in 24 hours; increase to 1 mg, as tolerated. Slightly higher doses may be given on alternate days.

Amphotericin, cream, lotion, or ointment.

Amphotericin, 50 mg vials.

VII. ANTIPARASITICS

ANTIMALARIALS

Quinine

Quinine has been a very important drug, though today others are often used instead; but quinine is used for analgesia and antipyresis, and mainly as an antimalarial, for suppression of either *Plasmodium vivax, P. malariae,* or *P. falciparum.* However, other antimalarials are preferred. In overdosage or hypersusceptibility, cinchonism gives symptoms particularly distressing to hearing and vision, which are treated with stomach lavage, tannic acid to precipitate the alkaloid, cardiac tonics, oxygen, blood transfusion, and other symptomatic measures.

Dosage: for suppression of malaria give 600 mg a day. Also, as an alternate procedure, 1000 mg three times a day for 2 days before the chill, and then 600 mg three times a day for 5 additional days.

Quinine, 180 or 300 mg capsules.

Quinine hydrochloride, powder, for individualized prescriptions, in bottles containing 30 or 150 g.

Quinine dihydrochloride, 2-ml ampoules with 500 mg or 5-ml ampoules with 1000 mg.

Quinine sulfate, tablets, 120 or 300 mg.

Quinine sulfate, 120, 180, 200, or 300 mg.

Chloroquine

Brand names: Aralen, Resochin. Chloroquine is prescribed for suppression or for the acute attack of malaria due to *Plasmodium (vivax, malariae, ovale,* and *falciparum*—except for some strains and the gametocytes of the latter).

Chloroquine phosphate cannot prevent relapses with the first two (*P. vivax* and *P. malariae*), for which two types it cannot even be used prophylactically. For the sensitive strains of *P. falciparum* it can be used as a radically curative agent. Resistant strains will be treated with quinine. In addition to this, chloroquine phosphate is as good an amebicidal agent as emetine. It is contraindicated in patients with ophthalmic problems.

Dosage: for suppression treatment give 500 mg once a week. For acute attacks of malaria give 100 mg as the initial dose; after 8 hours, 500 mg; thereafter, 500 mg daily, for 3 days. Gametocidal therapy (*P. vivax* and *P. malariae*): as for the acute attack. Radical cure (sensitive strains of *P. falciparum*): as for the acute attack.

Chloroquine phosphate, 125 or 200 mg tablets.

Chloroquine hydrochloride, 250 mg ampoules (5 ml).

Quinacrine

Brand names: Atabrine, Mepacrine. Quinacrine hydrochloride is used for the same purposes as chloroquine.

Dosage: for suppressive treatment give 100 mg once a week. For acute attack of malaria give 200 mg as the initial dose; after 8 hours give 100 mg, and thereafter 100 mg daily, for 3 days. Gametocidal therapy (*P. vivax* and *P. malariae*): as for the acute attack. Radical cure (sensitive *P. falciparum* strains): as for the acute attack.

Quinacrine hydrochloride, injectable, a powder for solution, 200 mg in 7 ml of sterile, distilled water, for intramuscular injection.

Quinacrine hydrochloride, 50 or 100 mg tablets.

Primaquine

From pamaquine, several other drugs were developed strongly active against *P. falciparum* and *P. vivax*. In *P. vivax* malaria the curative effect is well marked, and primaquine is the *drug of choice* for radical cure. When it is given at recommended dosage, the side effects are of little consequence. Otherwise, there may be methemoglobinemia with cyanosis, or leukopenia. Blacks may be too sensitive to primaquine. In most instances primaquine should be associated with chloroquine or amodiaquine, for administration.

Dosage: for radical cure give primaquine base, 15 mg a day for 14 days (with chloroquine, 1500 mg of base in 3 days). The dosage of primaquine base but without chloroquine may be used during the latent periods of the disease. This schedule is recommended in temperate zones; otherwise, 30 to 45 mg of primaquine base should be given, but in these instances there is less risk of hemolytic reactions if 60 mg of primaquine base is given with 300 mg of chloroquine once a week, for 8 weeks (only 6% failures!).

Primaquine phosphate, 15 mg of base (26.3 mg of the salt) in each tablet.

Chloroguanide

Brand names: Paludrine, Guanatol, Proguanil. Chloroguanide seems active against both *P. vivax* and *P. malariae* (not *P. falciparum*). Side effects are usually of little consequence; only hematuria or diarrhea, if no high doses are given.

Dosage: for prophylactic use, in endemic areas give 100 mg daily, for nonimmune persons; at times, for those residing in dangerous areas, 200 mg may be needed. Semi-immune persons will get 300 mg once a week, or, better, 200 mg twice a week. For the acute attack give 300 to 600 mg to start, followed by 300 mg daily, as long as needed; but for no less than 5 to 10 days.

Chloroguanide, 25, 100, or 300 mg tablets.

Pyrimethamine

Brand name: Daraprim. Pyrimethamine is prescribed for prophylaxis of malaria due to sensitive plasmodia, and for conjoint use to start transmission control and suppressive cure. Together with a sulfa, pyrimethamine is used for the treatment of toxoplasmosis; large doses are required, which may cause megaloblastic anemia, leukopenia, other blood dyscrasias, convulsions, and other symptoms of stimulation of the central nervous system. Folinic acid is the basic treatment for this toxicity.

Dosage: for preventive use, give 25 mg once a week. For the acute attack (only for sensitive strains), 50 mg daily, for 2 days. For toxoplasmosis (together with a sulfa), 50 to 75 mg a day—if tolerated—for 1 to 3 weeks; thereafter, half the initial dosage for 4 to 5 additional weeks.

Pyrimethamine, tablets, 25 mg each.

AMEBICIDES

Emetine

Emetine is effective against both intestinal and extraintestinal amebiasis, controls amebic symptomatology very rapidly, and can cure amebiasis in other organs, namely liver and brain; but unfortunately it does not kill amebic cysts in the intestinal tract, and cannot accomplish a radical cure.

Also, local irritation of the digestive tract precludes the oral route for its administration. Other side effects may occur, as diarrhea, vomiting, acute lesions of the liver, weakness, tenderness, aching and stiffness, and disturbances of the cardiovascular system, as hypotension, anginal pain, tachycardia, and EKG changes.

Emetine is recommended for the treatment of extraintestinal amebiasis: amebic hepatitis and amebic abscesses; also for the treatment of balantidiasis (which responds better to oxytetracycline), and infestations with lung and liver flukes. It is not recommended for intestinal amebiasis except in cases of severe diarrhea and acute amebic dysentery; doses should not be larger than 60 mg in 24 hours and should be given for periods no longer than 10 days. Always watch for intolerance!

Dosage: only by deep subcutaneous or intramuscular injection; 30 mg each dose, every 12 to 24 hours; do not use emetine for more than 10 days, and give no more than 600 mg total. Underweight or debilitated patients will receive only 30 mg a day. A second treatment should be delayed until 6 weeks after terminating the previous one.

Emetine, 30, 60, or 65 mg in 1-ml ampoules (never use emetine intravenously!).

Chloroquine

Brand names: Aralen, Resochin. For the treatment of extraintestinal amebiasis, chloroquine is almost as effective as emetine, particularly against *Entamoeba histolytica* in amebic hepatitis and abscesses, which may respond after failing to do so with emetine. Other extra intestinal forms of amebiasis also respond well. No amebic resistance against chloroquine ever develops.

Dosage: for oral treatment give 1000 mg a day, for 2 days; thereafter, 500 mg a day for 14 to 21 days. For parenteral treatment give only to patients unable to tolerate oral administration; 200 to 250 mg injected daily for 10 to 20 days (change to the oral route as soon as possible).

Chloroquine phosphate, 125 or 250 mg tablets.

Chloroquine hydrochloride, 250 mg in 5-ml ampoules.

Carbarsone

This pentavalent arsenical is an amebicide effective against *Entamoeba histolytica,* when the trophozoites are in the lumen or in shallow ulcers of the colon; not to be used in amebic hepatitis. Patients should be watched for possible accumulation, noted because of increased gastrointestinal symptomatology, or development of nausea, vomiting, cramps, and diarrhea if not previously present. Carbarsone is considered one of the safest arsenicals in use; nevertheless, among its toxic possibilities are neuritis, visual disturbances, exfoliative dermatitis, hemorrhagic encephalitis, and hepatic damage (jaundice), possibly leading to liver necrosis.

Dosage: 250 mg every 8 to 12 hours for no more than 10 days. If therapy has to be continued, a pause of 10 to 14 days will be observed, before second course of medication is given.

Carbarsone, 250 mg capsules.

OTHER ANTIPROTOZOAL AND ANTHELMINTHIC DRUGS

These drugs will be reviewed in the following pages. Of course, some of them have been dealt with previously, such as the sulfonamides, pyrimethamine, and quinacrine, q.v. above.

Pentamidine

Brand name: Lomidine. Pentamidine is recommended in the treatment of leishmaniasis and trypanosomiasis and is also effective against fungi, particularly *Blastomyces;* but the use of amphotericin B is preferred for the treatment of blastomycosis.

Pentamidine may provoke disturbing but not alarming reactions, as dyspnea, tachycardia, vomiting, or fainting, possibly due to hypotension or intravenous administration.

Dosage: for the treatment of trypanosomiasis (only to start within the first 21 to 28 days in infections caused by *Trypanosoma rhodisiense,* and not to be given if caused by *T. cruzi*) give 4 mg for each kilo of body weight in 24 hours, once a day or at longer intervals, by intramuscular injection; also can be given intravenously, but no more than 10 injections. For prophylaxis of trypanosomiasis, in endemic areas give 3 to 5 mg for each kilo of body weight, two or three times a year, by the intramuscular route. For the treatment of leishmaniasis give the same dosage as for trypanosomiasis, but only in courses of 12 to 15 injections; after an interval of 1 or 2 weeks, the course may be repeated.

Pentamidine, 200 mg ampoules.

Antimony Compounds

Trivalent antimonials are used in schistosomiasis, leishmaniasis, filariasis, mycosis fungoides, and granuloma inguinale; particularly antimonium potassium tartrate, antimonium sodium tartrate, the dimercaptosuccinate, and stibophen. Untoward effects are: emesis, shock, cough, pneumonia, articular pain, myalgia, bradycardia (which calls for immediate discontinuance of the medication), headache, dyspnea, edema, hepatitis (also requiring cessation of therapy), and hemolytic anemia. Contraindications are: hepatitis, myocarditis (cardiac insufficiency), and nephritis.

Tartar emetic (antimony potassium tartrate) is used for schistosomiasis, fungoides, and granuloma inguinale. Tartar emetic still seems to be the most effective agent against *S. japonicum,* though other less toxic drugs are used in other schistosomiases.

When one is injecting tartar emetic, the procedure has to be very slow, to prevent possible severe reactions (!), and with extreme care to avoid leakage into perivascular tissues.

Dosage: starting dose is 40 mg (8 ml of the 0.5% solution, or 4 ml of the 10 mg/ml ampoule); if it is well tolerated, increase by 20 mg (4 ml of the 0.5% solution) each successive dose, until a maximum of 140 mg (28 ml of the 0.5% solution) is reached, and a total of 1800 mg (360 ml of the 0.5% solution) is given. Injections are given on alternate days.

Antimony potassium tartrate, 10 mg in each ml in 50-ml vials.

Antimony potassium tartrate, 0.5% solution, for injection.

Antimony sodium tartrate is to be used in the same way as the potassium salt. Some say it is less toxic.

Sodium antimony dimercaptosuccinate, less toxic than stibophen, is very effective against schistosomiasis. It is given parenterally, by intramuscular or very slow intravenous injection. Toxic reactions may be dermatological (rashes), gastrointestinal (vomiting), neurological (asthenia), or febrile. In case of trouble, stop therapy, especially in herpes simplex or herpes zoster, bacterial infections, or hepatic, cardiac, or renal insufficiency. It is not recommended with massive intestinal helminthiasis, or if any other antimonial has been used within the previous 60 days.

Dosage: a total dose of 30 to 50 mg for each kilo of body weight, not to exceed a maximum of 2500 mg, will be divided into five injections, to be given at a rate of two a week.

This medication is not available in the United States, but is sold in other countries under the name of Astiban.

Sodium antimony dimercaptosuccinate, 2000 mg of the powder in vials to be completed with 20 ml of sterile water (10% solution).

Stibophen (Fuadin). This compound, among the least toxic in the group, is perhaps the most widely used for the treatment of schistosomiasis. Toxic reactions that demand stopping the administration of the drug include vomiting, severe articular pain, progressive albuminuria, intercurrent febrile infections, blood dyscrasias, and insufficiency of the liver, the kidney, or the heart.

Stibophen is active against schistosomiasis, though in the case of infections with *S. japonicum* the doses have to be high and are risky to the patient. It is also useful for the treatment of granuloma inguinale.

Dosage: for intensive therapy give 17 mg (2 ml), 34 mg (4 ml), and 51 mg (6 ml), respectively, the first three days, followed by 68 mg (8 ml) daily for 11 days; but with this dosage schedule most patients will present some toxic reactions. For conservative slow therapy give somewhat smaller amounts: 12.75 mg (in 1.5 ml) the first day, 29.75 mg (3.5 ml) the second day, 42.5 mg (5 ml) the third day, and six more injections at 2- or 3-day intervals; the course to be repeated a second time after 7 to 14 days. For conservative rapid therapy, give on the first day 17 mg (2 ml) in the morning, 34 mg (4 ml) at midday, and 34 mg (4 ml) in the afternoon; followed by 34 mg (4 ml) given three times a day the second and the third days; the course to be repeated a second time after 7 to 14 days.

Stibophen is marketed in the form of a 6.3% aqueous solution for strict intramuscular injection (carefully avoid entering a vein).

Stibophen, 42.5 mg of the drug in 5-ml ampoules.

After opening the ampoule, discard unused portion.

Do not store for a long time.

Suramin

Brand names: Antrypol, Germanin, Bayer 205. This is not an official drug in the United States, but has been used successfully in the treatment of onchocercosis, pemphigus, and trypanosomiasis (but not for *T. cruzi*). Toxic reactions are: shock, vomiting, colic, urticaria, late rashes, photophobia, and paresthesias. Blood dyscrasias, as agranulocytosis and hemolytic anemia, may also occur.

Dosage: for trypanosomiasis and pemphigus give early in the disease by slow intravenous injection *only* after 24 hours of a diagnostic lumbar puncture; starting dose, 200 mg to test for sensitivity; thereafter, give 100 mg, also in slow i.v., on days 3, 7, 14, and 21; and, if needed, an additional 1000 mg once a week, for 5 weeks. For prophylaxis of trypanosomiasis give (when it is known that the patient tolerates suramin), an intravenous injection of 1000 mg, which will afford protection for about 3 months. For onchocercosis and following an initial treatment with diethylcarbamazine (q.v.) give an initial 200-mg trial dose to be followed by 1000 mg 5 days later, and repeated every 5 days for a total of six doses (6000 mg in toto).

Wherever suramin is marketed, it is available as:

Suramin, 1000 mg ampoules; prepare freshly in 10% solution for intravenous use.

Brand names: Arsobal, Mel B. Because of its diffusion into the nervous system, melarsoprol is the *drug of choice* for the treatment of meningoence-phalitic trypanosomiasis. It is also very effective in the hemolymphatic stage, but is preferably employed for the treatment of the late stage. If patients in a late stage prove refractory to melarsoprol, nitrofurazone can be tried.

Melarsoprol should be used only under hospital supervision because of its very common side effects, such as reactive encephalopathy (the most common) and hypersensitivity reactions (controlled by slowly increasing dosage); other blood dyscrasias and hepatic disturbances may occur, but are not frequent.

Dosage: give by strict intravenous injection (avoid leakage into surrounding tissues!); adults over 50 kilos (110 lb.) and with less than 40 mg% of protein in the spinal fluid will receive 72 mg (2 ml of a 3.6% propylene glycol solution) the first day, 90 mg (2.5 ml) the second day, 108 mg (3 ml) the third day; then a pause of 7 days to be continued by 3 consecutive days with 126 mg (3.5 ml), 144 mg (4 ml), and 180 mg (5 ml); another 7-day pause, and again 3 consecutive days with 180 mg (5 ml). Debilitated adults will receive about 3.6 mg for each kilo of body weight as a maximal final dose.

Melarsoprol, ampoules with 36 mg (3.6%) in each ml.

Lucanthone

Brand names: Miracil, Nilodin. Lucanthone frequently causes side effects, which may be serious, particularly if there is a kidney impairment, a condition that would prohibit its use. Most recipients will complain of symptoms from the gastrointestinal tract; others, of vertigo, insomnia, sweating, or convulsions. Perhaps the simultaneous administration of atropine or an antihistaminic will ameliorate these reactions.

Lucanthone (not used for *S. japonicum*) can be given by mouth, an advantage particularly helpful for mass treatment in endemic areas.

Dosage: For the treatment of schistosomiasis: the total dose varies according to the country involved; in South America (*S. mansoni*) the total dose will be 100 mg for each kilo of body weight, or even a somewhat higher amount; a total dose between 100 and 200 mg for each kilo of body weight in the lands of the Old Testament; and lower doses, 60 to 100 mg, in Africa; in each instance, the individual dose will be about 5 mg for each kilo of body weight; and longer periods of treatment will be preferred to the shorter ones.

Lucanthone (hydrochloride), 200 mg tablets.

Diethylcarbamazine

Brand names: Banocide, Hetrozan. The filaricidal effect is marked on microfilariae and less noticeable in adult worms, but it undoubtedly happens with at least a few varieties (*W. bancrofti, W. malayi,* and loa-loa). It gives a radical cure in cases of parasitism by the aforementioned three in single or multiple courses. In onchocercosis, good control can be obtained after a short interrupted course of administration.

In regular dosage schedules the side effects are frequent, but minimal, usually disappearing soon, even during continuance of treatment. Among the disturbances are: headache, asthenia, articular pains, vomiting, lymphadenitis, edema, fever, the latter more marked in cases with onchocercosis, mostly subsiding in less than one week.

Dosage: For the treatment of *W. bancrofti* and *W. malayi,* give 2 mg for each kilo of body weight; take after meals three times a day, for no less than 21 days. A mass treatment for these infections consists of 2 mg per kilo of body weight, after meals, three times a day for 7 days. The treatment of loa-loa infections requires larger doses, of from 2 to 4 mg for each kilo of body weight, after meals three times a day, for 10 days; successive courses, to obtain cure, will not be given until after pauses of 20 to 30 days. To treat onchocercosis, check for eye complications, give no more than 0.5 mg for each kilo of body weight, once the first day, twice the second; then increase to 1 mg for each kilo of body weight, three times a day for 1 day, followed by 2 mg for each kilo three times a day to a total of 21 days.

Important notice: Extensive infections may cause severe symptoms due to the number of killed parasites. Decrease or stop medication in such a case.

Diethylcarbamazine citrate, 50 mg tablets.

Diethylcarbamazine citrate, syrup, containing 30 mg in each ml.

Thiabendazole

Brand name: Mintezol. Thiabendazole is reported to be a good larvicide in cases of infections with trichina or ascaris. In trichinosis, treated cases have shown highly acceptable results, even though post-treatment muscle biopsies have shown larvae still living.

Dosage: 25 mg for each kilo of body weight in 24 hours, in two installments, for 5 to 10 days.

Thiabendazole, suspension containing 500 mg in each 5 ml, in containers of 120 ml each.

VIII. ANTISEPTICS

These drugs are used to control the spread of germs from localized sites and for the elimination of systemic infections. Of course, sulfas and antibiotics have cut down sharply on their use. Pharmacological action of antiseptics may be achieved by disruption of metabolic processes of the germ, interference with cell multiplication, or any other change incompatible with survival.

Alcohol

Perhaps the most widely used disinfectant is ethyl alcohol, called alcohol by antonomasia, an aliphatic alcohol, used in beverages, with well-known effects on the nervous system and on respiration, the cardiovascular system, the gastrointestinal tract, the liver, and the kidneys. On the skin, alcohol is also used as a solvent for topical medications, and as a bactericidal disinfectant when used at the optimal concentration of 70%. Concentrations below 60% or over 90% are less bactericidal. Rubbing alcohol contains, in addition, acetone, ketones, coal-tar colors, perfume, and water, and also has a 70% concentration.

> Alcohol, 70% concentration.

> Rubbing alcohol.

Hydrogen Peroxide

Hydrogen peroxide is not a good germicide because of its selective, evanescent, and weak chemical quality and lack of diffusive power. Its main use is for dressing wounds and as a cleanser in Vincent's angina and other superficial infections. Because of gas expansion, do not inject it into cavities.

> Hydrogen peroxide solution containing 10 or 20 vol. of H_2O_2 in water; dispensed in bottles of varied sizes, e.g., 120 ml, 240 ml, or larger.

Silver Compounds

These compounds are used locally.

Silver nitrate usage is correlated with concentration and length of application; silver nitrate may be used in solid form or in solution. As a solid it is presented in the form of pencils to remove warts and to cauterize wounds and granulation tissue. Solutions vary in strength, from 1 : 10,000 to 1 : 10 (10%)—the weaker for washing urethra and bladder, the stronger to treat, very carefully, infected ulcers of the mouth. Silver picrate or lactate is also used.

Silver nitrate, pencil.

Silver nitrate, 1% solution (ampoules).

Silver nitrate, 1% ophthalmic solution.

Silver picrate, powder, for individualized prescriptions.

Chlorine Compounds

Chlorine compounds are powerful disinfectants, but too irritant to tissues. Hypochlorite solutions, chlorinated lime, and halazone are used for disinfection of water, or wounds. They are seldom used for human therapeutic purposes.

Halazone, tablets.

Iodine

Tincture of iodine, also among the most widely used disinfectants for skin abrasions and wounds, is perhaps the best skin disinfectant at our disposal.

Iodine, 0.5 to 1% water solution for wounds, abrasions, and other dermal uses.

Iodine, 0.1% water solution for irrigations.

Iodine, 2% glycerin solution, to use on mucosal surfaces.

Iodine, tincture U.S.P., 7½% for skin infections (bacteria, fungi).

Dyes

Coal-tar dyes may be used against protozoa, as wound cleansers, and as general antiseptics.

Phenazopyridine (brand name: Pyridium) is an azo dye with little germicidal action, but useful as a urinary analgesic.

Scarlet red is another azo dye used in ointment or oily solutions for cleansing wounds, and promoting epitheliazation (4 to 8% concentrations).

Fluorescein is presently used for diagnostic purposes (corneal ulcers). A 2% ophthalmic solution is a good antibacterial.

Phenolphthalein is mainly a diagnostic agent.

Gentian violet and *crystal violet* are rosaniline dyes used for superficial and fungal infections, and also as anthelmintics.

Methylene blue may be somewhat effective in rickettsial infections or in herpes simplex in conjunction with white light.

Pyridium, tablets, 100 or 200 mg.

Scarlet red, 5% ointment.

Fluorescein, 2% ophthalmic solution.

Gentian violet, 1% solution.

Gentian violet, powder, for individualized prescriptions.

Methylene blue, 1% solution, 1 or 10 ml.

Methylene blue, tablets or powder.

Surface-Active Agents

According to definition, surface-active agents are those that "alter the energy relations at interfaces." They are used as antiseptics for skin and mucous membranes, and as disinfectants.

Soap is not a member of this group, and even antagonizes the action of cationic surface-active agents; but it is the simplest of all cleansers for the skin. The bactericidal action is negligible.

Hexachlorophene (brand names: Hexachlorophene Liquid Soap U.S.P., Phisohex, or Soy-Dome cleanser) should not be applied to large areas or to abraded skin because of its very rapid absorption and tendency to reach toxic blood levels. Also, a recent discovery is the development of resistant strains after its use as a bacteriostatic skin cleanser. Stop its use at the first sign of cerebral irritability.

Hexachlorophene, liquid soap U.S.P., in different sizes (240 ml).

Hexachlorophene, powder, in different sizes (240 g).

Benzalkonium chloride (brand names: Zephiran, Cetylicide) is used in aqueous solution, tincture, and spray for antiseptic cleansing of skin wounds, preservation of topical medications, and irrigation of cavities.

Benzalkonium chloride, 12.8, 17, or 17.5% concentrate, in bottles.

Benzalkonium chloride, 1:750 aqueous solution.

Benzethonium chloride, methylbenzethonium chloride, and *cetyl-pyridinium chloride* are used in the same way that benzalkonium chloride is used.

Dosage for the above agents: 1:1000 tincture may be used on the un-abraded skin; 1:10,000 to 1:2000 solutions aqueous may be applied to mucous membranes and abraded skin; 1:5000 to 1:2000 solutions are to be used for instillation in the eye and vagina; 1:10,000 to 1:5000, for irrigation of large areas of abraded skin; 1:20,000, for irrigation of the bladder, or 1:40,000 if the solution is to be retained; 1:1000, for deep lacerations; 1:3000, for infected deep wounds.

Furan Derivatives

The antibacterial action of furan derivatives has a broad spectrum of activity, extending to gram-positive and gram-negative microorganisms. It is extremely rare that resistance to furans develops. *Nitrofurantoin* is used for the treatment of urinary infections (q.v. below). *Nitrofurazone* (Furacin) is used for the treatment of infections of the skin, by local application of 2% ointment or solution. *Furazolidone* (Furoxone) is recommended for the treatment of gastrointestinal infections caused by *Shigella, Salmonella, S. cholerae asiaticae, Giardia lamblia, E. coli,* staphylococci, and *Aerobacter aerogenes.*

It is advisable to drink no alcohol during furazolidone therapy, and for 4 days thereafter; nor should monamine oxidase inhibitor drugs be given simultaneously. A mixture of furazolidone and nifuroxime is used for vaginal infections (trichomonas, candidas, monilia).

Nitrofurazone, 0.2% solution.

Nitrofurazone, 0.2% topical cream.

Furazolidone, 100 mg tablets (one every 6 hours).

Furazolidone, 5 mg, plus nifuroxime, 7.5 mg, in the form of suppositories; and equivalent proportions for a powder form.

Mercury Compounds

Mercuric chloride is used as 1:1000 to 1:2000 solution to wash the hands, gloves, or nonmetallic surfaces. *Insoluble mercury compounds* are made into ointments for antisepsis and for their ecto-parasiticidal action (yellow oxide of mercury ointment). *Merbromin* (Mercurochrome) is not a potent germicide and has poor diffusion into tissues, but is not irritant to them.

Mercuric chloride tablets, blue (corrosive sublimate, 0.5 g; citric acid 2.50 mg). One tablet in 500 cc water makes 1:1000 solution.

Mercuric chloride, powder for individualized prescriptions.

Yellow mercury oxide, 0.5 or 2% ophthalmic ointment.

Merbromin, 2% aqueous solution.

Phenols

Phenol is a weak antiseptic advised for cauterization (full strength liquefied phenol) of small wounds caused by bites (dog, snake), and as an antipruritic. For this purpose only 2% or lesser concentrations will be used in aqueous solutions.

Phenol, 1 or 2% ointment.

Liquefied phenol.

Substitute Phenols

Many of these substances possess a better bactericidal action than phenol itself. *Cresol* is used as a mixture of the three alkyl isomers (Saponated Cresol Solution), active against most pathogenic microorganisms. Other substitute phenols are the following: guaiacol, an expectorant, rarely used as an antiseptic; hexylresorcinol, better known as an anthelmintic agent; and resorcinol, less potent than phenol. Also belonging to this group are creosote, thymol, and picric acid. Hexachlorophene is a chlorinated bio-phenol, which has been discussed with the "surface-active agents," q.v.

Cresol, solution.

Urinary Antiseptics

Mandelic acid is rapidly excreted into the urine, and shows bactericidal activity depending on its concentration and on the urine pH (below 5.5). A restricted water intake is advised to increase concentration. Sensitive bacteria do not become resistant, but there are resistant strains of *Proteus* and *Pseudomonas*.
Dosage: 3000 mg every 6 hours.

Mandelic acid, 120 or 150 g flasks, to prepare individualized prescriptions.

Methenamine mandelate (brand name: Mandelamine) is a compound of mandelic acid and methenamine. For more details, see above information on mandelic acid.
Dosage: 1000 mg after breakfast, lunch, and dinner and at bedtime.

Mandelamine, 250, 500, or 1000 mg tablets.

Nitrofurantoin (brand name: Furadantin) is a furan derivative mainly used for the treatment of urinary infections caused by *E. coli,* enterococci, staphylococci (not all strains), *Proteus* (not all strains), *Pseudomonas* (not all strains), *Klebsiella* (not all strains), and *Aerobacter* (not all strains). A test for sensitivity is advised in most instances. Sensitive bacteria rarely become resistant. Watch for renal damage, blood dyscrasias, and peripheral neuropathy.
Dosage: 50 to 100 mg every 6 hours, with meals. Administer by the intramuscular or intravenous route in patients over 55 kg (120 lb), giving 180 mg in 500 ml infusion every 12 hours.

Nitrofurantoin, 50 or 100 mg tablets.

Nitrofurantoin, oral suspension containing 25 mg per 5 ml.

Nitrofurantoin, 25, 50, and 100 mg capsules.

Nitrofurantoin, 180 mg in 20-ml vials.

Nalidixic acid (brand name: NegGram Caplets) is a very weak organic acid with an acceptable bactericidal effect, particularly active against urinary infections caused by *E. coli, Proteus, A. aerogenes, Klebsiella,* and *Pseudomonas* (not all strains). During therapy with nalidixic acid, as with other urinary antiseptics, care should be taken for the possibility of liver or kidney damage, gastrointestinal or visual disturbances, psychotic symptoms or convulsions.
Dosage: 1000 mg every 6 hours for 1 or 2 weeks; if treatment has to be prolonged, dosage can be reduced one half, to 500 mg every 6 hours.

Nalidixic acid, suspension, with 250 mg in each 5 ml.

Nalidixic acid, 250, 500, or 1000 mg "caplets."

Phenazopyridine (brand name: Pyridium) is presently used only as a pain reliever for the lower urinary tract. Simultaneous antibacterial treatment should be started in most instances.
Dosage: 200 mg every 8 hours taken after meals.

Phenazopyridine, 100 or 200 mg tablets.

Note: Phenazopyridine is also marketed in preparations combined with antibacterial drugs.
Trimethoprim plus sulfamethoxazole (brand names: Bactrim, Septra) is a combination of a pyrimidine derivate and a sulfa, used in the United States only for urinary infections, but also for other generalized infections in other parts of the world. Watch for hypersensitivity reactions, blood dyscrasias, and renal damage. Use for cystitis, pyelitis, or pyelonephritis due to *E. coli, Proteus, Enterobacter,* and *Klebsiella.* Nevertheless, a test for sensitivity should always be run.
Dosage: one double-strength or two regular tablets, every 12 hours. A 5-ml dose of the oral suspension is equivalent to one regular tablet. It is advisable to check the creatinine clearance and give only one daily dose if it is found between 15 and 30. A value below 15 warns against administration of the drug.

Tablets, regular strength.

Tablets, double strength.

Oral suspension.

IX. CANCERICIDALS

Surgery still is the procedure of choice for the treatment of most neoplastic diseases. Only when radical removal of the new growth proves to be impossible, or the spread of metastases appears likely, do we readily resort to radiotherapy or chemotherapy. Up to the present time no true cancericidal agent has been found. Only Hodgkin's disease and other lymphomas and lymphosarcomas usually respond well to chemotherapy. Also, corticoids and ACTH may favorably influence the course of some lymphomas and leukemias; and estrogens show a good effect on prostatic cancer, as do estrogens or androgens on mammary carcinoma.

Good specialized literature on this subject is available; therefore in this brief review only a summary of the basic facts will be presented. As usual, we shall consider indications, side effects, dosage, and available marketed preparations.

Also, with respect to the use of any of these products, the following requirements will always be kept in mind:

1. Need for adequate function of bone marrow, kidney, and liver prior to the use of a chemotherapeutic agent.

2. Absence of any concomitant disabling disease which might increase the risks of using these potent drugs.

3. Maintenance of a close watch, with periodic laboratory examinations, on the condition of the bone marrow and the level of uric acid in the blood (which should not increase), or for evidence of any other form of toxicity which might require stoppage of chemotherapy.

4. Careful evaluation of pros and cons when treating frail elderly persons, particularly those over 80 years of age.

Mechlorethamine (Nitrogen Mustard)

Brand name: Mustargen. This drug is recommended in the first instance for Hodgkin's disease, following the administration of radiotherapy. Only secondarily will it be considered for the treatment of other lymphomas, Wilm's tumor, seminoma, chorioepithelioma, neuroblastoma, and carcinomas of the breast, the ovary, or the nasopharynx.

Prominent side effects are anorexia, nausea and vomiting, bone marrow depression, and local phlebitis. Keep a constant watch for the response of the bone marrow to medication.

Dosage: a daily dose of 0.1 mg for each kilo of body weight by the intravenous route for 4 days. The total 4 day dose might be given in only one injection or in several consecutive shots. It is preferable to administer the injection at night, preceded by the administration of a dose (10 to 20 mg) of prochlorperazine. Repeat the same schedule every 6 weeks, always prefering an infusion lasting only a few minutes. Intracavity administration may also be given. For patients over 79 years of age it is better to give no more than 0.1 mg daily for each kilo of body weight for only 2 days.

Mechlorethamine, 20-ml vials containing 20 mg per vial. Prepare fresh with 10 ml of water.

Cyclophosphamide

Brand name: Cytoxan. This drug is also indicated for the treatment of Hodgkin's disease and other lymphomas, lymphosarcomas, and reticulum cell sarcoma, and, in addition, for myeloma, leukemia, mycosis fungoides, neuroblastoma, adenoma of the ovary, and retinoblastoma.

The use of cyclophosphamide should be avoided in cases of leukopenia, thrombocytopenia, impaired liver or kidney function, or bone marrow tumors, and should not, without consideration, follow the use of radiotherapy or any other cytotoxic agents (see below for precautions if so used).

Frequent side effects produced by the drug are leukopenia, thrombocytopenia, anorexia, nausea, vomiting and other gastrointestinal disturbances, alopecia, darkening of the skin, pulmonary fibrosis, and particularly a hemorrhagic cystitis, which may be very severe and may be prevented by the use of plenty of water.

Dosage: Initial therapy consists of a total of 40 to 50 mg for each kilo of body weight, given intravenously in several installments for 4 to 5 days; orally 1 to 5 mg for each kilo of body weight every day. The dosage will be cut in half if a cytotoxic drug or radiotherapy has been used previously. Maintenance therapy consists of 1 to 5 mg for each kilo of body weight once a day, by mouth; or intravenous injections of 3 to 5 mg for each kilo every 7 to 10 days.

Cyclophosphamide, tablets, 25 or 50 mg.

Cyclophosphamide, vials, 100, 200, or 500 mg, to be prepared with sterile water or 5% glucose. Not to be stored!

Uracil Mustard

Uracil mustard is recommended for the treatment of Hodgkin's disease and other lymphomas and lymphosarcomas. It is also used for reticulum cell sarcoma, myeloma, leukemia, mycosis fungoides, neuroblastoma, retinoblastoma, and ovarian adenoma.

Side effects are almost the same as with other nitrogen mustards, but the advantage is that alopecia is less frequent when using uracil mustard than it is with the others. Nausea, vomiting, and diarrhea are frequent.

Dosage: 1 or 2 mg a day, for 3 weeks; stop for 1 week, and then repeat the same dosage. An alternate procedure is to give 3 to 5 mg a day for 7 days, and thereafter 1 mg a day for 7 weeks.

Uracil mustard, 1 mg capsules.

Chlorambucil

Brand name: Leukeran. This drug is mainly prescribed for chronic lymphocytic leukemia, but also is used for Hodgkin's disease and lymphomas.

The outstanding side effect is bone marrow depression, which should be checked for very frequently. To minimize complications, try to avoid its use after radiotherapy or the use of other chemotherapeutic agents.

Dosage: 0.1 to 0.2 mg for each kilo of body weight is the daily dose, which will be maintained for 3 to 6 weeks. This dosage will be readjusted as needed. For Hodgkin's disease, give 0.2 mg for each kilo of body weight every day, as above; but in cases of lymphomatous infiltration of bone marrow, use small amounts in all instances.

Chlorambucil, 2 mg tablets.

Busulfan

Brand name: Myleran. Busulfan is used in the treatment of chronic myelocytic leukemia—not for cure, which it cannot provide, but for controlling symptoms and to prolong life. It can be used regardless of previous treatment with radiation or chemotherapy.

Side effects are: thrombocytopenia, hyperuricemia (use allopurinol to avoid this), the usual gastrointestinal complaints, and alopecia.

Dosage: 4 to 8 mg a day, depending on the severity of the disease and the leukocyte count. When the latter falls below 10,000 on monthly check, stop therapy. Start again when the count rises over 50,000. Those patients whose remissions last less than 3 months should be kept on a maintenance dosage of 1 to 3 mg a day.

Busulfan, 2 mg scored tablets.

Melphalan

Brand name: Alkeran. A total of 30 to 50% of patients treated for multiple myeloma respond favorably, though response is slow and at times takes months to be seen.

Marked bone marrow depression may occur, as well as the usual gastrointestinal symptoms. It should not be given following the administration of other chemotherapeutic drugs or radiotherapy.

Dosage: 6 mg a day, for 2 or 3 weeks, then a pause, and thereafter a maintenance dosage of 2 mg a day. Several other schedules have also been employed.

Melphalan, 2 mg scored tablets.

Triethylenemelamine, TEM

TEM is used like other nitrogen mustards; the side effects are also similar, but less marked on the gastrointestinal tract.

Dosage: During the first week give 2.5 mg every other day, together with 2 g of sodium bicarbonate; thereafter, give 2.5 to 5 mg a week until a response is seen. Then stop therapy until relapse is noted. A continuous maintenance dosage can be given as long as a careful observation of the bone marrow is carried out.

TEM, 1 or 5 mg tablets.

Triethylenethiophosphoramine, ThioTEPA

Brand name: Thiotepa. Good results have been obtained in the treatment of adenocarcinoma of the breast or ovary, Hodgkin's disease and other malignant lymphomas, bronchogenic carcinoma, and intracavity effusions due to neoplasms. Favorable results have been obtained in cancer of the bladder.

As with similar drugs, gastrointestinal side effects may occur as well as local pain at the site of the injection, febrile reactions, bleeding, hyperuricemia, thrombocytopenia, and other evidences of bone marrow depression.

Dosage: For older people, 45 mg is sufficient when used locally, and no more than 30 mg if given intravenously. Maintenance dosages, individualized, will be at 1- to 4-week intervals. Topical applications are used for vesical cancer, instilling a solution with 60 mg or less in 30 to 60 ml of water, to be retained for about 2 hours.

ThioTEPA, 15 mg vials to be prepared with 1.5 ml of distilled water (if stored, keep at 2° to 8°C).

Methrotexate

Used either by mouth or by injection, methrotexate is prescribed among older people for squamous cancer of the head or neck, leukemia, and lymphosarcomas; also, for mycosis fungoides and psoriasis. It is mainly recommended for maintenance treatments.

Because the toxicity of methrotexate is high, the dosage will be kept at the lowest limits, and careful evaluation of the decision to use or not to use will be observed according to the nature of the disease (psoriasis, for instance) and the personal condition of the patient. Watch for ulcerative stomatitis as well as for the usual side effects of these drugs.

Dosage: Several different schedules have been recommended. Average maintenance dosage will be about 5 to 6 mg (3.3 mg for each square meter of body surface) every day, for 4 to 6 weeks. In other instances, 10 to 20 mg a day may be given orally for 4 to 8 days, with pauses of no less than 1 week. Summarizing: check for appropriate dosage in each particular instance of treatment with methrotexate.

Methrotexate, 2.5 mg tablets.

Methrotexate, 2-ml vials containing 2.5 or 25 mg each.

Fluorouracil

Brand names: Efudex, Fluoroplex. Fluorouracil is presented in the form of topical preparations, namely, solutions or creams, to be used in patients with superficial basal cell carcinoma; also, those with actinic keratoses. Given by injection, it is used for the palliative treatment of carcinoma (rectum, breast, ovary, stomach, bladder, pancreas, lung), and in cases of head and neck squamous cancer.

It is recommended that the administration of fluorouracil be stopped in the presence of any of the following side effects: stomatitis, pharyngitis, esophagitis, rapidly developing leukopenia, thrombocytopenia, vomiting, diarrhea, and bleeding. Since its margin of safety is very narrow, special care should be taken with giving this drug to those of advanced years.

Dosage: For local application, solutions usually give better results; cover the lesions twice a day until frank ulceration appears. For basal cell carcinoma a 5% solution strength is advised, to be used for about 3 to 6 weeks, or more, until lesions are obliterated. Only intravenous injections will be given, if it is used parenterally. In this instance give 12 mg of the drug for each kilo of the ideal weight (if the patient is overweight), daily for 4 successive days. In no instance will a dosage over 800 mg be given. When there is good tolerance, therapy will be continued with half the above-indicated dosage, given on days 6, 8, 10, and 12. Frail elderly persons will receive only 6 mg daily for each kilo of body weight for 3 days; and 3 mg on days 5, 7, and 9. Maintenance is achieved by repeating the same schedules after 1-month pauses.

Fluorouracil, in bottles containing 1, 2, or 5% solution.

Fluorouracil, 1% in cream dispensers.

Fluorouracil, 10-ml ampoules containing 500 mg.

Mercaptopurine

Brand name: Purinethol. This drug is given for the treatment of acute leukemias, though elderly persons react poorly to its administration. It should also be tried in cases of chronic myelocytic leukemia because there is good response in some instances—unfortunately, only a few.

Side effects are usual, but special care should be taken to discontinue it at the first evidence of a reduction in the leukocyte count. Do not forget that these side effects may appear late, in many instances.

Dosage: will be carefully individualized. The daily dose will be between 100 and 200 mg (about 2.5 mg for each kilo of body weight). If there is no evident response after 1 month of treatment, increase the dosage to a double amount. If allopurinol is also given to control hyperuricemia, the dose of mercaptopurine will be reduced to one third or one fourth of the usual amount. Keep elderly persons at the lowest possible dose.

Mercaptopurine, 50 mg scored tablets.

Cytarabine

Brand name: Cytosar. This drug is recommended for the treatment of adult leukemia, particularly the acute granulocytic type.

Side effects are leukopenia and thrombocytopenia, frequently.

Dosage: only given parenterally, by subcutaneous or intravenous injection or infusion (better tolerated are rapid intravenous injections). There is daily administration of 2 mg per kilo of body weight, for 10 days. If there is good tolerance, double the dose, and administer it until results (pro or con) are obtained.

Cytarabine, 100 or 500 mg vials to be reconstituted with 5 or 10 ml of bacteriostatic water for injection.

Actinomycin D

Brand name: Cosmegen. This drug is given for the treatment of metastatic testicular carcinoma, together with chlorambucil or methrotexate.

Usual side effects are anorexia, nausea, vomiting, glossitis, diarrhea, proctitis, alopecia, and other common side effects of the chemotherapeutic agents.

Dosage: 0.000015 mg. (15 μg) for each kilo of body weight as a daily intravenous injection, for 5 days. If it is tolerated, repeat the same schedule every 2 to 4 weeks.

Actinomycin D, vials containing 0.5 mg.

Mithramycin

Brand name: Mithracin. Mithramycin is recommended for the treatment of testicular cancer when surgery or radiation is not advisable.

Manufacturers strongly recommend hospitalization of patients to carry out treatment, since severe thrombocytopenia with bleeding and even death may result.

Dosage: The drug is given by intravenous administration, slow infusion (4 to 6 hours), diluted in 1 liter of 5% dextrose. It will be given at the amount of 0.000025 mg (25 mg) for each kilo of body weight every day for 8 to 10 days. Additional courses after pauses of 1 month can be given.

> Mithramycin, vials containing 2.5 mg of the powder, to be reconstituted with 4.9 ml of sterile water. Discard the unused portions.

Vincristine

Brand name: Oncovin. This drug is recommended for the treatment of acute leukemia; also in combination with similar drugs, for Hodgkin's disease, lymphosarcoma, other sarcomas, neuroblastoma, and Wilm's tumor.

Side effects, particularly hyperuricemia, are of the same type as with other chemotherapeutic agents, perhaps with less toxicity, though overdosage may cause serious and even fatal reactions.

Dosage: Several different schedules are advised, mostly using 1.4 mg for each square meter of body surface (average adult will receive about 2.5 mg). This dose is given intravenously once a week (even small leaks will cause marked irritation).

> Vincristine, vials containing 1 or 5 mg of the powder, to be dissolved in Bacteriostatic Sodium Chloride for injection.

Vinblastine

Brand name: Velban. This drug is advised for palliation in cases of Hodgkin's disease and other lymphomas, lymphosarcoma, reticulum cell sarcoma, neuroblastoma, and mycosis fungoides. It is less effective in cases of carcinoma of the breast or the testis.

Leukopenia and other common reactions are frequent findings when using this drug.

Dosage: strict intravenous injection (severe irritation if leaked) once a week, starting with 0.1 mg for each kilo of body weight; increasing 0.05 mg for the successive injections, up to a maximum of 0.3 mg for each kilo of body weight. Other schedules are also recommended.

> Vinblastine, ampoules containing 10 mg of powder.

Procarbazine

Brand name: Matulane. This drug is given only to cases of Hodgkin's disease resistant to other forms of therapy, and when other cancers are similarly resistant. Some amelioration of symptoms is usually obtained.

Side effects are the usual ones, perhaps more marked on the central nervous system.

Dosage: give 100 to 200 mg a day, preferably in divided doses, for 1 week. Thereafter, increase to 300 mg a day until leukopenia is noted. Stop until a satisfactory recovery occurs. Then, start again at a lower dosage, 50 to 100 mg a day.

Procarbazine, 50 mg capsules.

Other Recommended Chemotherapeutic Agents

The number of agents found in the search for more active and less toxic medication for the treatment of malignancies is continually increasing. Among these other agents, the following are frequently prescribed, in addition to those mentioned in more detail in the preceding lines.

Lomustine (Brand name: CeeNU) is used together with other antineoplastic drugs in Hodgkin's disease and brain tumors. Dosage: 130 mg for each square meter of body surface (average adult, 230 mg), given by mouth every 6 weeks.

Lomustine, 10, 40, or 100 mg capsules.

Floxuridine (Brand name: FuDR) is very toxic and to be given only to hospitalized patients with carcinomas not responsive to other agents. Dosage: 0.1 or 0.2 mg for each kilo of body weight, daily. Repeat until adverse reactions appear.

Floxuridine, 5-ml vials containing 500 mg.

Streptonigrin has been recommended for breast cancer, head and neck squamous cell carcinoma, cancer of the ovary, Hodgkin's disease, and other lymphomas. Stop its use if bone marrow depression occurs. Dosage: 0.1 to 0.2 mg for each kilo of body weight, daily by mouth; or 0.000005 mg (5 μg) in a 1-liter infusion, the dosage distributed over 5 days.

Bleomycin (Brand name: Blenoxane) is recommended for squamous cell carcinoma, testicular carcinoma, Hodgkin's disease, and lymphosarcomas. Dosage: start with 2 units or less, once or twice a week by injection (intravenous, intramuscular, or subcutaneous). If there is no adverse reaction, increase to 10 or 20 units. Maintenance therapy will be achieved with 1 to 5 units a week.

Bleomycin, ampoules with 15 units each.

Dexorubicin (Brand name: Adriamycin) is recommended for the treatment of leukemias, Hodgkin's disease, lymphomas, sarcomas, and cancer of the lung, the breast, or the female genital organs. Cardiac toxicity must be carefully watched for. With intermittent injections this danger is somewhat minimized. Dosage: should be kept below 200 mg a day for the average adult (120 to 150 mg to be preferred), given in three divided doses, once a day. Repeat every 3 or 4 weeks.

Dexorubicin, vials containing 10 or 50 mg.

Other cancericidals frequently recommended are the following: *thioguanine,* for acute leukemia (40 mg tablets), to give 2 mg for each kilo of body weight, to increase to 3 mg if after 1 month there is no adverse reaction; *mitomycin* (brand name, Mutamycin), for its use together with other cancericidals in cancer of the stomach or the pancreas (vials containing 5 mg), using doses below 20 mg for each square meter of body surface (average adult will receive 35 mg); and also *daunomycin* and *demecolcine* for leukemias.

Hormones

See section XXVI.

Radioisotopes and Radiotherapy

Because the expert must be skillful, competent, and fully familiar with the management of radioisotopes and radiation equipment for their use in either diagnosis or therapy, and because these methods are not within the reach of the practicing physician, only a few lines will be devoted to this type of therapy.

Soon after the discovery of both X-ray apparatus and radium, their use for the treatment of tumors began. Since the late thirties and early forties, ^{32}P and ^{131}I have been used for the treatment of polycythemia and thyroid diseases. Later on, the use of radioactive gold, cobalt, strontium, cesium, and other metals started, mostly with only modest success.

Better results of radiotherapy—usually associated with surgery—have been obtained in the treatment of cancer of the skin, the breast, and the rectum and sigmoid. But up to the present time, complete reliance for cure can be placed only on an early excision.

Sodium iodide ^{131}I, U.S.P. and sodium phosphate ^{32}P, U.S.P. are, perhaps, the most frequently used radioisotopes. The latter is employed in the treatment of chronic granulocytic leukemia (for which disease busulfan is preferred), chronic lymphocytic leukemia, and the palliation of polycythemia vera. The radioactive iodide has been recommended for the treatment of metastatic thyroid cancer, but the results have been disappointing. These radioisotopes are dispensed by specialized centers (such as the Nuclear Regulatory Commission), as follows.

Sodium iodide ^{131}I, U.S.P., in ampoules containing 250 microcuries in 10 ml, or 1000 microcuries in 40 ml. There are other presentations also available.

Sodium phosphate ^{32}P, U.S.P., solution containing 2 microcuries in 1 ml, for oral use. Also, for injection, 2 microcuries in 1 ml.

X. ANALGESICS AND ANTIPYRETICS

Morphine

Morphine is a phenanthrene derivative extracted from opium. It increases pain threshold and decreases the natural reactions of alertness, anxiety, and fear, so that analgesia results in most body structures. Also, morphine causes sleepiness, depression with euphoria, slowing of respiration and functions of the digestive system (particularly causing constipation), and miosis; it checks cough and diarrhea, but increases the tone of the smooth muscle of the biliary tract, the ureters, and the urinary bladder, thus leading to urinary retention. Nausea and vomiting may occur after its administration.

This alkaloid is rapidly absorbed when administered by mouth or by injection. The analgesic effect usually lasts 4 hours, but with advancing years this effect may be somewhat prolonged. Nevertheless, regarding this resistance to opiates, it is not advisable to increase dosages, since the resultant respiratory depression may become a serious problem because many older patients of a lesser size and weight are subject to constipation and urinary retention. Another problem: after a few days of using morphine, tolerance develops, which is rapidly extended to codeine and other opium alkaloids.

The use of morphine is reserved for the treatment of pain not responsive to other analgesics, principally pain caused by cancer, traumatic accidents, pericarditis, and pleurisy; and possibly in cases with biliary or renal colic, vascular occlusions (coronary, peripheral, or pulmonary), internal hemorrhage, heart failure, thyrotoxicosis, or diseases interfering with sleep.

Dosage: from 10 to 20 mg every 4 hours, by subcutaneous injection. For more rapid action, it may be dissolved in 5 ml of saline and injected very slowly into a vein. In asthenic patients, try lower amounts first.

Morphine sulfate, hypodermic tablets, 5, 8, 10, 15 or 30 mg.

Morphine sulfate, 15, 30, or 60 mg capsules.

Morphine sulfate, injectables, 8, 10, 15, 20, or 30 mg in each ml; in 1-ml ampoules and 10- or 20-ml vials.

Morphine poisoning will cause three symptoms, which are almost pathognomonic: coma, shallow respirations, and pinpoint pupils. Treatment must be given as soon as possible with a patent airway maintained and the administration of either nalorphine or levallorphan.

Nalorphine HCl (Nalline), 10 mg in 2-ml ampoules; to give 5 to 10 mg intramuscularly, repeating every 10 to 15 minutes if no response is obtained, not to exceed 40 mg in a 3-hour period; the series may be repeated at 3- to 4-hour intervals.

Levallorphan tartrate (Lorfan), 1 mg in 1-ml ampoules, to inject intravenously; followed by 0.5 mg at 3-minute intervals, for one or two injections.

Meperidine

Brand name: Demerol. This drug is a crystalline powder which shares properties corresponding to both morphine and atropine, for which reason it is better indicated for pain of spastic origin. Meperidine may lead to addiction because of its euphoric and sedative effects. It is rapidly absorbed when given by mouth or by injection. Analgesia is rapidly obtained, but lasts only about 3 hours because of the drug's very rapid excretion. The main side effects are dryness of the mouth, flushing of the face, and sweating; but there may also occur nausea, vomiting, tremors, incoordination, blurring of vision, and syncope. As with morphine, respiratory depression is very important. Cerebral excitation will indicate overdosage. Meperidine has to be given very cautiously to patients with hypotension, and not at all to those in shock, because these conditions would be exaggerated owing to vasodilation.

Meperidine relaxes the smooth muscles of the lower gastrointestinal tract, the bronchi, the urinary bladder, and the uterus; and contracts the upper gastrointestinal tract and the gall bladder. It is, therefore, recommended for the relief of pain in the lower gastrointestinal tract, the urinary bladder, or the uterus, if the pain is due to spasm of these muscles. Pulmonary depression is rarer with this drug than with morphine.

Dosage: from 50 to 150 mg, average 100 mg; never use more than 200 mg in one dose, but stay at the lower ranges of action. Meperidine in combination with other drugs, as it is found so frequently on the market, is not to be recommended for the elderly.

Meperidine HCl, 50 or 100 mg tablets.

Meperidine HCl, elixir, 50 mg in each teaspoonful.

Meperidine HCl, powder, in bottles containing 15 g for individual prescriptions.

Meperidine HCl, ampoules of 1, 1½, or 2 ml, or vials containing 10, 20, or 30 ml, with 50 mg in each ml; also 75 mg per ml in disposable units.

Meperidine HCl, 1-ml ampoules or disposable units, and 10- or 20-ml vials, with 100 mg per ml.

Methadone

Brand name: Dolophine. This drug's analgesic effects start quickly and last about 4 hours. These effects are similar to those of morphine; it is recommended for painful chronic conditions, and used as an antitussive; but mainly it is used for the treatment of morphine addiction. Since the actions, side effects, and toxicity are essentially the same as for morphine, the reader is referred to the above information.

Dosage: 5 to 10 mg if given by mouth, and a little less if by injection; repeating three or four times a day, only if needed. Do not give large doses by injection, since they are irritating to tissues.

Methadone HCl, tablets containing 2.5, 5, 7.5, and 10 mg.

Methadone HCl, elixir, with 5 mg in 4 ml (teaspoonful).

Methadone HCl, syrup, containing 1.7 mg in 4 ml.

Methadone HCl, suppositories containing 10 mg.

Methadone HCl, injectable, containing 10 mg in each ml, in 1-ml ampoules and 20-ml vials.

Opium Preparations

Paregoric elixir, or camphorated tincture of opium, is administered at a 4-ml dosage repeated several times a day, principally for the management of intestinal colic.

Laudanum, or tincture of opium, is given at a lower dosage of 0.5 ml, also several times a day, for gastrointestinal pains or for diarrhea.

Powdered opium at a dosage of 50 mg, several times a day, has been used for diarrhea; and in suppositories also containing extract of belladonna and tannic acid, for the treatment of hemorrhoids.

Because these pharmaceutical preparations are not excessively powerful, they might be used for elderly people; nevertheless, similar *cough preparations,* usually containing the equivalent of 1 mg of morphine or dihydromorphinone, are better avoided for these persons.

Pantopon contains half its weight of morphine (20 mg of pantopon contains 10 mg of morphine); but it should be considered as morphine itself when administered to older people, in spite of the claims that combining morphine with the other opium alkaloids enhances its activity and lessens the side effects.

Codeine (Methylmorphine)

Codeine, which is obtained by methylation of morphine, is mainly used in the form of the more soluble phosphate or sulfate. Its actions are similar to those of morphine, but markedly weaker, rarely causing addiction and principally recommended for the treatment of mild to moderate pain, or cough. The drug is rapidly absorbed when given by mouth or by injection; the analgesic effect usually lasts less than 4 hours. This drug could be given to older people but only if its administration proves not to cause constipation, dizziness, or drowsiness, which are prone to occur in the frail or the debilitated.

Dosage: Small repeated doses are better, namely, 15 to 30 mg; for cough, 5 to 10 mg may suffice.

Codeine phosphate, 15, 30, or 60 mg tablets.

Codeine phosphate, 15, 30, or 60 mg capsules.

Codeine phosphate, injectables, 1-ml ampoules containing either 15, 30, or 60 mg; or 20-ml vials containing 30 mg in each ml.

Papaverine

This opium derivative belongs to a different chemical group from that of morphine—that is, the benzylisoquinoline group. It is deprived of the dangerous side effects of morphine except when it is administered intravenously, which should be done very slowly, since a rapid injection may result in cardiac arrhythmias and even death. To minimize this untoward reaction, dilute the drug with saline or glucose infusions so as to give 100 mg in about 10 minutes. Other side effects are: gastrointestinal distress, drowsiness, malaise, sweating, and headache; these may force stoppage of medication.

Its principal activity is on the smooth muscle, which is relaxed by an antispasmodic direct action, thus alleviating pain indirectly in cases of biliary, urinary, or gastrointestinal colic; or in conditions causing contraction of blood vessels. It is usually indicated for the treatment of angina pectoris, myocardial infarction, peripheral arterial embolism, pulmonary embolism, mesenteric thrombosis, cerebral thrombosis, and impaired circulation to the brain.

Dosage: no more than 100 mg repeated three to five times a day; or even more, if so required and given with adequate care. Given by mouth, up to 200 mg three to five times a day may be required. In cases of pulmonary embolism it is advisable to give it in association with atropine, 1 mg, or with digitalis or quinidine whenever these drugs are indicated.

Papaverine HCl, 30, 60, 90, 100, 180, or 200 mg tablets.

Papaverine HCl, 150 mg sustained-release capsules.

Papaverine HCl, powder for individual prescriptions in bottles containing 30, 120, or 150 g.

Papaverine HCl, injectable, in 1- or 2-ml ampoules containing 30 mg in each ml; also 60 mg in 2-ml ampoules; or 10-ml vials, with 30 mg in each ml.

Propoxyphene Hydrochloride

Brand name: Darvon. This is a synthetic, nonnarcotic analgesic related to methadone, with effects lasting for about 6 hours. Side effects are of little consequence, and it does not produce respiratory depression; but it may cause drowsiness or dizziness, nausea or vomiting. It is recommended for the treatment of headache, migraine, toothache, arthritis, fibrositis, and hemorrhoids. Large doses may depress circulation and respiration, or cause convulsions or coma; so they will be avoided for depleted persons.
Dosage: 65 mg four times a day; better if in combination with acetylsalicylic acid.

Propoxyphene, capsules containing 32 or 65 mg.

Pentazocine

Brand name: Talwin. This drug is recommended by the manufacturers as a substitute for morphine for all types and degrees of pain.

Pentazocine HCl, tablets, 50 mg.

Pentazocine lactate, injectable, each ml containing 30 mg, in ampoules of 1, 1½, or 2 ml, or in 10-ml vials.

Indomethacin

Brand name: Indocin. This drug possesses anti-inflammatory, antipyretic, and analgesic properties, but is not chemically related to corticoids or salicylates. It is recommended for the treatment of gout, rheumatoid arthritis, ankylosing spondylitis, and osteoarthritis of the hip. Apparently, indomethacin works better if given together with acetylsalicylic acid. In general, this drug is less risky than phenylbutazone, corticoids, gold, and the drugs employed for rheumatic diseases; but it should not be given to patients with latent or active peptic ulcer, asthma, ulcerative colitis, regional enteritis, epilepsy, parkinsonism, or any other condition in which corticoids are contraindicated. Many patients may react with diarrhea and gastrointestinal bleeding; others will develop a pre-pyloric gastric ulcer—not to be taken for a malignancy, but this will not be sufficient reason to withdraw indomethacin from the armamentarium against rheumatic diseases, particularly gout.

Dosage: 25 mg two or three times a day, not to exceed 200 mg a day, but this larger amount should very rarely be given to frail and small people. It is recommended that these patients be given a 100-mg dose at night; but a 25-mg twice-a-day regimen is frequently effective for prolonged medication.

Indomethacin, 25 or 50 mg capsules.

Acetylsalicylic acid (Aspirin)

This is the acetic acid ester of salicylic acid, with analgesic and antipyretic effects lasting for about 4 hours. Antipyresis is evident only if the body temperature is elevated, probably due to a "resetting" to normal of the regulatory nervous mechanism in the hypothalamus. The analgesic effect, which is inferior to that of codeine, is more marked against integumental than against visceral pain, but it does not cause anesthesia or any mental change when given in therapeutic doses.

Large doses, as those given for rheumatic fever, may cause hyperventilation with subsequent alkalosis ending in acidosis, which is more noticeable among the elderly. Gout may require large doses to respond. Intolerance to the medication is frequently found, such as nausea, vomiting, urticaria, and edema; but most important are gastric bleeding and nephritis, among the elderly. Intoxication is noted by ringing in the ears, more marked gastrointestinal distress, sweating, and mental confusion. In these cases, decrease the concentration of salicylate in the blood, and give sodium lactate.

Acetylsalicylic acid is recommended for the treatment of headache, arthritis, neuralgia, and other pains. For the relief of rheumatic fever and gout, as stated above, large doses are needed, which may induce undesirable side effects.

Dosage: by mouth, give 300 to 600 mg each time, repeating every 2 to 4 hours. Frail, small patients will do better with only 300 mg; but the large doses required for rheumatic fever and gout, 5 to 10 g or more a day, should be given with caution, and an attempt made to get along with smaller amounts, as 6 g, usually given for maintenance. It will be advisable always to give this medication on a full stomach or after meals. Tablets containing buffers, or coated for intestinal release, are recommended to avoid gastric irritation; the concomitant use of sodium bicarbonate to counter the drug's acidity will require the use of larger doses to compensate for the chemical change.

Acetylsalicylic acid, tablets, 60, 75, or 300 mg.

Acetylsalicylic acid, buffered tablets, 300 mg.

Acetylsalicylic acid, enteric coated tablets, 300 or 600 mg.

Acetylsalicylic acid, 300 or 600 mg capsules.

Acetylsalicylic acid, suppositories, 60, 200, 300, or 600 mg.

Compounds of Acetylsalicylic Acid. There are innumerable compounds of acetylsalicylic acid (ASA) containing other medications. Some of these compounds are mentioned here, as an example.

ASA, 300 mg, with chloropheniramine maleate, 2 mg, and caffeine, 30 mg (Coricidin); take four tablets a day.

ASA, 325 mg, with propoxyphene hydrochloride, 65 mg (Darvon with ASA), pulvules; take three or four a day.

ASA, 300 mg, with prednisolone, 0.5 mg (Cordex), or prednisolone, 1.5 mg (Cordex-Forte); take one or two tablets, four times a day; these are presented either plain or buffered.

ASA, 200 mg, with meperidine hydrochloride, 30 mg, phenacetin, 150 mg, and caffeine, 30 mg (APC with Demerol); take one or two tablets, three or four times a day.

Sodium Salicylate

Sodium salicylate is rapidly absorbed from the gastrointestinal tract, reaching high blood concentrations in less than 2 hours. Intolerance may be either local, as when following closely its administration, or central, when delayed. Intoxication presents the same symptomatology as with acetylsalicylic acid, which is described above.

Dosage: for rheumatic fever up to 15 g a day may be given in divided doses every 4 hours; tolerance may be increased by giving small amounts of thyroid extract (30 mg a day) and adding to each dose some sodium bicarbonate or aluminum hydroxide, or by using enteric coated tablets. Central intolerance will not be helped by coating the tablets or giving antacids. To diminish any bleeding tendency, particularly among the elderly, give menadione (1 mg per g of sodium salicylate). For mild pain, dosage is 300 mg every 3 or 4 hours, to be increased to about 1 g every 4 hours if severe. These dosages are usually given by mouth; the parenteral route is rarely used.

Sodium salicylate, tablets containing 300, 500, or 600 mg.

Sodium salicylate, enteric coated tablets containing same dosages.

Sodium salicylate, injection, 200 mg in each ml, in 5-ml ampoules or 10-ml vials.

Methylsalicylate (Oil of Wintergreen)

This is an oily liquid used topically for muscle and joint pains.

Methylsalicylate, in bottles containing 500 ml or 2.5 liters for individualized prescriptions.

Salicylamide

This drug is rapidly absorbed with effects lasting about 6 hours or less. Uses and intolerance are as for other salicylates.
Dosage: 2 g every 4 to 8 hours for rheumatic conditions.

Salicylamide, tablets containing 300 mg.

Salicylamide, powder, in bottles of 120 g, 500 g, or 2.5 kg, for individualized prescriptions.

Salicylsalicylic Acid

Two molecules of salicylic acid are formed from one of salicylsalicylic acid, a change that occurs in the intestines because it is poorly soluble in water. Being slowly hydrolyzed, it shows retarded and prolonged activity. Uses and intolerance are as for other salicylates.
Dosage: 300 to 600 mg two or three times a day, usually administered together with aspirin.

Salicylsalicylic acid, 485 mg, plus 160 mg of acetylsalicylic acid, in tablets.

Acetaminophen

Brand names: Tylenol, Tempra, Apamide. This drug, which is acetylparaaminophenol, is a synthetic product closely related to acetophenetidin. It is rapidly absorbed and capable of relieving pain in 15 to 30 minutes after ingestion, the effect lasting for 2 or 3 hours. Only moderate pain will respond to the medication, such as headache, myalgia, arthralgia, and similar discomforts.
Dosage: 300 to 600 mg every 4 hours; but it is better to follow indications given by manufacturers, since the medication is frequently mixed with other drugs, codeine, for instance.

Acetaminophen, 300 mg in tablets.

Acetaminophen, 300 mg in effervescent tablets.

Acetaminophen, liquid, 120 mg in each ml (1 teaspoonful); or as solution of 100 mg per ml.

Acetophenetidin (Phenacetin)

This drug is rapidly absorbed, peak concentrations in the blood are reached in 1 to 2 hours, and effects last only about 3 hours, as antipyresis and analgesia. The drug is mainly used for headaches, joint and muscle pains, peripheral nerve irritation, and other mild discomforts. When it is given to elderly persons, watch particularly for methemoglobinemia and nephritis. Intoxication will cause cyanosis, dyspnea, virtigo, anginal pain, and final circulatory failure, shock, coma, and death; and thus must be promptly treated with stomach lavage, blood transfusion, inhalation of oxygen, and all needed supportive measures.

Dosage: doses below the average 300 mg and given at shorter intervals than every 3 hours are equally effective and less toxic.

Acetophenetidin, 120, 200, or 300 mg tablets.

Acetophenetidin 150 mg, with acetylsalicylic acid, 230 mg, and caffeine, 30 mg, in tablets.

Antipyrine

A pyrazolon derivative, antipyrine is a drug widely used in the past, rapidly absorbed from the gastrointestinal tract, with effects lasting for about 4 hours. The main use is for antipyresis and analgesia. Skin eruptions are frequent side effects, but it rarely affects the blood.

Dosage: 300 mg, once or twice every 4 hours.

Antipyrine, 300 mg tablets.

Aminopyrine (Pyramidon)

This drug is a derivative of antipyrine, with almost identical properties, but with the rare disadvantage that it may cause agranulocytosis.

Dosage: 300 to 600 mg every 4 hours.

Aminopyrine, 300 mg tablets.

Phenylbutazone (Butazolidine)

One of the main drugs used in the treatment of gout, phenylbutazone is not capable of reaching full blood concentration in less than 3 days. Its metabolism and excretion are slow, and detectable amounts remain in the blood for 1 week after it is discontinued.

Its pharmacologic effects are anti-inflammatory, analgesic, and antipyretic. The principal uses are for the treatment of arthritis, particularly of the gouty or rheumatoid variety, ankylosing spondylitis, psoriatic arthritis, osteoarthritis (in this case only for acute exacerbations not responsive to other medications), post-traumatic inflammations (as in the case of surgery), acute superficial thrombophlebitis, cancer, Hodgkin's disease, and inflammatory ocular conditions.

Phenylbutazone is prone to cause local irritation, which may be avoided or minimized by the use of sodium-free antacids, belladonna alkaloids, or both, and by giving it with milk or after meals. It may reactivate a peptic ulcer, and care should be taken when it is given to patients with hypertension, drug allergy, blood dyscrasias, or diseases of the heart, liver, or kidney, and particularly those prone to edema. Other undesirable side effects are the possibility of its causing severe blood dyscrasias, such as aplastic anemia, thrombocytopenic purpura, agranulocytosis, or leukopenia; or less severe complications, such as gastrointestinal distress, hepatitis, skin rashes, pruritus, polyuria, or nervous symptoms; for which reasons phenylbutazone should be reserved only for selected cases not responding to usual therapy. Special care will be taken with older patients who may also react with fluid retention.

Dosage: start with 300 to 600 mg a day, in divided doses; when some improvement occurs after 1 week of treatment, resort to the minimum maintenance dosage, which should not exceed 400 mg a day, always in three or four installments; if no improvement occurs, discontinue the administration of phenylbutazone. For the treatment of gouty arthritis, a slightly higher schedule is advised, namely, 400 mg initially, followed by 100 mg every 4 hours, not to exceed 1 week of treatment. Watch the frail elderly patients very carefully.

Phenylbutazone, 100 mg tablets.

Phenylbutazone, 100 mg, plus dried aluminum hydroxide gel 100 mg, magnesium trisilicate, 150 mg, and homatropine methyl-bromide, 1.25 mg, in capsules (Butazolidin Alka).

Cinchophen or Phenylcinchoninic Acid (Atophan)

The analgesic effect starts about 3 hours after ingestion and lasts for 3 or 4 hours.

Cinchophen is acidic and causes burning sensations in the stomach; it may even encourage the development of peptic ulceration. The addition of sodium bicarbonate may prevent not only gastric irritation but also the precipitation of urates in the urine. Intoxication presents a symptomatology similar to that produced by salicylates, such as allergic reaction in the skin, including angioneurotic edema, and hepatotoxic reactions. Intoxication is rare if the drug is administered judiciously and avoided in patients with liver or kidney damage.

The pharmacologic effects are similar to salicylate activity; but the diuretic action is greater, which makes it particularly indicated in gout. It is also used in rheumatic fever and other arthritic conditions, though less toxic drugs will be preferred in these cases.

Dosage: Cinchophen will be given only by the oral route, never injected, in amounts of 300 mg to 1 g every 3 to 4 hours; but in the acute attack of gout the best dosage will be 500 mg every 3 hours, for four or five doses; and in chronic cases 500 mg every 8 hours for only 5 days each week. A combination of cinchophen and colchicin gives better results in many cases than either drug given alone.

Cinchophen, 300 or 500 mg tablets.

Neocinchophen

Pharmacologically, the activity of neocinchophen is identical with that of cinchophen, except for a lesser diuretic action, lack of irritative power against the gastrointestinal tract, and an overall lower toxicity. It is a crystalline powder practically insoluble in water, a property which may make gastrointestinal absorption incomplete.

The main indication is for the treatment of gout, but it may also be used for other forms of arthritis.

Dosage: as for cinchophen, shown above.

Neocinchophen, 300 or 500 mg tablets.

Hydroxyphenylcinchoninic Acid

Brand names: Oxinophen, Fenidrone. This drug only slowly reaches adequate blood concentrations.

It is used for the treatment of rheumatic fever, rheumatoid arthritis, scleroderma, and gout; but because it has not proved superior to salicylates and is poorly tolerated, it is not in general use, except in some cases of gout and scleroderma.

Dosage: ranges from 10 to 20 mg for each kilo of body weight in 24 hours, the total amount given in four or five installments.

Hydroxyphenylcinchoninic acid is not yet available in the United States.

Colchicine

The meadow saffron yields a pale yellow powder, an alkaloid soluble in water, very rapidly absorbed, which stays in the body for prolonged periods of time. This substance, colchicine, is highly toxic, the first symptoms being gastrointestinal in nature. It is very irritant to tissues.

Colchicine has been used as an antimitotic agent, but its main indication is for the acute gouty attack, for which it seems to be the drug of choice, though it should be given together with ACTH.

Dosage: 1 mg every 2 to 3 hours, for no more than five doses; stop at the first gastrointestinal warning. It is given strictly by intravenous injection (irritant when extravasated), no more than 4 mg, with 1 mg initially and 0.5 mg in subsequent injections every 6 hours. Use of combined ACTH and colchicine requires continuing with colchicine after withdrawal of ACTH. For prolonged treatment, the dosage is 0.5 to 2 mg daily or every other day (better given at night), adjusting the amount to the patient's need.

Colchicine, tablets, containing 0.5 or 0.6 mg.

Colchicine, injectable, containing 0.5 mg per ml in 1-ml ampoules.

Colchicum Official Preparations

Prefer colchicine, but any of the following offer equally effective therapeutic applications.

Colchicum corm, fluid extract, in bottles of 500 ml for individualized prescriptions; dosage is 0.25 ml.

Colchicum corm, strong tincture, in bottles of 500 ml for individualized prescriptions; dosage is 0.6 to 2 ml of the 10% tincture.

Colchicum seed, fluid extract, in bottles of 500 ml and of 4 liters for individualized prescriptions; dosage is 0.12 to 0.25 ml.

Colchicum seed, tincture, in bottles of 500 ml and of 4 liters for individualized prescriptions; dosage is 0.3 to 1 ml of the 40% tincture.

Quinine

This alkaloid is a microcrystalline white powder, soluble in water and alcohol. Several of its salts are soluble and used instead of pure quinine. All are rapidly absorbed from the gastrointestinal tract, but blood concentration is not more rapid after injection. The rectal route is not used. Quinine is rapidly metabolized and eliminated from the bloodstream (no accumulation), and finally excreted in the urine. Its main use is for the treatment of malaria.

It also produces analgesia and antipyresis, in a way similar to that of salicylates. It is useless in severe pain, but shows good results in the treatment of pain in muscles or joints. Regarding antipyresis, it is remarkable in the case of fever of malarial origin, but almost negligible in other fevers. Other pharmacological actions of quinine are of great importance (cardiovascular, oxytocic, muscular, and so on). It is also used for the treatment of certain myopathies, night cramps, headaches, and neuralgias. Cinchonism is a clinical syndrome similar to salicylism (q.v.), particularly distressing to hearing and vision. Treatment includes stomach lavage, the use of alkaloid precipitants (tannic acid), cardiotonics, oxygen, blood transfusion, and other symptomatic measures. The drug should be avoided for patients sensitive to it (skin rashes), and patients with tinnitus or optic neuritis.

Dosage: 300 to 600 mg, not to exceed 2 g in 24 hours. Quinine salts, e.g., quinine dihydrochloride or quinine sulfate, are given in identical amounts. The treatment of malaria requires a special dosage, i.e., 600 mg a day, for suppression of either *Plasmodium vivax, P. malariae* or *P. falciparum,* or 1 g three times a day for 2 days, before the chill, and then 600 mg three times a day for 5 days (other agents are preferred).

Quinine, capsules containing 180 or 300 mg.

Quinine powder, bottles containing 30 or 150 g for individualized prescriptions.

Quinine dihydrochloride, powder, bottles containing 30 or 150 g for individualized prescriptions.

Quinine dihydrochloride, injectable, containing 500 mg in 2-ml ampoules and 100 mg in 5-ml ampoules.

Quinine sulfate, tablets containing 120 or 300 mg.

Quinine sulfate, capsules, containing 120, 180, 200, or 300 mg.

Other quinine preparations dispensed in bottles containing 30 or 150 g of the powder are: ethylcarbonate, glycerophosphate, hypophosphite, hydrochloride, phosphate, salicylate, and hydrobromide.

XI. LOCAL ANESTHETICS

Cocaine

Cocaine is an alkaloid, benzoylmethylecgonine, a white crystalline powder with a hydrochloride salt soluble in water, the base soluble only in organic solvents, absorbed slowly because of the vasoconstriction that it induces, and not active when given by mouth because of hydrolysis in the gastrointestinal tract. Excretion and detoxification are still slower, thus easily allowing drug intoxication.

It acts by blocking nerve conduction, stimulating the central nervous system (first the cortex and later the medulla), and on the cardiovascular system it provokes bradycardia followed by tachycardia and vasoconstriction accompanied by hypertension. Cocaine induces local anesthesia, vasoconstriction, and mydriasis, and may cause corneal ulceration when used in the eye. Toxic symptoms are: nervous irritability, restlessness, anxiety, confusion, and headache, rapidly leading to delirium, convulsions, and final respiratory arrest. These symptoms may follow a dose of 20 mg, and over 1 g is ordinarily fatal. Sometimes death occurs instantaneously. The treatment of choice is the intravenous administration of a short-acting barbiturate (sodium pentobarbital, for instance). Other helpful measures are artificial respiration and the application of a tourniquet, if possible, proximal to the site of injection. Cocaine may induce tolerance and addiction.

Use only for surface anesthesia: for application to the cornea, 1 to 4% solutions, preferably with epinephrine (1 : 100,000); 10 to 20% solutions, also with epinephrine, for nose or throat anesthesia.

Cocaine, powder or crystals, in bottles containing 4, 8, 30, or 150 g.

Cocaine, granules, in bottles containing 4, 8, or, for individualized prescriptions, 30 g.

Cocaine hydrochloride, to prepare solutions, in bottles containing 4, 8, 30, or 150 g.

Procaine (Novocaine)

This drug is not to be confused with the more toxic cocaine. Procaine is a synthetic white crystalline powder, mainly used as the hydrochloride salt, freely soluble in water, very rapidly absorbed from the injected site (a vasoconstrictor, epinephrine, is usually added to retard absorption), and rapidly hydrolyzed to paraaminobenzoic acid and diethylaminoethanol, both excreted in the urine. Blocking of sensitive nerves is the most important pharmacological action of procaine, but some generalized analgesia, maximal in 20 minutes and lasting for about 1 hour, may follow systemic administration. The well-known procaine-sulfonamide antagonism should be kept in mind. It is perhaps the most widely used local anesthetic; but it has also been recommended for the treatment of urticaria, delayed serum sickness, and cardiac arrhythmia, although not always with better results than with more appropriate drugs.

Dosage: for infiltration on small nerves, 1% solution may suffice; large nerves may require 4% solution. Also, 0.5% solutions may be used. For each cm use 1 ml of the solution.

Procaine, powder, in bottles containing 30 or 120 g, or 2, 10, or 20 kg.

Procaine, tablets, N.F. preparations; also tablets for local action on mouth or throat.

Procaine, solution, at a concentration of 1 or 2% in vials containing 30 or 100 ml.

Procaine, injectable, 1 or 2% solution, in ampoules or vials containing 1, 5, 10, 30, 50, or 100 ml.

Procaine, solution, at a concentration of 1 or 2%, together with epinephrine, in vials containing 30 ml; also 2.3-ml ampoules.

Procaine, injectable, at a concentration of 1 or 2%, together with epinephrine, in vials containing 30 ml and ampoules containing 2.3 ml.

Procaine, injectable, at a concentration of 4%, in ampoules containing 2.3 ml.

Tetracaine (Pontocaine)

This drug has the disadvantage of a higher toxicity than that of procaine; its advantage is absorption through mucous membranes, making it useful for surface anesthesia. It is rapidly absorbed on injection, and its effects are somewhat more prolonged than those of procaine.

Tetracaine, ophthalmic solution, in bottles containing 15 ml.

Tetracaine, base, in bottles containing 10 g, for individualized prescriptions.

Tetracaine hydrochloride, 0.5% ophthalmic solution, in bottles containing 1 or 15 ml.

Tetracaine hydrochloride, injectable, containing 500 mg in 2 ml or in 7.5 ml.

Tetracaine, injectable, 0.15% solution.

Tetracaine hydrochloride, containing 250 mg together with zinc sulfate, 100 mg, in 7.5-ml vials.

Tetracaine hydrochloride, powder, in bottles containing 15 or 30 g.

Tetracaine, 1% cream and ointment, and 0.5% ophthalmic ointment.

Tetracaine, tablets, containing 100 mg.

Dibucaine (Nupercaine)

This drug is a potent local anesthetic, but also very toxic. Toxicity is lower when it is used in high solution, which does not impair adequate and prolonged activity. It has been used for all types of local anesthesia, but because some vasodilation occurs from the injection of low concentrations, epinephrine should be added.

Dibucaine, 1% ointment, in jars of 2.2 kg.

Dibucaine, 0.5% cream, in tubes of 30 g.

Dibucaine hydrochloride, suppositories, containing 20 mg.

Dibucaine hydrochloride powder, in bottles containing 10, 25, 30, or 120 g.

Dibucaine hydrochloride, injectable, containing 5 mg in 2-ml ampoules (0.25%).

Dibucaine, lozenges, for oral use, containing 1 mg each.

Lidocaine (Xylocaine)

Surface and deep anesthesia are well obtained with lidocaine, which may be used without a vasoconstrictor; but the effects are less prolonged and the toxicity increases. It should be used when epinephrine is contraindicated (hypersensitivity).

Lidocaine, viscous, an aqueous 2% solution, for oral administration, in bottles containing 100 or 450 ml (average dose, 1 tablespoonful for adults, 1 teaspoonful for children, not to exceed eight doses in a day).

Lidocaine, 2% jelly, in 30-ml tubes for mucous membranes.

Lidocaine, 2.5 or 5% ointment, in 15- or 35-g collapsible tubes.

Lidocaine, suppositories, containing 100 mg each.

Lidocaine, injectable, at concentrations from 0.5 to 1, 1½, and 2%, in ampoules or vials, 2, 5, 10, 20, 30, 50, or 100 ml [available either plain or with epinephrine, the latter 1:50,000 (for dental use), 1:100,000, or 1:200,000].

Lidocaine, solution, 4%, in 5-ml ampoules or 50-ml bottles.

Lidocaine, for spinal anesthesia, at a concentration of 5%, containing 50 mg per ml, in 2-ml ampoules.

Diperodon (Diothane)

Because of its toxicity, this long-acting local anesthetic is used practically only in suppositories or ointment for hemorrhoidal pain.

Diperodon, powder, in 5-g bottles.

Diperodon, ointment, 1% in 30-g tubes or 2.2-kg jars.

Diperodon, 1%, suppositories.

Alcohol (Ethanol)

Alcohol has been used for pain relief by injection, intravenously, by which route it also acts as a sedative, a nutrient, and a vasodilating agent, so that care should be taken in cases of impending or actual shock. Nerve injection block is carried out for the treatment of trigeminal neuralgia, sciatica, or cancer, or even in cases of angina pectoris, thromboangiitis obliterans, or lumbar paravertebral block.
Dosage: for relieving pain, 2 to 4 ml of alcohol injected around the involved nerve. If used intravenously, no more than 10 ml of alcohol per hour should be given (200 ml of a 5% solution).

Alcohol, 95% by volume, in 5- or 50-ml vials.

Alcohol, solution, containing 5% alcohol and 5% glucose, in 1000-ml bottles.

Dehydrated alcohol, 100% by volume, in 2-ml ampoules.

Other Local Anesthetics

Butamben picrate (Butesin picrate), which is related to procaine, is a long-acting surface anesthetic because of its poor absorption from the site of application. Also, because of its picric acid content, it shows some antiseptic properties. It is a useful drug for minor burns and abrasions. Only in rare cases, it may cause dermatitis. It should not be given to patients sensitive to procaine and its analogues. Because of its yellow color, it stains skin and clothes.

Butamben picrate ointment (with Metaphen) in tubes.

Butamben picrate ointment, in 30- or 60-g jars.

Ethylaminobenzoate (Benzocaine) is also related to procaine, and, because of its poor absorption, is indicated for surface anesthesia, for superficial abrasions and minor burns. It does not stain tissues or clothes.

Ethylaminobenzoate, crystals, for individualized prescriptions.

Ethylaminobenzoate, 1% otic solution, in bottles containing 15 or
30 ml.

Ethylaminobenzoate, 5% ointment (also 20% in water-soluble
base).

Ethylaminobenzoate, suppositories, containing 120, 180, or 500
mg.

Guaiacol is obtained either as a natural derivative of hardwood tar or
synthetically. It is used for topical anesthesia: 12 ml of guaiacol mixed with
18 ml of olive oil, as:

Guaiacol, liquid, in bottles containing 30, 120, or 500 ml or 2.5
liters.

Eugenol is employed in dentistry as an antiseptic and weak anesthetic, for
the treatment of caries.

Eugenol, liquid, in bottles containing 30, 120, or 500 ml.

Chlorobutanol (Chloretone) is a local anesthetic not irritant to the gastric
mucosa, recommended for gastralgia and for vomiting. Also, dentists use
chlorobutanol as a surface anesthetic in "toothache drops."

Chlorobutanol, powder, 1 or 5% for prescription.

Chlorobutanol, substance, anhydrous or hydrous, in bottles containing 120 or 500 g for individualized prescriptions.

Chlorobutanol, 25% in olive oil, for toothache.

Phenazopyridine (Pyridium) is recommended by the manufacturers as a
mild analgesic to the urinary tract, for the relief of symptoms of pain, burning, and urgency, in cases of cystitis.

Pyridium, tablets, containing 100 mg.

Technic for the Use of Local Anesthetics

The use of local anesthetics falls within the domain of the anesthetist, who is
familiar with the many preparations marketed. Other physicians or surgeons
should follow the advice of the American Medical Association recommend-
ing that: (1) very special care be taken not to confuse cocaine and procaine,
an error which has caused fatalities, since cocaine is much more toxic than
procaine; (2) cocaine not be used for purposes other than surface anesthesia;
(3) butacaine not be used except for surface anesthesia; (4) the user not
exceed a total amount of 100 mg of cocaine, that is, 0.5 ml of a 20% solution,
1 ml of a 10% solution, or 10 ml of a 1% solution, and one should use only

solutions containing 1 or 2% procaine for injection; and (5) there should not be passed into the urethra any anesthetic solution if there is inflammation, stricture, or trauma.

Local surface anesthesia may be used on wounded skin or intact, diseased mucosae; also, for instrumentation or surgery of the latter. Cocaine preparations may be used for this purpose.

Procaine is probably the most widely used local anesthetic, but because the easily soluble procaine hydrochloride is not absorbed by mucous membrane, it is not adequate for surface anesthesia. More toxic, and absorbable, anesthetics must be used on the surface of mucous membranes, but necessary precautions should be kept in mind. Preparations to use are dibucaine, lidocaine, tetracaine, and diperodon.

In spite of its high toxicity, dibucaine is well tolerated for the above-mentioned surface anesthesia. Lidocaine is widely used for surface anesthesia because it is more potent than procaine, and of about the same toxicity when used topically or in low concentrations. The advantage of tetracaine consists in its longer duration of action, but its high toxicity must be taken into consideration. Diperodon is employed when a prolonged effect is the most desirable action of the anesthetic preparation.

Infiltration and block anesthesia are frequently used forms for local anesthesia. Infiltration of the intradermal tissues is followed by superficial anesthesia; subcutaneous injection exerts its effects upon more extensive areas of the skin or the adjacent mucosae. In block anesthesia, the local effect is obtained by interruption of transmission when the anesthetic solution is injected in the vicinity of a nerve. Different techniques are employed according to the nerve involved, and are best handled by specialists in such procedures.

Infiltration is the procedure of choice for minor operations. The slow introduction of the needle preceded by instillation of a drop of the anesthetic at the site of injection is practically painless. Then, the amount of solution to be introduced depends on the extent of the area to be manipulated, about 1 ml per each 2 square centimeters (average concentrations). Injecting a circle around the operative area (ring block) and a quantity at a deeper level may spare anesthetic solution. Care should be taken, always, not to inject into a blood vessel. A *finger* is anesthetized by injecting on each side of the corresponding metacarpal, at its midpoint, and then advancing the needle to the interdigital web. The *hand* is anesthetized by blocking the median, the ulnar, and the radial nerves at the wrist. To block the brachial plexus, for anesthesia of both *arm* and *forearm,* the supraclavicular or the axillary route is followed. The first is risky; the second, somewhat easier. The *foot* is anesthetized by injecting around the posterior tibial nerve just on the medial aspect of the tendon of Achilles. The *leg* is anesthetized by injecting around the sciatic nerve. The *thigh* is anesthetized by injecting around the femoral nerve. Blocking both the sciatic and femoral nerves gives good anesthesia for operations from *below the knee* to the foot. Adequate agents are procaine, lidocaine, and also alcohol, in special cases of neuralgia.

Spinal anesthesia and other forms of local anesthesia, such as paravertebral, epidural, and caudal, are extremely useful in surgery, but are better carried out by anesthetists who are familiar with the advantages and the risks in each particular case.

XII. SEDATIVE AND RELAXANT DRUGS

BARBITURATES

The absorption of barbiturates is rapid, no matter what route of administration is employed. Soon they can be found in all tissues and fluids. The more soluble it is in lipids, the more rapid and the shorter-acting is the barbiturate concerned. Depression of the central nervous system is their main effect, ranging from shallow to deep and depending upon the nature of the chemical, its dose, route of administration, the greater or lesser irritability of the nervous system, and tolerance of the drug, as well as circumstances at the moment of administration and the age of the patient. Induction of hypnosis and sedation are the main indications for use. These drugs also depress respiration and the activity of the cardiovascular system. Higher doses may depress blood circulation and the functions of the urinary excretory pathways. Barbiturates are anticonvulsants. Tolerance and dependence arise after prolonged use.

Toxic symptoms will appear with amounts from five to ten times the hypnotic dose; and doses over fifteen times the hypnotic dose may very seriously endanger life. Either accidentally or on purpose, barbiturates may be injected in quantities that will provoke barbiturate poisoning. Under these circumstances, symptoms of central nervous system and cardiovascular depression occur, but the diagnosis is not always easily made (confusion with alcohol intoxication), except when chemical identification of the barbiturate in the body fluids is carried out. The treatment of barbiturate poisoning is better done at a hospital with adequate facilities (monitoring pCO_2 and pH, maintenance of blood pressure, hemodialysis, and the use of analeptic agents).

Tolerance is poor among the elderly, who will be closely watched when treated with barbiturates, especially those patients who have been sensitized to the drugs or who have reacted abnormally to them on a previous occasion. Barbiturates will be avoided in those who have chronic pulmonary diseases, because of the depression of respiration, and in those with porphyria. Phenobarbital and all other barbiturates mainly excreted through the kidney will also be avoided in patients with renal impairment. Rashes may occur, particularly when the medication is followed by deep X-ray therapy. Care must be taken in giving barbiturates to persons with suicidal or addictional tendency and to frail elderly persons, particularly those over 70 to 80 years of age.

Physicians should familiarize themselves with three or four different barbiturates to use concurrently in their practice.

Phenobarbital

Brand name: Luminal. Sedation and hypnosis are the main therapeutic properties of phenobarbital, which is also used to treat convulsive seizures. In some patients, excessive sedation or hypnosis may interfere with epileptic seizure treatment. Side effects are: excitement, pain, allergic reactions, and a sort of "hang-over," which might appear after the depressive effect is over, characterized by digestive symptoms, vertigo, or lassitude.

Why phenobarbital depresses nervous functions or interferes with synaptic transmission of impulses is not well known. It is still the most widely used barbiturate.

Dosage varies considerably from case to case, but as a general rule, we may consider adequate dosage for starting a treatment as 30 mg three times a day. A high dosage would be 100 mg three times a day; nevertheless, such dosages are frequently needed to control seizures in resistant patients. The proper dose must be adjusted for the individual patient and use.

Phenobarbital, powder to be used in individual formulations.

Phenobarbital, elixir containing 4 mg per ml.

Phenobarbital, tablets containing 15, 30, 60, or 100 mg.

Phenobarbital sodium, powder for individual formulations.

Phenobarbital sodium, tablets containing 30 or 100 mg. It may be possible to obtain other sizes.

Phenobarbital sodium, injectables in solutions containing 75 or 150 mg per ml, or in ampoules containing 120 or 300 mg each.

Phenobarbital sodium, suppositories, containing 30, 60, 90, and 120 mg.

Amobarbital

Brand name: Amytal. This barbiturate is mainly used for the treatment of convulsive disorders (epilepsy, chorea, eclampsia, tetanus, meningitis, or toxic reactions), and for sedation because of anxiety, mania, or other similar conditions. Since it is a moderately long-acting medication, particular care should be observed in giving it to frail people, especially if they have impaired liver and renal function, or advanced forms of atherosclerosis.

Dosage: must be evaluated for each patient and purpose. For sedation use 15 to 150 mg two to four times a day; preferably not over 50 mg for each dose. For hypnosis give 100 to 200 mg at bedtime. Be careful with injectables; reject all that are not absolutely clear, or which form precipitates. Do not give more than 1 mg a minute intravenously (apnea of hypotension); do not exceed an amount of 1 g or inject more than 500 mg intramuscularly at one site.

Amobarbital, powder (U.S.P.) in bottles containing 30, 120, or 480 g, for division into individual prescriptions.

Amobarbital, elixir containing 132 mg in each tablespoonful.

Amobarbital, tablets containing 15, 30, 50, or 100 mg.

Amobarbital, capsules containing 60, 180, or 200 mg.

Amobarbital, ampoules containing 125, 250, or 500 mg.

Pentobarbital Sodium

Brand name: Nembutal. This short-acting barbiturate is used for sedation or hypnosis. Care should be taken as for other barbiturates.

Dosage: 20 to 30 mg every 6 or 8 hours; as a hypnotic, 100 mg before going to bed. A dose of up to 150 or 200 mg can be given by injection.

Pentobarbital, elixir containing 20 mg in 5 ml (teaspoonful).

Pentobarbital, capsules containing 30, 50, or 100 mg each.

Pentobarbital, long-acting tablets (Gradumets) with 100 mg each.

Pentobarbital, ampoules containing 50 mg in each ml (2-, 5-, and 50-ml vials).

Thiopental

Brand name: Pentothal. This drug is mainly used for brief surgical procedures as the sole anesthetic, for the induction of anesthesia prior to the administration of other anesthetics, for the supplementation of weaker anesthetics, for psychiatric aid in both diagnosis and treatment of some diseases, and for the control of convulsive seizures. There are authorities who prefer thiopental to phenobarbital for the control of convulsions of some intensity, when the medication is to be administered by vein.

Dosage is a matter of personal adjustment. Start with 25 to 50 mg, up to 125 mg or more for convulsions, as needed and tolerated. The rectal suspension will not be administered to patients with lesions of the lower bowel.

Pentothal sodium, for intravenous use, supplied in 500-mg or 1-g ampoules; also in multiple-dose 5-g, 6.25-g, 10-g, and 12-g ampoules.

Pentothal sodium suspension, for rectal use, supplied in syringes, each with four detachable rectal applicators dispensing 200 mg per applicator.

Mephobarbital

Brand name: Mebaral. This drug is mainly used as an anticonvulsant capable of controlling both grand mal and petit mal seizures. It is also used as a sedative and an antispasmodic against tension, anxiety, and other hyperreactive conditions of the central nervous system.
Dosage: 100 to 200 mg three times a day.

Mephobarbital, tablets containing 32, 50, 100, and 200 mg.

Metharbital

Brand name: Gemonil. Metharbital is used for the treatment of myoclonic seizures and symptomatic seizures from organic brain damage. The side effects due to metharbital are mild and infrequent, generally similar to those due to the use of other barbiturates.
Dosage: for frail or elderly people, 50 mg three times a day, to be increased to 100 or 200 mg three times a day, whenever necessary.

Metharbital, tablets, providing 100 mg each.

Secobarbital

Brand name: Seconal. This is a rapidly acting sedative and hypnotic drug, with effects of short duration. Large doses may cause anesthesia.
Side effects are as for the barbiturates, and accentuated among the elderly, who will always receive the lower recommended doses.
Dosage: For insomnia, give 30, 50, or 100 mg, whichever is the lowest effective oral dosage for a given person; by the rectal route, try 30 or 60 mg first, and try to avoid larger doses such as 120 or 200 mg. Injectables will be used only for the treatment of tetanic convulsions, at a dosage of about 5 mg for each kilo of body weight, repeated every 3 or 4 hours, as needed and tolerated.

Secobarbital, capsules containing 30, 50, or 100 mg.

Secobarbital, elixir containing 22 mg in each 5 ml.

Secobarbital, suppositories containing 30, 60, 120, or 200 mg each.

Secobarbital, 20-ml ampoules for intravenous or intramuscular injection, containing 50 mg in each ml; and 2-ml ampoules containing 100 mg of the active drug.

Butabarbital

Brand name: Butisol. This is another fast-acting sedative and hypnotic drug of short duration. It will be carefully used when anticoagulants are also given, particularly with older and debilitated patients.

Dosage: 15 to 30 mg, three or four times a day, for sedation; or 50 to 100 mg for hypnosis. Always try to give the lower dosage.

Butabarbital, tablets containing 15, 30, 50, or 100 mg; also, capsules with same amounts of active drug.

Butabarbital, elixir containing 30 mg in each 5 ml.

Barbital

Brand name: Veronal. Its main interest is that barbital was the first barbiturate, used during the first years of this century. Its pharmacologic activity is similar to that of other barbiturates.

Primidone

Brand name: Mysoline. The primidone structural formula is that of a pyrimidine derivative resembling the basic formula for barbituric acid. It is intended for the control of grand mal and psychomotor seizures. In general, the side effects provoked by primidone are minor and infrequent, and tend to disappear after continued use. Rarely, megaloblastic anemia may occur, which is controlled with folic acid without discontinuing the treatment.

Dosage: 125 to 500 mg, three times a day. An amount over 2000 mg a day is not advised. Adjust the dosage carefully.

Primidone, 50 and 250 mg tablets.

Primidone, suspension containing 50 mg per ml (250 mg in 5 ml or 1 teaspoonful).

OTHER SEDATIVE DRUGS

Besides the barbiturates, there are, of course, other sedative drugs currently used in medical practice. Most of them will be mentioned briefly in the following lines. They include chloral hydrate, bromides, paraldehyde, piperidinedione derivatives (glutethimide and methyprylon), hydantoins (diphenylhydantoin, ethotoin, and mephenytoin), succinimides (ethosuximide, methsuximide, phensuximide), oxazolidinediones (trimethadione, paramethadiones), one of the glutarimides (aminoglutethimide), acetylureas (phenacemide and pheneturide), and several of the muscle relaxants and other sedatives and anticonvulsant drugs, such as the following: mephenesin, carisoprodol, chlormezazone, methocarbamol, phenyramidol, chlorzoxazone, trihexyphenidyl, cycrimine, biperidin, benztropine, orphenadrine, ethopropazine, methocarbamol, meprobamate, diazepam, chlordiazepoxide, ethchlorvynol, methaqualone, curare, acetazolamide, dextroamphetamine, quinacrine, methotoin, carbamazepine, and magnesium sulfate.

Chloral Hydrate

Brand names: Noctec, Aquachloral, Felsules. This drug is also marketed by other manufacturers under the generic name. It is one of the safer hypnotics and sedatives to be given to older people. Nevertheless, it should not be given to those receiving anticoagulants or other depressant drugs, including alcohol.

Dosage: 500 to 1000 mg, to induce sleep; 250 mg every 8 hours, as a sedative.

Chloral hydrate, 250 or 500 mg capsules.

Chloral hydrate, elixir or syrup containing 500 mg in each 5 ml.

Bromides

The bromides were the first antiepileptic drugs ever used, but are effective almost solely against grand mal seizures. The risk in the use of bromides for therapeutic purposes among the elderly is bromide intoxication, particularly in its chronic form, in which the symptoms may be: mental disturbances (impaired thought and memory); irritability, and even hallucinations, mania, or lethargy; tremors, incoordination, dermatitis (bromide rash, ordinarily in the form of acne); gastrointestinal disturbances; loss of weight; conjunctivitis; and perhaps other less frequent symptoms.

It is advisable not to use bromides in the elderly unless a close observation of the patient can be carried out, including frequent checks of bromide content of the blood. The bromides are contraindicated in cases of renal insufficiency, in neurological or psychological disorders suggesting bromide intoxication, or in those suffering from cerebral arteriosclerosis, depression, alcoholism, or any form of organic damage.

The N.F. includes ammonium and potassium bromide, and the Three Bromides (tablets and elixir), the last consisting of equal parts of ammonium, potassium, and sodium bromide. Sodium bromide may also be prescribed.

Ammonium bromide must be kept in well-closed containers, since it becomes yellowish in air.

Dosage: from 320 mg three times a day up to 1000 mg three times a day, and even 10 g a day, whenever necessary.

Ammonium bromide in powder, to prepare solutions, or capsules.

Potassium bromide has the same dosage as ammonium bromide; but higher dosages may be given, up to 12–15 g per day.

Three Bromides is a preparation that includes equal amounts of three different bromides, namely, ammonium, potassium, and sodium. To give 1, 2 or more tablets, three times a day; one or two tablespoons, three times a day.

Three Bromides, tablets with 150 or 300 mg of each bromide.

Three Bromides, elixir, with 400 mg of each bromide.

Sodium bromide is also available for prescriptions; its use is similar to that of the other bromides, including the dosage.

Sodium bromide, tablets, 300 and 600 mg.

Sodium bromide, elixir, containing 200 mg in each ml.

Paraldehyde

This drug is a prompt hypnotic because of its rapid absorption. It is very safe, though the unpleasant odor it imparts to the breath is an important drawback.

Paraldehyde does not depress respiration or blood pressure; only high dosage may depress these functions. Principal uses today are for hypnotic purposes, for the control of convulsive seizures, and for analgesia under certain circumstances. It is a popular remedy for nervous tension from drunkenness. This drug is supplied in liquid form to be administered by mouth, rectally, or by intramuscular or intravenous injection (the latter being reserved only for intractable convulsive seizures).

Dosage: by mouth or rectal administration, from 1 to 8 ml a day. Some persons may tolerate up to 10 ml a day. Subcutaneous injections are extremely painful; intramuscular injections may provoke sterile abscesses. Do not inject intravenously (pulmonary edema).

Glutethimide

Brand name: Doriden. This is a rapidly acting nonbarbiturate hypnotic, usually well-tolerated by the aged. Prolonged use may induce withdrawal symptoms on discontinuance (gastrointestinal or of a nervous nature).

Skin rashes may be a warning to stop the drug. Blood reactions will be kept in mind.

Dosage: strictly individualized; give 250 to 500 mg at bedtime.

Glutethimide, 250 or 500 mg tablets.

Methyprylon

Brand name: Noludar. This drug is recommended for the induction of sleep in cases of insomnia. Usual measures of care will be maintained while using this medication.

Dosage: strictly individualized, starting with 50 mg and increasing gradually to 200, 300, or rarely 400 mg before retiring.

Methyprylon, tablets containing 50 or 200 mg.

Methyprylon, capsules, containing 300 mg each.

Diphenylhydantoin

Brand name Dilantin. This drug exerts its anticonvulsant action causing very little depression of the central nervous system. It is well absorbed, but slower in action than soluble barbiturates. The duration of its action is long, and it is excreted through the intestinal tract and the kidney. Diphenylhydantoin is one of the more effective drugs for the treatment of grand mal and psychomotor seizures, with a less marked narcotic side effect than the barbiturates have. It can also be used for the treatment of conditions other than epilepsy, such as Parkinson's disease or chorea, to control involuntary movements.

Dosage will be adjusted for each patient, to control seizures without provoking undesirable side effects, particularly muscular incoordination, but also gastric disturbances, dizziness, and hypertrophy of gums. Regular dosage will be 100 mg three times a day to a maximum of 200 mg three times a day. Gastric disturbances due to the alkalinity of the drug can be avoided by drinking at least half a glass of water with each dose or by taking it during or after meals.

Diphenylhydantoin, 30 and 100 mg capsules.

Diphenylhydantoin in oil, capsules containing 100 mg.

Diphenylhydantoin, suspension, 100 mg in each 4 ml.

> Diphenylhydantoin, 50 mg tablets.

There are also capsules available containing diphenylhydantoin with phenobarbital, and with phenobarbital and desoxyephedrine. Diphenylhydantoin is also available for injection.

> Diphenylhydantoin, vials containing 100 and 250 mg, with solvent to adjust pH, 12 and 50 mg per ml.

The high alkalinity of the solution to be injected is to be noted. It is capable of producing tissue damage if injected extravascularly. The injection is used for the treatment of severe seizures, at a speed of 50 mg per minute up to 150 or 250 mg per dose. A subsequent dose of 100 to 150 mg may be given after 30 minutes if the seizure is not controlled. When an injection is given, signs of respiratory or circulatory depression should be watched for. Injection of diphenylhydantoin is also used in neurosurgery for the control of induced seizures.

Ethotoin

Brand name: Peganone. This is a drug of low potency, to be used in conjunction with more potent agents for the treatment of grand mal and psychomotor attacks, though in some instances, it may be used for the treatment of petit mal seizures. It is not advisable to use ethotoin conjointly with phenacemide.

Because of its low potency, the side effects are also minimal: rashes, gastrointestinal disturbances, and drowsiness.

Dosage: Amounts under 2 g are usually ineffective; but in all instances adjust the dose to the patient's needs and response.

> Ethotoin, 250 and 500 mg tablets.

Mephenytoin

Brand name: Mesantoin. This drug is closely related to diphenylhydantoin; it is not only anticonvulsant but also a sedative. It may be, in some instances, superior to diphenylhydantoin; but as with ethotoin, the greater the potency the greater the side effects and toxicity. It causes less gum hypertrophy and other changes also produced by diphenylhydantoin. In general, it must be considered dangerous, particularly because of the possibility of inducing blood dyscrasias, hepatic damage, and skin rashes.

Dosage: 100 mg three times a day, up to 400 mg three times a day.

> Mephenytoin, 100 mg tablets.

Ethosuximide

Brand name: Zarontin. The third succinimide to appear, presently it is preferred for the treatment of petit mal seizures. It cannot control grand mal seizures. No contraindications have been pointed out for its use, except in patients with grand mal attacks if it is not given with drugs adequate to control the seizures. The side effects may be of some importance: rashes, leukopenia or even agranulocytosis, aplastic anemia, and, much more frequently, gastrointestinal disturbances, headache, dizziness, and other symptoms that ordinarily are transient and subside with prolonged treatment.

Dosage: Individual adjustment will be made, but the average will be from 250 mg three times a day up to 500 mg four times a day.

Ethosuximide, 250 mg capsules.

Methsuximide

Brand name: Celontin. This drug is also intended for the treatment of petit mal and psychomotor attacks; but it seems that results are not as favorable as with ethosuximide and other drugs mentioned. Also, care must be taken that the drug be withdrawn on the appearance of behavioral alterations, particularly aggressiveness or depression. The more important side effects are symptoms of the central nervous system, as drowsiness or ataxia, dermal rashes, and gastrointestinal disturbances (nausea and anorexia).

Dosage: Adjust optimum dosage for each patient, which will be about 300 mg twice a day, up to 600 mg four times a day.

Methsuximide, 150 or 300 mg capsules.

Phensuximide

Brand name: Milontin. This drug is also intended for the treatment of petit mal seizures, being a very effective medication, but perhaps is more toxic than ethosuximide and methsuximide. Its effective dosage may cause nausea and dizziness. Nevertheless, the side effects are relatively mild and transient.

Dosage: 500 mg twice a day up to 1000 mg four times a day.

Phensuximide, 250 and 500 mg capsules.

Phensuximide, suspension providing about 250 mg in each 5 ml or teaspoonful.

Trimethadione and Paramethadione

Brand names: Tridione and Paradione, respectively. These were the first drugs to show a selective activity for the treatment of petit mal seizures, and are practically identical in properties and side effects. They are anticonvulsants that provoke little effect on respiration and circulation of blood. Only large amounts may provoke unconsciousness and depression of respiration. They are slightly analgesic.

Their administration provokes sedation and hemeralopia, the latter due to local action of the drugs (the appearance of scotomata indicates the necessity to discontinue them). More serious side effects are rarely seen, such as skin rashes, hepatitis, kidney damage, and the provocation of grand mal seizures.

Trimethadione is indicated for the control of petit mal seizures, but does not control (or may precipitate) grand mal seizures. It is worth noting that skin rashes may herald exfoliative dermatitis or erythema multiforme. The occurrence of any dermatologic symptom may indicate the discontinuance of the drug.

Dosage for trimethadione is 300 mg twice a day up to 600 mg three times a day.

Trimethadione, 150 mg tablets.

Trimethadione, 300 mg capsules.

Trimethadione, solution, 40 mg per ml.

Paramethadione merely is a trimethadione homologue, causing the same benefits and side effects.

Dosage: as for trimethadione, 300 mg twice a day, up to 600 mg three times a day.

Paramethadione is supplied in capsules and solution for oral use. The solution contains 65% alcohol, and must be diluted before its administration.

Paramethadione, 150 and 300 mg capsules.

Paramethadione, solution containing 300 mg in each ml.

Aminoglutethimide

Brand name: Elipten. This drug has been used for all types of convulsions, but is not preferred for petit mal seizures. The low activity of the product and its high incidence of side effects (morbilliform rash, in the first place) do not recommend its use, unless it is needed because of failure of other anticonvulsants.

Dosage: 750 to 1500 mg per day, followed by a gradual increase, if needed.

Aminoglutethimide, tablets of 125 and 250 mg.

Phenacemide

Brand name: Phenurone. This is one of the more toxic anticonvulsants, to be used only when other drugs fail to control psychomotor and other seizures. The principal untoward effects are: blood dyscrasias, hepatitis, kidney damage, gastrointestinal disturbances, rashes, and, most important, psychological troubles such as depression, aggressiveness, or suicidal tendency.

Dosage: 500 mg three times a day. Increase slowly up to 3000 mg three times a day; only rarely will higher doses be given, more rarely with elderly patients, to reach 6000 or 8000 mg in 24 hours.

Phenacemide, 500 mg tablets.

Pheneturide

This drug is used in Europe similarly to the way phenacemide is used, but it is not available in the United States.

Mephenesin

Mephenesin is used to induce muscular relaxation in rheumatic diseases and other spastic conditions, whenever abnormal hypertonicity is present. Parenterally, it has been used as an adjuvant to general anesthesia. Side effects are of little importance in most cases; but intravenous administration of solutions of over 2% concentration may cause thrombosis.

Dosage: from 1 to 3 g, three to five times a day, by mouth; by intravenous injection, given very slowly, 500 mg to 3 g, depending on needs.

Mephenesin, 250 or 500 mg tablets.

Mephenesin, 250 or 500 mg capsules.

Mephenesin, elixir, containing 100 mg per ml (500 mg per teaspoonful, 5 ml).

Mephenesin, injectable, containing 20 mg per ml, in 50- or 100-ml ampoules.

Carisoprodol

Brand names: Soma, Rela. This drug has muscle-relaxant activity and has been recommended for the treatment of muscle spasm and stiffness with pain occurring in musculoskeletal dyskinesias (traumatic, inflammatory, or degenerative), neurologic disturbances, or muscular dyskinesias. Side effects are of minor importance.

Dosage: up to 350 mg four times a day.

Carisoprodol, 250 or 350 mg tablets.

Chlormezazone

Thus drug is also recommended for the treatment of skeletal muscle spasm in rheumatic diseases, low back pain, disc syndrome, torticollis, bursitis, and the like. Side effects may occur occasionally, drowsiness being the most important.

Dosage: 200 mg three or four times a day.

Chlormezazone, 100 or 200 mg tablets.

Phenyramidol

This drug produces muscle relaxation and analgesia, and has been recommended as an analgesic for common pains. Gastrointestinal side effects may occur.

Dosage: 200 to 400 mg every four hours.

Phenyramidol, 200 or 400 mg tablets.

Phenyramidol, elixir, containing 100 mg per teaspoonful (5 ml).

Chlorzoxazone

Chlorzoxazone reduces muscle spasm and pain.

Dosage: 250 to 500 mg, three or four times a day; maintenance dosage is smaller.

Chlorzoxazone, 250 mg tablets.

Trihexyphenidyl

Brand names: Artane, Tremin. This drug inhibits parasympathetic impulses and relaxes smooth muscles, similarly to atropine, but perhaps with fewer side effects. It is indicated for the treatment of parkinsonism, either alone or in combination with levodopa. It may also help in the treatment of extra-pyramidal disorders caused by certain drugs (phenothiazines, thioxanthenes, etc.).

It is to be used very carefully—or avoided if possible—in patients with glaucoma, hypertension, or disorders of the liver, the heart, or the kidneys. All patients over 60 years of age have to be supervised for untoward reactions of an allergic type; hypersensitivity of any kind; psychiatric, gastrointestinal, or urinary reactions; or increased intraocular tension.

Dosage: strictly individualized; start with 1 mg the first day, and increase with care to a daily total of 6 mg—very rarely 10 mg. It is better not to use the long-lasting "sequels" with patients over 60 years of age.

Trihexyphenidyl, 1 or 5 mg tablets.

Trihexyphenidyl, elixir, containing 2 mg in each 5 ml.

Cycrimine

Brand name: Pagitane. Cycrimine is prescribed for the symptomatic relief of parkinsonism. Its general activity is of the belladonna type, and may cause cerebral stimulation. Patients over 60 years of age, particularly those with atherosclerotic changes, have to be carefully evaluated at all times.

Dosage: from 1.25 to 2.5 mg four times a day; dosage to be increased, if needed, up to a total of 20 mg a day. Postencephalitic patients may have up to 45 mg a day.

Cycrimine, 1.25 or 2.5 mg tablets.

Biperidin

Brand name: Akineton. Biperidin is used as an adjunct therapy in all forms of parkinsonism and other extrapyramidal disorders induced by drugs (phenothiazines, reserpine).

Caution will be used with all patients over 60 years of age regarding intraocular tension, renal and bladder function, and other atropine-type reactions.

Dosage: strictly individualized; start with 2 mg and gradually increase up to 6 mg a day—rarely 8 mg. For drug-induced symptoms, injections of 2 or 4 mg may be given, also carefully evaluating the dosage.

Biperidin, 2 mg tablets.

Biperidin, 5 mg in 1-ml ampoules.

Benztropine

Brand name: Cogentin. Benztropine has an activity similar to that of atropine and is mainly used for the treatment of parkinsonism and other extrapyramidal disorders.

The same warnings as for similar drugs are to be given regarding the therapeutic use of benztropine, particularly when it is prescribed for older patients.

Dosage: strictly individualized; start with 0.5 mg a day, gradually increasing to a total of 4 mg—rarely 6 mg. The medication can be given by mouth or by injection.

Benztropine, 0.5, 1, and 2 mg tablets.

Benztropine, 1 mg ampoules.

Orphenadrine

Brand name: Disipal. Orphenadrine is another drug provided with parasympatholytic and antitremor activity, specially recommended for the treatment of parkinsonism. Warnings are the same as for all other similar drugs in use.

Dosage: start with 50 mg a day, and increase up to a total of 150 mg—rarely 250 mg in 24 hours.

Orphenadrine, 50 mg tablets.

Ethopropazine

Brand name: Parsidol. This drug seems to be of value for the treatment of parkinsonian tremors. Since it is a phenothiazine derivative, it has anticholinergic activity.

Dosage: start with 10 mg four times a day, and increase as needed and tolerated, even to a total of 1000 mg a day.

Ethopropazine, 10, 50, or 100 mg tablets.

Methocarbamol

Brand name: Robaxin. This is not exactly a muscle relaxant drug, but is mainly indicated for the treatment of acute painful muscle disorders (usually as an adjunct to rest and other measures), and may be used in the symptomatic relief of tetanus.

Side effects are of the allergic type and may present congestion of the nose or head and blurred vision.

Dosage: 1000 to 1500 mg, three or four times a day; maintenance could be about 1000 mg four times a day, if tolerated. Regular treatment is by the oral route. For tetanus, use the intravenous or intramuscular routes.

Methocarbamol, 500 or 750 mg tablets.

Methocarbamol, 10-ml vials containing 100 mg in each ml.

Intravenous injections will be at a maximum rate of 3 ml a minute; better to use a 5% glucose solution.

Meprobamate

Brand names: Equanil, Miltown. This is a popular mild tranquilizer used successfully in the relief of anxiety and nervous tension. Also, it has given some results in the treatment of petit mal seizures, but may provoke grand mal seizures if given alone to patients with mixed attacks. There are no contraindications to its use, except for allergy to the drug; and the other adverse reactions are minimal in most instances. Serious reactions have been reported only very rarely.

Dosage: may go up to 2400 mg, after careful adjustment. Each individual dose will be 200 to 800 mg.

Meprobamate, 200 or 400 mg tablets.

Diazepam

Brand name: Valium. This drug is a central nervous depressant mainly used for the treatment of anxiety and tension. It is also useful for the treatment of muscle spasms and convulsions, including the complex situation of status epilepticus.

Injected diazepam may cause cardiac arrest, dyspnea, and local thrombosis when given to elderly persons, for which reasons extreme care will be taken when this procedure is advisable. Do not inject to comatose or other intensely depressed patients, or to those intoxicated with alcohol or treated with narcotics.

Dosage: from 2 to 10 mg, three or four times a day, by the oral route. By intravenous (large veins only!) or intramuscular injection (not subcutaneous!) 2 to 20 mg may be given, carefully evaluating tolerance when giving the drug to the elderly.

Diazepam, 2, 5, or 10 mg tablets.

Diazepam, 2-ml ampoules or 10-ml vials, containing 5 mg in each ml.

Chlordiazepoxide

Brand name: Librium. This is also a nervous system depressant mainly used in the treatment of anxiety and tension. It is a secondary drug for the treatment of petit mal seizures and psychomotor crises. It can also be used for the treatment of grand mal seizures. Chlordiazepoxide can be used by either the oral or the parenteral route. Side effects and precautions are as for diazepam (see above paragraph).

Dosage: by mouth, up to 40 to 80 mg a day in divided doses (average 20 to 40 mg a day). By injection (i.m. or i.v.), the starting dose is 50 to 100 mg, to be repeated every 2 to 4 hours, up to a maximum of 300 mg in a 6-hour period.

Chlordiazepoxide, 5, 10, or 25 mg tablets.

Chlordiazepoxide injectable, in ampoules containing 100 mg of the dried product (2 ml of diluent in a second ampoule).

Ethchlorvynol

Brand name: Placidyl. This is a different chemical with hypnotic properties, of relatively rapid induction and short duration.

This drug should not be given to depressed patients or to those with renal impairment or porphyria. Avoid its use together with similar depressant drugs; also avoid it with those in anticoagulant therapy. In short, the elderly will receive the smallest possible amounts.

Dosage: 500 to 750 mg at bedtime.

Ethchlorvynol, 100, 200, or 750 mg capsules.

Methaqualone

Brand names: Quaalude, Sopor, Parest. This is one more of the independent sedative and hypnotic drugs.

Precautions will be of the same nature as those for the use of similar sedative and hypnotic medication.

Dosage: 150 to 300 mg, at bedtime, for hypnosis; 75 mg three or four times a day for sedation.

Methaqualone, 150 or 300 mg scored tablets.

Methaqualone, 200 or 400 mg capsules, delayed release.

Curare

Curare induces a selective paralysis of motor-end plates in skeletal muscle. At a proper dosage, curare will produce only a relaxation, not a paralysis. The drug is employed for the prevention of fractures in shock therapy, for the treatment of muscle spasm that follows rheumatic or similar illnesses, and for the treatment of spastic or convulsive disorders. It is contraindicated in patients with myasthenia gravis, and others with allergic disorders.

Dosage: 3 mg per 20 kg of body weight strictly by the intramuscular route, always keeping a close watch.

Curare (dimethyltubocurarine or similar salts), injectable, containing 1 mg per ml in 10-ml vials.

Other Antiepileptic Drugs

There are drugs not primarily intended for the treatment of convulsions, but which may be of some help in these conditions. Belonging to diverse pharmacological groupings, these drugs include acetazolamide (a diuretic), quinacrine (an antimalarial), dextroamphetamine (a sympathomimetic) and a few others which are listed below.

Acetazolamide (brand name: Diamox), used principally as a diuretic, may be of some help in treating periodic crises, since the drug induces some form of tolerance, forcing its discontinuance after a period of administration.

Acetazolamide is contraindicated in patients with decreased concentrations of sodium and/or potassium in the blood, with severe kidney damage or liver disease, with hyperchloremic acidosis, and with adrenal insufficiency. Other adverse reactions are those that occur with all sulfonamide derivatives.

Dosage: start with 500 mg given in four divided doses, thereafter adjusting the final doses to the patient's needs. If the drug is given with other anticonvulsants, the starting dose will be only 250 mg once a day, with subsequent adjustment. The dosage can be increased to 1000 mg a day.

Acetazolamide 125 or 250 mg tablets.

Acetazolamide injectable, in vials of 500 mg.

Acetazolamide Sequels, 500 mg.

Dextroamphetamine is presently used less frequently than amphetamine. Dextroamphetamine is active when given by the oral route, causing symptoms due to the stimulation of the sympathetic system.

Dextroamphetamine is recommended as a coadjuvant to phenobarbital for the treatment of grand mal seizures; at the same time it may improve the depressive side effects of the barbiturate (larger doses may be given together with amphetamine). Dextroamphetamine may be used alone or in combination with a succinimide for the treatment of petit mal seizures.

Dosage: 5 mg t.i.d. or q.i.d., up to 15 mg slow-release capsules b.i.d. Higher dosage can also be given with adequate control.

Dextroamphetamine, 5 mg tablets.

Dextroamphetamine elixir, containing 5 mg per teaspoonful.

Dextroamphetamine slow-release product, containing 5, 10, or 15 mg per capsule.

Quinacrine (brand name: Atabrine) is a drug mainly used for the treatment of malaria. It has given good results in the treatment of petit mal seizures not responding to the primary drugs.

Dosage: 100–200 mg per day followed by a maintenance dose of 100 mg a day for periods of 2 or 3 months.

Quinacrine HCl, 100 mg tablets.

Methetoin (brand name: Deltoin) is an analog of diphenylhydantoin useful for the treatment of grand mal seizures. It has the advantage of less severe side effects, including less gum hypertrophy; but the drug has not been so extensively evaluated as the parent product.

Carbamazepine (brand name: Tegretol) has been used as an adjunct medication for the treatment of grand mal seizures.

Magnesium sulfate, when given by intramuscular or intravenous injection, has a central depressant activity capable of controlling seizures, particularly those due to acute nephritis.

Side effects are noted as a sharp fall of blood pressure and the danger of respiratory paralysis. In such instances, intravenously inject calcium preparations, which should be always at hand when injecting magnesium.

Dosage: intramuscularly, about 0.2 ml of a 20% solution for each kilo of body weight; intravenously, give up to 4 g (even more, if needed and tolerated) in 250 ml of 5% glucose.

Magnesium sulfate, a 50% solution, in 2 ml or 10 ml ampoules.

XIII. STIMULANT DRUGS

Amphetamine

Brand name: Benzedrine. Actually, this is a complex of levo- and dextro-amphetamine sulfates, indicated only for the treatment of obesity and to treat narcolepsy.

Extreme irritability of the nervous system is a frequent side effect caused by the use of this drug, for which reason it will be avoided as much as possible when treating patients of advanced age or any others prone to react in such a way or to become addicted to the use of stimulants. It is never to be used for prolonged periods; avoid its use as much as possible for elderly patients.

Dosage: Start with a low dosage, such as 5 mg, to be increased even to 60 mg a day in several installments, if needed and tolerated.

Amphetamine, 5 or 10 mg tablets.

Amphetamine, 15 mg capsules, prolonged effect.

Dextroamphetamine

Brand name: Dexedrine. There are no substantial differences between this drug and its congener, described in the above paragraph. It is used to treat narcolepsy and obesity, but not to be used for prolonged periods.

Side effects are the same: extreme irritability of the nervous system, arrhythmias, hypertension. Elderly patients should never use this sort of stimulant drugs.

Dextroamphetamine, 5 mg tablets,

Dextroamphetamine, elixir, containing 5 mg in each 5 ml.

Dextroamphetamine, 5, 10, or 15 mg capsules.

Ephedrine

Brand names: Ectasule minus Sr. & Jr. and III, Slo-Fedrin 30 & 60. Ephedrine is mainly used in formulations for the relief of nasal congestion and similar conditions, usually in combination with other related drugs. Given alone, it is intended for the relief of allergic nasal congestion, asthmatic conditions, emphysema, and hypotension. Thus drug should not be given to apprehensive subjects, or those with prostatic problems, glaucoma, cardiovascular disorders, porphyria, diabetes, or hyperthyroidism.

Adverse reactions may be gastrointestinal, cardiovascular erethism, nervousness, and other manifestations of general irritability.

Dosage: 15 to 30 mg, only rarely 60 mg every 12 hours in slow-release capsules.

Ephedrine, 15, 30, or 60 mg capsules in slow-release form.

Chlorphentermine

Brand name: Pre-Sate. Chlorphentermine is prescribed almost entirely for the treatment of obesity, to reduce appetite. The drug will be used with caution when given to the elderly, and will be avoided in cases of glaucoma or arteriosclerosis and particularly if monoamine oxidase inhibitors have been given previously or are in use at the time (reactive hypertension). Do not use for long periods.

Side effects are the usual symptoms of generalized hyperirritability as noted with similar drugs.

Dosage: 65 mg taken after breakfast.

Chlorphentermine, 65 mg tablets.

Diethylpropion

Brand names: Tepanil, Tenuate. This drug is also dispensed by the generic name by some manufacturers. It too is prescribed almost exclusively for obesity, and is to be given cautiously to the elderly, like other similar drugs. Treat patients with diethylpropion only for limited periods of time.

Dosage: 25 mg, taken 1 hour before each of the three principal meals; if the long-acting capsule is used, give only one, in midmorning.

Diethylpropion, 25 mg tablets.

Diethylpropion, tablets for long-lasting effect containing 75 mg each.

Methylphenidate

Brand name: Ritalin. Methylphenidate is one of the frequently recommended drugs for the treatment of narcolepsy and mild depression, and for the aged suffering from withdrawn senile behavior.

Like other stimulant drugs, it will not be used in cases of tension or anxiety; and is better avoided in patients with severe depression, blood hypertension, or seizures; or when nervousness, insomnia, skin rashes, and other evidence of adverse reactions occur.

Dosage: 20 to 30 mg every 8 or 12 hours, preferably half an hour before meals. Reduce or increase the dosage according to response and tolerance.

Methylphenidate, 5, 10, or 20 mg tablets.

Pentylenetetrazol

Brand name: Metrazol. Elderly persons are somewhat benefited from this drug for the treatment of senile depression and slowness of physical activity. For this purpose it is usually given by mouth. By injection it is given to treat respiratory depression due to drug effect.

This is a well tolerated drug, with very few side effects when given in ordinary doses.

Dosage: 100 or 200 mg, two or three times a day, as needed and tolerated.

Pentylenetetrazol, 100 mg tablets.

Pentylenetetrazol, powder for individual prescriptions.

Pentylenetetrazol, ampoules containing 100 mg in each ml; also 30-ml vials containing 100 mg in each ml.

Nikethamide

Brand name: Coramine. Main indications for nikethamide are nervous depression, respiratory depression, and circulatory failure, particularly when due to the effect of depressant drugs.

Side effects are relatively frequent because of overdosage, felt as a burning or itching retronasal sensation, flushing, sweating, and other forms of nervous irritability. The drug is not to be injected in the arteries, since spasm and thrombosis are a frequent consequence.

Dosage: Intravenous administration is the preferred route; the solution used (25%) contains 250 mg in each ml, and is given in doses of 5 to 10 ml. Orally, for maintenance effects, the dose is 3 to 5 ml every 4 to 6 hours.

Nikethamide, ampoules containing 250 mg in each ml; each 1.5-ml ampoule contains 375 mg of the active drug.

Nikethamide, solution for oral use, also containing 250 mg in each ml.

Bemegride

Brand name: Megimide. This is an analeptic mainly recommended for the treatment of severe depression due to the use of drugs.
Side effects may include convulsive reactions.
Dosage: 100 to 200 mg, or even more to comatose patients.

Bemegride, 10-ml ampoules containing 5 mg in each ml. Give 50-mg doses intravenously, repeating as needed and tolerated.

Aromatic Spirits of Ammonia

This solution may be used as a reflex stimulant.
Dosage: 2 ml, diluted in generous amounts of water.

Aromatic ammonia spirits, solution.

Picrotoxin

This is only used for the treatment of nervous depression due to the administration of active drugs.
Do not forget that picrotoxin is very toxic, causing extreme irritability of the nervous system.
Dosage: Use the lowest possible dose, and repeat these intravenous injections as frequently as needed.

Picrotoxin, injectables containing 3 mg in each ml.

Caffeine

This alkaloid is specially recommended for stimulation of the central nervous system, particularly when depressant drugs are overactive. Do not give it to patients with peptic ulcer, and allow only small amounts to hypertensives or irritable patients.
Dosage: 500 mg tablets containing citrate; and i.m. injectables, benzoate salts, 500 mg per ampoule.

Caffeine citrate, 60 or 120 mg tablets.

Caffeine benzoate, 2-ml vials containing 500 mg each, for intramuscular injection.

Coffee beverages usually contain from 100 to 150 mg of caffeine in a cup. Cocoa (chocolate) may give 50 mg in a cup. A cola drink (12 ounces or 350 ml) will provide 35 to 55 mg of caffeine.

Theophylline

Among the main indications for use is the need for relaxation of the bronchial smooth muscle; it is also used for symptoms of heart failure (congestive crises, dyspnea), angina pectoris, coronary thrombosis, and to induce diuresis. In some instances, it is used for the pains of biliary colic and headache.

Inject it very slowly into the veins. Local injection (muscle) is very painful. Excessive dosage is followed by vomiting, thirst, and agitation, and if very toxic levels are reached, by convulsions and shock. Death may be the consequence.

Dosage: 500 mg by vein, for bronchial asthma; followed by oral administration, 250 mg three times a day.

Theophylline, 100 or 200 mg tablets.

Theophylline, ampoules consisting of the ethylendiamine salt (aminophylline), reviewed in the following paragraph, q.v.

Aminophylline

This is a combination of theophylline with ethlendiamine, perhaps the most frequently used preparation of this type. It is marketed in tablets, suppositories, or ampoules, to be used like theophylline itself.

Aminophylline, 100 or 200 mg tablets.

Aminophylline, suppositories containing 125, 250, or 500 mg.

Aminophylline, ampoules containing 250 mg in the 10-ml ampoule, and 500 mg in the 20-ml ampoule (for intravenous use).

Phenelzine

Brand name: Nardil. This is a potent monoamine oxidase inhibitor (MAOI), recommended for the treatment of depression, particularly in those cases that are nonendogenous or neurotic, and those caused by anxiety. It is advisable not to use phenelzine as the first drug, but rather when other more frequently used ones fail.

Do not give it to those who react allergically to it, or to those with pheochromocytoma, heart failure, liver disease, or who are taking other drugs; and watch for hypertension or hypotension(!), convulsions, hyperthermia, nervous manifestations, suicidal tendencies, mania, schizophrenia, dizziness, constipation, glaucoma, or sexual disturbances.

Dosage: 15 mg three times a day is an adequate start; increase if needed and tolerated to about 60 mg in 24 hours. Maintenance dosage may be only 15 mg a day.

Phenelzine, 15 mg tablets.

Isocarboxacid

Brand name: Marplan. This is also a potent MAOI recommended for many different forms of depression; it presents similar activity, contraindications and warnings as phenelzine, q.v. above.

Dosage: Start with 10 mg three times a day; and because this drug has cumulative effects, as soon as results are noted, decrease to maintenance dose of 5, 10, but no more than 20 mg a day.

Isocarboxacid, 10 mg scored tablets.

Tranylcypromine

Brand name: Parnate. This is a rapidly acting MAOI usually recommended for hospitalized patients who have not responded to other medications. Warnings, contraindications, and precautions are the same as with phenelzine, q.v. above.

Dosage: Start with 10 mg twice a day; if there is a poor or no response in a few days of therapy, increase to 10 mg three times a day; after obtaining satisfactory results, decrease to a maintenance dosage of 10 or 20 mg a day.

Tranylcypromine, 10 mg tablets.

Pargyline

Brand name: Eutonyl. Since this drug is promoted solely for the treatment of hypertension, it will be reviewed in the appropriate section of this book.

Desipramine

Brand names: Pertofrane, Norpramin. Desipramine, a dibenzazepine derivative, is recommended by the manufacturers for the treatment of depression with symptoms of sadness, fatigue, pessimism, feelings of inferiority, insomnia, related anxiety, anorexia, suicidal drive, and others.

Contraindications, warnings, and adverse reactions: it is not to be used at the same time as MAOI, after myocardial infarction, with hyperpyretic or allergic reactions, or in cases of reactivated psychoses of all kinds, glaucoma, anginal pains, other cardiovascular reactions, convulsions, hypertension, or suicidal trends; adverse reactions are usually of a mild nature (liver, skin, blood).

Dosage: 25 mg two or three times a day is an adequate starting schedule for the elderly, who rarely will need more than 100 mg in 24 hours.

Desipramine, 25 or 50 mg capsules.

Nortriptyline

Brand name: Aventyl. This drug is also prescribed for the treatment of depression, particularly when of endogenous origin.

Contraindications, warnings, and adverse reactions are similar to those advised for desipramine, as quoted in the above paragraph.

Dosage: Start with the conservative amount of 10 mg, three times a day; a maximum of 50 mg in 24 hours seems to be advisable with the elderly.

Nortriptyline, 10 or 25 mg capsules.

Nortriptyline, liquid containing 10 mg in each 5 ml.

Amitriptyline

Brand names: Elavil, Endep. Amitriptyline is also a dibenzazepine derivative recommended for the treatment of depressive conditions, particularly when of endogenous origin; and when depression is accompanied by anxiety.

Do not give it to patients allergic to it; avoid its use when there are hyperpyretic reactions, convulsions, recent myocardial infarction or other cardiovascular problems, glaucoma, hyperthyroidism, schizophrenia, or mania; and watch for hematological, gastrointestinal, neurological, urinary, and endocrinological reactions.

Dosage: 10 mg three times a day, and 20 mg at bedtime are the adequate amounts for elderly persons. Changes will not be noticed for 2 weeks.

Amitriptyline, 10, 25, 50, 75, or 100 mg tablets.

Amitriptyline, injectable containing 10 mg in each ml in 10-ml vials.

Imipramine

Brand names: Presamine, Tofranil. This is another derivative of dibenzazepine, with almost the same activity as amitriptyline, q.v. above.

Dosage: Because of less intense effects, doses can be a little higher, namely starting with 75 mg a day, at bedtime, and increasing to a maximum of 150 mg (rarely 200 mg) in one or two daily installments. Doses over 150 mg a day should be avoided for older people.

Imipramine, 10, 25, or 50 mg tablets.

Imipramine, 75, 100, 125, or 150 mg capsules.

XIV. PSYCHOTROPIC DRUGS

Only for the last 20 years have drugs been available that have marked activity on intellectual functions, and are used for the treatment of psychiatric disturbances. At this time, physicians are prescribing very large amounts of these drugs, namely, the phenothiazines, Rauwolfia derivatives, meprobamate, the monoamine oxidase inhibitors (MAOI), and other similar products with adequate activity. Some are listed here; others (such as MAOI) that were reviewed in the preceding chapter, on stimulant drugs, are also intimately related to psychotropic therapy.

PHENOTHIAZINES

Regarding phenothiazines, the first warning must be that these drugs impair psychological functions and may cause physical illness when given to the elderly. Thus extreme caution will always be observed when treating these patients, strict individualized dosages will be calculated for each particular person, and the lower amounts must be given in each instance. Never give them to older people with previous brain damage.

Patients receiving phenothiazines will be watched for the following: in the first place, for the occurrence of extrapyramidal symptoms, particularly those of parkinsonian type, but also any sort of dyskinesia, dystonia, hyperreflexia, oculogyric crises, opisthotonos, akathisia, and other manifestations of that kind. Other nervous disturbances may be of the convulsive type, cerebral edema, intensification of the effects of depressant drugs and of psychotic conditions, headache, catatonia, and possibly death due to failure of cough reflexes. Other undesirable effects are dryness of the mouth, nasal congestion, nausea, constipation (with the possibility of adynamic ileus), blood dyscrasias of several kinds (notably agranulocytosis and purpura), and dermatological and allergic reactions. The occurrence of markedly elevated temperature is not exceptional with several of the phenothiazines.

The main uses of phenothiazines are for the management of psychiatric patients, for treatment of nausea and vomiting, as antihistaminics, and to correct parkinsonism, for which reasons they are recommended in cases of psychoses, neuroses (anxiety and tension), behavioral disorders of the aged (senility, arteriosclerosis), nausea, and vomiting.

Chlorpromazine

Brand names: Chlor-P2, Thorazine; also marketed by its generic name. Chlorpromazine is a very useful medication for the treatment of psychotic disorders, particularly of the manic crises types, excessive anxiety and tension, and marked agitation; it is also useful for the control of nausea and vomiting, hiccups, intermittent porphyria, and symptoms of alcohol withdrawal; and helpful in the treatment of severe pain and tetanus.

Side effects are prone to occur among the elderly, who will always be treated with the smallest possible dose. They will be closely watched for reactive hypotension, extrapyramidal reactions of the parkinsonian type, dyskinesias, convulsions, and the like. Other frequent side effects are drowsiness, jaundice, blood dyscrasias (including agranulocytosis), and skin and ocular changes.

Dosage: Always use the smallest dose for each elderly patient under treatment; start with 10 mg, two, three, or four times a day, by mouth; increase the dosage only if the symptoms are severe and not controlled with the low dosage. Injections will be given intramuscularly, or by intravenous infusions only in selected cases. For any parenteral injection, give 25 mg; doses are to be increased only if needed and tolerated.

Chlorpromazine, 10, 25, or 50 mg tablets.

Chlorpromazine, 30, 75, 150, or 200 mg capsules (slow release).

Chlorpromazine, containing 25 mg in each ml, in ampoules with 1 or 2 ml, and vials with 10 ml.

Chlorpromazine, also available in syrup, suppositories, and concentrate.

Promazine

Brand name: Sparine. Its effects are entirely similar to those of other phenothiazines, but the extrapyramidal, antiemetic, and sedative activity is only moderate; the hypotensive effect is marked; and the dosage is among the higher ranges.

Dosage: Single intramuscular injection of 50 to 200 mg can be given; the usual antipsychotic dose ranges between 500 and 1000 mg.

Promazine, 10, 25, 50, 100, or 200 mg tablets.

Promazine, syrup containing 2 mg in each ml (10 mg per teaspoonful).

Promazine, concentrate containing 30 or 100 mg for each ml, to be diluted.

Promazine, injectable containing 25 mg in each ml, in ampoules of 1 or 2 ml, and vials of 10 ml. There are also vials containing 50 mg in each ml in sizes of 2 or 100 ml.

Mesoridazine

Brand name: Serentil. This is one of the phenothiazine tranquilizers recommended for the treatment of anxiety, tension, and other manifestations of psychological stress. It is also used in schizophrenia, behavioral problems, and alcoholism.

Side effects are those usually present with this kind of drug, for which reason it is not advisable to prescribe it for the depressed or debilitated elderly patient.

Dosage: It is always advisable to prescribe the lowest effective amounts, especially when dealing with the older patient; start with 10 mg three times a day, and increase slowly to a maximum of 50, 100, or 150 mg total. Larger doses are used for schizophrenia, if tolerated.

Mesoridazine, 10, 25, 50, or 100 mg tablets.

Mesoridazine, 1-ml ampoules containing 25 mg each.

Mesoridazine, concentrate containing 25 mg in each ml (graduated dropper).

Triflupromazine

Brand name: Vesprin. This drug is only indicated for the treatment of psychotic disorders, and for nausea and vomiting.

Side effects are similar to those of chlorpromazine (q.v. above), but the incidence of reactional elevated temperature is more frequent (treat with total-body ice-packing).

Dosage: Try not to exceed a daily amount of 30 mg, and never more than 100 mg. By injection, doses of only a few mg (10 mg as a maximum, for the elderly) will be given.

Triflupromazine, 10, 25, or 50 mg tablets.

Triflupromazine, suspension containing 10 mg in each ml (50 mg per teaspoonful).

Triflupromazine, injectables containing 20 mg in each ml, in 10-ml vials; also 1-ml ampoules with 10 mg.

Fluphenazine

Brand names: Permitil, Prolixin. Fluphenazine is recommended only for the management of psychotic disorders.

Contraindications and precautions are the same as for other phenothiazines.

Dosage: In all instances the smallest individual dose will be given; it will range from 1.25 mg twice a day to a maximum of 2.5 mg three or four times a day, by intramuscular injection. By mouth, the dosage will be about the same.

Fluphenazine, 1, 2.5, 5, or 10 mg tablets.

Fluphenazine, elixir containing 0.5 mg in each ml.

Fluphenazine, injections containing 2.5 mg in each ml, in 10-ml vials.

Perphenazine

Brand name: Trilafon. This phenothiazine is mainly prescribed for the treatment of neuroses, and for severe nausea and vomiting.

As with similar drugs, its use will be watched carefully, and it will not be given to patients with blood dyscrasias, convulsive disorders, or hypotension, or those reacting with skin rashes or elevated temperatures.

Dosage: will be carefully individualized, ranging from 2 mg twice a day to an upper limit of 8 mg three or four times a day, by mouth. The long-lasting tablets (8 mg) will be given twice a day (one or two tablets for each dose, as needed and tolerated). By intramuscular injection no more than 5 mg (1 ml) will be tried at first, increasing to an amount of 15 mg in 24 hours.

Perphenazine, 2, 4, 8, or 16 mg tablets.

Perphenazine, tablets of prolonged action, 8 mg.

Perphenazine, concentrate containing 16 mg in each 5 ml.

Perphenazine, injectables containing 5 mg in 1-ml ampoules.

Prochlorperazine

Brand name: Compazine. Prochlorperazine is used for the management of severe nausea and vomiting, psychotic disorders, and anxiety, tension, and agitation (particularly when associated with somatic conditions).

Warnings and precautions are the same as for other phenothiazines.

Dosage: Try always to use the lower dosages; 5 mg three or four times a day, by mouth; by intramuscular injection, about the same doses. Intravenous infusions of less than 20 mg in each 1000 ml can be given. Rectally, somewhat higher doses could be given, up to 25 mg twice a day.

Prochlorperazine, 5 or 10 mg tablets.

Prochlorperazine, slow-release capsules, 10, 15, or 30 mg.

Prochlorperazine, injectables in ampoules containing 2 ml (5 mg in each ml) or vials containing 10 ml (5 mg in each ml).

Prochlorperazine, concentrate containing 10 mg in each ml.

Prochlorperazine, suppositories containing 25 mg.

Thioridazine

Brand name: Mellaril. This phenothiazine is promoted for the treatment of psychotic disorders, depression, anxiety, and alcohol withdrawal syndrome, to help in the treatment of pain, and for senile manifestations. Nevertheless, when depression originating in the central nervous system is of a severe nature, the drug is contraindicated. It is also contraindicated in cases of marked heart disease, particularly when accompanied by either hyper- or hypotension. All other warnings and side effects common to the phenothiazines are to be kept in mind when using thioridazine.

Dosage: strictly individualized, starting with 50 mg three times a day, not to exceed 500 or, at most, 800 mg a day, in divided doses. For less severe conditions, use even smaller amounts, namely, 25 mg t.i.d.

Thioridazine, tablets containing 10, 25, 50, 100, 150, or 200 mg.

Thioridazine, concentrate containing 30 or 100 mg in each ml.

Trifluoperazine

Brand name: Stelazine. This drug is indicated for the treatment of psychotic disorders, anxiety, tension, and agitation. It is to be used following the usual precautions, as for other phenothiazines.

Dosage: strictly individualized, starting with no more than 1 or 2 mg twice a day; rarely 4 and never more than 5 mg twice a day for elderly persons, the last amount (10 mg a day) only to be given in exceptional cases.

Trifluoperazine, 1, 2, 5, or 10 mg tablets.

Trifluoperazine, concentrate containing 10 mg in each ml.

Trifluoperazine, injectable containing 2 mg in each ml, in 10-ml vials.

OTHER PSYCHOTROPIC DRUGS

Rauwolfia

Brand name: Raudixin. The whole root of *Rauwolfia serpentina* has a particular effect in decreasing elevated blood pressure, but it also has sedative and tranquilizing activity; thus it is recommended for the treatment of hypertension and the relief of psychotic symptoms. For this last purpose it may be given to those who do not tolerate phenothiazines.

Rauwolfia powder should not be given to markedly allergic patients or to those with depression, peptic ulcer or ulcerative colitis, gall bladder diseases (mainly with stones prone to cause biliary colic), or kidney insufficiency—or, if it is really needed, administration has to be extremely cautious with continuous watchfulness for any complications. Other adverse reactions are: gastrointestinal hyperactivity, ocular reactions (glaucoma, uveitis), arrhythmias, dermatological symptoms, nasal congestion, or diverse aches.

Dosage: Start with 50 mg, two or three times a day, increasing to a maximum of 300 or 400 mg in 24 hours. Advanced age is an indication for the lowest dosage.

Rauwolfia serpentina, 50 or 100 mg tablets.

Reserpine

Brand names: Serpasil, Rav-sed, Ravloydin, Raurine, Reserpaid, Sandril, Serfin, Serpate, Vio-Serpine. Reserpine is the main alkaloid derived from the root of various species of *Rauwolfia*. Indications, contraindications, and dangers are the same as for Rauwolfia serpentina powder, mentioned in the preceding paragraph, q.v.

Dosage: Start with 0.125 mg; then give an active dose of 0.5 mg, decreasing it for maintenance to 0.125 mg again. Doses of 1 mg should be avoided for the aged. The dosage mentioned is intended for 24 hours.

Reserpine, 0.25 mg tablets.

Deserpidine

Brand name: Harmonyl. Deserpidine is another alkaloid obtained from the roots of various species of *Rauwolfia*. Its actions are essentially identical with those of other Rauwolfia alkaloids, particularly reserpine. For information, please see the above paragraph devoted to Rauwolfia serpentina.

Dosage: Start with 0.75 mg once a day, to a maximum of 1 mg; but frequently a lesser amount is used for maintenance. Adjustments take about 2 weeks to become noticeable.

Deserpidine, 0.1 or 0.25 mg tablets.

Alseroxylon

Brand name: Reauwiloid. Alseroxylon is another of the Rauwolfia alkaloids, this one mainly indicated for the treatment of hypertension.

All warnings, precautions, and contraindications are the same as for similar Rauwolfia derivatives, as described in the above paragraph.

Dosage: start with 2 or 4 mg, once a day, and keep a maintenance dosage of 2 mg. For the elderly, it is better to use the 2-mg dose.

Alseroxylon, 2 mg tablets.

Haloperidol

Brand name: Haldol. Haloperidol is a tranquilizer of the butyrophenone series, useful for the management of psychotic disorders and the control of tics and of vocal utterances in some cases of Gilles de la Tourette's syndrome.

The drug is contraindicated in all sorts of depressive conditions, in parkinsonism, and for patients allergic to butyrophenones. Elderly people using halperidol will be watched for bronchopneumonia, dehydration, ocular changes, cardiovascular disorders (anginal pain, tachycardia, or hypotension), extrapyramidal reactions in varied manifestations (parkinsonism and other dyskinesias), leukopenia (even agranulocytosis), and other dermic, gastrointestinal, endocrinological, hepatic, and respiratory reactions.

Dosage: Initial treatment may require from 0.5 to 5 mg, two or three times a day. Elderly persons will always be kept at the lowest possible doses.

Haloperidol, 0.5, 1, 2, or 5 mg tablets.

Haloperidol, concentrate containing 2 mg in each ml.

Haloperidol, injectables containing 5 mg in each ml, in ampoules containing 1 ml, or 10-ml vials.

Chlorprothixene

Brand name: Taractan. A thioxanthene derivative, this drug is recommended for the treatment of psychotic disorders.

Contraindications include depressive conditions (collapse, coma) and allergic reactions to thioxanthenes. Precautions are the same as for phenothiazines, q.v.

Dosage: Start with 25 mg, orally, three or four times a day; increase, if needed and tolerated, up to 50 mg per dose, not to exceed 400 or 500 mg in 24 hours. Injections should be of about 25 mg, intramuscularly; only in selected cases will 50 mg be given.

Chlorprothixene, 10, 25, 50, or 100 mg tablets.

Chlorprothixene, concentrate containing 100 mg in each 5 ml (20 mg in each ml).

Chlorprothixene, injectable in 2-ml ampoules containing 25 mg each (12.5 mg in each ml).

Meprobamate

Brand names: Equanil, Miltown, SK-Bamate. This drug is also marketed under the generic name by other manufacturers. Its activity as a tranquilizer has been questioned lately. Nevertheless, it seems to be useful for the treatment of anxiety and tension, particularly when these conditions interfere with sleep.

Contraindications and warnings: Porphyria, liver and kidney diseases, convulsive conditions, depressive conditions and reactions, leukopenia and agranulocytosis, other blood dyscrasias, and allergic reactions. Watch for any other unusual reaction.

Dosage: 400 mg, three times a day, but no more than 2000 mg in 24 hours.

Meprobamate, 200 or 400 mg tablets.

Meprobamate, 400 mg capsules.

Chlordiazepoxide

Brand name: Librium. This and the next tranquilizer listed, diazepam, are among the most widely used at the present time, perhaps abused in many instances. They are recommended for the treatment of anxiety and tension, and in many other instances when anxiety or tension is a problem.

Contraindications, warnings, and precautions: depressive conditions of any kind, allergic reactions, dermic changes, extrapyramidal symptomatology, blood dyscrasias, liver reactions, hypotension, tachycardia, or any other undesirable consequences.

Dosage: The elderly should always be kept at the lowest possible dosages, usually 5 mg two or three times a day, by mouth; by injection, because of acute situations, give 25 mg intramuscularly or intravenously, to be repeated as needed and tolerated. Doses double those mentioned above are to be given only in selected cases.

Chlordiazepoxide, 5, 10, or 25 mg tablets.

Chlordiazepoxide, 5, 10, or 25 mg capsules.

Chlordiazepoxide, ampoules containing 100 mg of the drug, to be completed with a solvent.

Diazepam

Brand name: Valium. Diazepam and chlordiazepoxide are almost interchangeable regarding indications and precautions, but there are patients who tolerate one better than the other, more frequently favoring the less potent chlordiazepoxide. In general, diazepam is indicated for the same situations as its congener, chlordiazepoxide, but diazepam is also used for the relief of muscle spasms and convulsions.

Contraindications, warnings, and precautions: allergic reactions, glaucoma, depressive conditions, nervous symptomatology, kidney or liver diseases, blood dyscrasias, skin reactions, and any other adverse symptomatology. Ataxia and oversedation may occur with older patients, particularly if dosage is not at the lowest limit.

Dosage: 2 or 5 mg, two, three, or four times a day. Doses of 10 mg are too potent for the elderly, particularly when they are frail or debilitated. These doses are intended for oral use. By injection, either intramuscularly or intravenously, dosage should range from 2 to 5 mg, repeated when needed and tolerated. Larger doses, up to 10 mg, may be needed to control seizures (these can be increased, in some instances!).

Diazepam, 2, 5, or 10 mg tablets.

Diazepam, injectable, containing 5 mg in each ml, in 2-ml ampoules and 10-ml vials.

Hydroxyzine

Brand name: Atarax. Hydroxyzine is another tranquilizer and muscle relaxant, though rarely employed for this latter purpose. It is recommended for the treatment of anxiety, tension, and agitation, particularly when due to emotional stress as well as to organic disturbances. Among these indications, the treatment of senile disturbances is of interest.

Caution will be taken when using hydroxyzine for allergic patients in cases of depression (either as a nervous symptom or a drug reaction); but in general this drug is fairly free of adverse reactions.

Dosage: Start with 25 mg three times a day, increasing dosage whenever needed and tolerated to 50 mg three or four times a day. Try to avoid doses of 100 mg except when needed. Do not give it more than three times a day for the elderly.

Hydroxyzine, 10, 25, 50, or 100 mg tablets.

Hydroxyzine, syrup containing 10 mg in each 5 ml.

Chlormezanone

Brand name: Trancopal. Chlormezanone is recommended for the treatment of anxiety and tension.

It will not be given to those who are allergic to the drug; and patients will be watched for drowsiness, skin rashes, depression, nausea, flushing, difficulties with micturition, or jaundice.

Dosage: start with a 100-mg dose, repeated three times a day; increase to a 200-mg dosage, three times a day, only if it is strictly needed and well tolerated. Mood changes will not be noted in less than 2 weeks.

Chlormezanone, 100 or 200 mg scored tablets.

XV. SYMPATHOMIMETIC DRUGS

Epinephrine

Brand name: Adrenalin. In most countries the hormone secreted by the adrenal medulla is called adrenalin. It stimulates most of the functions of the sympathetic system (except for sweat glands and arteries of the face). Consequently, it is indicated as life-saving in cases of anaphylactic shock, as well as in functions more minor, as for the relief of nasal congestion. Major uses are for the following: bronchospasm, allergic reactions to most allergens, cardiac arrest, hemostasis, angioneurotic edema, hives, serum sickness, open-angle glaucoma, relaxation of the uterus, and prolongation of local and intraspinal anesthesia.

Do not use it in narrow-angle glaucoma, shock, organic brain damage, coronary insufficiency, or cardiac dilatation, during labor, or in injections to fingers and toes; and use it very cautiously, or not at all, for the elderly, diabetics, hypertensive patients, hyperthyroidism, cardiovascular diseases, or persons treated with digitalis or diuretics or many other drugs. Repeated or excessive doses may cause palpitation, anxiety, or necrosis at the site of injections.

Dosage: Epinephrine ampoules contain 1 mg in each ml (1 : 1000 solution); it is administered in doses of 0.1 to 0.5 ml, either by itself or diluted in intravenous infusions. Solutions of 1 : 10,000 are made for application to the eye or mucosae.

Epinephrine, ampoules containing 1 mg in 1 ml. Also provided in 5-, 10-, and 30-ml vials. Reject colored solutions.

Epinephrine, solution for inhalation (1 : 100 in oil) will never be used for injection.

Norepinephrine or Levarterenol

Brand name: Levophed. L-arterenol activity is very similar to that of epinephrine, but its use is practically limited to restoration of decreased blood pressure when the acute hypotension is due to anesthesia, myocardial infarction, poliomyelitis, septicemia, drug reactions, surgery for pheochromocytoma or sympathectomy, blood transfusions, or cardiac arrest.

The drug is not to be given if hypotension is due to blood volume deficit unless emergency treatment is needed to maintain coronary and cerebral blood supplies (while blood replacement is being done). Neither is it to be administered to patients with thrombosis, unless it may be a life-saving procedure. Certain anesthetics are incompatible with it (cyclopropane, halothane). It is to be very carefully used with patients on MAOI therapy, or those with reactive hypertension or its precursor headache or bradycardia; and watch the site of injection continuously for vasoconstriction or extravasation (free flow or blanching).

Dosage: Use an infusion with 5% dextrose (either water or saline) with 4 ml of levarterenol in each liter, at a flow rate of 2 or 3 ml a minute, which will be carefully evaluated for response and adjustment. Place in site an intravenous plastic catheter through a needle well advanced centrally and securely fixed (avoiding catheter tie-in technique). Therapy will be continued until blood pressure and tissue perfusion become adequate.

Levarterenol, 4-ml ampoules containing 4 mg.

Isoproterenol

Brand name: Isuprel. This amine is related to epinephrine; nevertheless, it is used almost exclusively for dilation of the bronchial tree in asthma, emphysema, and similar diseases.

Do not give it to patients with arrhythmias, other cardiac disorders, diabetes, hyperthyroidism, or any other condition associated with sympathetic stimulation, or in status asthmaticus.

Dosage: It is mainly used by inhalation, repeated 5 to 15 times, with a 1:200 solution. Use of the 1:100 solution has to be carefully evaluated if it is needed for older patients. The tablets are recommended for heart block, at an initial dose of 10 mg; monitoring is needed to adjust subsequent dosage.

Isoproterenol, 10 or 15 mg tablets.

Isoproterenol, solution 1:200 or 1:100.

Ephedrine

Brand names: Ectasule Minus SR (60 mg), Ectasule Minus JR (30 mg), Ectasule Minus III (15 mg); Slo-Fedrin 60, Slo-Fedrin 30. It is also marketed under the generic name. It is indicated almost exclusively for bronchial dilation, like proterenol, q.v. above. Warnings, precautions, and so on, are also similar.

Dosage: If brand-name preparations are used, give one capsule every 12 hours, preferably administering 30 mg to the elderly. For non-sustained-action tablets, use 22.5 or 45 mg, repeating as needed and tolerated.

Ephedrine, 15, 30, or 60 mg capsules.

Ephedrine, 22.5 or 45 mg tablets.

Ephedrine, injectables, 25 or 50 mg each.

Amphetamine and Dextroamphetamine

Brand names: Benzedrine and Dexedrine, respectively. These drugs were discussed under "Stimulant Drugs." They are indicated almost exclusively for obesity and narcolepsy. The main side effect is nervous irritability. For more details, refer to the earlier discussion of the drugs.

Dosage: for both, start with 5 mg and increase, if needed and tolerated, to 60 mg in 24 hours. Discontinue therapy as soon as possible.

Amphetamine, 5 or 10 mg tablets.

Amphetamine, 15 mg capsules, prolonged effect.

Dextroamphetamine, 5 mg tablets.

Dextroamphetamine, 5, 10, or 15 mg tablets, prolonged effect.

Dextroamphetamine, elixir with 5 mg per 5 ml.

Methamphetamine

Brand names: Dexoxyn, Fetamin, Phelantin, and many others. This drug is indicated for obesity.

As all derivatives of amphetamine and methamphetamine cause nervous irritability, they should not be given to hypertensive patients, those who have had MAOI or insulin therapy, or patients with glaucoma; also, watch for tachycardia, gastrointestinal disturbances, impotence, or allergic reactions.

Dosage: Start with 5, 10, or a maximum of 15 mg a day. Do not extend therapy for more than 2 months' duration.

Methamphetamine, 2.5 or 5 mg tablets.

Methamphetamine, 5, 10, or 15 mg slow-release tablets.

Hydroxyamphetamine

Brand name: Paredrine. This derivative of amphetamine has been recommended for the treatment of postural hypotension and for heart block. At the present time, only preparations with hydroamphetamine and boric acid are being promoted by the manufacturers for pupil dilatation.

Warnings are given against its use for patients who are or have been on MAOI, reserpine, or guanthidine therapy. Watch for possible tachycardia, arrhythmias, hypertension, respiratory distress, irritability, or similar symptoms.

Dosage: Start with 20 mg a day, and increase if needed and tolerated to 60 mg in 24 hours. Higher doses have been given, but are not recommended for old people.

Hydroxyamphetamine, tablets containing 20 mg.

Mephentermine

Brand name: Wyamine. This preparation, like the former one, is not being promoted by the manufacturers at the present time. It has been recommended for hypotensive conditions.

Dosage: 10 to 30 mg subcutaneously or intramuscularly. Tablets are also available.

Mephentermine, injectables, in vials containing 1, 2, or 10 ml. Solutions may contain 15 or 30 mg in each ml.

Mephentermine, 12.5 or 25 mg tablets.

Metaraminol

Brand name: Aramine. This sympathomimetic amine is a potent drug recommended for hypotensive conditions due to brain tumor or trauma, hemorrhages, or reactions to medications and anesthesia.

It is not recommended for use with cyclopropane or halothane anesthesia, patients using digitalis or MAOI, those with liver cirrhosis, heart disease, hyperthyroidism, or diabetes, or those with hypertension, tachycardia, arrhythmia, tissue necrosis, abscesses, or any other source of toxemia.

Dosage: Intramuscular or subcutaneous injections will be given only at selected sites, to avoid undesirable reactions and in amounts of 2 to 10 mg. Do not repeat injections in less than 10 minutes. Intravenous therapy will be by means of infusions of 15 to 100 mg in 500 ml of 5% glucose, adjusting the speed to the level of blood pressure obtained. In very severe shock a direct intravenous injection of 0.5 to 5 mg can be given.

Metaraminol, injectable containing 10 mg in each ml, in vials containing 10 ml, or in 1-ml ampoules.

Phenylephrine

Brand name: Neo-Synephrine. This drug, chemically related to epinephrine and ephedrine, is recommended for the treatment of hypotension due to shock or any similar cause, and for local use in cases of ocular congestion, pupil dilatation, and rhinitis or nasal allergies.

Warnings and precautions are as for similar agents, q.v. above.

Dosage: By subcutaneous or intramuscular injection give from 1 to 5 mg, or 10 mg in selected cases (but never this amount for the first dose); by intravenous injection do not exceed 5 mg in any case—start with 1 or 2 mg, usually. For infusions, give 10 mg in 500 ml of 5% glucose solution. Successive doses depend on the initial response, the amount depending on blood pressure levels. Ophthalmic use should be preceded by instillation of a suitable anesthetic; then apply one drop of any of the concentrated solutions. The weakest nasal solutions will be preferred in most instances; spraying may be repeated about every 4 hours.

Phenylephrine, 1-ml ampoules containing 10 mg in each ml.

Phenylephrine ophthalmic solution, containing 2.5 or 10%; and a viscous solution also containing 10%.

Phenylephrine, nasal spray containing solutions of 0.125, 0.25, 0.5, or 1%.

Nilidrin

Brand name: Arlidin. Nilidrin is prescribed to increase blood supply in cases of arteriosclerosis, thromboangiitis obliterans, Raynaud's phenomenon and disease, thrombophlebitis, ischemic ulcers, diabetic vasculopathies, cramps, and other vasospastic conditions. It is used for circulatory disturbances of the inner ear.

It is not recommended for cases with myocardial infarction or progressive anginal state, hyperthyroidism, paroxysmal tachycardia or other arrhythmias, or heart failure, or for those who develop nervous irritability, palpitations, hypotension, or other symptoms of autonomic dysfunction.

Dosage: 6 mg three or four times a day; 12 mg may be given in selected cases.

Nilidrin, 6 or 12 mg tablets.

Isoxsuprine

Brand name: Vasolilan. This drug is indicated for the treatment of cerebral vascular insufficiency and other peripheral vascular diseases, as advised for nilidrin, q.v. above.

Do not inject it intravenously or for low blood pressure or tachycardia. Other warnings and precautions are similar to those referred to above.

Dosage: Intramuscular injections of 5 or 10 mg, to start with in severe cases. By mouth, 10 to a maximum of 20 mg, three or four times a day.

Isoxsuprine, 10 or 20 mg tablets.

Isoxsuprine, injectables in 2-ml ampoules containing 5 mg per ml.

Naphazoline

Brand name: Privine. This drug is indicated only for the relief of nasal congestion. Reactions to its use will occur occasionally.
Dosage: two drops of the nasal solution or spray into each nostril.

Naphazoline, nasal solution (0.05%).

Naphazoline, nasal spray (0.05%).

Tuaminoheptane

Brand name: Tuamine. This drug is also indicated only for the relief of nasal congestion, but it is no longer promoted by the manufacturers. Reactions were reported occasionally.
Dosage: one or two gentle inhalations, or one or two drops in each nostril.

Tuaminoheptane, 1 or 2% solution.

Tuaminoheptane, inhaler.

Xylometazoline

Brand name: Otrivin. This is another sympathomimetic amine intended for the relief of nasal congestion.
It is not to be used in patients with glaucoma, hypertension, heart diseases (particularly angina), arteriosclerosis, hyperthyroidism, or those who react allergically to it or become irritable or show arrhythmias, or any other undesirable side effect.
Dosage: Apply one or two drops in each nostril, or one or two inhalations.

Xylometazoline, 0.1% nasal solution.

Xylometazoline, nasal spray (0.1%).

Phenylpropanolamine

Brand name: Propadrine. This medication is still marketed in capsules containing 25 or 50 mg, but is not actively promoted by the manufacturers.

Phenylpropanolamine, 25 or 50 mg capsules.

Phenmetrazine

Brand name: Preludin. This drug and the following sympathomimetic amines are used principally as anorexigenics. For better results and to avoid side effects, the drug will be administered only for a few weeks.

It is contraindicated for hypertensive patients and those with arteriosclerosis, glaucoma, arrhythmias, and any of the well-known undesirable effects caused by sympathomimetic agents.

Dosage: It is advisable not to give old or debilitated persons more than 50 mg a day, in two or three doses before meals. One long-acting tablet containing 50 mg may be given to cover a 12-hour span.

Phenmetrazine, 25 mg scored tablets.

Phenmetrazine, long-acting tablets, 50 or 75 mg.

Phendimetrazine

Brand name: Plegine. This drug also is indicated for the control of appetite. All warnings are the same as for phenmetrazine.

Dosage: Use the lowest possible amount; give no more than 35 mg before the two main meals of the day.

Phendimetrazine, 35 mg scored tablets.

Diethylpropion

Brand names: Tepanil, Tenuate. Diethylpropion is another of the drugs used for the management of obesity, given to curb excessive appetite. All warnings and precautions are the same as those previously indicated for similar medications.

Dosage: 25 mg before the two or three principal meals.

Diethylpropion, 25 mg tablets.

Diethylpropion, 75 mg long-acting tablets.

Benzphetamine

Brand name: Didrex. All directions given for the foregoing medications intended for the management of obesity also apply here.

Dosage: 25 mg before the two largest meals of the day; larger doses, namely 50 mg, will be avoided for the aged.

Benzphetamine, 25 mg tablets; or scored tablets of 50 mg.

XVI. SYMPATHOLYTIC DRUGS

Ergotamine

Brand name: Gynergen. Ergotamine controls sympathetic irritability in a relatively broad sense, but at the present time is recommended solely for the treatment of vascular headache, particularly migraine.

Its use should be avoided in cases of coronary heart disease, hypertension, peripheral vascular disease, and for those patients who react with hypersensitivity, who have renal or liver impairment, or arrhythmias, or who present numbness or any other paresthesia of fingers, toes, nose, or tip of the tongue, any other unusual reaction.

Dosage: Each dose will be of no more than 1 mg; and a weekly intake will not exceed 10 mg, preferably given by mouth; by injection, the dosage will be 0.5 mg or less. Try to determine the lowest effective dosage for each patient.

Ergotamine, 1 mg tablets.

Ergotamine, 1-ml ampoules containing 0.5 mg.

Dihydroergotamine

Brand name: D.H.E. 45. This drug has the same indications, contraindications, and warnings as for ergotamine, q.v. above.

Dosage: Intramuscularly give 1 mg, which may be repeated every hour to a total of 3 mg. By intravenous injection do not give over 2 mg.

Dihydroergotamine, injectable containing 1 mg per ml, in 1-ml ampoules.

Dihydroergocornine, Dihydroergocristine, and Dihydroergokryptine

Brand name: Hydergine. These three ergot derivatives are used together for the treatment of depression, unsociability, confusion, and other similar symptoms occurring in elderly people.

No serious side effects have been reported, since these derivatives do not show the vasoconstrictor activity of other natural ergot alkaloids. Nevertheless, some gastrointestinal symptoms may occur.

Dosage: A total of 1 mg of these derivatives is the average amount to be taken sublingually, three times a day.

Dihydroergocornine, dihydroergocristine, dihydroergokryptine—0.175 or 0.333 mg tablets.

Methysergide

Brand name: Sansert. This is an ergot derivative recommended only for the treatment of vascular headache occurring one or more times every week, or when it is so severe that it does not respond to other therapy.

Long-term treatment will always be avoided because of the frequency of fibriotic reactions; but in all instances care will be taken in arteriosclerosis, cardiovascular diseases, pulmonary diseases, collagenosis, or impaired liver or kidney function, or in the development of paresthesias of any kind, leg cramps, pains, or any other abnormal symptom.

Dosage: 4 to 8 mg a day, taken with meals.

Methysergide, 2 mg tablets.

Phenoxybenzamine

Brand name: Dibenzyline. This drug is said to cause "chemical sympathectomy" adequate for the treatment of hypertensive and sudoral pheochromocytoma crises, and possibly effective for vasospastic conditions of the Raynaud type, acrocyanosis, and frostbite sequelae.

It is contraindicated whenever blood pressure may fall dangerously, or tachycardia may develop; and is to be used with caution in cases of arteriosclerosis, kidney impairment, respiratory infections, or gastrointestinal reactions, or when ejaculation is inhibited.

Dosage: to be carefully evaluated for each patient, starting with about 10 mg a day; slowly increased by 10-mg stages, every 4 or 5 days; not to exceed 60 mg when given to the elderly (it is better to administer lower amounts).

Phenoxybenzamine, 10 mg capsules.

Tolazoline

Brand name: Priscoline. This drug is promoted for the treatment of vascular spasticity (Buerger's disease, arteriosclerosis obliterans, diabetic vasculopathy, Raynaud's disease, and other similar conditions).

It is contraindicated after cerebrovascular accidents, coronary disease, and peptic ulcer; and to be used cautiously in cases of gastritis, arrhythmias, angina, hypertension, and gastrointestinal derangements.

Dosage: should be individualized, starting with 25 mg four times a day, to be increased to a maximum of 50 mg four to six times a day (it is better not to exceed 200 mg a day when treating the elderly). Give similar doses by injection.

Tolazoline, 25 mg scored tablets, or long-acting 80 mg tablets.

Tolazoline, injectables containing 25 mg in each ml, in 10-ml vials.

Phentolamine

Brand name: Regitine. Phentolamine is one of the most effective drugs capable of controlling hypertensive crises in cases of pheochromocytoma. It is also used for the prevention or treatment of the necrotic reaction to extravasation of epinephrine, norepinephrine, or similar vasospastic drugs.

Do not use it in coronary patients, and watch for cerebrovascular spasms or shocklike reactions, tachycardia or other arrhythmias, hypotension, or gastrointestinal side effects.

Dosage: 20 mg three to six times a day, by mouth; for local injection, use 5 to 10 mg in 10 ml of saline.

Phentolamine, 50 mg scored tablets.

Phentolamine, 5 mg in an ampoule, to be reconstituted with 1 ml saline.

Azapetine

Brand name: Ilidar. Azapetine is similar to tolazoline, q.v. above. It too is used for the treatment of vascular spasticity.

Dosage: Start with 50 mg three or four times a day. Adjust individually, according to response.

Azapetine, 25 mg tablets.

Guanethidine

Brand name: Ismelin. Guanethidine is indicated for the treatment of moderate or severe hypertension, either idiopathic or renal.

It is not to be used in patients with pheochromocytoma, those treated with MAOI, or those suffering from a different form of heart failure (not due to hypertension); and it is to be cautiously given to those who react with hypotension (mainly the orthostatic type), or who have impaired renal function, coronary insufficiency, dizziness or syncopal reactions, gastrointestinal symptoms, fluid retention, inhibited ejaculation, dyspnea, or any other autonomic nervous side effect.

Dosage: Start with a small dose, 10 mg, to be increased gradually according to response and tolerance; following good control of blood pressure, give only one dose a day.

Guanthidine, 10 or 25 mg tablets.

Rauwolfia and Its Derivatives

In the section devoted to ''Other Psychotropic Drugs'' in the chapter on ''Psychotropic Drugs,'' a summary description of Rauwolfia products was given. These products are mainly recommended for the treatment of hypertension; but they will not be given to depressed patients or those who react unfavorably.

Rauwolfia serpentina, 50 or 100 mg tablets; give 50 mg two or three times a day to start.

Reserpine, 0.25 mg tablets; start with half a tablet.

Deserpidine 0.1 or 0.25 mg tablets; start with 0.75 mg once a day.

Alseroxylon, 2 mg tablets; start with a dose of 2 or 4 mg (better 2 mg for the elderly).

XVII. PARASYMPATHOMIMETIC DRUGS

Choline

Similar to, but much less active than, acetylcholine, this drug has been advocated for the treatment of liver diseases (cirrhosis, hepatitis), with little substantiation of therapeutic effects.

Choline dihydrogen citrate, 500 mg tablets or capsules.

Acetylcholine

Regardless of its very important physiologic activity, acetylcholine is rarely used for therapeutic purposes.
Dosage: 40 to 200 mg, orally; 10 to 100 mg intravenously.

Methacholine

This drug is used, at times, for paroxysmal tachycardia (other measures are now preferred), spastic vasculopathies, and glaucoma.
Dosage: Start with 50 mg, up to four or more times a day, by mouth. It may be injected subcutaneously.

Methacholine, 200 mg tablets.

Bethanechol

Brand names: Urecholine, Myotonachol. Bethanechol, a choline-like drug, is mainly indicated for the treatment of urinary retention due to neurogenic atony of the bladder or to a reaction to previous surgery.
This drug is contraindicated in cases of peptic ulcer, asthma, bradycardia, hypotension, coronary insufficiency, parkinsonism, epilepsy, weak gastroin-

testinal or bladder walls, and other similar conditions; and patients will be watched for any sort of adverse reactions.

Dosage: Start with 10 or 20 mg (rarely 30 mg) by mouth three or four times a day, to obtain a satisfactory response; by injection, 5 mg subcutaneously.

Bethanechol, 5, 10, or 25 mg tablets, scored.

Bethanechol, injectables in 1-ml ampoules of 5 mg each.

Carbachol

This drug has been used for glaucoma, but is seldom employed now. It is given by mouth or subcutaneously, and as an ophthalmic medication. Tablets contain 2 mg each, ampoules contain 0.25 mg in each ml, and ophthalmic ointment or solution is at concentrations of 0.75 or 1.5%.

Pilocarpine

This alkaloid causes marked miosis and is one of the preferred drugs for the medical treatment of glaucoma, particularly during the early stages of the wide-angle variety. It has a limited effect in combatting xerostomia.

Dosage: locally, one or two drops of the 4% ophthalmic solution (better if given together with physostigmine, 1%), for the acute attack; in chronic cases, use smaller dosages (0.5 to 3%).

XVIII. PARASYMPATHOLYTIC DRUGS

Belladonna

The alkaloids of belladonna are mainly represented by atropine, which is reviewed next. Belladonna extracts, tincture, and similar pharmacologic preparations are among the most effective and frequently used drugs. They are recommended, and usually of very good help, for the treatment of gastrointestinal spasms (peptic ulcer, spastic colitis, pylorospasm, and a variety of colics due to colonic or biliary problems), nervous diseases of the type of post encephalitic parkinsonism, motion sickness, or vagal irritability; and also in bronchial asthma, hypersecretions of the bronchial tree, renal colic, dysmenorrhea, or any other condition characterized by spasticity of the smooth muscles or by excessive hypersecretion.

Belladonna is especially contraindicated in cases with glaucoma or any other form of elevated intraocular pressure, impaired hepatic or renal function, allergic reactions to the drug, or prostatism with urinary retention; and must be carefully administered to older persons with constipation or delirium and those with dryness of the mouth, flushing of the face, or blurring of vision.

Dosage: Tolerance varies greatly from patient to patient; so dosage has to be individualized. Each ml of the tincture has about 0.3 mg of the alkaloids, or 0.0075 mg in a drop; the first trial should be by giving only 0.6 ml three times a day. The dosage will be increased only very slowly to reach an effective level. Remember, 1 ml = 40 drops.

> Tincture of belladonna, to be dispensed by dropper. Different manufacturers market belladonna products in the form of tincture, powder, or tablets, and in combination with other medications.

Atropine

Atropine is the active principle of belladonna, and its activities are essentially the same as for belladonna (q.v. above).

It is also indicated as an antispasmodic medication for gastrointestinal, biliary, ureteral, and similar spastic condtions. Atropine is also used pre-anesthetically (to lessen undesirable secretions) and in poisoning with organic phosphoric cholinesterase inhibitors (insecticides, "nerve gases"); locally, it is used for iritis, iridocyclitis, and keratitis.

Do not use it in cases with glaucoma or asthma.

Dosage: individualized, starting with 0.4 mg.

> Atropine sulfate, 0.4 mg tablets.

> Atropine sulfate, ampoules containing 0.4 mg in each ml.

> Atropine sulfate, ophthalmic ointment.

Homatropine

Brand names: Homapin, Mesopin, Novatrin. This drug has the same indications as belladonna or atropine, but is less active and less toxic than they are.

Dosage: 2.5 to 5 mg, three times a day, before meals.

> Homatropine methylbromide, 2.5, 5, and 10 mg tablets.

> Homatropine methylbromide, solution or elixir; the former with 1.25 mg in each ml, the latter with 2.5 mg in each 5 ml.

> Homatropine methylbromide, 1.1-ml ampoules of 5 mg each.

Scopolamine

This is also a belladonna alkaloid. The peripheral actions of the drug are similar to those of atropine, but the actions upon the central nervous system notably differ. It is recommended for sedation in cases of cerebral excitation (mania, delirium tremens, parkinsonism, paralysis agitans, spastic conditions, motion sickness) and is a potent mydriatic.

It is not to be given to patients with asthma or hepatitis; and is to be watched for causing other belladonna-like side effects.

Dosage: 0.3 to 1 mg given by mouth three or four times a day; similar dosage by injection (subcutaneous, intramuscular, intravenous).

Scopolamine hydrobromide, 0.3, 0.4, 0.6, or 1.2 mg tablets.

Scopolamine hydrobromide, 1-ml ampoules containing 0.3, 0.4, or 0.6 mg (also 20-ml vials).

Belladonna Substitutes

The effort to develop products more or less specifically active from the pharmacologic point of view, and at the same time less toxic, has led to the presentation of several drugs, some of them herein reviewed.

Most of these drugs have a similar therapeutic activity, being prescribed for the treatment of hyperacidity, peptic ulcer, and other spastic condtions of the gastrointestinal tract or the urinary tract, as well as for parkinsonism.

They are contraindicated in cases of glaucoma, obstructive diseases of the gastrointestinal tract or the urinary tract, prostatic hypertrophy, intestinal atony of the elderly, coronary insufficiency, ulcerative colitis, myasthenia gravis, and allergic reactions. Their use must be carefully controlled in all asthenic people, when visual troubles develop, or if there is weakness, nervous irritability, diarrhea, diminished sweating, impaired function of liver or kidney, impotence, or any other undesired side effect.

Oxiphenonium (brand name: Antrenyl). Dosage: 10 mg four times a day; decrease and adjust individually.

Oxiphenonium, 5 mg scored tablets.

Diphemanil (brand name: Prantal). Dosage: 100 mg every 4 to 6 hours, but strictly individualized.

Diphemanil, 100 mg scored tablets, or 100 mg long-acting tablets.

Isopropamide (brand name: Darbid). Dosage: Start with 5 mg twice a day, and adjust individually.

Isopropamide, 5 mg. tablets.

Methantheline (brand name: Banthine) and *Propantheline* (brand name: Pro-Banthine). With methantheline, give 50 mg before meals and 50 or 100 mg at bedtime, by mouth; or inject intramuscularly or intravenously 50 mg per dose, three or four times a day. With propantheline, give 7.5 or 15 mg with meals, and also at bedtime, by mouth; by intramuscular injection, give 30 mg. In all instances adjust dosage individually.

Methantheline, 50 mg scored tablets.

Methantheline, 1-ml ampoule containing 50 mg.

Propantheline, 7.5 or 15 mg tablets.

Propantheline, 30 mg long-acting tablets.

Propantheline, 1-ml ampoule containing 30 mg.

Hexocyclium (brand name: Tral). Dosage: also strictly individualized, starting with 25 mg four times a day, or 50 mg of a long-acting preparation in the morning, and 100 mg at bedtime.

Hexocyclium, 25 mg tablets.

Pipenzolate (brand name: Piptal). Dosage: 5 to 10 mg three times a day, before meals, and a dose upon retiring.

Pipenzolate, 5 mg tablets.

Tridihexethyl (brand name: Pathilon). Dosage: 25 to 50 mg three times a day, plus one dose at bedtime, by mouth; injectables will be given when needed or in acute cases, 10 to 20 mg every 6 hours.

Tridihexethyl, 25 mg tablets; also long-acting 75 mg tablets.

Tridihexethyl, 1-ml ampoules containing 10 mg.

Oxyphencyclimine (brand names: Daricon, Vio-Thene). Dosage: Start with 5 mg twice a day; may increase to 10 mg twice a day; individualize.

Oxyphencyclimine, 10 mg scored tablets.

Adiphenine (brand name: Trasentine). Recommended not only for gastrointestinal, but also for urinary problems. Dosage: 75 to 150 mg three times a day, before meals.

Adiphenine, 75 mg tablets.

Piperidolate (brand name: Dactil). Dosage: 4 mg before each meal and at bedtime.

Piperidolate, 4 mg tablets.

Dicyclomine (brand name: Bentyl). Dosage: 10 to 20 mg every 6 or 8 hours, by mouth; intramuscular injection, 20 mg every 4 to 6 hours.

Dicyclomine, 20 mg tablets.

Dicyclomine, 10 mg capsules.

Dicyclomine, syrup containing 10 mg in each 5 ml.

Dicyclomine, injectables containing 10 mg in each ml, in 2-ml ampoules or 10-ml vials.

Procyclidine (brand name: Kemadrin). This drug is not only promoted for the same indications that the above drugs are, but also for parkinsonism and other dystonias. Dosage: to be adjusted individually, starting with a trial dose of 2 mg three times a day.

Procyclidine, 2 or 5 mg scored tablets.

XIX. CARDIOTONICS

Digitalis

The dried leaves of digitalis contain mainly the alkaloid digitoxin, and also small amounts of gitoxin and gitalin. One U.S.P. unit is equivalent to 100 mg of digoxin.

The main indication for digitalis is congestive heart failure. It is also used for auricular fibrillation or flutter, heart dilatation, and supraventricular tachycardia, including the paroxysmal type.

Digitalis is contraindicated in ventricular tachycardia, except for the case in which congestive failure occurs and the patient has not yet been treated with these alkaloids. Care should be taken when arrhythmias or nausea and vomiting develop after starting digitalis therapy, or there is glomerulonephritis, rheumatic fever, heart block, potassium depletion, myocardial infarction, myxedema, constrictive pericarditis, bradycardia, confusion, acute abdomen, or allergy to the drug.

Dosage: Digitalization for those who had taken these alkaloids for at least 10 days or more may be carried out with 200 mg twice or three times a day until the adequate response is obtained or toxic symptoms appear. The average digitalization is obtained with about 1800 mg given in 3 days. Acute cases require 500 mg with subsequent doses of 200 mg every 6 hours until response or toxic symptoms are noted.

Digitalis, 30, 50, 60, or 100 mg tablets.

Digitalis, pills containing same amounts as above.

Digitalis, 60 or 100 mg capsules.

Digitalis tincture, 100 mg per ml.

Digoxin

Brand names: Lanoxin, SK-Digoxin; also marketed by the generic name. Indications, contraindications, and warnings are the same as for digitalis, q.v. above.

Dosage: Oral digitalization for those not previously treated may be accomplished with 0.5 to 0.75 mg as the starting dose, followed by 0.25 or 0.5

mg every 6 or 8 hours until a complete response is obtained, or toxic symptoms are noted; it usually requires a total amount of 1 to 1.5 mg. Maintenance dosage usually is 0.125 to 0.5 (0.25) mg a day. For rapid digitalization in acute cases, intravenous or intramuscular injections of 0.25 or 0.5 mg are usually given, with additional doses of 0.25 mg every 4 to 6 hours until complete response or toxic symptoms appear.

Digoxin, 0.125, 0.25 mg tablets; or 0.5 mg scored tablets.

Digoxin, injectables containing 0.25 mg in each ml; in 2-ml ampoules.

Digitoxin

Brand name: Crystodigin; also marketed by the generic name. Indications, contraindications, and precautions are the same as for digitalis, q.v. above.

Dosage: Digitalization is obtained by giving by mouth 0.2 mg twice a day for about 4 days, which is then followed by 0.05 to 0.15 mg a day; in more severe cases, a more rapid schedule is achieved with 0.6 mg to start, then 0.4 mg, and thereafter 0.2 mg every 4 or 6 hours, until response or toxic symptoms are noted.

Digitoxin, 0.05, 0.1, 0.15, or 0.2 mg tablets.

Digitoxin, injectables containing 0.2 mg in each ml, in 1-ml ampoules.

Lanatoside

Brand name: Cedilanid. This drug has the same indications, contraindications, and warnings as for digitalis, q.v. above.

Dosage: By mouth, give 3.5 mg the first day, 2.5 mg the second, 2 mg the third, and thereafter 1.5 mg until digitalization or toxic symptoms occur; maintenance dosage is usually about 1 mg. In severe or other special cases, use injections intramuscularly or intravenously to reach 1.6 mg in 12 hours (may use 0.8-mg portions).

Lanatoside, 0.5 mg tablets.

Lanatoside, injectable containing 0.2 mg per ml, in 2- or 4-ml ampoules.

Strophanthin

Brand name: Ouabain. This drug has the same indications, contraindications, and warnings as for digitalis, q.v. above; nevertheless, it must be borne in mind that strophanthin is much more rapid and potent.

Dosage: very slowly injected in all instances, only by the intravenous route, and no more than 0.25 mg per dose (except in very special cases, which may require 0.5 mg). Following this first injection, doses amounting to 0.1 mg may be given at hourly intervals until full digitalization or toxic symptoms occur. Strophanthin initial therapy must be followed by oral administration of cardiotonics.

G Strophanthin, injectables containing 0.25 mg per ml, in 2-ml ampoules.

XX. DRUGS FOR HYPERTENSION

Veratrum Alkaloids

These drugs, obtained from the roots of *V. viride* and *V. album,* have a relatively potent antihypertensive activity, but are extremely prone to cause nausea and vomiting, effects which have almost abolished their therapeutic application.

Cryptenamine (brand name: Unitensen) is manufactured in the form of tablets or injectables. The tablets are used for mild or moderate hypertension; the injectables, for short-term therapy in cases of hypertensive rises. The dosage must be carefully evaluated individually to obtain a good response and to avoid emesis. Care must be taken to avoid bradycardia, bronchoconstriction, or any other untoward reaction, particularly of the allergic or anginal type. Do not use cryptenamine together with digitalis, anesthetic and pre-anesthetic agents, and saluretic drugs.

Dosage: by mouth, from 1 mg four times a day up to 8 or 10 mg as a daily total (treatment may start with 2 mg after breakfast and at bedtime). Hypertensive crises will be treated with diluted intravenous or plain intramuscular injections only until control of the crisis is achieved, starting with 1 mg (0.5 ml) either intramuscularly or intravenously, and increasing gradually with very strict observation of the blood pressure.

Cryptenamine, 2 mg scored tablets.

Cryptenamine, injectable containing 2 mg (260 Carotid Sinus Reflex Units) in each ml, in 2-ml ampoules.

Veratrum viride, plain powdered extract in 15, 20, 30, or 100 mg tablets.

Rauwolfia Alkaloids

Besides their sedative and tranquilizing effects, Rauwolfia derivatives have a particular activity in decreasing elevated blood pressure. Nevertheless, because of their slow onset of action, they are used only for mild or moderate forms of the disease and should be avoided when some future surgery is expected to be performed. When aged persons are treated, the smaller doses should be considered.

Rauwolfia derivatives are contraindicated for markedly allergic patients, or those with depression, peptic ulcer or ulcerative colitis, gall bladder diseases (with stones causing colic), gastrointestinal hyperactivity, glaucoma, uveitis, arrhythmias, dermatological symptoms, nasal congestion, diverse aches, and kidney insufficiency—though in a few of the least severe of these last instances the medication can be given, but with extreme caution.

Rauwolfia serpentina (brand name, Raudixin). The regular treatment will start with 50 mg two or three times a day; increase to a maximum of 300 or 400 mg in 24 hours.

Rauwolfia serpentina, tablets of 50 or 100 mg.

Reserpine (brand names: Serpasil, Rau-sed, Rauloydin, Reurine, SK-reserpine, Reserpoid, Sandril, Serfin, Serpate, Vio-serpine). Dosage: Start with 0.125 mg; then increase to 0.5 mg until the full effect is obtained; thereafter give 0.125 mg for maintenance, as a daily schedule. Higher dosages (1 mg) are to be avoided for frail or elderly people.

Reserpine, 0.25 mg tablets.

Deserpidine (brand name: Harmonyl). Dosage: 0.75 mg, once a day, as starting dose, to a maximum of 1 mg a day. Adjustment of dosage to results takes about 2 weeks to be noticeable.

Deserpidine, 0.1 or 0.25 mg tablets.

Alseroxylon (brand name: Rauwiloid). For the elderly, an adequate starting dose is 2 mg, once a day; for maintenance, no more than 2 mg.

Alseroxylon, 2 mg tablets.

Rescinnamine (brand name: Moderil). Start with 0.5 mg twice a day; increase as needed and tolerated, but try to come to a maintenance dose of about 0.25 mg in 24 hours.

Rescinnamine, 0.25 or 0.5 mg scored tablets.

Syrosingopine (brand name: Singoserp). Initial amounts will be 1 or 2 mg, in one or two doses a day; for maintenance, 0.5 to a maximum of 3 mg a day.

Syrosingopine, 1 mg scored tablets.

Monoamine Oxidase Inhibitors (MAOI)

These drugs, mainly prescribed for the management of depression, were frequently found to cause orthostatic hypotension. They are not recommended for those who react allergically, or who have a pheochromocytoma, or heart, kidney, or liver disease, or who are taking other powerful drugs. Administration of the drugs will be watched for convulsions, hyperthermia, nervous manifestations, suicidal tendencies, mania, schizophrenia, dizziness, constipation, glaucoma, or sexual disturbances.

Pargyline (brand name: Eutonyl). This MAOI is primarily indicated for the treatment of hypertension, either moderate or severe, but not for the malignant variety. Its use is not advised in the presence of certain foods or beverages. Any unusual reaction will be immediately reported to the physician. Therapy is initiated with 10 or 25 mg once a day; changes in amount are made in less than 1 week of observation, and amounts must not surpass 150 or 200 mg in each 24-hour period; the older the patient, the lower the dosage.

Pargyline, 10, 25, or 50 mg tablets.

Thiazide Derivatives

Either used alone or together with other drugs, thiazides are effective agents for the treatment of hypertension and also for edema, particularly if due to heart failure, renal insufficiency, liver cirrhosis, or the use of certain drugs (corticoids or estrogens). Concerning hypertension, the types responsive to thiazides range from mild to severe; and some drugs, such as diazoxide, may control the malignant type.

As with all drugs, thiazides are contraindicated for patients who show allergic reaction to them, and for patients who suffer renal decompensation; and they should not be given when the hypertension is of the compensatory type, as in cases with aortic coarctation.

During administration of thiazides to elderly persons, care should be taken that a reasonable balance of electrolytes is maintained, and glucose metabolism should be checked, as diabetics may change in their insulin requirements. Also blood uric acid concentration may increase, and the PBI may decrease without symptoms or with hypothyroid reaction. Liver disease, cataracts, kidney disease, and lupus erythematosus have been reported, and other adverse reactions of the gastrointestinal tract, the central nervous system, the blood, the skin, and the cardiovascular system, such as shock, myocardial infarction, or arrhythmias, are to be watched for. Interactions with norepinephrine, other hypertensive drugs, adrenergic blocking agents, corticosteroids, ACTH, tubocurarine, and perhaps other drugs may occur.

Chlorothiazide (brand name: Diuril). Start with 500 mg per dose once or twice a day; to be increased if needed or tolerated, not to exceed 2 g in 24 hours; this is given by mouth. If injected, give intravenously about the same dosage as if by mouth, always trying to avoid extravasation.

Chlorothiazide, 250 or 500 mg scored tablets.

Chlorothiazide, suspension containing 250 mg in 5 ml.

Chlorothiazide, injectable containing 500 mg of the powder, to reconstitute with 18 ml of adjunct liquid.

Hydrochlorothiazide (brand names: Esidrix, HydroDiuril). The initial dosage should be 50, 75, or 100 mg, once or twice a day. Start the elderly on the smallest dose.

Hydrochlorothiazide, 25, 50, or 100 mg scored tablets.

Methyclothiazide (brand names: Aquatensen, Enduron). Individualize dosage by starting with 2.5 mg once a day; maintenance dose usually will be 2.5 to 5 mg once a day; never exceed 10 mg a day.

Methyclothiazide, 2.5 or 5 mg tablets.

Trichlormethiazide (brand names: Naqua, Metahydrin). Individualize dosage, starting with 2 mg twice a day; the maintenance dose will be 2 or 4 mg once a day.

Trichlormethiazide, 2 or 4 mg tablets.

Polythiazide (brand name: Renese). Give 2 to 4 mg a day, according to individual response and tolerance.

Polythiazide, 1, 2, or 4 mg tablets.

Benzthiazide (brand names: Aquatag, Exna). Individualized treatment will consist of 25 mg twice a day, up to 200 mg in 24 hours. Give the elderly the smaller doses.

Benzthiazide, 25 or 50 mg scored tablets.

Cyclothiazide (brand name: Anhydron). Best results are obtained with 2 mg given once, twice, or three times a day, according to individual response and tolerance.

Cyclothiazide, 2 mg scored tablets.

Hydroflumethiazide (brand names: Diucardin, Saluron). Average adult dosage varies from 50 to 100 mg in 24 hours, although there are patients who respond well to 25 mg, and others who need more—but do not exceed 200 mg in 24 hours, a dose not to be given in advanced age.

Hydroflumethiazide, 50 mg scored tablets.

Bendroflumethiazide (brand name: Naturetin). Usual starting dose is 5 mg given in the morning, which will be adjusted later for each particular case. A daily dose of 20 mg will rarely be used for aged people.

Bendroflumethiazide, 2.5, 5, or 10 mg tablets; the 5- and 10-mg tablets are scored.

Diazoxide (brand name: Hyperstat). Diazoxide in its oral form is prescribed for the treatment of hypoglycemia, not for hypertension; but the injectable is an emergency drug for the reduction of elevated blood pressure in cases of malignant hypertension, to be followed immediately by oral antihypertensive drugs as soon as the emergency situation is over. This form of therapy is to be instituted in hospitalized patients, and not to be carried out in those with pheochromocytoma. The adequate dose will be given rapidly by a peripheral vein, undiluted, and with extreme care to avoid extravasation, repeating the injection every 4 to 24 hours but not extending the treatment more than a few days, depending upon the individual's reaction to the treatment. The 300 mg of the ampoule will be injected in about 30 seconds.

Diazoxide, 20-ml ampoule containing 300 mg.

Sympatholytic Drugs

Some of the sympatholytic drugs, namely, phentolamine, tolazoline, azapetine, and phenoxybenzamine, are successfully employed for the control of hypertensive crises in cases of pheochromocytoma. Guanethidine is not to be used for these crises, but only in cases of moderate to severe hypertension, either idiopathic or renal. Also, these drugs may help in vasospastic conditions of the Raynaud type, acrocyanosis, frostbite sequelae, arteriosclerosis obliterans, diabetic vasculopathy, and other similar conditions. Phentolamine is also indicated for the management, prevention, or treatment of necrotic reactions due to extravasation of epinephrine, norepinephrine, or any other similar drug.

Sympatholytic drugs should be avoided in coronary patients, or those with arteriosclerosis, kidney impairment, respiratory infections, gastrointestinal reactions, inhibited ejaculation, cerebrovascular spasms or shocklike reactions, tachycardia and other arrhythmias, or hypotension (or dangerous fall of blood pressure), particularly of the orthostatic type, or for heart failure.

Phentolamine (brand name: Regitine). Give 50 mg three to six times a day, by mouth; for local injection, 5 to 10 mg in 10 ml of saline.

Phentolamine, 50 mg scored tablets.

Phentolamine, 5 mg in an ampoule to be reconstituted with 1 ml of saline.

Tolazoline (brand name: Priscoline). Give individualized dosage, starting with 25 mg four times a day, to be increased to a maximum of 50 mg four to six times a day (not to exceed 200 mg with elderly patients. Similar doses may be given with injectables.

Tolazoline, 25 mg scored tablets; or long-acting tablets, 80 mg.

Tolazoline, injectables containing 25 mg in each ml, in 10-ml vials.

Azapetine (brand name: Ilidar). Start with 50 mg three or four times a day, and adjust individually according to response and tolerance.

Azapetine, 25 mg tablets.

Phenoxybenzamine (brand name: Dibenzyline). Dosage has to be carefully evaluated for each patient, starting with about 10 mg a day; slowly increased by 10 mg each time, every 4 or 5 days; not to exceed 60 mg when given to the elderly.

Phenoxybenzamine, 10 mg capsules.

Guanethidine (brand name: Ismelin). Start with a small dosage, not over 10 mg, to be increased gradually according to response and tolerance with careful observation of the blood pressure. Give only one dose a day.

Guanethidine, 10 or 25 mg tablets.

Other Diuretics for Hypertension

Spironolactone (brand name: Aldactone). For the treatment of hypertension, spironolactone is usually prescribed together with other drugs, when the commonly used antihypertensives cannot be adequately administered to a particular patient. Because it is an aldosterone antagonist, it is recommended for primary hyperaldosteronism (short-term preoperative therapy, or long-term therapy in milder cases when surgery is not advisable). Other indications are: congestive heart failure, cirrhosis with ascites, nephrotic syndrome, and hypokalemia.
Contraindications: anuria, acute renal insufficiency or other forms of renal impairment, allergic reaction, and hyperkalemia. Warnings and precautions: excessive potassium intake, electrolyte imbalance, elevation of BUN, development of tumors, and gynecomastia.
Dosage: Give 25 mg, two to four times a day; adjustments will take about 2 weeks, and will be done individually.

Spironolactone, 25 mg scored tablets.

Chlorthalidone (brand name: Hygroton). The long-term effect and low toxicity make this an acceptable medication for moderate to severe hypertension, heart failure, cirrhosis, nephrosis, and other forms of renal impairment with edema. Contraindications: anuria or other severe forms of renal impairment, also hepatic malfunction, or any allergic reaction. Warnings and precautions: as stated above for spironolactone. Dosage: strictly individualized, starting with 50 mg every other day, and adjusted according to response and tolerance.

Chlorthalidone, 50 or 100 mg tablets.

Hydralazine

Brand names: Apresoline, Dralzine; also marketed under the generic name. This drug is indicated for the treatment of hypertension, from moderate to severe. It is contraindicated for patients with coronary insufficiency, rheumatic heart disease, or those who present any form of allergic reaction to it.

Warnings and precautions to be observed are the occurrence of a lupus erythematosus–like reaction, anginal symptoms, previous cardiovascular diseases, renal insufficiency, peripheral neuritis, blood dyscrasias, headaches, palpitation, nausea, or diarrhea.

Dosage: adjusted individually, starting with 10 mg four times a day and increasing gradually once a week, when given by mouth; severe cases are treated parenterally with 20 to 40 mg, the dose repeated if so needed (intravenously or intramuscularly).

Hydralazine, 10, 25, 50, or 100 mg tablets.

Hydralazine, 1-ml ampoules containing 20 mg per ml.

Methyldopa

Brand name: Aldomet. Used for the treatment of hypertension, this drug is contraindicated in cases with hepatic disorders or allergic reactivity.

Warnings and precautions: Watch for frequent blood dyscrasias (do blood counts at regular intervals), liver disease, dyskinetic reactions, or any other untoward reaction of the nervous system, heart, blood vessels, or gastrointestinal tract.

Dosage: by mouth, 250 mg two or three times a day, to be adjusted individually; in the case of severe crises, give the medication intravenously, 100 mg in 5% glucose solution, in slow infusion, or increase up to 250 or 500 mg at 6 hour intervals, according to response and tolerance.

Methyldopa, 125, 250, or 500 mg tablets.

Methyldopa, 5-ml vials containing 250 mg.

Propranolol

Brand name: Inderal. Mainly designed for the treatment of cardiac arrhythmias, this drug is also effective for hypertension, angina of the sclerosis type, hypertrophic subaortic stenosis, and pheochromocytoma. For hypertension it is better given together with a thiazide.

Contraindications: asthma and other allergic diseases, and allergic reactivity; bradycardia, cardiogenic shock, and other forms of heart failure; and patients treated with MAOI or other drugs.

Warnings and precautions: Withdraw medication and digitalize the patient as soon as any symptoms of heart insufficiency appear; watch especially the hyperthyroid patient, those with allergic reactions, or diabetics.

Dosage: For hypertension give 80 mg as the starting dose, to be adjusted individually according to response and tolerance. Other diseases require a different dosage.

Propranolol, 10, 40, or 80 mg scored tablets.

Propranolol as the injectable medication is not used for hypertension, but for acute arrhythmias.

Clonidine

Brand name: Catapres. Clonidine is indicated for the treatment of hypertension, against which it is mild to moderate in potency, but very rapid in activity. Better results are obtained when it is given together with other antihypertensives or diuretics.

Not too much emphasis is given to contraindications, warnings, and precautions; but in general the same care will be taken as with any of the other drugs considered in this chapter.

Dosage: individualized, starting with 0.1 mg twice a day, and changing according to response and tolerance. It is recommended that the dosage be decreased gradually when the medication is to be withdrawn.

Clonidine, 0.1 or 0.2 mg scored tablets.

Nitroprusside

Brand name: Nipride. This drug is indicated for emergencies related to hypertension, but to be used in hospitalized patients.

Trimethaphan

Brand name: Arfonad. This drug is recommended only for hospitalized patients.

Prazosin

Brand name: Minipress. Since it is prone to cause syncopal reactions, it is better not to use this drug with frail elderly persons.

XXI. ANTIARRHYTHMIC DRUGS

Quinidine

Brand names: Cardioquin, Quinaglute, Quinidex, Quinora, SK-Quinidine; it is also marketed under the generic name. Quinidine and procainamide are the drugs favored for the treatment of arrhythmias as atrial fibrillation and flutter, paroxysmal tachycardias (both atrial and ventricular), and premature systoles. Paroxysmal A-V junctional rhythm as well as maintenance of correction after electrical conversion of fibrillation or flutter are helped. Some prefer digitalis for the elderly in cases of arrhythmia.

Contraindications: all forms of A-V block, thrombocytopenia, hypotension, abnormal rhythm due to escape mechanism of ventricular origin, renal insufficiency, congestive heart failure, and digitalis intoxication.

Precautions: Watch for ventricular tachycardia, allergic reactions, and symptoms of intoxication, such as tinnitus, vertigo, headache, visual disturbances, or gastrointestinal reactions. Advanced age is an indication for hospitalization, in order to maintain continuous monitoring.

Dosage: must be individualized for patients and diseases. For atrial fibrillation start with 200 mg every 3 hours, increasing the daily amount until normal rhythm is restored or toxic symptoms appear. For atrial flutter, first digitalize the patient, then treat as for fibrillation, according to response and tolerance. For other forms, 200 or 300 mg three or four times a day, which is a good maintenance dose. Long-acting formulations are mainly intended for use after conversion, giving about 300 or 600 mg every 8 or 12 hours. Injections will be prescribed when a rapid effect is needed or the oral route is not easily used: test tolerance first, with 200 mg intramuscularly; adequate therapeutic doses are 600 mg to be followed by 400 mg even every 2 or 3 hours—always under strict monitoring of response. Intravenously, the salt will be diluted—most patients will respond to about 300 mg; some will need 500 to 700 mg.

Quinidine, 200 or 300 mg tablets.

Quinidine, 200 mg capsules.

Quinidine, ampoules containing 80 mg per ml, in 10-ml vials.

Quinidine, 300 mg long-acting tablets.

Procainamide

Brand name: Pronestyl; it is also marketed as procaine amide hydrochloride. Good responses are usually obtained in ventricular arrhythmias (premature contractions or tachycardia), except those cases due to digitalis intoxication. It is also effective in atrial fibrillation and paroxysmal atrial tachycardia. The injectable is mainly indicated for arrhythmias initiated by anesthetics during surgery.

Contraindications: myasthenia gravis, allergy, complete block, and partial block unless an electrical pacemaker is operative in this last instance.

Precautions: Watch for hypotension, appearance of other arrhythmias, gastrointestinal disturbances, dermic reactions, and blood dyscrasias (mainly agranulocytosis); and carry out careful monitoring, being alert to reactions with untoward arrhythmic effects, some requiring digitalization.

Dosage: For fibrillation and paroxysmal atrial tachycardia give 1250 mg as the starting dose, followed by 750 mg after 1 hour if no changes occur, and then 500 to 1000 mg every 2 hours until a positive response is obtained or toxic symptoms appear. Maintenance dosage is 500 to 1000 mg every 4 to 6 hours. Other arrhythmias require between 250 and 500 mg every 3 hours (50 mg for each kilo of body weight, in 24 hours). Injections of up to 1000 mg (intramuscularly or intravenously) are to be given only in emergencies, but special care will be taken if reactional hypotension or widening of the QRS occurs.

Procainamide, 250, 375, or 500 mg tablets.

Procainamide, 250, 375, or 500 mg capsules.

Procainamide, injectables containing 100 mg in each ml, in 10-ml vials; or 500 mg in each ml, in 2-ml ampoules.

Digitalis Preparations and Strophanthin

In the case of auricular flutter, digitalis is one of the best therapeutic approaches to solving the problem. For atrial fibrillation, it will not halt the arrhythmia but only restore the efficiency of the heart beats. Paroxysmal tachycardia responds well to either quinidine or digitalis. Strophanthin is more potent and rapid than digitalis.

The treatment of arrhythmias requires an average digitalization, for which reason the reader is referred to the chapter on cardiotonics, where adequate information will be found.

Propranolol

Brand name: Inderal. This is an effective medication for the control of arterial hypertension; supraventricular arrhythmias paroxysmal tachycardia, steady tachycardia (including thyrotoxicosis tachycardia), extrasystolia, fibrillation, and flutter; ventricular arrhythmias—tachycardia (except when due to digitalis or catecholamines), extrasystolia; tachyarrhythmias persisting after causative digitalis is discontinued or those due to excessive catecholamine action during surgical anesthesia; the tachycardia due to pheochromocytoma before or during surgery; and other symptoms due to hypertrophic subaortic stenosis.

Contraindications: allergic conditions, including asthma, rhinitis; heart block; heart failure; and the previous use of most psychotropic drugs. Special care will be taken if propranolol has to be given to anginal patients; those with thyrotoxicosis, diabetes, hypoglycemia, or Wolff-Parkinson-White syndrome; and those subject to surgery. Watch for any sort of allergic reaction, blood dyscrasias, bronchospasm, or nervous disturbances.

Dosage: should be individualized; but, generally speaking, for arrhythmias give 10 or 20 mg every 6 or 8 hours, before meals (the last dose at bedtime). For pheochromocytoma the dosage is 20 mg every 8 hours, either as a maintenance dose or for 3 days prior to surgery. In acute crises, use propranolol intravenously, 1 mg in 1 minute, repeating after 2 minutes if there is no response (do not repeat in the next 4 hours).

Propranolol, 10, 40, or 80 mg tablets.

Propranolol, injectables containing 1 mg in each ml, in 1-ml ampoules.

Lidocaine

Brand name: Xylocaine. Good results are obtained in the management of ventricular arrhythmias, as those due to myocardial infarction or during cardiac surgery.

Contraindications: heart blockade of any kind, or cases of allergic reaction to the drug.

Precautions: During administration of lidocaine for arrhythmias, a constant monitoring of the heart function will be carried out (to stop administration when PR or QRS waves widen or the arrhythmia worsens), and a careful watch observed for nervous, cardiovascular, or respiratory adverse reactions, particularly in the presence of kidney or liver diseases, shock, convulsions, hypotension, collapse, bradycardia, or any other untoward side effect.

Dosage: Inject in the vein 25 or 50 mg in 1 minute; and a second dose after 5 minutes in case there is no response; but no more than 200 mg—or less—to be given in a 1-hour period. If the arrhythmia has a tendency to recur, use an infusion with 5% glucose solution at a rate of 2 or 3 ml a minute (20 to 40 μg for each kilo of body weight a minute). As soon as possible, change to an oral antiarrhythmic drug.

Lidocaine, ampoules containing 100 mg in 5 ml.

Isoproterenol

Brand names: Isuprel, Proterenol. Isoproterenol is recommended for the management of shock, cardiac standstill, cardiac arrest, Stokes-Adams syndrome, ventricular arrhythmias (including fibrillation and tachycardia), and bronchospasm during anesthesia.

Contraindications: tachycardia due to digitalis intoxication. Care will be observed when treating patients with coronary insufficiency, those receiving epinephrine (do not use these two medications at the same time, but give them alternatively, if actually needed), patients with diabetes or hyperthyroidism, or patients showing any allergic reaction to the drug. Watch for tremors, flushing, palpitation, or any untoward reaction.

Dosage: For cardiac standstill or arrest use the injectable; for arrhythmias, use the injectable, if needed, or the sublingual form. Subcutaneously or intramuscularly, the dose is 0.2 mg, to be followed by 0.02 to 0.1 mg according to response and tolerance; intravenously, use diluted solutions, to give no more than 0.02 to 0.06 mg, repeating a dose of 0.01 to 0.2 mg; by infusion, 2 mg in 500 ml of 5% glucose, give 5 μg a minute.

Isoproterenol, sublingual (or rectal) tablets containing 10 or 15 mg.

Isoproterenol, injectable containing 0.2 mg in each ml, in 1-ml ampoules (0.2 mg) or 5-ml ampoules (1 mg).

Other Antiarrhythmic Drugs

A relatively large number of drugs not specifically indicated for the treatment of arrhythmias may be of help in special circumstances. A few will be mentioned here.

Potassium salts are mainly helpful in the treatment of digitalis intoxication, mostly accompanied by arrhythmias.

Disodium edetate is useful in 50 to 60% of all arrhythmias due to digitalis intoxication, either atrial or ventricular, when given by injection (an infusion with 50 mg for each kilo of body weight).

Quinine derivatives have been recommended for atrial fibrillation and flutter, and for premature systoles; but quinidine is to be preferred.

Chloroquine is indicated as an alternate to quinidine for arrhythmias (see description under "Antimalarials").

Finally, let us just mention that antiarrhythmic properties have been ascribed to *choline, reserpine, quinacrine,* and some antihistamines.

XXII. VASODILATOR AND VASOCONSTRICTOR DRUGS

In spite of doubts regarding their mechanism of action, nitrites are still among the most widely used and well-accredited antianginal drugs, particularly the rapidly acting amyl nitrite and nitroglycerin, the favorites in the management of anginal pain. Also, the less popular long-acting nitrites (and nitrates) are frequently used for the prophylactic therapy of angina pectoris.

Generally speaking, nitrites are prescribed for anginal crises or for their prevention; but a distinction must be made in using the rapidly absorbed drugs for the acute crises, and the long-acting ones only for prevention.

When giving nitrites, the more important contraindications are a recent myocardial infarction or its prodromal phase, the possibility of cerebral hypertension or hemorrhage, and the occurrence of allergic reactions. Be alert to the presence of glaucoma, orthostatic hypotension, severe flushing, headache, or nausea and vomiting.

As a general measure, keep containers tightly closed at all times, to protect the stability of nitrites.

Following the nitrites, other well established drugs for vasodilation will be briefly reviewed here: papaverine, dipyridamole, propranolol, cyclandelate, nicotinyl tartrate, nilidrin, isoxsuprine, and dioxyline.

The chapter closes by dealing with vasopressor drugs, namely, metaraminol, methoxamine, dopamine, levarterenol, ergotamine, and dihydroergotamine.

NITRITES AND RELATED DRUGS

Amyl Nitrite (Vaporole)

Also marketed by its generic name, this is a rapidly absorbed and short-acting drug for the relief of anginal attacks. Other drugs are preferred, such as nitroglycerin, to abort anginal pains, being less troublesome to administer than amyl nitrite, which requires breaking a pearl and inhalation of the vapor. The amount of medication to use will be decided by response and tolerance.

Amyl nitrite, pearls containing 0.2 or 0.3 ml.

Nitroglycerin

Tablets containing 0.12, 0.15, 0.3, 0.4, 0.6, 1.2, 1.5, 3, or 6 mg of the drug are available (doses over 1 mg use the oral solid for extended release).

An average dosage consists of 0.4 or 0.6 mg; but this varies considerably from patient to patient, and at different times for the same patient. The rapidly released small dosages are intended for the acute attack; the larger doses, for prophylaxis.

Nitrospan: long-acting capsules containing 2.5 mg, to be given every 12 hours, only as prophylactic therapy.

Nitrobid: long-acting capsules containing 2.5 or 6.5 mg; to be given every 12 hours. There is a 2% Nitrobid ointment, to apply on the skin, every 3 or 4 hours, but preferably at bedtime (dose applicator).

Nitroglyn: another brand of long-acting tablets, containing 1.3, 2.6, or 6.5 mg; one every 12 hours taken for prophylaxis.

Nitrong: 2.6 mg long-acting tablets, for prevention of anginal attacks.

Nitrostat: sublingual tablets intended for the treatment of acute anginal attacks—and even subacute myocardial infarction; given in doses of 0.3, 0.4, or 0.6 mg (which are the amounts often furnished in different mixtures).

Pentaerythritol

All preparations in this list are intended for prophylaxis of anginal attacks, and not for the acute crisis. All are contraindicated in early myocardial infarction; and the general indications for their use are the same as for other nitrites, q.v. above. It is recommended that they be taken on an empty stomach.

Peritrate: tablets containing 10 or 20 mg each, one or two to be taken three or four times a day (a maximum of 160 mg a day should not be exceeded). Long-acting tablets contain 80 mg each; take one every 12 hours. As usual, dosage must be individualized for better results.

Antora: long-acting capsules containing 30 mg; take one every 12 hours.

Duotrate: long-acting capsules containing 45 mg; take one every 12 hours.

Pentritol: long-acting capsules containing 60 mg; take one every 12 hours.

SK-Petn: tablets containing 10 or 20 mg; one or two tablets taken every 6 to 8 hours, preferably on an empty stomach.

Erythritil (Cardilate)

This drug is not intended for the treatment of acute anginal crisis, but for prophylaxis and long-term therapy.

Precautions are the same as for other nitrites, q.v. above. More rapid absorption is obtained with the sublingual or the chewable preparations, but oral administration is to be preferred.

Dosage: 10 mg taken orally, every 8 hours; if the chewable preparation is used, give the same amounts; but only one-half for the sublingual. In all instances dosages must be individualized.

Erythritil, 5, 10, or 15 mg scored tablets for oral or sublingual use.

Erythritil, 10 mg chewable tablets.

Isosorbide Dinitrate (Isordil, Isobid, Sorbitrate)

The sublingual and chewable forms are recommended for acute anginal attacks; the oral presentation is intended for long therapy. Other precautions are the same as for regular nitrites, q.v. above.

Dosage: The oral medication should be taken on an empty stomach, in amounts of 5 to 30 mg every 6 hours. Sublingual and chewable forms are given in an average dose of 5 mg (2.5 to 10 mg), also every 6 hours. Individualize dosage, and avoid large doses for older patients.

Isordil, 5, 10, or 20 mg scored, oral tablets; sublingual tablets, 2.5 or 5 mg; 40 mg long-acting tablets or capsules (these to be taken every 12 hours).

Isobid, 40 mg long-acting capsules.

Sorbitrate, 5 or 10 mg scored, oral tablets; 2.5 or 5 mg sublingual tablets; 5 mg scored, chewable tablets.

Mannitol Hexanitrate (Nitranitol)

This is a nitrate (not nitrite) mainly recommended for hypertension because it is too slow to relieve anginal pains. Cautions are the same as for other nitrites, plus the possible incidence of methahemoglobinemia. Average dosage: 15 to 60 mg every 4 to 6 hours.

Mannitol hexanitrate, 15 or 30 mg tablets.

Trolnitrate (Metamine, Nitretamin; triethanolamine trinitrate biphosphate)

This drug is useful for prophylaxis of anginal pains, but not for the acute attack. Doses over 20 mg may be given in a 24-hour period. Methemoglobinemia and other nitrate-induced reactions may occur.

Dosage: strictly individualized, according to response and tolerance, starting with 2 mg every 6 hours and increasing in a reasonable way. Give the medication on an empty stomach.

Trolnitrate, 2 or 10 mg tablets.

Trolnitrate, 10 mg long-acting tablets.

OTHER VASODILATORS

Papaverine (Cerespan, Pavabid, Vasal, Cerebid, Pavakey, and others)

There are also many preparations marketed under the generic name.

Because of its activity on smooth muscle, this drug is indicated for therapy in cases of vascular spasm, as in cerebral or peripheral ischemia, and for the treatment of myocardial ischemia, particularly if complicated by arrhythmias.

For more information, see the chapter on "Analgesics and Antipyretics."

Papaverine HCl 30, 60, 90, 100, 150, or 200 mg tablets.

Papaverine HCl, injectables containing 30 mg in each ml, in 1- or 2-ml ampoules or 10-ml vials.

Dipyridamole (Persantine)

This pirimidine is intended for long-term therapy of angina pectoris, and is not suitable for acute attacks.

Warnings refer to peripheral vasodilation following excessive doses, this caution to be observed when treating hypotensive patients, and the possibility of headaches, asthenia leading to syncope, gastrointestinal symptoms, and rare individual reactions of the allergic type.

Dosage: one or two tablets every 8 hours, preferably 1 hour before meals. It may be 2 or 3 months before a good response is noted.

Dipyridamole, 25 mg tablets.

Propranolol (In deral)

Propranolol has been reviewed in the chapter devoted to antihypertensive drugs, q.v.

Cyclandelate (Cyclospasmol)

Also active against smooth muscle spasm, this drug is recommended as a vasodilator for the treatment of arteriosclerosis obliterans, intermittent claudication, leg cramps, Raynaud's phenomenon, and selected cases of cerebral ischemia, and for the control of vasospasm and muscle ischemia in cases of thrombophlebitis.

The drug will not be given to patients sensitive to it, and its effects must be carefully controlled in patients with glaucoma, those with severe obliterative vascular condtions of the heart or the brain, and those who complain of gastrointestinal symptoms, flushing, asthenia, headache, or tachycardia.

Dosage: It is advisable to start with high doses; nevertheless, if this is done with older patients, a very careful watch must be kept at all times. Doses ranging from 200 to 400 mg before meals and at bedtime can reach a total of 1200 mg; but no more than 1600 mg is permitted in each 24-hour period. Decrease dosage as soon as possible, but always decide according to response and tolerance.

Cyclandelate, 100 mg tablets.

Cyclandelate, 200 or 400 mg capsules.

Nicotinyl Tartrate (Roniacol)

Because it relaxes the smooth muscle of peripheral vessels, nicotinyl tartrate is advisable for conditions with deficient blood circulation, such as peripheral vascular disease, ulcers (varicose or decubitus), Meniere's syndrome and other forms of vertigo, and chilblains.

Side effects may be flushing, headache, gastrointestinal symptoms, rashes, or other allergic symptoms.

Dosage: 50 to 100 mg every 8 hours; or a long-acting tablet every 12 hours.

Nicotinyl tartrate, 50 mg scored tablets.

Nicotinyl tartrate, elixir containing 50 mg in each 5 ml.

Nicotinyl tartrate, 150 mg long-acting tablets.

Nylidrin (Arlidin)

This drug is recommended in vascular disease of the type of arteriosclerosis obliterans, thromboangiitis obliterans, thrombophlebitis, diabetic vasculopathy, leg cramps, Raynaud's phenomenon and disease, ulcers of the ischemic or the decubitus type, acrocyanosis, acroparesthesia, frostbite and coldness of the extremities, and diseases of the inner ear with ischemic reactions.

Do not give it to patients with a progressive anginal syndrome or myocardial infarction, paroxysmal tachycardia, or thyrotoxicosis; and be careful if nervousness, tremors, palpitations, or gastrointestinal symptoms are noted, and particularly if the patient presents congestive heart failure, arrhythmias (mainly tachycardia) or any other untoward reaction.

Dosage: from 3 to 12 mg, every 6 to 8 hours, according to response and tolerance.

Nylidrin HCl, 6 or 12 mg scored tablets.

Isoxsuprine (Vasodilan)

Indications and cautions are very similar to those stated above for nylidrin, q.v.

Dosage: by mouth, 10 or 20 mg three times a day; by injection, 5 or 10 mg twice a day; in both instances according to response and tolerance.

Isoxsuprine HCl, 10 or 20 mg tablets.

Isoxsuprine, injectable containing 5 mg in each ml, in 2-ml ampoules.

Dioxyline (Paveril)

This drug is recommended for angina pectoris and other diseases with vascular spasm or spasm of other smooth muscles.

Caution will be observed if there is nausea, flushing, abdominal cramps, sweating, dizziness, or oversedation.

Dosage: 100 to 400 mg three or four times a day, according to response and tolerance.

Dioxyline, 100 or 200 mg scored tablets.

Other Preparations

A few other preparations have been recommended for increasing blood flow, mainly to the skin, and also for lowering blood pressure, thus helping in cases of acrocyanosis, acroparesthesia, Buerger's disease, vascular spasm, skin ulcers, chilblains, intermittent claudication, cramps, Raynaud's disease and phenomenon, Meniere's syndrome, arteriosclerosis, thrombophlebitis, thromboangiitis obliterans, causalgia, endarteritis, gangrene, and other diseases with impaired blood supply to any segment of the body.

Nicotinic acid or niacin may cause a flush from clavicles upward, and also to other areas of the skin.

Phenoxybenzamine also increases blood supply to the skin, and lowers increased blood pressure.

Sodium nitrite may also help in the treatment of angina pectoris.

Tolazoline exerts an action on the skin vessels, particularly of the fingers and toes, and perhaps to a somewhat limited extent on the skeletal muscle circulation.

Nicotinic acid, 25, 50, or 100 mg tablets.

Nicotinic acid, 25, 50, or 100 mg capsules.

Phenoxybenzamine, 10 mg capsules.

Sodium nitrite, granules; or 60 mg tablets.

Tolazoline, 25 mg tablets; or 80 mg sustained-release-action tablets.

VASOCONSTRICTORS

Metaraminol (Aramine)

Metaraminol is indicated for the management of acute hypotensive conditions due to hemorrhage, shock (brain damage from tumors or trauma), reactions to drugs (including anesthetics) and surgery, cardiogenic shock, or septicemia.

Advise the use of metaraminol together with cyclopropane; and be careful of rapid increases of blood pressure, arrhythmias, pulmonary edema, cardiac arrest, the simultaneous use of digitalis, MAOI or sympathomimetics, the presence of cirrhosis of the liver, ventricular arrhythmias, cardiopathies, hypertension, or the need of plasma expanders when plasma volume is diminished.

Dosage: Inject through large veins or in subcutaneous and intramuscular areas with good vascular circulation. Intravenous drip is used with 15 to 100 mg in 500 ml 5% glucose solution, adjusting speed to response and tolerance. When it is used subcutaneously or intramuscularly, inject from 2 to 10 mg. In severe shock, inject from 0.5 to 5 mg directly into a vein; then follow with an infusion.

Metaraminol, injectables containing 10 mg in each ml; in 1-ml ampoules or 10-ml vials.

Methoxamine (Vasoxyl)

Similar to metaraminol, this is a sympathomimetic amine, with the main indications for its use being the maintenance of blood pressure during anesthesia (including the use of cyclopropane) and suppression of supraventricular paroxysmal tachycardia. It is not to be mixed with local anesthetics to prolong their action.

Care must be taken not to cause an undesirable increase of blood pressure by giving excessive dosage or using ergot derivatives; nor should it be given to the hypertensive patient, the hyperthyroid, one with myocardial insufficiency, or those who react with hypertension, bradycardia, headache, or vomiting.

Dosage: By vein, slowly inject 3 to 5 mg, followed by intramuscular administration of a supplementary amount, 10 to 15 mg. Do not give a second dose until some 15 minutes has elapsed.

Methoxamine, injectables containing 20 mg in each ml, in 1-ml ampoules or 10-ml vials.

Dopamine (Intropin)

This precursor of norepinephrine is used for the therapy of shock, myocardial infarction, or heart insufficiency. It is also useful in renal insufficiency, trauma, septicemia, and hypotension due to inadequate cardiac output and the consequent poor organic perfusion.

Dopamine is not to be prescribed for patients with pheochromocytoma, tachycardia, ventricular fibrillation, hypovolemia, decreased pulse pressure, extravasation, and occlusive vascular disease of any kind.

Dosage: Under continuous monitoring give adequately diluted infusions in

5% glucose, always in large veins. Regulate speed according to the desired response, starting with 0.4 or 0.8 mg a minute.

> Dopamine injectable, containing 40 mg in each ml, in vials of 5 ml (one vial added to 500 ml of the solution to be infused will provide 0.4 mg in each ml; if added to 250 ml, it will provide 0.8 mg).

Levarterenol (Levophed)

This is *l*-norepinephrine, a very potent peripheral vasoconstrictor and coronary vasodilator. It is widely used for the control of hypotensive situations and also cardiac arrest. It is particularly effective in myocardial infarctions, blood transfusion or drug reactions, septicemia, or surgical procedures causing dangerously lowered blood pressure.

As with similar vasoconstrictor drugs (see above), care must be taken to avoid hypotension due to blood volume deficit; first replace the lost blood if time permits and cerebral and coronary perfusion can be maintained. All other indications and warnings are essentially the same, q.v. above. Nevertheless, this drug is perhaps favored by many physicians because it appears to be relatively safer than others.

Dosage: In general, add 4 mg to each liter of 5% glucose for infusion, and control speed according to desired response and tolerance, starting at a rate of 2 or 3 ml a minute. For maintenance, a dose of 0.5 to 1 ml a minute is acceptable in most instances. Nevertheless, individual fluctuations make it necessary to provide an individualized dose. In rare instances much larger doses are needed for adequate control.

> Levarterenol, injectables containing 1 mg per ml, in each 4-ml ampoule.

Ergotamine (Gynergen)

Ergotamine is recommended for the treatment of migraine (not for other headaches) and a miscellaneous group of diseases and symptoms such as itching, thyrotoxicoses, neuroses, and others. It is contraindicated in cases of sepsis, toxemia, coronary heart disease, obliterative vascular disease, and impaired liver or kidney function.

Dosage: 0.5 to 1 mg by injection, or 1 mg by tablet. Do not give more than 2 ml a week, or six tablets in each migraine attack. Individualize dosage.

> Ergotamine, 1 mg tablets.

> Ergotamine, injectables containing 0.5 mg in each ml, in ampoules of ½ or 1 ml.

Dihydroergotamine (D.H.E. 45)

This drug is recommended for patients who do not tolerate ergotamine. The indications and warnings are the same as for ergotamine.

Dosage: Individualize treatments with doses more or less similar to those of ergotamine.

Dihydroergotamine, injectables, 1 mg in each ml, in 1-ml ampoules.

XXIII. ANTI-ATHEROSCLEROTIC DRUGS

Atherosclerosis has been largely linked to some sort of lipid error of metabolism involving cholesterol and triglycerides. Management of diet, the substitution of polyunsaturated vegetable fat for the animal saturated ones, has seemed to play a relatively favorable role in its prevention or improvement. The use of amino acids has been encouraged, including methionine, inositol ("Methischol, Lufa-Methischol"), and nicotinic acid; also cholesterol analogs (triparanol) or hormones, particularly thyroid and estrogens, have been given. Heparin has also been found to decrease levels of triglycerides when given parenterally in doses of 100 to 200 mg. Presently, clofibrate is most frequently prescribed for this anti-atherosclerotic purpose.

Clofibrate (Atromid-S)

Clofibrate is an antilipidemic agent recommended as an adjunct therapy for the reduction of hypercholesterolemia and hypertriglyceridemia (in all types except type I). But the influence of this reduction on atherosclerosis is not yet known with respect to the long-term course of the disease.

Watch carefully liver and kidney functions, since patients with cirrhosis may react with increased cholesterolemia. Frequent rechecking of cholesterolemia, triglyceridemia, and concentration of transaminases is advisable for patients receiving clofibrate. Side effects may be cardiac arrhythmias, leukopenia, reactivation of peptic ulcers, symptoms of the type of influenza (myalgias, principally), and other reactions from the cardiovascular, dermic, gastrointestinal, hematologic, genitourinary, neurologic, or musculoskeletal systems.

Dosage: 500 mg four times a day.

Clofibrate, 500 mg capsules.

Nicotinic Acid (Nico-span)

This amino acid not only increases blood circulation to peripheral sites of the skin, but is also capable of decreasing the production of very low-density lipoproteins, namely, in the management of hyperlipidemias corresponding to types IIB, IV, and V, in which lipids are elevated.

Watch for excessive peripheral dilation of blood vessels (nose, fingers, toes), itching, or gastrointestinal disturbances.

Dosage: Start with 100 mg three times a day; increase as needed and tolerated, to a total of 5, 6, or 7 g per day, with meals.

Nicotinic acid, 25, 50, or 100 mg capsules.

Cholestyramine (Questran)

This is an anion exchange resin said to help in the management of hyper-cholesterolemia due to type IIA hyperlipidemia, but not to be given to patients with any other of the hyperlipidemic types. It is also prescribed for the relief of itching due to partial biliary obstruction.

Do not give it to patients with complete biliary obstruction, or to those who show an allergic reaction to its ingestion. Be careful that there is no interference with fat absorption (including fat-soluble vitamins); and that it does not cause a bleeding tendency, hyperchloremic acidosis, constipation, or side effects referred to the gastrointestinal, hematologic, neurologic, renal, cardiovascular, musculoskeletal, or visual systems. Do not give this medication in a dry form, or together with other drugs whose absorption may be impaired.

Dosage: 4 g three times a day, before meals; individualize the final amount according to response and tolerance. Always mix the medication with water or any other fluid, without stirring, until the powder is well hydrated—then stir to obtain a uniform suspension. Four grams three times a day is an average maintenance dose.

Cholestyramine, in 9-g packages containing 4 g of the active medication.

Sitosterols (Cytellin)

These plant sterols are used as the above cholestyramine is, to inferfere with the intestinal absorption of cholesterol in the management of hypercholesterolemia and hyperbetalipoproteinemia. The same precautions and warnings as for cholestyramine are to be observed.

Dosage: 3 g before meals, to be increased whenever needed and tolerated, but not to exceed 24 g a day.

Sitosterols, suspension containing 3 g in 15 ml.

Thyroid and Estrogens

These drugs are discussed in the chapter devoted to hormones, q.v.

XXIV. DIURETICS

Urea (Ureaphil)

Urea is mainly used for the relief of intracranial pressure (cerebral edema) and elevated pressure within the eye.

It is contraindicated in patients with impaired renal or hepatic function, marked dehydration, or intracranial bleeding. Patients will be carefully watched for electrolyte imbalance, extravasation of the infusion, headache, syncope or disorientation, or any other untoward reaction. Do not use hypothermia, or the same catheter for urea and for blood transfusion. Do not use veins of the lower extremities with the elderly because of the risk of thrombosis or phlebitis.

Dosage: About 1 g of urea each minute seems to be an adequate infusion speed (60 drops of a 30% solution made by dissolving the drug in 5 or 10% glucose solution) to give a total of 1 to 1.5 g for each kilo of body weight in 24 hours (not to exceed 120 g a day).

Urea in containers of 40 g each, mixed with 105 ml of the diluent to provide 30% solution.

Mannitol (Nitranitol)

This drug was briefly reviewed in the chapter devoted to vasodilators, q.v.

Mercurial Diuretics

Mercurial diuretics are mainly recommended for the treatment of cardiac edema, nephrotic edema, the nephrotic stage of glomerulonephritis, and the ascites due to hepatic cirrhosis or portal obstruction.

Contraindications are acute or subacute nephritis, ulcerative colitis, allergic reactions to mercury, or evidence of dehydration. Also contraindicated is use of the venous route for administration of organic mercurial diuretics. During mercurial therapy care must be taken to avoid electrolyte imbalance, dehydration (which occurs easily with the elderly), fever, flushing of the face, chills, gastrointestinal disturbances, skin rashes, and other untoward reactions which may indicate discontinuance of the treatment.

In all instances, dosage is an individual problem which will depend on response and tolerance; try, of course, to use the smallest amount of the drug.

Chlormerodrin (*Neohydrin*) is used orally and is recommended for a continuance of therapy after the use of injectable forms. The average dosage ranges from 55 to 110 mg in 24 hours.

Chlormerodrin, 18.3 mg tablets.

Merethoxylline (Dicurin Procaine) adds the contraindications and warnings for procaine and theophylline, used to stabilize the product. Injections can be given subcutaneously or intramuscularly, starting with 0.5 ml or less, and giving no more than 2 ml in 24 hours.

Merethoxylline, injectable in 10-ml vials.

Mercaptomerin (Thiomerin) is recommended for use either subcutaneously or intramuscularly in doses ranging from 0.2 ml to no more than 2 ml in 24 hours.

Mercaptomerin, injectable, 125 mg in each ml in 2-ml ampoules.

Thiazide Diuretics

These drugs were reviewed in the chapter devoted to drugs for hypertension, q.v. Included are chlorothiazide, hydrochlorothiazide, methyclothiazide, trichlormethiazide, polythiazide, benzthiazide, cyclothiazide, hydroflumethiazide, bendroflumethiazide and diazoxide.

Carbonic Anhydrase Inhibitors

The carbonic anhydrase inhibitors are indicated for the treatment of edema due to congestive heart failure or to the effect of drugs, for epilepsy (petil mal or unlocalized seizures), and in open-angle glaucoma, and also in secondary glaucoma and postoperatively in acute angle closure.

Contraindications include depletion of sodium and potassium, hyperchloremia, severe kidney and liver disease, hypoadrenalism, and other forms of glaucoma (particularly angle closure). Watch carefully for the appearance of fever, skin reactions, renal calculus, blood dyscrasias (particularly agranulocytosis), paresthesias, drowsiness, visual disturbances, and other untoward reactions.

Acetazolamide (Diamox) is prescribed in doses of 250 to 375 mg a day for edema (if it is drug-induced, stop after 2 days of therapy, to resume therapy if needed), and also for heart failure; higher doses are given for glaucoma, even to 1000 mg a day; also higher doses for epilepsy. In cases of emergency, inject 500 mg.

Acetazolamide, 125 or 250 mg, scored tablets.

Acetazolamide, 500 mg long-acting tablets.

Acetazolamide, injectables containing 500 mg, to add 5 ml water.

Dichlorphenamide (Daranide): 50 mg tablets, give one or two a day.
Methazolamide (Neptazane): 50 mg tablets, give one or two a day.
Ethoxzolamide (Cardrex): 125 mg tablets.

Sulfonamide Derivatives

This group of sulfonamide derivatives is recommended for the therapy of hypertension as well as for edema. Chlorthalidone was briefly reviewed in the chapter on antihypertensive drugs. Responsive forms of edema are due to heart failure, liver cirrhosis, and nephrosis; also to renal failure and other nephropathies such as acute glomerulonephritis, and edema caused by steroid therapy with corticoids or estrogens.

Contraindications are those usual for diuretics, namely, anuria and allergic reactions to the drug. A careful watch must be kept at all times for the development of severe renal or liver damage, and for any electrolyte imbalance (mainly hypokalemia, which may lead to hepatic coma), an increased need for insulin, any sort of interaction with other drugs, and the development of symptoms from the gastrointestinal or central nervous systems, blood dyscrasias, rashes, or orthostatic hypotension.

Chlorthalidone (Hygroton) is given at doses of 50 to 100 mg a day—not to exceed 200 mg in 24 hours.

Chlorthalidone, 50 or 100 mg tablets.

Quinethazone (Hydromox) dosage is 50 to 100 mg in 24 hours.

Quinethazone 50 mg scored tablets.

Metolazone (Zaroxolyn) dosage has to be individualized (do not forget that this is a good precaution for the administration of any diuretic). Give from 5 to 10 mg once a day for cardiac edema, or up to 20 mg in the case of renal edema. For hypertension, doses are lower: 2.5 to 5 mg once a day.

Metolazone, 2.5, 5, or 10 mg tablets.

Xanthines

Caffeine, theophylline, and aminophylline were briefly reviewed in the chapter devoted to stimulant drugs. But these drugs also have more or less marked diuretic properties.

Caffeine is used at times in acute circulatory failure, but mainly as a cerebral stimulant and secondarily as a heart stimulant. The safety margin is ample, and the secondary effects are of relatively little importance. Oral dosage, as caffeine citrate, goes from 60 to 120 mg; by injection, in acute poisoning, 500 to 1000 mg may be given.

Caffeine citrate, 60 or 120 mg tablets.

Caffeine with sodium benzoate, injectables containing 250 mg in each ml, in 2-ml ampoules and 10-ml vials.

Theophylline is mainly prescribed for relaxation of bronchial smooth muscle, and for cardiac diseases such as failure, congestive crises, anginal pains, and coronary thrombosis; also for biliary colic, headache, and the induction of diuresis. Excessive dosage may be followed by agitation and vomiting, and later by convulsions and shock. Dosage: 250 mg three times a day, by mouth; the injection of 500 mg by vein is reserved for bronchial asthma (aminophylline).

Theophylline, 100 or 200 mg tablets.

Aminophylline is used as the above drugs are.

Aminophylline, 100 or 200 mg tablets.

Aminophylline, suppositories, 125, 250, or 500 mg.

Aminophylline, ampoules containing 250 mg in 10-ml vials or 500 mg in 20-ml vials (for intravenous use).

Theobromine might be a less active but a longer-acting diuretic drug, and is used in larger doses than its congeners.

Theobromine (sodium salicylate), 500 mg tablets.

Spironolactone

This drug was reviewed in the chapter devoted to drugs for hypertension, q.v.

Ammonium Chloride

Ammonium chloride is often used with mercurial diuretics, which are thus potentiated, or with methenamine in urinary infections because the acid urine helps the release of formaldehyde. Other uses are as an expectorant, for the therapy of alkalosis, and in Ménière's disease.

It causes gastrointestinal side effects (less marked with enteric-coated tablets) and should not be given in acidotic patients.

Dosage: 4 to 12 g a day, in divided doses (average, 8 g). Best diuretic results are obtained by giving the drug for 3 or 4 days, pausing for a few days, and then resuming therapy. For Ménière's disease give 3 g three times a day for 3 days, pause 2 days, then give 3 days of therapy, and so on.

Ammonium chloride, 300 mg tablets.

Ammonium chloride, 300 or 500 mg coated tablets.

Other Diuretics

Amisometradine (Rolicton) and *aminometradine* (Mincard) are intended for the treatment of moderate edema due to congestive heart failure, cirrhosis, and nephrosis; but since they are diuretics of little potency, they are not recommended to initiate therapy but for maintenance.

Gastrointestinal disturbances, electrolyte imbalance, skin rashes, and other minor side effects have been recorded, and should be watched for.

Dosage: Start with 400 mg four times a day; maintenance therapy is usually achieved with half this dosage.

Amisometradine, 400 mg scored tablets.

Furosemide (Lasix) is indicated for hypertension and for edema due to heart failure, cirrhosis, or nephrosis; also acute pulmonary edema, which requires rapid action.

Contraindications: anuria, oliguria, increased BUN, hepatic coma, electrolyte depletion, and allergic reactions. Patients are to be watched for dehydration, electrolyte imbalance, hyperuricemia, hypoglycemia, blood dyscrasias, gastrointestinal reactions (particularly small bowel lesions), hypotension, ototoxicity, and reaction when given together with other drugs. When elderly persons are treated with furosemide, great care will be observed for the development of thrombosis or embolism.

Dosage: The oral route is to be preferred, giving 20 to 80 mg once a day, but individualizing each case; for hypertension give 40 mg twice a day. Rapid action is obtained with injections of 20 to 40 mg.

Furosemide, 20 mg tablets; or 40 mg scored tablets.

Furosemide, injectable containing 10 mg in each ml, in 2-ml ampoules or 10-ml vials.

Ethacrynic Acid (Edecrin) is indicated for edema due to heart failure, cirrhosis, nephrosis, and ascites; also for lymphedema and pulmonary edema (in this last instance treatment is carried out with rapid-acting injections).

Contraindications: anuria, electrolyte imbalance, severe diarrhea, severely decompensated myocardium, and also severe cases of cirrhosis. Elderly persons will be carefully watched for the development of thrombosis, which may occur if there is a rapid hemoconcentration; in all instances watch for electrolyte imbalance and hypokalemia, gastrointestinal disturbances (mainly small bowel lesions), asthenia, cramps, paresthesias, hypotension (particularly if a drug is also given for this purpose), vertigo, tinnitus (deafness!), blood dyscrasias, renal reactions, and hyperglycemia. Anticoagulant doses have to be very carefully determined for each patient.

Dosage: Always give the lowest possible amount, and make therapy intermittent (50 to 100 mg a day—never to exceed 200 mg a day). Intravenously, give 50 mg (or 0.5 to 1 mg/kg/day).

Ethacrynic acid, 25 or 50 mg tablets.

Ethacrynic acid, injectable containing 50 mg in a 50-ml vial.

Triamterene (Direnium) is indicated for edema due to heart failure, cirrhosis, nephrosis, treatment with steroids, and hyperaldosteronism.

Contraindications: kidney diseases, liver damage, hyperkalemia, and reactional allergy to the drug. Watch for blood dyscrasias, liver or kidney damage, electrolyte imbalance, hypotension, gastrointestinal disturbances, asthenia, headache, and rashes. Do not mix with spironolactone.

Dosage: individualized at about 100 mg twice a day; do not exceed 300 mg in 24 hours.

Triamterene, 100 mg capsules.

XXV. ANTICOAGULANTS

Heparin (Liquaemin, Lipo-hepin, Panheprin, heparin sodium)

Many preparations are marketed under the generic name of heparin. It represents the prototype of anticoagulant injectable therapy, indicated for the prevention and treatment of thrombosis, pulmonary embolism, chronic coagulopathies, and the prevention of cerebral thrombosis in cases of stroke; also for coronary occlusion and as an adjunct therapy in surgery. Small amounts—not enough to induce anticoagulation—are recommended to prevent "residuals" of glomerulonephritis.

Contraindications: uncontrollable bleeding, allergic reactivity to the drug, and situations in which the patient cannot be carefully controlled. Watch for possible tendency to hemorrhages, as in endocarditis, atherosclerosis, hematologic conditions (like hemophilia), gastrointestinal ulcers, or any other tendency to bleed. Be careful not to give barbiturates to elderly persons receiving anticoagulant therapy with heparin or any other drugs that might interfere with clotting such as salicylates, digitalis, tetracyclines, and antihistamines.

Dosage: individualized by continuous monitoring of coagulation (clotting time to be 2.5 to 3 times greater than the control value); usually achieved with 8000 to 10,000 units every 8 hours or 15,000 to 20,000 units every 12 hours given subcutaneously.

Heparin is supplied in a great variety of preparations; the physician will become familiar with a few reliable ones.

The Coumarins

Development of the oral use of coumarin anticoagulants was a good therapeutic achievement. These drugs will usually be given for chronic administration, once a more rapid action has been initiated with injectable heparin. The final indications are essentially the same for both.

Contraindications are also essentially the same, but care will be observed because of the possible accumulation of effects. Drugs particularly to be watched if used simultaneously (better to avoid them!) are the barbiturates, meprobamate, steroids, the butazones, chloral hydrate, and many others. Thus, it will be advisable to check coagulation each time a drug is added or discharged from the list of current anticoagulant therapy.

Dosage: individualized by continuous monitoring of the prothrombin time (when heparin is given, allow time to check coagulation), to maintain 2.5 to 3 times the control value.

Warfarin sodium (Panwarfin, Coumadin) is to be adjusted at about 50 mg (40 to 60 mg) as the initial dose (half this amount for the very old or debilitated) followed by 5 to 10 mg a day, always under strict control of prothrombin time.

Warfarin sodium, 2, 2.5, 5, 7.5, 10, and 25 mg tablets.

Acenocoumarol (Sintrom) requires an initual 16- to 28-mg dose, followed by 8 to 16 mg the second day and finally 2 to 10 mg daily.

Acenocoumarol, 4 mg tablets.

Ethyl biscoumacetate (Tromexan) is less potent, requiring administration of 1500 mg during the first 24 hours, followed by 600 to 900 mg a day.

Ethyl biscoumacetate, 150 or 300 mg scored tablets.

Indandione Derivatives

The actions, indications, and warnings with indandione derivatives are similar to those of the coumarins, perhaps with a more rapid effect. Among these products there are an anisindione, a phenindione, and a diphenadione.

Anisindione (Miradon) is given at an initial dosage of 300 mg the first day, 200 mg the second day, and 100 mg the third day; individually adjust the dosage between 25 and 250 mg a day thereafter.

Anisindione, 50 mg scored tablets.

Phenindione (Danilone, Hedulin, Indon, P.I.D.) is given at a dosage of 100 or 150 mg twice a day, the first day, to stay at a maintenance dose of about 75 mg a day, through strict monitoring of the prothrombin time. For elderly and frail patients give the smaller dose.

Phenindione, 20 or 50 mg tablets.

Diphenadione is marketed under the trade name Dipaxin.

XXVI. HORMONES

Pituitary Hormones

ACTH (Acthar) is the physiologic stimulant for corticoids released by the adrenal gland; thus, its actions are essentially the same as those of the natural corticoids. Nevertheless, therapeutically it is recommended only for acute gout, acute rheumatic carditis, pemphigus, Stevens-Johnson syndrome, herpes zoster, iritis, uveitis, sympathetic ophthalmia, tuberculous meningitis with subarachnoid block, and trichinosis. It may be indicated as well for certain collagen diseases, a few forms of rheumatic disorders, and allergic states.

Contraindications: osteoporosis, systemic fungal infections, peptic ulcer, ocular herpes simplex, scleroderma, hypertension, congestive heart failure and allergic reactivity. Watch for adrenal overstimulation, development of cataracts, glaucoma, reactivation of tuberculosis, and hypothyroidism. Check for water and electrolyte balance.

Dosage: Regular doses are 40 to 80 units of the repository form every 24 to 72 hours; or 20 units of the regular form every 6 hours.

> ACTH, regular form, in 1-ml ampoules or 5-ml vials, containing 25, 40, or 80 units in each ml.

> ACTH, repository form, 40 or 80 units for intramuscular use.

Chorionic gonadotropin (A.P.L. and Follutein) is the natural stimulant to the gonads and contains both luteinizing and follicle-stimulant fractions. It is indicated for the induction of ovulation (of no use after the menopause), for cryptorchidism, and for other instances of male hypogonadism. This preparation is of little use for the elderly.

Pitressin or vasopressin is used almost solely for the treatment of diabetes insipidus. It is not advisable to give it to patients with coronary problems (if it is absolutely needed, be very cautious); also watch for water retention and for the reactions of epileptics, asthmatics, patients with heart failure, chronic nephritis, drug allergy, or other individual symptomatology of intolerance.

Dosage: only by intramuscular administration (never in veins!); give 1.5 to 5 units of the tannate in oil.

> Pitressin tannate, in oil injectable containing 5 units per ml, in 1-ml ampoules.

Oxytocin has no indication in this group of older patients.

Thyrotropin (Thytropar) is the thyrotropic hormone used for diagnostic purposes (hypothyroidism, evaluation of thyroid therapy, detection of thyroid cancer remnants) and for the treatment of cancer of the gland and its metastases.

Contraindications: hypoadrenalism when untreated, coronary thrombosis, and allergic reactivity. Watch for anginal reactions, heart failure, hypotension, tachycardia, fibrillation, and any other general reaction.

Dosage: regularly, 10 units for no more than 8 days.

Thyrotropin injectable containing 10 units in powder form, to be dissolved in 2 ml of diluent.

Thyroid Preparations

Thyroid extracts (Proloid, SPT, Thyroid Strong), as well as any other of the thyroid preparations that follow, are indicated for the treatment of hypothyroidism in all its different clinical manifestations (hypothyroidism, myxedema, cretinism), many different types of goiter, thyroiditis, and other conditions such as hypercholesterolemia. Synthetic products may substitute for extracts when the patient reacts allergically to the latter, and in some cases of thyroiditis.

Contraindications valid for all thyroid preparations are: untreated hypoadrenalism (Addison's disease), severe cardiopathies (coronary), or any other clinically insurmountable form of intolerance. Special care should be taken when thyroid preparations are given to cardiac patients; those with nephrosis, hypogonadism, or tachycardia; digitalis users (perhaps other drugs as well); or patients with any other form of hyperthyroid reactivity.

Dosage: Start low (30 to 180 mg) and increase according to personal reactions, since the administration of thyroid must be strictly individualized. Concentrated preparations will require only 66% of the regular extract.

Thyroid extract, 15 or 30 mg (¼ or ½ grain) tablets.

Thyroid extract, 60, 90, 120, 180, or 300 mg tablets.

Thyroid extract, 60, 120, 180, or 300 mg capsules.

Thyroid concentrated extract, 30, 60, 120, or 180 mg tablets.

Thyroxine (Cholixin) is mainly promoted for the management of hypercholesterolemia, but its clinical use is identical to that of thyroid preparations, as stated above for the extract. Treatment may be initiated by giving from 4 to 8 mg, but dosage must be stricly individualized.

Thyroxine, 1, 2, 4, or 6 mg scored tablets.

Triiodothyronine (Cytomel) has the same indications, contraindications, and warnings as for the extract. The dosage has to be strictly individualized after starting with 0.005 to 0.025 mg in 24 hours.

Triiodothyronine, 0.005 mg tablets; and 0.025 or 0.05 mg scored tablets.

Tetraiodothyronine or levothyronine (Letter, Synthroid, Levoid) has same indications and precautions as for the extracts, q.v. The dosage will start with 0.025 mg and will be individualized.

> Tetraiodothyronine, 0.025, 0.05, 0.1, 0.15, 0.2, 0.3, or 0.5 mg scored tablets.

> Tetraiodothyronine, injectables containing 0.5 mg in a 10-ml vial (to be reconstituted) or 0.1 mg in each ml in a 10-ml vial.

Liotrix (Euthroid, Thyrolar) is a mixture of triiodo- and tetraiodothyronine in a ratio of 1:4. The indications and other precautions are the same as for the extract, q.v.; but it is more strongly indicated in cases of thyroiditis and when there is intolerance to the extracts. Start the treatment with a dose of 12.5 to 50 μg (0.0125 to 0.05 mg) and individualize in all instances.

> Liotrix, 6.25 to 25 μg, 12.5 to 50 μg, 25 to 100 μg, 37.5 to 150 μg, or 62.5 to 250 μg tablets.

Parathyroid

Parathyroid hormone is indicated for the treatment of tetany (acute or chronic hypoparathyroidism), usually with a prompt response, but also with a refractoriness developing soon.

Intravenous injections should be avoided at all times, as well as the use of this hormone when there is some sort of hypercalcemia or cardiac or renal disease. Allergic reactions occur very frequently.

Dosage: For acute tetany, inject intramuscularly from 20 to 40 units; repeat every 12 hours whenever needed.

> Parathyroid hormone, injectable containing 100 units in each ml, in 5-ml vials.

Insulin

This pancreatic hormone represents the rational approach to the management of patients with diabetes mellitus, both the chronic condition and its acute acidotic episodes (diabetic coma). The only dangers in using it are the production of hypoglycemia (which will be accentuated with insulin) and not-too-rare allergic reactivity.

In general, the dosage of insulin is a matter of individual need. Insulin administration is the best example of individualized treatment. One patient will respond to about 10 units, while another will require 100. Also, the timing of injections must be suitable; it is usually given about 30 minutes before meals (breakfast, lunch, dinner), but always with consideration of the particular type of insulin to be used. The type used may be rapid in action or lower in effect; thus, the insulin preparation used can be varied.

Regular insulin starts rapidly and is short-lived in activity; usually, therefore, several injections have to be given every day before each meal. Try to use the insulin prepared from beef; resort to pork insulin in case of allergy.

> Regular insulin, U-40, U-80, or U-100 (the number of units in each ml) in 10-ml vials.

Globin insulin is of slow onset and long-lasting in effects; hence, no more than two injections a day are usually needed, before breakfast and supper.

> Globin insulin, U-40, U-80, or U-100 in 10-ml vials.

NPH insulin: the onset occurs between the onsets of the regular and globin types; its effects are also maintained for a longer time. Usually it is needed once, but no more than twice, a day.

> NPH insulin, U-40, U-80, or U-100, in 10-ml vials.

Protamine zinc insulin starts slowly, like globin insulin, but acts for longer periods of time. It is usually given once a day; but not more than twice.

> Protamine zinc insulin, U-40, U-80, or U-100 in 10-ml vials.

Semilente insulin is similar to regular insulin regarding the onset and prolongation of effects.

> Semilente insulin, U-40, U-80, or U-100 in 10-ml vials.

Lente insulin shows intermediate rates for onset and prolongation of effects (similar to globin or NPH).

> Lente insulin, U-40, U-80, or U-100 in 10-ml vials.

Ultralente insulin shows some similarity to protamine zinc insulin regarding onset and prolongation of effects.

> Ultralente insulin, U-40, U-80, or U-100 in 10-ml vials.

Oral Hypoglycemiant Drugs

Two main groups represent the drugs able to help diabetics to manage their condition without the inconveniences of the daily injections: the biguanides and the sulfonylureas. These drugs can be recommended only in responsive forms of diabetes, namely, the stable, maturity-onset types not responsive to diet alone. Patients nonresponsive to sulfonylureas will present a similar intolerance to any representative in the group, but may respond to biguanides and perhaps also to tolinase.

The biguanides are contraindicated in cases of cardiovascular diseases, gangrene, infections, diseases of the liver or the kidney, and acidosis (particularly lactic acidosis, or patients prone to or who already have had this form of acidosis). The sulfonylureas are contraindicated in practically all similar situations (except for lactic acidosis). In all instances great care will be taken for symptoms of hypoglycemia, gastrointestinal reactions, and allergic reactivity, and for those receiving chlorpropamide for jaundice or very late hypoglycemic reactions. Patients receiving other sulfas will have enhanced the antidiabetic effect; and those receiving a thiazide, the effect of acetohexamide.

Phenformin (Meltrol, DBI-TD and DBT) is the best example of the biguanides. The dose will be 50 or 100 mg a day, in one or two doses, never to exceed 100 mg in 24 hours.

Phenformin, 25 or 50 mg tablets.

Phenformin, 50 mg long-acting capsules.

Chlorpropamide (Diabinese) will not be given to elderly patients in doses greater than 100 or 125 mg; it is not to exceed 500 mg in 24 hours. As usual, dosage will be strictly individualized.

Chlorpropamide, 100 or 250 mg scored tablets.

Acetohexamide (Dymelor) is given in doses of 1000 mg once a day, or 750 mg twice a day; not to exceed 1500 mg in 24 hours. Individualize each dose.

Acetohexamide, 250 or 500 mg scored tablets.

Tolazamide (Tolinase) may be used when other oral antidiabetics fail; the dose is 100 to 250 mg once a day, according to individual response.

Tolazamide, 100, 250, or 500 mg scored tablets.

Tolbutamide (Orinase) is perhaps the least dangerous of antidiabetics when given to elderly persons at a dose of 1000 to 2000 mg a day.

Tolbutamide, 500 mg scored tablets.

Glucagon

This is another pancreatic hormone, with an action opposite to that of insulin. It is recommended for hypoglycemic conditions (post insulin, post oral antidiabetics) only if there is a remnant of liver glucogen. Patients with diabetes of the juvenile type need infusion of glucose. Avoid giving glucagon to those who react against it. Dosage: 0.5 to 1 unit by subcutaneous, intramuscular, or intravenous injection; doses to be repeated every 5 to 20 minutes if the patient does not wake up after the injection (give intravenous glucose if glucagon fails to act).

Glucagon, powder in ampoules containing 1 or 10 units, to be dissolved in the accompanying diluent.

Epinephrine and Norepinephrine

Both have been reviewed in the chapter devoted to sympathomimetic drugs, q.v.

Cortisone

Cortisone is recommended for the treatment of adrenal insufficiency (Addison's disease), and also for rheumatic fever and other forms of arthritis as well as iritis, iridocyclitis, uveitis, herpes zoster, leukemia, trichinosis with myocardial invasion, hypopituitarism, allergic diseases, lupus erythematosus, periarteritis nodosa, dermatomyositis, scleroderma, sarcoidosis, pemphigus, atopic dermatitis, psoriasis, pulmonary fibrosis, nephrosis, hepatitis, mutliple sclerosis, Sjogren's syndrome, and any other disease responsive to corticoids. It causes sodium retention with edema, hyperglycemia, acne, hirsutism, cutaneous striae, cervico-thoracic hump, and rounded facies.

Dosage: from 30 to 300 mg in 24 hours, the last instance only if severity warrants the risk of the high dosage. This is the case in some inflammatory diseases of the eye. For cortisone, as well as for all other corticoids, elevated doses are to be cut down to the lowest effective amount as soon as symptoms are under control. Stoppage must be very gradual.

Cortisone, 5, 10, or 25 mg tablets.

Cortisone, injectable, in solution containing 25 mg in each ml (20-ml vials).

Hydrocortisone (Cortef)

Hydrocortisone is more powerful than cortisone on a grainage basis, but the effects of the two are essentially the same. The physician is obliged to watch carefully for side effects: sodium retention with edema, hyperglycemia, acne, hirsutism, and all other consequences listed for cortisone, q.v. It is also recommended for the same purposes as cortisone, and in addition, for ulcerative colitis, injections into joints or bursae, and pulmonary or meningeal tuberculosis. In all other instances, hydrocortisone will be used only in cases resistant to cortisone or any other less active corticoid. Accordingly, side effects are worse, and may reach undesirable levels, particularly for sodium retention and edema. Infection may be aggravated, and its spreading enhanced. Effective dosage depends upon the disease concerned.

Dosage: Start with 20 to 500 mg (average: 100 to 200 mg) in 24 hours, in divided doses. Maintenance will be achieved with 10 to 60 mg every 24 hours. Stoppage of the drug should be carried out slowly and followed closely because of the suppression of adrenal glands.

Hydrocortisone, 5, 10, or 20 mg tablets.

Hydrocortisone, oral suspension with 10 mg for each 5 ml.

Hydrocortisone, ointment containing 1 or 2.5%.

Hydrocortisone, injectable containing 50 mg in each ml.

Desoxycorticosterone (Percorten)

Desoxycorticosterone is mainly recommended for adrenal insufficiency and salt-losing adrenogenital syndrone. Injections and pellets are for implantation under the skin.

Desoxycorticosterone, 5 mg in each ml, in 10-ml vials.

Desoxycorticosterone, i.m. repository, 25 mg in 4-ml vials.

Desoxycorticosterone, pellets containing 125 mg.

Prednisone (Deltasone)

Prednisone is four or five times more potent as an anti-inflammatory agent than hydrocortisone, and produces little or no retention of sodium. It is indicated in thyroiditis, acute gout, acute rheumatic carditis, tuberculous meningitis with subdural-arachnoid block, leukemia, Stevens-Johnson syndrome, pemphigus, herpes zoster, inflammatory diseases of the eye, or any other disease responsive to cortisone.

Dosage: from 10 to 80 mg in 24 hours, to start; to be reduced as soon as possible to lower, effective levels, these ranging from 2.5 to 20 mg in 24 hours.

Prednisone, 2, 2.5, or 5 mg tablets.

Prednisone, powder, for individualized prescriptions.

Prednisolone (Delta-Cortef)

Prednisolone is entirely comparable to prednisone, perhaps minimally more active, but to be used for the same indications and in the same dosages.

Prednisolone, 1, 2.5, or 5 mg tablets.

Prednisolone, powder, for individualized prescriptions.

Prednisolone acetate, 25 or 50 mg in each ml, in 10-ml vials (also 30-ml vials, 25 mg per ml).

Dexamethasone (Hexadrol, Decadron)

Dexamethasone is still stronger than prednisone and prednisolone, and is used in smaller amounts but for the same indications, q.v.; but especially avoid its use in systemic fungal diseases. The equivalent dosage is 0.75 mg of dexamethasone for 4 or 5 mg of prednisone or prednisolone.

Dexamethasone, 0.25, 0.5, 0.75, 1.5, or 4 mg tablets.

Dexamethasone, 4 mg in each ml, vials containing 1, 5 or 25 ml.

Triamcinolone (Aristocort, Kenacort)

Triamcinolone is a derivative of prednisolone, their indications and warnings being the same (4 mg triamcinolone equals 5 mg of prednisone or prednisolone, of 0.75 mg of dexamethasone).

Triamcinolone, 1, 2, 4, or 8 mg tablets.

Triamcinolone, syrup, containing 4 mg per ml.

Triamcinolone, for deep intramuscular injection only, containing 40 mg in each ml, in 1-ml, 5-ml, or 10-ml vials.

Triamcinolone is also available for topical use in the form of ointment, cream, lotion, and spray, in different concentrations.

Betamethasone (Benisone, Celestone)

Betamethasone, on a grainage comparison basis, is the most powerful of the corticoids presently in use. The 0.6-mg tablet is equivalent to the 0.75-mg tablet of dexamethasone. For this corticoid, indications and warnings are the same as for others.

Betamethasone is marketed in the form of tablets, syrup, a 0.2% cream for dermatological use, and an injectable suspension, which has the advantage that it can be administered to muscles, dermis, bursae, joints, and other bodily locations.

Betamethasone, 0.6 mg tablets.

Betamethasone, syrup, containing 0.6 mg per ml.

Betamethasone, 0.2% cream.

Betamethasone, injectable suspension, containing both 3 mg of a rapid-absorption salt and 3 mg of a slow-absorption salt in each ml, in 5-ml vials.

The injectable is recommended in doses of 0.25 to 1 or 2 ml for small to large joints. For local application the dose is from 0.25 to 1 ml.

Other Corticoids

A few other corticoids are also available.

Methylprednisolone, 2, 4, or 16 mg tablets; cream (0.25 or 1%); and sustained-action capsules containing 2 or 4 mg each.

Paramethasone, 1 or 2 mg tablets.

Estrogens

In the case of elderly persons, estrogens are mainly recommended for the management of the climacterium, senile vaginitis and kraurosis vulvae, hypoestrogenic osteoporosis, and some cases of breast cancer (resistant to radiotherapy, inoperable, and starting at least 5 years after the menopause). For men, estrogens are prescribed for inoperable prostatic cancer.

Breast cancer is a contraindication for the use of estrogens, except in the cases mentioned above; other contraindications are cancer of the uterus, any thromboembolic condition, and an impaired liver function.

The list of precautions and wide effects which may occur during estrogen therapy is a very long one, but it essentially refers to the following situations: cancer (uterine or at any other location), thrombotic conditions of any kind (limbs, retina), gastrointestinal reactions, reactions of the central nervous system (including epilepsy, migraine, headache), cardiac and renal diseases, rashes, edema, allergic reactivity, or any other untoward reaction referable to estrogen therapy, for which a constant watch will be maintained at all times.

Conjugated estrogens (Premarin; also marketed under the generic name) and all other estrogens are preferently given in relation to the menstrual cycle, except for the treatment of cancer. Indications, contraindications, and precautions are those described above. Regular dosage is 1.25 mg or less a day for 20 or 28 days; with adequate pauses; for prostatic cancer, 1.25 to 2.5 mg three times a day, without pauses.

Conjugated estrogens, 0.3, 0.625, 1.25, or 2.5 mg tablets.

Conjugated estrogens vaginal cream (0.625 mg per g).

Esterified estrogens(Evex, Menest, SK-estrogens) are very similar to the conjugated estrogens with respect to indications, contraindications, warnings, and dosage.

Esterified estrogens, 0.3, 0.625, 1.25, or 2.5 mg tablets.

Ethinyl estradiol (Estinyl) has essentially the same indications and precautions as the conjugated estrogens, q.v. The recommended dosage for the climacterium is 0.02 mg every other day; and for cancer 0.5 mg daily.

Ethinyl estradiol, 0.02, 0.05, or 0.5 mg tablets.

Diethylstilbestrol also has the same indications and warnings as those given above. Dosage: for prostatic cancer, 1 to 3 mg a day; for breast cancer, 15 mg a day; for kraurosis of the vulva, 5 mg a week in suppository form plus 0.5 to 2 mg orally. For inoperable cancer there is a high-dosage tablet containing 50 mg (and an injectable with 250 mg in 5-ml ampoules, to start intensive therapy with intravenous infusions), to administer three tablets a day and increase dosage if tolerated.

Diethylstilbestrol, 0.1, 0.25, 0.5, 1, or 5 mg tablets.

Diethylstilbestrol, concentrated tablets, 50 mg.

Diethylstilbestrol, injectable containing 250 mg in each 5-ml ampoule, to dilute for infusion.

Chlorotrianisene (Tace) has the same indications and warnings as the preceding estrogens, but is mainly recommended for cancer therapy (prostatic), at a dose of 12 to 25 mg once a day. For the climacterium and senile vaginitis use the same dosage, but in cyclic courses.

Chlorotrianisene, 12 or 25 mg capsules.

Progesterone

The second ovarian hormone, progesterone, is of little use for older women; it is given only in rare cases of mastodynia, adenosis, residual cystic mastitis, and cervical cancer; but in all these instances its use is still considered experimental, and its value is not yet proved. Progesterone is the natural hormone; medroxyptogesterone, norethynodrel, norethindrone, and ethisterone are synthetic derivatives.

Progesterone, injectables in 2, 5, 10, 25, 50, or 100 mg ampoules or vials; also in sublingual tablets containing 10, 20, or 25 mg each, or in 25 or 50 mg vaginal tablets.

Ethisterone, 5, 10, or 25 mg tablets; or sublingual tablets of 10 mg.

Testosterone

In the upper age bracket, the testicular hormone is used for the treatment of male climacteric symptoms, and among women for the treatment of inoperable breast carcinoma. It may be of some use in the treatment of impotence.

This hormone is contraindicated in cancers of the breast and of the prostate among males, and for all patients in decompensation of the heart, the liver, or the kidney and in those showing hypercalcemia. Caution will be observed for sexual overstimulation or gynecomastia (hirsutism when given to females), jaundice (from cholestatic hepatitis), acne, edema, or allergic reactivity.

Testosterone (Oreton, Delatestryl, Perandren, Depo-testosterone) is manufactured as the propionate, enanthate, phenyl acetate, or other salts, most of them of equal pharmacologic value by weight. Regular dosage is of about 10 to 40 mg a day (one half of this dose if given sublingually); for breast cancer, up to 200 mg a day.

> Testosterone, 10 or 25 mg tablets; also tablets for sublingual administration, 10 mg.

> Testosterone, pellets for subcutaneous implantation, containing 75 mg each (to implant from two to six tablets every 3 or 4 months).

> Testosterone, injectables containing 25, 50, 100, or 200 mg in each ml; 1-, 5-, and 10-ml containers. The 200-mg dose is to be administered once a month (no more than 400 mg, intramuscularly).

Dromostanolone (Drolban) is a synthetic androgen recommended for the treatment of breast cancer. Dosage: 100 mg three times a week, intramuscularly.

> Dromostanolone injectable containing 50 mg in each ml, in 10-ml vials.

Fluoxymesterone (Halotestin, Ora-testryl, Ultandren) is a testosterone derivative presented in the form of tablets to be swallowed.

> Fluoxymesterone, 2.5 or 10 mg tablets.

Methandriol (Methylandrostenediol, Stenediol) is related to methyltestosterone, and is to be administered orally.

> Methandriol tablets, 5 or 25 mg (there is also an injectable form).

Nandrolone (Durabolin, Deca-durabolin) is a synthetic androgen, mainly indicated for the treatment of breast cancer, and also recommended (experimentally) for the treatment of refractory anemias.

> Mandrolone, injectable containing 25 or 50 mg in each ml, in 1-, 2-, or 5-ml containers.

Norethandrolone (Nilevar) is another synthetic androgen to be administered in tablets, liquid, or injections.

Norethandrolone, 10 mg tablets.

Norethandrolone, liquid containing 0.25 mg in each drop.

Norethandrolone, injectable containing 25 mg in each 1-ml ampoule.

Stanolzol (Winstrol) is also related to methyltestosterone and used similarly.

Stanolzol, 2 mg tablets.

XXVII. ANTI-HORMONES

Still a poor chapter in pharmacology, the list of drugs capable of controlling excessive secretion of hormones by the corresponding glands is growing little by little, with a few effective ones for the control of hyperthyroidism, phenoxybenzamine active against large amounts of nor- and straight epinephrine in the blood, danazol to inhibit the output of gonadotropins from the pituitary, spironolactone active against aldosterone, and some others still under study. To this we may add that papers were published abroad and in the United States in past years regarding the use of bismuth compounds to inhibit thyroid function, and toxins from *Necator americanus* or *Ancylostoma duodenale* to inhibit pituitary activity.

Danazol (Danocrine)

This is a synthetic androgen with weak androgenic activity, but it is an inhibitor of gonadotropin from the pituitary gland. Therefore, it is used for the treatment of endometriosis when patients cannot tolerate other medication or do not respond to it. It is of little use for older women.

Propylthiouracil

This is a thiocarbamide compound prescribed for the treatment of hyperthyroidism; it is not to be used if there is an allergic reaction to it.

Be alert for any evidence of adverse reaction, particularly agranulocytosis, bleeding tendency, skin rashes, gastrointestinal problems, jaundice, or adenopathy.

Dosage: 300 mg a day is the usual initial amount, but in severe cases 600 to 900 mg a day will be required. Maintenance dose of 150 to 200 mg will suffice.

Propylthiouracil, 50 mg scored tablets.

Methimazole (Tapazole)

Indications and precautions are essentially the same as with propyl-thiouracil, q.v. in the paragraph immediately above.

Dosage: Most cases will respond to an initial therapy with 30 to 40 mg a day in three installments. Less severe cases or frail patients will receive no more than 15 to 20 mg, while severe cases may require up to 60 mg in a 24-hour period. A daily dose of 5 to 15 mg will be enough for maintenance.

Methimazole, 5 or 10 mg scored tablets.

Methylthiouracil (Methiacil)

Indications and precautions are essentially the same as with propyl-thiouracil, perhaps with more side effects.

Dosage: Start with 50 mg four times a day, but do not exceed 300 mg in 24 hours. Maintenance dosage will be established according to tolerance and response.

Methylthiouracil, 50 mg scored tablets.

Iothiouracil (Itrumil sodium)

The indications and precautions are the same as with propylthiouracil, but it will be noted that it may also induce thyroidal involution (because of its iodine content), causes less vascularization, and is less goitrogenic. Nevertheless, it is not really superior to propylthiouracil.

Dosage: Start with 100 mg three times a day; but use lesser amounts for mild cases or frail patients. If there is no response, the dose may be slightly increased, never surpassing 300 mg in 24 hours. For prolonged maintenance therapy, decrease the dose to a lesser effective amount.

Iothiouracil sodium, 50 mg scored tablets.

Iodine

Iodine for years has been the principal inhibitor substance of thyroid activity, advised for the prophylaxis of goiter and the treatment of hyper-thyroidism. It is presently used together with propylthiouracil to prepare patients for surgery.

Contraindications and warnings refer to tuberculosis, laryngeal edema, swelling of the salivary glands, sialorrhea, and instances of skin reactivity against iodides.

Dosage: Lugol's solution is the preferred preparation, given in doses of 0.1 to 0.3 ml in water after meals (three times a day). Thyroid crises are treated with a higher dosage, up to 1 ml three times a day.

Lugol's solution, the desired amount in a bottle.

131I

Radioisotopes, among them ^{131}I, are dispensed by specialized centers, such as the Atomic Energy Commission; this particular one is used for the treatment of hyperthyroidism or thyroid cancer. These radioisotopes are to be used only by authorized personnel.

Sodium iodide ^{131}I, U.S.P., in ampoules containing different amounts (microcuries) in 10- or 40-ml vials.

Note: [125]I is also being used by some physicians for the treatment of hyperthyroidism.

Spironolactone (Aldactone)

This substance is a pharmacologic antagonist of the adrenal hormone aldosterone and is used for the treatment of hyperaldosteronism, essential hypertension, edema (heart failure, nephrosis, or cirrhosis), and hypokalemia. For more details see the chapter devoted to antihypertensive drugs.

Spironolactone, 25 mg scored tablets.

Phenoxybenzamine (Dibenzyline)

This drug was reviewed in the chapter on antihypertensive drugs. It opposes the actions of both nor- and straight epinephrine, for which reason it is advised for the treatment of pheochromocytoma and for some other diseases with vasopastic reactions. For more details, see the mentioned review.

Phenoxybenzamine, 10 mg capsules.

XXVIII. ANTIANEMICS

Iron

In treating the anemias, the amount of iron in the regular diet cannot cope with the deficiency in iron reserves encountered. Supplementary iron is necessary, and no special contraindications have to be considered. However, do not administer iron with the tetracyclines, and remember that gastrointestinal reactions such as cramps, loose stools, or constipation may occur when it is given by mouth. Massive infusions by parenteral administration may cause symptoms resembling hemochromatosis, and, of course, injected substances can be locally irritant.

Ferrous sulfate (usually prescribed by name, but also known under brand names such as Feosol, Fer-in-sol, Fernalox, Mol-iron, and others) is given in daily amounts of about 200 mg, in either tablets, elixir, or capsules of the slow-release variety. In cases of severe anemia, larger doses may be given, such as 400 mg, if tolerated.

Ferrous sulfate, 200 mg tablets. (Other forms are also available.)

Ferrous fumarate (Ircon, Ferro-Sequels, Feostat, Fumaral) is given at a daily dosage of about 300 mg, or more if tolerated.

Ferrous fumarate, 300 mg tablets.

Ferrous gluconate (Fergon, Simron) is claimed by manufacturers to be better utilized and tolerated than other iron salts. It can be given in doses of about 400 mg (yielding about 50 mg of elemental iron, as compared with the sulfate, which yields some 22 mg for each 100 mg, but which is not so well tolerated).

Ferrous gluconate, 300 mg tablets or 400 mg capsules.

Ferrous polysaccharide (Hytinic, Niferex, Nu-iron) is provided in capsules releasing 150 mg of elemental iron; also in syrup form.

Ferrous polysaccharide, 150 mg capsules.

Ferric hydroxide in a dextran base (Imferon) is given solely by intramuscular injection (intravenously only if the muscle is not a suitable site for absorption). It should not be given if there is liver impairment. There is a risk of carcinogenesis. The proper dosage is to be calculated from a formula or checked in a special table. It is presented in 2-, 5-, and 10-ml containers (ampoules or vials).

Vitamins

Vitamins B_{12}, folic acid, pyridoxin, and riboflavin are used for the treatment of anemias, but these products will be dealt with in a special chapter devoted to vitamins.

Liver Extract

Actually, vitamin B_{12} is the active component of liver extract, its potency measured in terms of its cyanocobalamin content. It is indicated in the treatment of macrocytic anemias, particularly pernicious anemia.

There are no real contraindications to the use of liver extract, but at times allergic reactions—possibly severe ones—may occur, and also local disturbances may follow injection.

Dosage: The equivalent of 10 μg of cyanocobalamin is injected intramuscularly daily for 3 days, thereafter once every 10 days, until normal blood values are restored.

Liver extract, equivalent to 10 or 20 μg of cyanocobalamin for each ml, in 10- or 30-ml vials.

XXIX. ANTIHISTAMINICS

Since antihistaminics interfere with the action of histamine upon cells, these drugs are intended for the treatment of many allergic conditions, such as seasonal hay fever, nasal allergies, asthmatic coughing, serum sickness, urticaria, angioneurotic edema, and drug reactions—particularly those due to antibiotics and sulfas. Other uses are for atopic and contact dermatitis, insect bites, and the itching accompanying most of these situations; also allergic conjunctivitis, dermographism, and motion sickness. And they have helped the movements of parkinsonism and drug-induced extrapyramidal reactions when given to older people who cannot tolerate other drugs.

Contraindications are very few: particularly included is a specific reaction against the given antihistamine, extending to others in the same structural group. A different antihistaminic may be tolerated in these instances. This holds true also for the side effects, which may vary from patient to patient and from drug to drug. Do not use antihistaminics for the treatment of asthma or other clinical reactions involving the lower respiratory tract, or when MAOI or depressants are in use. Watch for untoward reactions when they are given to patients with glaucoma (narrow angle), peptic ulcer, duodenal obstruction, hypertension, or hyperthyroidism. Watch very carefully for dizziness, sedation, reactional hypotension, prostatic hypertrophy, and bladder neck obstruction, especially among the elderly. Check for agranulocytosis, anemia, arrhythmias, confusion, restlessness, or urinary difficulties.

Diphenylhydramine

Brand names: Benadryl, Dramamine, SK-Diphenhydramine. Indications, contraindications, and precautions are as stated above. Dosage: It is effective in about 1 hour, lasting up to 6 hours. The regular dose is 50 mg three or four times a day. If it is prescribed for motion sickness, start some 30 minutes prior to exposure.

Diphenylhydramine, 25 or 50 mg capsules.

Diphenylhydramine, elixir containing 12.5 mg in each 5 ml.

Diphenylhydramine, injectables containing 10 mg in each ml in 5-, 10-, or 30-ml vials; and 50 mg in each ml, in 1-ml ampoules or 10-ml vials.

Diphenylhydramine, 50 mg scored tablets.

Diphenylhydramine, suppositories containing 100 mg.

Diphenylpyraline

Brand names: Hispril, Diafen. Indications, contraindications, and precautions are as above. Dosage: one capsule every 12 hours; tablets, accordingly to dose.

Diphenylpyraline, 5 mg capsules, slow-release.

Diphenylpyraline, 2 mg scored tablets.

Tripelennamine

Brand names: Pyribenzamine, PBZ-SR. Indications, contraindications, and precautions are as above. Dosage: The regular dosage is 25 or 50 mg every 4 to 6 hours; at times a double dose is used, but it is not advised for the elderly. Slow-release preparations will be given every 12 hours.

Tripelennamine, 25 or 50 mg scored tablets.

Tripelennamine, 50 or 100 mg slow-release tablets.

Tripelennamine, elixir containing 37.5 mg in 5 ml.

Tripelennamine, 2% ointment or 2% cream, for local application for the relief of itching.

Metapyrilene

Brand names: Histadyl, Thenylpyramine. Indications, contraindications, and precautions are as above.

Dosage: 25 to 50 mg by mouth every 4 hours; elderly patients should not have the highest allowed maximum of 100 mg four times a day. By intravenous injection, no more than 10 or 20 mg to start, a dose that could be increased, if tolerated, to 40 mg. Always inject slowly. Intravenous drip in 250 ml of saline will reduce the side effects. Intramuscularly or subcutaneously, amounts to 20 or even 40 mg may be given, every 4 to 6 hours.

Metapyrilene, 25 or 50 mg capsules.

Metapyrilene, injectibles containing 20 mg in each ml, in 1-ml ampoules or 10-ml vials.

Pyrilamine

This antihistaminic is mainly used in mixed formulas of different kinds.

Chlorpheniramine

Brand names: Histaspan, Chlor-trimeton, Teldrin. In general, indications, contraindications, and precautions are the same as for most other antihistaminic drugs.

Dosage: 4 mg every 4 to 6 hours is the regular amount, or 8 to 12 mg of the long-acting preparation every 12 hours; by injection, no more than 40 mg will be given in a 24-hour period, 10 to 20 mg as a single dose. Do not use the intravenous route.

Chlorpheniramine, 4 mg tablets.

Chlorpheniramine, 8 or 12 mg slow-release capsules.

Chlorpheniramine, syrup containing 2 mg in 5 ml.

Chlorpheniramine, injectables containing 10 mg in 1-ml ampoules, or 100 mg in 2-ml vials.

Carbinoxamine

Brand names: Clistin. Indications, contraindications, and precautions are as above. Dosage: 4 mg three or four times a day; up to 8 mg per dose, if needed and tolerated.

Carbinoxamine, 4 mg tablets.

Tripolidine

Brand name: Actidil. Uses and precautions are as above. Dosage: 2.5 mg every 8 or 12 hours.

Tripolidine, 2.5 mg scored tablets.

Tripolidine, syrup containing 2.5 mg in 5 ml.

Dexchlorpheniramine

Brand names: Polaramine, Dextro Chlorpheniramine. Uses and warnings are essentially the same as above. Dosage: 1 or 2 mg repeated three or four times a day is the average dosage; or the long-acting tablets every 12 hours (the 6-mg dose only for resistant and tolerant cases).

Dexchlorpheniramine, 2 mg scored tablets.

Dexchlorpheniramine, 4 or 6 mg long-acting tablets.

Dexchlorpheniramine, syrup containing 2 mg in each 5 ml.

Brompheniramine

Brand names: Dimetane, Parabromdylamine maleate. Brompheniramine is used like other regular antihistaminics, but the injectable is particularly promoted for allergic reactions to infusions of blood or plasma.

Dosage: Give 4 or 8 mg three or four times a day; or the long-acting preparations, one every 12 hours. By injection, give from 5 to 20 mg (average, 10 mg) once or twice a day, with a maximum of 40 mg in 24 hours. Individualize dosage.

Brompheniramine, 4 mg scored tablets.

Brompheniramine, 8 or 12 mg long-acting tablets.

Brompheniramine, elixir containing 2 mg in 5 ml.

Dexbrompheniramine

Brand name: Disomer, Dextro Brompheniramine maleate. Uses and precautions are as above. Dosage: Give 6 mg in long-acting preparations twice a day.

Dexbrompheniramine, 6 mg long-acting tablets.

Dimethindene

Brand names: Forhistal, Triten, Dimethpyrindene maleate. The usual indications and warnings are as for other antihistaminics. Dosage: Give 1 or 2 mg from one to three times a day; but always try to individualize administration.

Dimethindene, 1 mg scored tablets.

Cyproheptadine

Brand name: Periactin. There are the usual indications and precautions, as stated above. Dosage: Individual dosage can be estimated to be 0.5 mg for each kilo of body weight in 24 hours. Most people will receive from 4 to 20 mg per day (starting with 4 mg three times a day).

Cyproheptadine, 4 mg scored tablets.

Cyproheptadine, syrup containing 2 mg in 5 ml.

Methdilazine

Brand name: Tacaryl. This drug is indicated particularly for the relief of urticarial pruritis. Contraindications and warnings are as for other antihistaminics. Dosage: 8 mg two to four times a day.

Methdilazine, 8 mg scored tablets.

Methdilazine, chewable 4 mg tablets.

Methdilazine, syrup containing 4 mg in 5 ml.

Promethazine

Brand names: Phenergan, Zipan. Indications and warnings are as above.
  Dosage: For allergic reactions give 25 mg at bedtime, or half this amount before meals and at bedtime; then adjust doses. For motion sickness, give 25 mg twice a day. For nausea and vomiting give 25 mg or less by injection or suppositories. For sedation smaller doses will suffice.

Promethazine, 12.5, 25, or 50 mg scored tablets.

Promethazine, syrup containing 6.25 mg in 5 ml, or 25 mg in 5 ml.

Promethazine, suppositories containing 12.5, 25, or 50 mg.

XXX. DERMATOLOGICALS

Protectants, Emollients, Demulcents

Most of the components of this group are only vehicles for the principal medications they carry, although a few may be used alone on account of their actions—emollient, protectant, or demulcent. The following are the main preparations.
  Petrolatum U.S.P. Both emollient and protective, it is presented in the form of liquid petrolatum, or a less viscous light liquid petrolatum. There is also a white petrolatum which will not take up water.

Liquid petrolatum.

Light liquid petrolatum.

Yellow ointment or *white ointment U.S.P.* are similar in use to petrolatum, but are generally preferred to the latter because of a slightly better absorption of water. Any of them may be used as a dressing for blisters or superficial ulcers. Both ointments are made with petrolatum and wax.

Yellow ointment.

White ointment.

Lanolin lotion is recommended as an emollient; it is also a frequently used vehicle for medications.

Lanolin lotion.

Lanolin (wool fat) is used mainly for mixtures, but may also be applied directly to the skin.

Lanolin, plain or anhydrous.

Calamine is used in the form of liniment, ointment, or lotion. It is emollient and protective. The alcoholic calamine lotion is soothing and protective and may also be used as a drying agent.

Calamine lotion.

Calamine alcoholic lotion.

Calamine ointment.

Calamine liniment.

Glycerin (Cornhusker's) lotion is also soothing and a help for dry skin.

Glycerin lotion (Cornhusker's lotion).

Wintergreen oil (methyl salicylate) is used topically in the form of liniment or ointment in cases of lumbago, rheumatic conditions, neuritis, and other painful states. Do not apply it to burned areas or to extensive ulcerated surfaces. Use it in 10 to 25% concentrations.

Wintergreen oil ointment.

Wintergreen oil liniment.

Zinc oxide and talc lotions are useful for mixing substances and as cooling and drying agents; the alcoholic lotion is apparently more active.

Zinc oxide and talc, alcoholic lotion.

Zinc oxide and talc, aqueous lotion.

Collodion is rarely used at the present time for protection, particularly of minor wounds.

Collodion, plain or flexible.

Acetic acid and sodium acetate are to be used as an ointment instead of the well-known boric acid.

Acetic acid and sodium acetate, ointment.

Paraaminobenzoic acid (*PABA*) is a good protectant for skin areas to be exposed to sunlight.

PABA, 10% ointment.

PABA, 10% solution in 70% alcohol.

Silicone (Dimethicone) in 20 or 30% ointment is protective against water and corrosive chemicals, for the treatment of dermatitis due to soap or water, decubitus ulcers, or surgical procedures (colostomy). Apply two or three times a day to clean, dry skin.

Silicone, 20 or 30% ointment.

Titanium dioxide in lotion or ointment is also a good protective against sunlight.

Titanium dioxide, lotion.

Titanium dioxide, ointment.

Oatmeal is prescribed for pruritus in most sorts of dermal reactions. The powder is mixed with tapwater (1 cup in 2 cups of water); or it may be used as an ointment for dermal reactions.

Oatmeal powder; or oatmeal ointment.

Starch is used like oatmeal, similarly prepared and prescribed for the same conditions.

Starch.

Anti-inflammatory Agents

Treating the cause of inflammation involves the care of inflammation itself. But not rarely there is a need for symptomatic agents, such as enzymes and corticoids.

Fibrinolysin and *desoxyribonuclease* (brand name: Elase) are prescribed in a mixture of both enzymes. Fibrinolysin liquifies fibrin, and thus destroys blood clots. Desoxyribonuclease acts upon desoxyribonucleic acid, thus reducing the extent of the polynucleotic chains to limits that make them more diffusible. Together they are used as debriding agents for wounds, ulcers, burns, abscesses, or fistulas.

Fibrinolysin and desoxyribonuclease, solution containing 0.83 unit of the first and 500 units of the second in each ml, in 30-ml containers.

Fibrinolysin and desoxyribonuclease, ointment containing 1 unit and 666.6 units respectively in each g, in 10- or 30-g containers.

Hyaluronidase (brand names: Alidase, Diffusin, Hyazyme, Wydase). Its main use is to promote better and more speedy absorption of subcutaneously injected drugs, for instance, penicillin.

Hyaluronidase, 150 units in each ml, in vials containing 1 or 10 ml.

Streptokinase and *streptodornase* (brand name: Varidase, a combination of both) are employed together in the removal of clotted blood and other accumulations of fibrinous or purulent material from injuries or inflammation. The local activity of this combination is very rapid, and it does not work on living cells; the only drawback is that it is antigenic. It may be used in empyema, osteomyelitis, infected sinuses, thrombophlebitis, abscesses, and cellulitis. It is administered by topical application, intramuscular injection, or oral administration. Do not use it on bleeding sites.

Streptokinase-streptodornase, for topical use, in a 125,000 unit vial of 15 ml.

Streptokinase-streptodornase, for intramuscular injection, 25,000 unit vial.

Streptokinase-streptodornase, 10,000 unit tablets, to take four a day for 4 to 6 days.

Trypsin (brand names: Parenzyme, Tryptar). Its use is essentially the same as for streptokinase-streptodornase, q.v.

Trypsin, 25 mg in a vial; also, vials containing 50,000, 125,000, and 250,000 units.

Trypsin, suspension containing 25 mg in each 5 ml.

Trypsin, 5 mg tablets.

Chymotrypsin (brand names: Chymoral, Avazyme, Orenzyme) is used in the same way as trypsin and streptokinase-streptodornase, q.v. These drugs are also marketed in a combined form in tablets.

Chymotrypsin tablets, containing 50,000 units.

Corticoids

Corticoids possess a powerful anti-inflammatory activity, which is helpful in many infectious diseases, including skin inflammatory reactions. For their systemic effects the reader is referred to the chapter on hormones. They will act symptomatically, but are not curative in the great majority of instances, particularly in reference to dermatoses. The conditions that react when corticoids are applied locally, and then are reactive according to the concentration reached in the skin, are as follows: the eczematous group, in the first place; atopic dermatitis, seborrhea, neurodermatitis, anogenital pruritus, and other similar skin conditions. Keep in mind that the following conditions will *not* respond to topical corticoids: urticaria, pemphigus, collagen diseases, psoriasis (occlusive application), and lichens, either planus or simplex. But many of these conditions will react to intralesional injections.

Very few persons will become sensitized to topically applied corticoids; but remember that on infected lesions it is better not to use corticoids. They are positively contraindicated in cases of herpes simplex (particularly if the ocular area is involved), varicella, vaccinia, and tuberculosis of the skin.

Apply these agents in thin films over the affected skin, using either lotions, ointments, creams, or aerosols.

Hydrocortisone (brand names: Cortef, Hydrocortone, Cortril, Cort-Dome, Cortifan, and others) may be significantly absorbed if applied to the genitourinary tract; thus, do not use the medication for more than a week. Use concentrations of 0.5% to no more than 2.5%; and when this higher amount is used, decrease the concentration to about 1% as soon as possible.

Hydrocortisone, lotion; 0.125, 0.25, 0.5, 1, 2, or 2.5%.

Hydrocortisone, ointment; 0.25, 0.5, 1, or 2.5%.

Hydrocortisone, cream; 0.125, 0.25, 0.5, 1, or 2%.

Hydrocortisone, aerosol, 0.5%.

Prednisolone (brand names: Meti-derm, Metimyd, Optimyd) at a concentration of 0.5% is applied locally one to four times a day. The aerosol form is far less concentrated and is suitable for extended lesions.

Prednisolone, lotion, 0.5%.

Prednisolone, ointment, 0.5%.

Prednisolone, cream, 0.5%.

Prednisolone, aerosol, 0.033%.

Methylprednisolone (brand name: Medrol) is used similarly, but at lower concentrations.

Methylprednisolone, ointment, 0.25 or 1%.

Fludrocortisone (brand names: F-Cortef, Florinef, Alflorine) is used in still smaller concentrations than the above agents.

Fludrocortisone, lotion, 0.1%.

Fludrocortisone, ointment, 0.1%.

Fluocinolone (brand names: Fluonid, Synalar, Synemol) is very active and should not be given at high concentrations.

Fluocinolone, ointment, 0.025%.

Fluocinolone, cream, 0.01 or 0.025%.

Flurandrenolone or fluandrenolide (brand name: Cordran) is also one of the very active topical corticoids.

Flurandrenolone, ointment, 0.05%.

Flurandrenolone, cream, 0.05%.

Flurandrenolone, tape (to be applied to a clean, dry skin for periods of 12 hours).

Dexamethasone (brand names: Decadron, Aeroseb-Ex) is presented in the form of a cream or an aerosol.

Dexamethasone, cream, 0.1%.

Dexamethasone, aerosol, 0.011%.

Fluorometholone (brand name: Oxylone) is marketed as a cream.

Fluorometholone, cream, 0.025%.

Triamcinolone (brand names: Arsitocort, Kenalog, Tramacin) is to be applied in small amounts two, three, or four times a day.

Triamcinolone, lotion, 0.1%.

Triamcinolone, ointment, 0.1%.

Triamcinolone, cream, 0.1 or 0.5%.

Triamcinolone, aerosol, 0.007%.

Triamcinolone, foam, 0.1%.

Sulfa Drugs and Antibiotics Used Locally

For general information, please refer to the chapters on sulfonamides and antibiotics.

Sulfisoxazole (brand name: Gantrisin) is indicated for conjunctivitis, corneal ulcer, or any other superficial infection of the eye; and for adjunct therapy in the treatment of trachoma, as presented in the form of ophthalmic ointment or solution. A cream is used for *Haemophilus vaginalis* vaginitis.

Sulfisoxazole, ophthalmic ointment, 4%.

Sulfisoxazole, ophthalmic solution, 4%.

Sulfisoxazole, cream, 10%.

Triple sulfa cream (brand name: Sultrin) is mainly prescribed for *Haemophilus vaginalis* vaginitis.

Triple sulfa cream (containing sulfathiazole, sulfacetamide, and sulfabenzamide).

Mafenide (brand name: Sulfamylon) is presented as a cream mainly advised for second and third degree burns, as an adjunct therapy.

Mafenide, cream, 8.5%.

Other sulfonamides, but mostly several of the above-mentioned ones, are presented in different mixtures aimed for local use. The list is extensive, and the secondary helpers are manifold.

Tetracycline (brand names: Achromycin, Steclin, Tetracyn, Panmycin, Polycycline) is mainly recommended for impetigo, infected ulcers, sycoses barbae, or any other susceptible infection of the skin. Apply locally two or three times every day to clean, dry skin.

Tetracycline, ointment, 3%.

Tetracycline, solution, 0.1 or 0.5%.

Oxytetracycline (brand name: Terramycin) is used like tetracycline, above.

Oxytetracycline, solution, 0.1 or 0.5%.

Chlortetracycline (brand name: Aureomycin) responds to the same indications as other tetracyclines.

Chlortetracycline, ointment, 3%.

Chlortetracycline, solution, 0.1 or 0.5%.

Chlortetracycline, ophthalmic ointment, 1%.

Chloramphenicol (brand name: Chloromycetin) is recommended for almost all susceptible skin infections. Apply locally three or four times a day, on clean, dry skin.

Chloramphenicol, ointment, 1%.

Chloramphenicol, cream, 1%.

Chloramphenicol, ophthalmic ointment, 1%.

Chloramphenicol, otic solution, 0.5%.

Bacitracin is used in many different mixtures; and should be preferred to other antibiotics because very rarely is it used systemically.

Bacitracin, ointment with 500 units per g.

Bacitracin, solution, with 250, 500, or 1000 units per ml.

Erythromycin (brand names: Erythrocin, Ilotycin) is applied on clean, dry skin, two or three times a day, for the skin infections due to susceptible germs.

Erythromycin, ointment, 1%.

Erythromycin, ophthalmic ointment, 0.5%.

Neomycin seems to be effective in superficial infections due to *K. pneumoniae* and *H. influenzae,* as well as *Pseudomonas* and *Proteus.* For trophic ulcers solutions are preferred. Apply locally two or three times a day. Neomycin is very frequently incorporated into complex formulas, of which there are a large number.

Neomycin, solution for topical use, 0.5%.

Neomycin, lotion, 0.5%.

Neomycin, ointment, 0.5%.

Polymyxin B (brand name: Aerosporin) is used for gram-negative organisms, but seems to be particularly effective against *P. seruginosa.*

Polymyxin B ointment, 20,000 units per g.

Polymyxin B solution, 10,000 or 20,000 units per ml.

Fungicides

This subject has been duly treated in chapter VI, devoted to antifungals, q.v.

Nystatin (brand name: Mycostatin) is mainly antifungal and effective against *Candida albicans* infections, for which it is particularly prescribed.

Nystatin, ointment, 100,000 units in each g.

Nystatin, dusting powder, 100,000 units per g.

Nystatin, cream, 100,000 units per g.

When given by mouth, it is presented as a suspension or tablet, to administer from 400,000 to 600,000 units (oral suspension) or 500,000 to 1,000,000 units (tablets), to a total of about 1,500,000 to 2,000,000 units a day.

Nystatin, 500,000 or 1,000,000 units per tablet.

Nystatin, oral suspension, 100,000 units in each ml.

Griseofulvin (brand names: Fulvicin U/F, Grisactin, Gris-Peg, Grifulvin V) is not intended for *C. albicans* infections, but for ringworm infections of the nails, the hair, and the skin, that is, tinea caused by different *Trichophyton* species, *Microsporum,* and *Epidermophyton.* Care will be taken with patients with liver dysfunction, porphyria, or allergic reactions to the drug. A dose of 500 mg a day, in one or two installments, will be satisfactory except in cases with infected feet or nails, which may need 500 mg given twice a day. Individualize the dosage.

Griseofulvin, 125, 250, or 500 mg tablets.

Griseofulvin, 125, 250, or 500 mg capsules.

Cupric sulfate is employed as a wet soak against fungal infections.

Copper sulfate, solution (1:4000 to 1:1000 concentration).

Gentian violet or methylrosaniline chloride is effective against yeasts, molds, and *C. albicans,* as well as other skin infections.

Gentian violet, solution (1 to 3% concentration) to be applied with a cotton swab twice a day.

Sodium hyposulfite or sodium thiosulfate is recommended for ringworm infections as well as tinea versicolor. The 25% solution is applied topically twice a day, for 2 or 3 months.

Sodium hyposulfite, 25% solution.

Zincundecate (undecylenic acid and zinc undecylenate) is applied twice a day on a clean dry skin for the treatment of tinea, tinea versicolor, *C. albicans* infections, dermatomycosis, and epidermophytosis in general.

Zincundecate, ointment.

Zincundecate, powder.

Ectoparasiticides

Gamma benzene hexachloride (brand names: Lindane, Kwell, Gexane) is a very effective scabicide and pediculicide, which works mostly after a single application. At times, more applications are needed for a complete cure. Do not allow it to come close to the eyes or other mucosae. If it is applied to the head, wear a towel over it for about 1 hour; and do not wash or bathe the treated parts until after 24 hours. If a second application is needed, wait at least a week. Use no more than 30 ml.

Gamma benzene hexachloride, 1% lotion.

Gamma benzene hexachloride, 1% ointment.

Copper oleate is recommended for the treatment of pediculosis, by rubbing onto the affected area 3 or 4 tablespoonfuls of the solution, or the adequate amount to the extent of the infected surface. Allow it to remain for 15 minutes, and then wash the area thoroughly with soap and water. Do not use it on irritated areas, or use it again in less than 2 days.

Copper oleate, solution.

DDT (dichlorodiphenyltrichloroethane) is extremely active against lice and bedbugs; but it is a toxic substance to be used with care. Use it in powder form for the body, and a kerosene solution for furniture. (Banned in the U.S.)

DDT, powder, 10% concentration, in talc.

DDT, 10% solution.

Crotamiton (brand name: Eurax) is antipruritic and also useful for the prevention and treatment of scabies. For the latter purpose it is massaged into the skin of the entire body, except for the face. Attention is paid to the particular sites lodging the parasite. Repeat the application after 24 hours. Finally, take a bath 48 or 72 hours after the second treatment. Change the entire clothing, personal and bed.

Crotamiton, 10% lotion.

Crotamiton, 10% ointment.

Local Anesthetics and Antipruritics

Local anesthetics have been dealt with in chapter XI, on local anesthetics, q.v. for more information.

Vinegar and water is a mixture easy to prepare at home with an acceptable antipruritic effect, but with the drawback of its bad odor. Small amounts spread over the itching area may soothe the discomfort for a little while.

Cyproheptadine (brand name: Periactin) seems effective, in addition to its antihistaminic properties, in the relief of itching due to urticaria, insect bites, drug reaction, allergic dermatoses, contact dermatitis, and chicken pox. Do not use it when antihistaminics are contraindicated or if warned against their use. Dosage should be individualized, usually between 4 and 20 mg in 24 hours (0.23 mg for each kilo of body weight in 24 hours).

Cyproheptadine, 4 mg scored tablets.

Cyproheptadine, syrup, 2 mg in 5 ml.

Dibucaine lotion (0.5% concentration) is mainly recommended for the relief of itching. The ointment is used for superficial anesthesia.

Dibucaine, lotion, 0.5%.

Camphor is used alone or in combination with phenol or menthol for the relief of itching.

Camphor, liniment in oil.

Camphor in water, or camphor in alcohol.

Trimeprazine (brand name: Temaril) is given orally for the relief of itching due to neurodermatitis, atopic dermatitis, contact dermatitis, lichenified lesions, drug eruptions, tinea, insect bites, diabetes, leukemia, Hodgkin's disease, jaundice, and other sources of itching. Contraindications and warnings are about the same as for most tranquilizers, q.v. Dosage must be less than 80 mg in 24 hours (in severe cases, if tolerated) in doses of 2.5 to 5 mg during the day, and 5 to 10 mg at bedtime. Give elderly persons the lowest possible amount.

Trimeprazine, 2.5 mg tablets.

Trimeprazine, 5 mg long-acting tablets.

Trimeprazine, syrup containing 2.5 mg in 5 ml.

Astringents and Keratolytics

Acetic acid lotion also called back lotion, is used for the prevention of bed sores by toughening the skin. Apply once a day.

Acetic acid, lotion.

Burow's solution and ointment, an aluminum acetate preparation, is recommended as a topical astringent for the control of acute and subacute inflammatory conditions of the skin. The ointment, also emollient and mildly antiseptic, is employed in dermatologic ulcerative conditions. The solution is usually diluted with 10 to 40 parts of water. Apply to the affected areas several times a day.

Burow's solution.

Burow's ointment.

Salicylic acid, which is keratolytic and germicidal, is prescribed for hyperkeratosis of palms and soles, for removal of warts and calluses, and against some parasitic diseases. Use 1 to 3% concentrations in petrolatum or other preferred base, in senile, dry skin; as a dusting powder it is used against fungi, particularly on the feet.

Salicylic acid, 1 to 3% in petrolatum.

Anthralin is preferred to crysarobin for the treatment of psoriasis, chronic eczema, chronic dermatomycoses, and other chronic dermatoses. Since it is irritant, its use must be carefully checked, especially if used on the face (which it is better to avoid). Start treatment with lower concentrations, and increase to tolerance.

Anthralin, ointment, 1%.

Podophyllum resin may remove venereal warts (condyloma acuminatum) when locally applied while the adjacent skin is carefully protected from its action with petrolatum or collodion. It is applied and covered with a bandage for 12 to 24 hours, and then carefully washed.

Podophyllum resin, ointment, 1%.

Podophyllum, tincture, 25%.

Trichloroacetic acid is of help in the treatment of warts (flat), acne scars, lupus erythematosus, and lichenified lesions, and in the removal of xanthomatosis in the skin. It is also recommended for tinea versicolor, molluscum contagiosum, and chloasma. Use 20% concentrations for superficial lesions, and stronger ones—to 50%—for the removal of other lesions.

Resorcinol, either alone or in mixtures with sulfur, zinc oxide, salicylic acid, or other ingredients, is used in cases of acute and chronic eczematous reactions, acne, seborrhea, psoriasis, sycosis vulgaris, and other inflammatory diseases of the skin. A 5% lotion is applied with cotton two or three times a day, for acne and seborrhea; a 1 or 2% solution in 70% alcohol solution, for urticaria, acute eczema, and similar inflammations of the skin.

Resorcinol, lotion, 5%.

Resorcinol, alcoholic solution, 1 or 2%.

Coal tar has some use in the treatment of eczematous dermatitis of different varieties, psoriasis, and other similar diseases. Its use must be watched carefully because it is an irritant drug.

Coal tar, ointment, 1 to 5%.

Coal tar, solution, 2 to 5%.

Ichthammol (brand name: Ichthyol) is recommended for subacute exudative conditions and subacute eczema. Watch for staining of clothes.

Ichthammol, ointment, 10%.

Ichthammol, paste, 5%.

XXXI. GASTROINTESTINAL MEDICATIONS

Laxatives and Cathartics

Milk of magnesia, better called magnesia magma, is a suspension of magnesium dioxide to be used as an antacid or a laxative, depending on the dose given. As an antacid, give 1 or 2 teaspoonfuls; as a laxative, 1 or 2 tablespoonfuls. Do not use it if appendicitis is suspected.

Milk of magnesia.

Castor oil (brand name: Neoloid), also called oleum ricini, is given when a rapid and complete intestinal evacuation is needed. The taste is unpleasant, for which reason aromatic preparations are available as well as emulsions. Dosage ranges from 15 to 60 ml. Try to use the smallest working dose when giving it to the elderly. Do not use it if appendicitis or similar problems are suspected.

Castor oil, liquid or capsules, the latter containing 0.6, 1, 1.25, 2.5, or 5 ml.

Aromatic castor oil.

Castor oil emulsion, 30 or 50% concentration (36.4% for Neoloid).

Cascara sagrada is somewhat slower than castor oil to cause bowel movements, for which reason it is preferable for habitual constipation. Dosage: 300 mg taken at bedtime in tablet form, equivalent to 1 ml of the fluidextract; find the suitable dose for each individual.

Cascara, 120, 200, or 300 mg tablets.

Cascara sagrada, fluidextract.

Glycerin suppositories are to be inserted rectally for occasional relief of constipation; habitual use usually causes local irritation.

Glycerin suppositories for adults.

Liquid petrolatum or mineral oil helps in cases of constipation by keeping the feces well-lubricated; but its continuous use is not to be encouraged because of interference with bile or vitamin absorption. Dosage: 1 or 2 tablespoonfuls at bedtime.

Liquid petrolatum.

Bran, the meal obtained from the covering of cereals, is rich in cellulose, which may enhance bowel movements and alleviate constipation. It is one of the more popular remedies used in the United States for this purpose. There are several brands on the market.

Psyllium hydrophilic mucilloid (brand name: Metamucil), the powdered mucillaginous portion of psyllium seeds, is also helpful in relieving constipation, when thoroughly mixed with water at dosages ranging from 4 to 7 g (a little less than 1 or a little more than 2 teaspoonfuls). Dependency may occur.

Psyllium hydrophilic mucilloid, powder.

Magnesium sulfate, popularly known as Epsom salt, in addition to its internal administration for the relief of convulsions or its local application for inflammatory reactions, is also employed as a purgative when rapid action is needed (1 to 2 hours). For this purpose 15 g (1 tablespoonful—not heaped) is given in a glassful of iced water.

Magnesium sulfate.

Bisacodyl (brand names: Dulcolax, Fleet bisacodyl, Fleet bisacodyl enema, Bon-O-Lax; sold also by the generic name) is given either by mouth or rectally (suppositories, enemas) for the treatment of constipation. Dosage: 10 mg at bedtime (but not within 1 hour after taking milk or antacids); the suppositories will act in about 15 minutes.

Bisacodyl, 5 mg tablets.

Bisacodyl, suppositories, 10 mg.

Bisacodyl, enema containing 10 mg.

Dioctyl, either sodium or calcium salt (brand names: Colace, Doxinate, Surfak, Bu-lax, Comfolax, and others, as well as generic-name preparations) only softens feces without any stimulation to the rectal musculature. Dosage: 200 to 400 mg or more a day, preferably in divided doses; individual adjustment will be carried out.

Dioctyl, 50, 60, 100, 240, or 250 mg capsules.

Dioctyl, liquid, 10 mg in each ml.

Dioctyl, solution, 5 mg in each ml.

Dioctyl, syrup, 20 mg in 5 ml.

Antidiarrheals

Most parasympatholytic drugs (see chapter XVIII) are capable of diminishing peristaltic activity, particularly *belladonna* and *atropine,* but others as well. The reader is referred to that section for more information.

Also opium derivatives, such as *paregoric, laudanum,* and similar medications, will show a similar activity; see chapter X, on analgesics and antipyretics.

Attapulgite, particularly in its activated form (brand names: Claysorb, Pharmasorb), is given for symptomatic treatment of diarrhea, acting as an intestinal absorbent. Start dosage of the aqueous suspension with 4 g, to be continued with 2 g after each bowel movement until control of the symptom.

Activated attapulgite is usually presented together with pectin, providing 500 or 600 mg of the former in each 5 ml.

Kaolin has an activity similar to that of attapulgite, q.v. above. Dosages of about 5 g (1 teaspoonful) can be given several times a day.

Kaolin powder.

Charcoal, also activated, has an activity similar to that of the two above medications. Dosage ranges from 4 to 8 g, once or twice a day.

Charcoal, 300 mg tablets.

Charcoal, powder.

Antiemetics

Cyclizine (brand name: Marezine) has antiemetic properties but is mainly recommended when vomiting is due to motion sickness or drug induction. It is also given for the symptomatic relief of vertigo due to vestibular disease until true corrective treatment is started. Dosage: about 50 mg before meals, three or four times a day.

Cyclizine, 50 mg tablets.

Cyclizine, suppositories, 50 or 100 mg.

Cyclizine, injectable, 50 mg in 1-ml ampoules.

Dimenhydrinate (brand names: Dramamine, Meni-D; sold also by generic name) may also be used as an antiemetic, but the main use is for motion sickness and other similar situations, as described above, q.v. Dosage: For prevention give 50, 75, or 100 mg half an hour before departure and repeat before meals and at bedtime; for suppression, give 25, 50, or more mg, also before meals. When injections are needed, dilute the medication.

Dimenhydrinate, 50 mg scored tablets.

Dimenhydrinate, suppositories, 100 mg.

Dimenhydrinate, injectable, 50 mg in each 1-ml ampoule.

Dimenhydrinate, liquid, 15.6 mg in each 5 ml.

Meclizine (brand names: Antivert, Bonine; sold also by the generic name) has the same indications as the above medications, q.v. Dosage: a once-a-day dose of 25 to 50 mg will control most situations.

Meclizine, 25 mg tablets.

Meclizine, elixir, 12.5 mg in each 5 ml.

Meclizine, injectable, 25 mg in each 1-ml ampoule (together with pyridoxine).

Trimethobenzamide (brand name: Tigan) has an antiemetic activity similar to that of the phenothiazides. It is not too potent, but has very few side effects. The drug is given for nauseating conditions, with or without vomiting, caused by motion, drugs, radiation, or infection. Dosage: by mouth, 100 to 250 mg as many times as needed and tolerated, effects starting in about 15 or 30 minutes and lasting for no less than 2 hours; rectally, 200 mg will suffice, intramuscular injections of 200 mg are given four or more times a day, as needed and tolerated.

Trimethobenzamide, 100 or 250 mg capsules.

Trimethobenzamide, suppositories, 200 mg.

Trimethobenzamide injectable, 100 mg in each ml, in 2-ml ampoules and 10-ml vials.

Emetics

Apomorphine causes emesis 10 or 15 minutes after a subcutaneous injection of 5 or 10 mg. Do not use it in cases of shock or depression induced by drugs. Do not give a second injection if the first fails.

Apomorphine, for subcutaneous injection, 6 mg.

Ipecacuanha, more commonly called ipecac, requires from 30 to 60 minutes to cause emesis after its ingestion. It is also given as an expectorant. Dosage: For emesis give 8 to 15 ml of the syrup (low amounts for the debilitated) or 0.5 to 1 ml of the fluidextract; for expectoration, 1 or 2 ml of the syrup or 0.06 to 0.12 ml of the fluidextract.

Ipecac, syrup.

Ipecac, fluidextract.

Digestants

Hydrochloric acid helps discomfort and gastric inefficiency in cases of anachlorhydria and hypochlorhydria. The diluted solution contains 10% of the acid, but it must be further diluted by putting 2 to 8 ml in 25 to 50 times its volume of water, to be sipped during meals. Hydrochloric acid is also derived from glutamic acid hydrochloride (brand name: Acidulin) or from dehydrocholic acid (brand names: Decholin, Procholon).

Hydrochloric acid, 10% diluted.

Ox bile extract substitutes for natural bile when there is a dimunition of the secretion of bile. It is also offered in several different commercial products. Dosage: 300 mg in water, three times a day.

Ox bile extract, 200 or 300 mg tablets.

Pancreatic enzymes (brand names: Cotazym, Kuzyme, Arco-lase, Digolase, Kanalase, Gustace, Festal, Mallenzyme, Viokase, and others) are indicated for supplying insufficient or absent pancreatic secretions in cases of pancreatitis, steatorrhea, cystic fibrosis, post-pancreatectomy, or any other lack of pancreatic secretions. Beware of allergic reactions to the enzymes, and do not give amounts higher than needed. Dosages vary in accordance with the concentrations given in the different commercial products; most of them are tablets or capsules containing some 300 mg each, to take one or two with each meal.

Combinations of digestants offer pancreatic enzymes with pepsin (brand name: Entozym), or with pepsin and bile (brand names: Enzypan, Entozyme), pancreatic enzymes with simethicone (brand names: Phazyme, Tri-cone), or pepsin with hydrochloric acid (brand names: Muripsin, Normacid), to be given in accordance with the basic digestive symptoms. Dosages are to be adjusted according to indications for each particular brand.

Antacids

Sodium bicarbonate (brand names: Alka-Seltzer effervescent Antacid, Ceo-Two, baking soda) is the most frequently used drug for the relief of gastric acidity. It is also used (mostly together with salicylates) for the relief of gastric irritation. Other uses are: to make the urine alkaline, to help the elimination of sulfa drugs, and by injection to combat acidosis. Dosage: of the powder, half a teaspoon or less in water after the principal meals; tablets, from one to six, also after meals; for elimination of sulfas, some four to six tablets every 4 to 6 hours.

Bicarbonate of soda, powder.

Bicarbonate of soda, tablets, 300 or 600 mg.

Magnesium trisilicate is not only antacid, but also protectant and absorbent; it is prescribed for hyperchlorhydria and peptic ulcer, and at times as a mild laxative. Take 1 to 4 g between meals.

Magnesium trisilicate, 300 or 500 mg tablets.

Aluminum hydroxide is also used against acidity and in the treatment of peptic ulcer, but it may cause constipation; also it may cause phosphorus depletion in cases of diarrhea or pancreatic insufficiency. It is also used for enteritis and phosphate calculi. In tablet form, give one or two every 4 hours, or as needed; as a gel, 5 to 30 ml in half a glass of water every 4 hours as needed.

Aluminum hydroxide, 300 or 600 mg tablets.

Aluminum hydroxide, gel, dispensed in bottles.

Kaolin and *charcoal* (q.v. above) may also be used as antacids.

Other antacids are marketed by most of the pharmaceutical companies, combining two or more of the known medications; they may also help in the treatment of hyperchlorhydric conditions.

Antiflatulents

Kaolin and activated charcoal in an equal-part mixture may be useful in the treatment of mild cases of meteorism; but a well-balanced diet, the avoidance of gas-producing foods, and perhaps the restoration of a normal intestinal flora may be better.

Simethicone (brand names: Antifoam, Phazyme, Mylican, Silain, Mylanta, Kinesed, Maalox, Tri-Cone) is a defoaming substance, thus favoring expulsion of formed gases in the bowel. It offers only symptomatic treatment of flatulence, and is not always as effective as desired. Tablets, to a daily total of 200 or 400 mg, will be given after meals and at bedtime.

Simethicone, 40 or 50 mg tablets.

Note: This medication is also presented in a liquid or suspension form, or manufactured together with other adjuvants.

XXXII. RESPIRATORY MEDICATIONS

Emetics are very frequently used as expectorants, for which they are given at very low dosages, barely nauseating but able to increase bronchial secretions. Ipecac and tartar emetic have been widely recommended for this purpose, at dosages of one fifth or one tenth of the emetic dose. They serve as antitussives when viscid sputum and secondary coughing can be exhausting, and thus are of great help in saving energy, particularly with the frail patient.

Care will be taken to be sure that no damage is done when coughing is no longer useful for cleansing the upper respiratory tract.

Presently most pharmaceutical specialties, and frequently prescriptions written by physicians, mix several medications used for the same purpose. The market is actually overstocked with medicines of this kind.

Potassium iodide and other iodides are used as expectorants because of the low toxicity of the iodism that may follow their use in average cases, namely, 300 mg of a saturated solution for each dose, repeated as needed (e.g., every 2 hours) until the effect is noted, to be stopped when the effect is achieved. The numerous mixtures on the market will serve the purpose.

Terpin hydrate and glyceryl guaiacolate are used in formulas for expectorants and control of cough. There are many specialties of this kind.

Mucolytic agents given by aerosol are marketed as specialties in this field.

Codeine

This opium alkaloid is used either in the form of the free alkaloid or as codeine phosphate or sulfate. The phosphate is better for pharmaceutic manipulations because of its greater solubility.

Its more important role is as a bechic medication; also, it is advised for mild to moderate pain. Naturally, when coughing becomes painful, as it so frequently does, codeine becomes the drug of choice.

Dosage: Doses between 15 and 60 mg are prescribed. For pain, for instance, when 60 mg does not work, larger doses will usually also fail. The medication can be given by either the oral or the parenteral route, absorption being no problem. Even though codeine rarely causes addiction, that possibility should be kept in mind. When codeine is used as an antitussive medication, give 15 or 30 mg per dose, repeated as needed and tolerated; but at times the bechic effect is obtained with small doses. Up to 60 mg may also be given for each individual dose.

Codeine phosphate, 15, 30, or 60 mg tablets.

Codeine phosphate, 15, 30, or 60 mg capsules.

Codeine phosphate, 15, 30, or 60 mg in 1-ml ampoules; or 20 mg in each ml in 20-ml vials.

Codeine is similarly available as the sulfate.

Hydrocodone

The bitartrate is frequently used (mostly in combination with other drugs) as a bechic medication when the cough reflex is due to pharyngitis, tracheitis, or bronchitis, or any other infectious disease of the respiratory system.

Narcotics

Other narcotic drugs are also effectively used as antitussives, a list that could be made a relatively long one, starting with morphine and continuing with its numerous analogs. But perhaps codeine has made their administration useless, owing to its relative safety and effectiveness.

XXXIII. INFUSIONS AND ELECTROLYTES

Alkalinizing Solutions

Sodium bicarbonate is the most widely used medication against metabolic acidosis. In earlier chapters other uses of this substance were reviewed. Intravenous infusions will be given at a very slow pace, diluting a 7.5% 50-ml ampoule in a total of 250 ml of sterile water to have a 1.5% solution. The amount to be injected can be estimated as follows:

60 − plasma CO_2 × 1.76 body weight in kilos = ml of 1.5% solution.

If CO_2 is unknown, a total of between 1 and 2 liters of the 1.5% solution of sodium bicarbonate will be injected; to stop as soon as symptoms improve.

Sodium bicarbonate, ampoule containing 50 ml of a 7.5% solution.

Sodium lactate is recommended in acidosis caused by diarrhea, vomiting, diabetes mellitus, renal failure, acute infections, or starvation. A dosage using 1/6 molar solution will be estimated by the above formula. Give it at a rate of no more than 300 ml in 1 hour.

> Sodium lactate, 100, 150, 250, 500, or 1000 ml of a 1/6 molar solution in ampoules or vials.

Acidifying Solution

Ammonium chloride is the main drug for the treatment of metabolic alkalosis, but is used only in severe cases, since lesser severity usually responds to correction of water or sodium deficit by the administration of sodium and potassium chloride. Do not give more than 200 or 400 ml of a 2% solution.

> Ammonium chloride, 2% solution for infusion.

Replacement Solutions

Isotonic saline or 0.9% sodium chloride solution compensates for chloride losses in cases of vomiting due to gastrointestinal obstruction, diarrhea, or any other form of extracellular fluid losses. Doses of 1.5 to 2 or 3 liters may be injected in 24 hours.

> Isotonic saline, in ampoules or vials of 10, 20, 30, 100, 150, 250, 500, or 1000 ml.

Hypotonic sodium chloride or 0.45% solution increases water without increasing osmotic pressure and is useful in the initial treatment of extracellular fluid losses. Give a total of 3 to 8% of the body weight.

> Hypotonic sodium chloride, in ampoules or vials of 150, 250, or 500 ml.

Hypertonic sodium chloride 3% or, better, 5% solutions are to be given very slowly and only in small amounts—no more than 200 to 300 ml—to patients with very low blood concentrations of sodium in diabetic coma and Addisonian crisis.

> Hypertonic sodium chloride, 3 or 5% solutions in 250- or 500-ml bottles.

Glucose or dextrose is presented in varied concentrations, mainly to provide calories, as needed, to supply body water, and to protect against excessive production of ketones by the liver, excessive consumption of body proteins, and loss of electrolytes. The 5% solution is indicated for dehydration, shock, and provision of calories. The 20% solution is given intravenously in cases of edema or renal failure. The 50% solution helps in cases of shock, to decrease elevated intracranial pressure, and, together with insulin, for the management of diabetic coma. Glucose solutions are also used for the administration of other medicaments. Dosages vary according to individual needs.

Glucose, 5% solution in 150-, 250-, 500-, or 1000-ml flasks.

Glucose, 20% solution in 500- or 1000-ml flasks.

Glucose, 50% solution in 20-, 50-, or 100-ml vials.

Glucose solutions of 2.5 and 10% are also available.

Dextran is an acceptable blood expander useful for the treatment of shock, either traumatic or hemorrhagic, though not a substitute for blood when it is needed. There is a low incidence of side effects. Try not to elevate systolic blood pressure over 85 mm of Hg; to avoid secondary hemorrhages 20 to 40 ml can be infused every minute for a total of 15 to 30 minutes, repeating whenever necessary.

Dextran 70, 6% isotonic solution in flasks of 250 or 500 ml.

Ringer's solution has the same uses as the isotonic saline, q.v., with the advantage of producing less sodium retention and edema when the patient is hypoproteinemic. The dosage is similar to that of isotonic saline.

Ringer's solution, in flasks of 30, 500, or 1000 ml.

Ringer's lactate solution is given in cases of dehydration, particularly when there is some sort of acidosis, or when electrolytes are lost. The dosage has to be individualized from an average of 20 to 30 ml for each kilo of body weight.

Ringer's lactate solution, in containers of 10, 20, 100, 250, 500, or 1000 ml.

Potassium chloride is the elective therapy for hypopotassemia. This may be caused by diarrhea, vomiting, polyuria, adrenal hyperfunction, poor potassium intake, or other hypokalemic conditions, which include diabetic acidosis, some surgical conditions, or cases of uremia, corticoid therapy, or familial periodic paralysis. To avoid intoxication, check potassium levels frequently and monitor electrocardiographic tracings. The injection should not exceed a rate of 30 mEq per liter of fluid in 1 hour.

Potassium chloride, injectable, 2 mEq per ml, in 10- or 20-ml ampoules or vials.

Potassium chloride, injectable, 3 mEq per ml, in 10- or 50-ml vials.

Potassium chloride, injectable, 3.2 mEq per ml, in 12.5-ml vials.

Potassium chloride, injectable, 153 mEq per 1-liter container.

Protein hydrolysate (brand names: Amigen, Aminosol, CPH, Hyprotigen, Parenamine, Travamin) should be used according to the content of sodium (large amounts in Amigen, smaller in Aminosol), potassium (in Aminosol), or both (in Travamin). In severe illnesses protein hydrolysate will help to maintain a positive nitrogen balance and correct severe malnutrition, and also promote chelating of copper in Wilson's disease. Glucose is usually given together with the hydrolysate. The combination should not be given, that is, glucose with the hydrolysate, in acidosis, and a careful watch will be kept for side effects (gastrointestinal, cardiovascular, local at the site of the injection). Dosage will be individualized and regulated at about 1 or 2 liters of the 5% solution, together with 5% glucose, at a rate of 500 ml in 1 hour.

Protein hydrolysate, 5% solution in bottles containing 500 or 1000 ml. Also available with 5% glucose, in containers of 125, 250, 500, or 1000 ml.

Protein hydrolysate, 10% solution in containers of 500 or 1000 ml.

XXXIV. VITAMINS

Vitamin A

This vitamin is indicated for the treatment of vitamin A deficiency manifested by: hyperkeratosis of the skin, excessive dermic dryness, xerophthalmia, nyctalopia, keratomalacia, and metaplasia of mucosae (with lessened resistance to infections). Avoid overdosage (arthralgias, hepatomegaly, headache, nervous irritability, papilledema, drying and crackling of the skin). Give an average dosage of 10,000 to 25,000 units a day; larger doses, in severe cases, for a restricted time.

Vitamin A, 5000, 25,000, 50,000, or 100,000 units, capsules.

Vitamin A, drops, 50,000 units in each ml (three drops provide 5000 units).

Vitamin B$_1$ (Thiamine)

In the first place, thiamine is used for the treatment of thiamine deficiency (clinical picture of beri-beri, anorexia, asthenia, paresthesias of the extremities); but it is also recommended for neuritis (alcoholic, trigeminal, diabetic) and some cardiovascular and gastrointestinal disorders attributable to deficient intake of vitamin B$_1$. Injections of 100 or 300 mg are given for prompt correction of a severe deficit. Thereafter, an average of 0.5 to 1 mg a day will be enough to fulfill requirements.

Thiamine, 5, 10, 15, 25, 50, or 100 mg tablets.

Thiamine, 1-ml ampoules of 50 or 100 mg.

Vitamin B_2 (Riboflavin)

Cheilosis and excessive corneal vascularization are preferably treated with riboflavin, usually given with other members of the B complex. Adequate dosage is 5 to 10 mg a day. Injections are given only when adequate absorption is impaired.

Riboflavin, 1, 2, 5, 10, 25, or 50 mg tablets.

Riboflavin, injectable, 50 or 100 mg in 1 or 10 ml.

Vitamin B_6 (Pyridoxine)

Today, the main use is for the prevention of isoniazid peripheral neuritis. The administration of 25 or 50 mg a day is usually enough.

Pyridoxine, 10, 25, or 50 mg tablets.

Vitamin B_{12} (Cyanocobalamin)

Given by the parenteral route, cyanocobalamin is practically specific for the treatment of pernicious anemia, sprue, and nutritional macrocytic anemia. Patients sensitive to liver extracts can be treated with vitamin B_{12}. Sensory neuropathies may respond to massive doses of the vitamin, including trigeminal neuralgia, toxic neuritis (alcoholic), or diabetic neuritis. Dosages vary greatly according to the disease under treatment, from 15 μg a day to 500 μg two or three times a week.

Cyanocobalamin, 30, 60, or 100 μg per ml, vials or ampoules.

Folic Acid

Folic acid is effective for the treatment of megaloblastic anemias and sprue, but should never be given alone for the treatment of pernicious anemia. Dosage should start with 15 mg for several days, to resort to a maintenance dose of 5 to 10 mg a day.

Folic acid, 5 or 20 mg tablets.

Folic acid, injectable, 15 mg in each ml, in 1-ml ampoules or 20-ml vials.

Nicotinic Acid (Niacin)

Niacin, part of the vitamin B group, is specific for pellagra. It is also recommended for differentiating dietary from nondietary psychoses (dietary to be treated with niacin) and some cases with hypercholesterolemia. In the case of fully developed pellagra, 50 mg is given ten times a day (if injections are needed, 25 mg two or more times a day). Otherwise, a dosage of 10 to 25 mg a day will suffice.

Niacin, 25, 50, or 100 mg tablets.

Niacin, injectable, 100 mg in 10-ml vials.

Niacinamide, 25, 50, or 100 mg tablets.

Niacinamide, injectable, 100 mg in 2-ml ampoules or 3000 mg in 30-ml vials.

Vitamin C (Ascorbic Acid)

Vitamin C is specific for the treatment of scurvy. It is also given for idiopathic methemoglobinemia, and in the form of continuous administration (not sporadically!) for the prevention of common colds—though this is a well known controversial subject. Dosage: no less than 1000 mg a day until restoration of vitamin body reserves; for methemoglobinemia, 300 mg a day, in divided doses; also, 500 mg a day may be given.

Ascorbic acid, 25, 50, 100, 250, or 500 mg tablets.

Ascorbic acid, injectable, 50, 100, or 500 mg in each 1-ml ampoule.

Vitamin D (Calciferol)

This vitamin is recommended for the treatment of rachitis, in the first place, but also for hypocalcemia, particularly when due to parathyroid insufficiency. It is also employed in cases of osteomalacia, spasmophilia, and many cases of lupus vulgaris, which may respond well to large doses. The usual therapeutic dosage is about 1500 to 5000 units a day, few patients requiring larger amounts. In acute parathyroid tetany a dose of up to 1.5 million units is needed, with 100,000 to 200,000 units as the maintenance dose. This last dosage is the one used for lupus vulgaris. In all instances, check blood calcium at frequent intervals.

Vitamin D, 50,000-unit capsules.

Vitamin D, 50,000-unit tablets.

Vitamin D, injectable, 500,000 units in each ml in 10-ml vials.

Vitamin E (Tocopherol)

Vitamin E has been recommended for so many different diseases that it seems futile to name them here, since we can make no recommendations.

Vitamin E, 25-unit tablets.

Vitamin E, capsules of 25, 30, 37.5, 45, 50, 68, 90, 92.5, 100, 300, 400, or 800 units.

Vitamin E, drops in different concentrations.

Vitamin E, injectables.

Vitamin K

Vitamin K is used in the management of hemorrhages due to deficiencies in prothrombin, dosages ranging from 1 to 10 mg.

Vitamin K, 5 mg tablets.

Vitamin K, injectable, 1, 2.5, 5, or 10 mg in 1-ml ampoules.

Multivitamins

Innumerable preparations containing several vitamins—either only vitamins, or vitamins with minerals—are available on the market. Since a single vitamin deficiency is rare, because typical cases of pure avitaminoses are usually accompanied by noticeable deficiencies of other vitamins, it is recommended that a multivitamin supplementation be used whenever a deficient diet is to be followed by a patient.

Take one a day of any of the vitamin preparations containing a full, officially recommended daily adult dose of at least five of the most common vitamins.

Part Two

Diagnosis and Treatment

I. INTRODUCTION

APPROACHING THE SUBJECT

As we pursue the subject of gerontology it becomes increasingly apparent that we are attacking a problem of burgeoning importance to the future of the human race. Studying the report of the subjects of interest brought up at the 29th annual meeting of the Gerontology Society, held in New York City in 1976, makes it plain that the cry for help to the medical profession has become desperate. We see that there are 650,000 elderly persons in this country today, and at projected rates there will be a million in 25 years.

Doctors have expressed more interest in treating youthful patients because they have the challenge of returning them to the mainstream of productivity. Also recent reports from questionnaires sent to 114 medical schools, with answers from 87, show that only 3 of those offered a specialty in geriatrics; only 35 provided internships with the elderly. The aged are becoming segregated from the main body of society. They are attracting a diminishing proportion of the interest of the medical profession.

Many elderly patients in nursing homes have not seen a doctor in two months and have not had a social visit in a year. Often their ailments are not correctly diagnosed because symptoms of disease in the aged are not like those of young patients.*

Let us keep in mind this appeal from the aged.

* *Aging,* Nos. 268–269, Feb., Mar., 1977.

GENERAL PHYSIOLOGICAL FACTS

Changes are occurring continuously during life. Without any fixed chronology, in the later years some changes have to take place. Tissues become less elastic, particularly connective tissue, which degenerates at a more or less rapid rate, especially noted by the slower regenerative processes following any injury. The skin becomes progressively drier, inelastic, wrinkled, and pigmented. The hair loses its pigmentation. Sclerotic changes particularly affect the arteries, heart, eyes, and brain. The lens loses accommodation (presbyopia) and transparency (cataracts). Muscles weaken and slow down. This situation, together with decalcification and atrophy of bones, produces an insecure gait. Sensorial acuity diminishes (hearing, vision), and the voice loses its control and clarity. There is less power of mental concentration, poorer memory (particularly for recent events), and less alertness. Some older persons become egoistic and intolerant; by the same token, many become more tolerant and have better judgment and analytic power, showing improved comprehension backed by experience, with the ability to interrelate facts.

As stated previously, "ailing aging" may start at any age, because of inconsistency of biological chronology. Senescence and involution are individual patterns. According to recent statistics, the three main causes of death are heart disease, cancer, and stroke. This estimate is valid for 35 years of age and above. Accident is another item to be considered, and an important factor from conception to death. Following in frequency are arteriosclerosis, which also is usually considered the chief cause of heart disease, influenza followed by pneumonia, cirrhosis of the liver, senile dementia in advanced ages, diabetes, and emphysema; and for those over 75 years of age, hernia and intestinal obstruction, hypertension, nephritis, and gastritis. To be noted: suicide is among the ten leading causes of death from below age 14 to age 75. This list proves, again, that senescence and involution are really individual patterns.

The elderly may present any disease, including measles, but the latter would be a very rare contingency. Usually, diseases most frequently related to old age are as follows:

Coronary occlusion	Coronary thrombosis
Arrhythmias	Cerebral thrombosis
Peripheral vascular disease	Stroke
Cancer (all sites included)	Accidents
Atherosclerosis	Infections (flu and pneumonia)
Cirrhosis of the liver	Early senility (senile dementia)
Diabetes	Emphysema (chronic bronchitis)
Hypertension	Hernia
Intestinal obstruction	Gastritis

Pylorostenosis	Peptic ulcer
Colon diverticulosis	Colon polyposis
Nephritis	Senile pruritus
Retinopathy	Arthritis
Chronic asthma	Huntington's chorea
Thyroid diseases (hypo)	Hypoadrenalism
Obesity	Gout
Hypercholesterolemia	Other musculoskeletal diseases
Pernicious anemia	Parkinsonism
Depression	Brain syndromes

Skin diseases (mainly, vascular changes, atopic eczema, sebaceous adenoma, senile keratosis, leukoplasia, and basal cell carcinoma, among many others)

DIAGNOSIS OF THE ELDERLY

Diagnosis of the elderly presents many hazards, which increase in incidence as age progresses. For instance, the history given the physician is often misleading, depending on the temperament of the patient. Some individuals become complaining and hypersensitive, and exaggerate, often inventing pains and malfunctions to incite sympathy and gain attention. Others are self effacing and apologetic, hiding their discomforts and disabilities, so that in their martyrdom they prevent a correct diagnosis and proper treatment.

Also, the debilitated elderly lack the sthenic response of youth and might suffer a damaging infection without a proper rise in temperature, which would signal the onset of a disease or indicate its progress.

Additionally, many of our drugs with potent effect on the human vital complex can easily unbalance the frail and sensitive regulatory network governing the heart, lungs, and nervous and digestive systems of the aged. Thus warned, a therapist of the elderly will use special care in employing the same drugs and methods found adequate for those with a recuperative reserve. In the event of an accident, like a fall, check with relatives, neighbors, or witnesses for relevant facts.

The physical examination will be as accurate as possible. It will include weight, blood pressure, pulse rate and rhythm, the condition of the skin and the musculoskeletal system, and the regular inspection, palpation, and auscultation of the respiratory system, the examination of the reflexes, and the condition of the eyes, ears, nose, and throat. It will be not only appropriate, but mandatory in many instances, to have a urinalysis, complete blood count, blood chemistry, sedimentation rate, and in most cases an X-ray of the chest and spine; also an electrocardiogram and gastric analysis may prove helpful.

Symptoms most frequently complained of or present are:

Weakness (asthenia)	Confusion
Unconsciousness	Dyspnea
Pain	Tumor (a mass)
Dysuria	Abnormal defecation

Pain is not an informative symptom in the very old. For instance, myocardial infarction may cause no pain or, at most, be mentioned as just discomfort or moderate tenderness. Painless myocardial infarction occurs, as does silent appendicitis, with little discomfort and usually with a rapidly deteriorating general condition. The lack of reliability is also emphasized because these patients may consider a new pain as a result of a previous illness, and a part of any other chronic or minor ailment. Care will be taken to evaluate these complaints, to place them in the proper relation either to a former condition, or to a change from the former state, or as an entirely new disease. Also, we must be aware of heterotopic pains because even a fracture of the hip may cause pain in the knee, and chest pain may be due to abdominal diseases. Many of these instances require the help of a good radiologic study to complement a conscientious physical examination.

Mental confusion accompanies so many ailments of the aged that it is to be found in about 33% of all hospitalized patients, but it must not be assumed that senility is always the sole cause of the mental obfuscation. Keep in mind that mental confusion may be the initial symptom of *any* disease affecting the elderly. In the first place consider heart disease, which causes confusion or lethargy more frequently than dyspnea or pain. Check the blood pressure, physical characteristics of the pulse, and auscultation of the heart and lungs, and complement these findings with X-ray and electrocardiograms in the study of each patient.

The added care given to diagnosis of the aged should include realization that the history may contain exaggeration, concealment, insensitivity, or bias and that the physical findings could be altered due to general asthenia, suppressing inflammatory swelling, redness, and fever. The history must be especially complete as to recent illnesses, exposure to infection, travel, and injuries. The physical examination must include X-ray, as indicated, of the respiratory tract, sinuses, mastoids, and lungs; evaluation of the circulatory system, blood pressure, electrocardiogram, complete blood count and coagulation time, serology for syphilis, and blood chemistry (SMA12, culture). Toxic effects of drugs must be considered, as well as brain tumor, cerebral hemorrhage, diabetes, alcoholism, uremia, cardiac failure, adrenal insufficiency, and hypothyroidism.

Alarming symptoms are confusion and unconsciousness. Unfortunately these symptoms are not very informative because they can be due to a large number of causes. Unconsciousness in the elderly is often due to cerebral hemorrhage, thrombosis or embolism, trauma to the head or other parts, acute infections, heart disease, tumors, poisoning, vasovagal syncope, orthostatic hypertension, emotional or physical stress, or exhaustion from a terminal illness.

The diagnosis of tumor masses is often difficult because of the frequently found deformity of the skeletal structures. Often an existing kyphosis pushes the viscera of chest and abdomen toward the anterior of either chest or abdomen. For instance, a sclerotic aorta displaced by spinal curvature could be mistaken for an abdominal tumor. In the case of abdominal masses, it will be highly advisable to do a rectal examination, which will reveal a distended bladder or impacted feces, two extremely frequent conditions found in the elderly. It must be seriously considered when there is a history of dysuria or abnormal defecation. In the case of diarrhea, always consider the possibility of excessive use of laxatives or overindulgence in eating.

According to what has been said about diseases in the elderly, those which will be suspected most should be the following:

No. 1 Sclerosis (coronary, leading to angina or infarction; cerebral, leading to strokes or falls
No. 2 Cancer
No. 3 Rheumatism
No. 4 Diabetes
No. 5 Acute infections (influenza leading to pneumonia)
No. 6 Prostate or bladder disease
No. 7 *Any other disease*

But never forget that the elderly may have—as implied above—any disease, not only those usually attributed to old age.

THE PROPER USE OF DRUGS

The opening paragraphs of Part One summarized the problem of the use of drugs for treatment during old age. It has been mentioned that age may change susceptibility to drugs. Considerations are frailty, degeneration, simultaneous occurrence of more than one disease, and the slowing of gastrointestinal absorption, as well as sluggish elimination; tolerance is decreased for a large number of medicaments (cardiotonics, barbiturates, tranquilizers, etc.), and some side effects are increased.

With the frail, the small, and the ailing, the necessity of giving lower doses of many drugs becomes evident; and the advantages of using the simplest medications, avoiding the natural tendency to poly-pharmacy when good results are not immediately obtained, will also be noted.

In summary, the aims of geriatric therapeutics should be to cure where possible or, at least, to help, and to encourage always.

Make certain the patient is able to remember the timing of medication; keep a constant watch for the occurrence of side effects; avoid prolonged bed rest; regulate dosages carefully, preferring lower ones to be on the safe side at all times; and always be alert for drug interactions when altering the dose or adding a drug.

ON DYING

Death is unpredictable, even from the state of good health. Older people, perhaps, can die more easily—no matter that those more advanced in age will more probably reach 100 years than the younger ones.

Patients can be told the probable outlook for their illness within certain limitations. Some responsible member of the family must be taken into the doctor's confidence. The physician should understand the patient's ability or inability to face the reality of a terminal illness and should be as frank as is believed justified for the patient's welfare. The rapport between the patient and physician should take preference before all others. If not mentally capable of understanding the situation, the patient should be protected from judgments that might be traumatic to accept.

Concerning medication, there are important steps that will not be minimized. First, give the basic treatment at its full strength, as if a cure is to be expected, together with all needed symptomatic measures. And second, do not spare any help for the relief of pain, sleeplessness, and/or apprehension. In other words, pain relievers should be given to the point of actually controlling suffering; hypnotics, to the point of promoting a restful sleep; and tranquilizers, to the point of calming apprehension.

II. PAIN

GENERAL DIAGNOSIS OF PAIN

The elderly will either overemphasize or minimize their pains, or will even refer to them as a natural manifestation of a previous condition. Thus it will always be good to be on the alert and properly evaluate the real meaning of any pain, either small or great. A succinct review of diseases that may cause pain follows, not always corresponding to what is presented in more detail later on, but intended as a summary of the main factors.

Chest Pain

This is a very common clinical finding among older people as well as others. Any patient over 50 or 60 years of age complaining of pain or only discomfort in the chest will be checked, first for *myocardial infarction,* especially when a sudden retrosternal oppression or pain is accompanied by apprehension, fear, or confusion. *Acute pericarditis* is suggested by retrosternal pain (increased by certain positions or movements), shallow, rapid respiration, anxiety, weakness, and the characteristic friction rub heard during the complete cardiac cycle. *Pneumonia* may show stabbing, sharp pain on one side, intensified by motion, with a sudden onset of fever, a productive cough, chills, and prostration. In *bronchopneumonia* the picture is similar, but is gradual in onset, milder in symptoms, and frequently follows a previous respiratory disease. *Legionnaires' disease* affects older people with some sort of pneumonic syndrome. *Pulmonary infarction* is a severe disease with abrupt rise in temperature, substernal pain, dyspnea, and anxiety. *Pleuritis* shows a clinical picture resembling pneumonia with pleuritic rub and pain, which disappears on holding the breath or splinting the sides with adhesive. *Epidemic pleurodynia* shows sore throat, fever, headache, malaise, and muscle pain in the intercostal area, and no auscultatory evidence of pleuritis. *Heterotopic pain* may result from *subdiaphragmatic abscess* (pain in the lower part of the chest, radiating to the shoulder and showing elevation and immobility of the corresponding diaphragm); *hepatic abscess* shows similar symptomatology, often caused by amebic infections. *Cholecystitis* presents with a history of biliary colic. *Valvular heart lesions* may also be accompanied by chest pain, but this condition is more frequent with younger patients. In *aortitis* or *aortic aneurism,* the pain resembles angina, but is even less marked. *Mediastinal lesions* will also cause pain, particularly cancer, with a pleuritic type of pain. In *atelectasis* pain in the side is followed by dyspnea, cyanosis, fever, and shock; there are reduced respiratory movements, diminished breath sounds, and little coughing. In *pneumothorax* of traumatic origin or secondary to a previous disease the diagnosis is obvious: a dramatic onset with sharp side pain, severe dyspnea, and dry cough; in spontaneous pneumothorax the symptoms are the same, but there is not a previous clue. Diseases of the *mammary glands* may also cause localized pain. *Heterotopic pain* in the chest may be due to liver or gall bladder diseases, peptic ulcer, or renal colic. Pain in the walls of the thorax or *thoracalgia* is noted in diseases of the ribs or the sternum (fractures, osteomyelitis, tuberculosis, tumors), intercostal neuralgia, subdiaphragmatic abscess, and multiple myeloma (always think of it when dealing with the elderly).

Abdominal Pain

Abdominal pain may be acute or chronic, diffuse or localized. *Appendicitis* causes an acute continuous or variable pain of a colicky nature, aggravated by pressure over the right iliac fossa, usually accompanied by local muscle spasm, fever, and increasing leukocytosis. In *acute pancreatitis* pain is located at the left side of the epigastrium, constant and very severe, exaggerated by certain positions (lying supine) and by local pressure, and accompanied by local muscle rigidity; the patient may appear critically ill or even in shock. *Typhoid fever* starts with a gradual rise in temperature, malaise, intestinal inflammation, headache, and general pains. There may be stupor and bradycardia. The intestinal inflammation may become violent and lead to perforation, causing severe pain. The appearance of rose spots on the chest and the abdomen is typical. In *pyelitis* and *pyelonephritis* pain is referred to the bladder or appears on urination, there is a febrile syndrome, and pain is referred to the back. In *perirenal* abscess and carbuncle there is a sudden onset of fever, with chills, prostration, nausea, vomiting, and pain with tenderness in the costovertebral angle. *Renal colic* presents excruciating pain from the corresponding costovertebral area to the abdominal flank, and to the genitourinary organs, accompanied by fever, chills, and vomiting. *Tuberculosis of the urinary organs* shows dull pain in the corresponding costovertebral region and abdominal flank, with frequency and painful terminal dysuria. In *salpingitis* there is pain in the iliac fossa, more frequently on the right, with fever and sometimes peritoneal reaction; the diagnosis is helped by gynecological examination. *Abdominal tuberculosis* occurs in patients with a previous history of the infection. The complaints are crampy abdominal pains and diarrhea, with a constant sensation of discomfort in tuberculosis of the intestines; tenderness, ascites, and cachexia are present in tuberculosis of the peritoneum. In *peritonitis,* usually following an antecedent disease, there is an agonizing, constant pain in the abdomen, exaggerated with motion; the legs are flexed, and the hippocratic facies is pale with an anxious expression.

Perigastritis follows a peptic or duodenal ulcer, and is noted by an abdominal mass and febricula. *Diverticulitis* mimics an attack of appendicitis located in the left iliac fossa. *Crohn's disease* is a regional enteritis showing fever, crampy pains, diarrhea, weight loss, and a mass located in the right iliac fossa. *Cholecystitis* shows fever, dyspepsia, and vague aches in the right flank; a history of colic if there is lithiasis; and pain on pressure, increased by deep inspiration, at the right hypochondrium. In the case of *biliary colic* there is an acute sharp pain in the right upper abdomen. *Liver abscess* shows a combination of digestive and fever symptoms with pain in the right hypochondrium, irradiated to the shoulder and increased with movements; there are also hepatomegaly and hepatalgia. *Hepatitis* will start like a case of abdominal influenza with weakness, fever, hepatalgia, and other abdominal discomfort, and soon jaundice will be noted; serum hepatitis follows a blood transfusion, and infectious hepatitis behaves like a contagious disease. *Subdiaphragmatic abscesses* usually follow abdominal surgery, perforation, or an infective disease of the digestive system, and are characterized by pain in the upper abdomen and lower chest radiating to the corresponding shoulder, the pain increasing under local pressure.

The above diseases are usually accompanied by a variable fever, which is not usually present in the following instances. *Peptic ulcer,* gastric or duodenal, presents only moderate pain, with tenderness on palpation; the diagnosis is suspected on exacerbation of symptoms from a chronic lesion (heartburn, distention, nausea, etc.). *Intestinal colic* refers to an acute gastroenteritis, possibly related to eating noxious food. In *cystitis* there is not always fever, but hypogastric discomfort, urgent urination, and a persistent sensation of bladder fullness. *Prostatitis* is evidenced by perineal pain and a feeling of pressure, together with symptoms of cystitis. In *urethritis* there is burning on urination and urethral discharge of pus. *Bartholinitis* is characterized by a painful nodule in the inferior portion of one of the labia minora. *Lymphogranuloma venereum* is to be strongly suspected on finding the combination of joint or abdominal pains, headache, fever, chills, conjunctivitis, splenomegaly, marked enlargement of the inguinal glands, and exaggerated edema of the sex organs. *Orchitis* and *orchoepididymitis* start with epididymitis followed by fever and swelling of the scrotum.

Headache and Pain in the Face

Headache cannot be a specific help in diagnosis since even a common cold with a minimal febricula can be accompanied by an annoying headache, particularly among the elderly. Nevertheless, it is always of some diagnostic value.

Headache reaches very severe proportions in *variola,* usually diagnosed with ease as soon as the characteristic umbilicated, one-stage, pustular rash develops. In *varicella* the rash closely resembles variolic dermic lesions, but the diagnosis is determined by the presence of different crops of vesicles, the lack of umbilication, and most frequently the mildness of headache and other symptoms. *Herpes zoster* is similar to varicella, but vesicles appear along the path of a sensory nerve, and usually the area is very painful. The *common cold* should not be mistaken for more severe diseases, in spite of the nonspecific syndrome of headache, mild (or absent) fever, coughing, sneezing, and general malaise. *Influenza* is a more severe disease, with sudden febrile onset with headache, muscle pains, intense malaise, weakness, and upper respiratory and occasionally gastrointestinal symptoms. In *herpangina* the diagnosis is made by finding headache, fever, and the characteristic herpetic stomatitis (papulovesicular rash on the tonsils, spreading in the form of large lesions to the rest of the mouth). In *epidemic pleurodynia* there are headache, sore throat, and pain in the muscles of the intercostal area with no auscultatory signs of pleuritis.

Aseptic meningitis is diagnosed by the failure to find any specific causative virus or larger germ in the presence of the symptoms of meningitis. *Colorado tick fever* cases are found in the western states and usually appear from March to August, with headache, muscle pains, fever, and a rash, all subsiding to reappear after 2 or 3 days. In *dengue fever* pains reach disabling proportions, with headache, fever, malaise, and a rapidly evanescent rash. *Bacteremia* is suspected when a previously known infection assumes septic symptoms with more intense fever, chills, general pains, purpuric or petechial rash, and the development of symptoms from additional affected areas. In *scarlet fever* the characteristic pink-red rash gives the best clinical clue to diagnosis. *Salmonellosis* shows a gradual increase in temperature and a few gastrointestinal symptoms: during the second week there will be diarrhea ("pea-soup"), and toxic stupor will supervene. Watch for pharyngeal, respiratory, renal, and other abnormal changes. *Malaria* presents with a sudden elevation of temperature, shaking chills, sweating, and headache as a secondary effect. The symptoms repeatedly recur after regular remissions of a few days. *Plague* shows a rapid onset, high fever, chills (headache may be absent in bubonic plague), tachycardia, hypotension, and enlarged lymph nodes; there is rapid deterioration of the general condition.

Glanders (farcy) starts abruptly following exposure to horses; there are headache, fever, chills, prostration, and a painful ulcer at the site of contagion. *Tularemia* follows exposure to wild animals, particularly rabbits, and shows headache, fever, nausea, severe malaise, and profuse sweating. Initially the site of infective contact presents a papule, which turns into a pustule and ulcerates. The regional lymph nodes are enlarged. *Brucellosis* begins with headache, fever, joint pains, sweating, and gastrointestinal upset. Lymphadenopathy, splenomegaly, and fever of the undulant type are characteristic. *Yellow fever* is suggested by fever, jaundice, and the presence of albuminuria. The diagnosis is backed by hematemesis ("black vomit") and other hemorrhages. *Leptospirosis* is suspected after exposure to animals (dogs) or infected soil (sewers, swimming), principally during summertime. It is heralded by sudden pains, fever, and conjunctival congestion. There may also be jaundice or a meningeal syndrome. *Relapsing fever* shows ups and downs of symptoms, with a history of louse or tick bites suffered in the western states. It starts abruptly with headache and general pains, fever, tachycardia, and an erythematous rash on the trunk and extremities, evolving into pink macules. All symptoms disappear after 3 to 10 days and come back after a similar interval. *Rickettsial diseases* usually show a common subsyndrome, consisting of high fever, malaise, headache, pains along the spine and legs, and conjunctivitis, which becomes more evident by the third day. *Epidemic typhus* shows a rash which turns petechial or purpuric and marked nervous symptoms; *murine typhus* shows a lesser tendency to hemorrhage, with the nervous and respiratory symptoms less marked; in *Rocky Mountain spotted fever* the rash appears first on the extremities, spreading to the trunk, and the symptomatology is severe; in *Q fever* there is no rash, but a rickettsial pneumonia appears to be more characteristic; and in *trench fever* the temperature curve shows two or three peaks separated by 12 to 24 hours.

Syphilis in the secondary stage shows headache and slight fever with a typical rash; cerebral syphilis manifests itself with a severe headache and fever; the diagnosis mainly depends on laboratory findings. *Lymphogranuloma venereum* shows fever, headache and other pains, and conjunctivitis, but the presence of a marked enlargement of lymph glands in the groins and a marked edema (elephantiasis) of sex organs will suggest the diagnosis. *Meningitis* is suggested in any person with fever, headache, and stiff neck. In *encephalitis* there are, in varied combinations, headache, convulsions, myoclonus, hemiplegia, and backache. *Sinusitis* is characterized by local pain, nasal discharge, and headache; the pain is increased by effort, bending the head, coughing, or percussion over the affected site. *Intracranial abscess* will be suggested by the combination of a previous known infection with symptoms of intracranial pressure. *Iritis* and *iridocyclitis* exhibit outstanding ocular symptoms with edema of the upper eyelid, lacrimation, photophobia, pain, myosis, congested corneal vessels, swelling of the iris, or cloudiness of the intraocular fluids.

Headache can occur *without fever,* even in the above-mentioned diseases. This situation is not rare, especially with the depleted vitality of the elderly.

Brain tumors and *cysts* may cause intense headache, projectile vomiting, papilledema, bradycardia, epileptic seizures, and behavioral changes. In *subdural hematoma* headache usually follows a trauma and shows a spastic hemiplegia. *Subarachnoid hemorrhage* follows some sort of exertion and shows stiff neck and convulsions. In *intracranial abscess* convulsions may precede the headache, and there are other signs of intracranial pressure. *Epilepsy* is readily diagnosed as soon as the first seizure is recognized.

Heart diseases are rarely accompanied by headache. Both *hypertension* and *hypotension,* particularly at the beginning of critical phases, do show headache, which will be related to the blood pressure findings. In *arteritis* there is also pain at the site of the temporal arteries, a condition which requires a prompt diagnosis to avoid blindness. *Heart failure* will be diagnosed because of dyspnea, rales heard in the lower lung fields, edema, and the other signs of failing circulation. Other causes of hypoxia are: all forms of *hypoventilation, high altitude syndrome, cerebral anoxia,* and *hemic abnormalities;* all present headache together with the other characteristic symptomatology.

Allergic headache is typical of *migraine* and *histamine headache,* both showing the classical hemicrania; *hay fever,* with the well-known rhinitis; and *anaphylactic shock* following the injection of an offending allergen. Toxic headache is related to the use and abuse of *tobacco, coffee* and *tea, carbon monoxide,* or other poisonous inhalants; or to the effects of *uremia, diabetes, hypoglycemia, acidosis,* or *alkalosis.* Diseases of the *gastrointestinal* system may cause headache, particularly liver disease; and, finally, headaches may be due to musculo-skeletal ailments such as *Paget's disease, endocranial hyperostosis* and *calcifications,* and strain of the muscles in the back of the head.

Pain in the face may be due to ophthalmic herpes zoster, trigeminal neuralgia, erysipelas, or sinusitis. *Ophthalmic herpes zoster* is characterized by pain along branches of the ophthalmic nerve, and vesicles at the same site. *Trigeminal neuralgia* consists of relatively brief attacks of pain involving one half of the face. *Erysipelas* is known by a red rash with elevated borders, usually around the mouth or the nose; and *sinusitis,* by local pain at the site of a sinus exaggerated by certain movements of the head, possible purulent discharge, and evidence of the disturbance as checked by transillumination or X-ray.

Mouth pain can be a symptom of the following conditions. In *dentoalveolar abscess* there is a previous condition of suppurative pulpitis, the gum is locally inflammed, and edema extends to the face. *Gingivitis* may be a symptom of diabetes, leukemia, pellagra, or Vincent's angina. *Gangrenous stomatitis* is a more severe disease; there is a grayish slough of the buccal mucosa—which swells and turns red and finally black. There is marked tissue destruction, with pain that is not as severe as the tissue damage, and an intolerable fetor. *Vincent's angina* starts as a common tonsillitis or gingivitis, with redness and swelling, but ulcerates and ends in necrotic tissue. *Glossitis* may be secondary to pellagra, smoking, or tuberculosis. In *tonsillitis* or *pharyngitis* there is pain increased by swallowing, local swelling and redness, and some exudate, at times. *Herpangina* is a sort of tonsillitis with local vesicular eruption. In *scarlet fever,* similarly, a somewhat severe tonsillitis or pharyngitis occurs; but the characteristic scarlet rash makes the diagnosis. *Infectious mononucleosis* occurs when sore throat is not accompanied by evident signs of tonsillitis, but by enlarged lymph glands, particularly in the neck. *Peritonsillar* and *retropharyngeal abscesses* are noted by fluctuation in the affected areas, together with pain increased by swallowing. *Neoplasms* are not rare in the mouth.

Eye pain is mostly caused by local infections, either primary or following generalized sepsis. *Dacryocystitis* is characterized by pain and swelling over the area of the lacrimal sac. *Conjunctivitis* may direct the attention of the physician toward local diseases (iritis, iridocyclitis) or general infections of the type of the common cold, coccidioidomycosis, or leptospirosis. In *keratitis* the cornea appears infiltrated or ulcerated. *Iritis* shows congestion of the blood vessels around the cornea, miosis, swelling and change of color of the iris, and edema of the upper eyelid. In *iridocyclitis* the symptoms are the same as in iritis but more severe, and the aqueous humor in the anterior chamber is clouded and shows precipitates. *Endophthalmitis, panophthalmitis,* and *orbital cellulitis* show notable deterioration of the patient presenting ocular symptoms, as chemosis and production of pus, with suppuration limited to the retina and the uveal tract at first, then spreading to the whole eye, then finally located in the orbit. *Optic neuritis* causes pain on eye motion. But *glaucoma* is the most important cause of pain in the eye, while internal pressure increases.

Herpes zoster with ear pain involves nervous tissue from the geniculate ganglion and the facial nerve, which nerve paths give rise to pain and vesicles. *Otitis media* usually follows infections of the nasopharynx, and its symptoms are fullness of the ear, deafness with tinnitus, and swelling and redness of the ear drum. *Mastoiditis* presents pain, increased by pressure, and edema over the mastoid area. Other causes of ear pain are *furunculosis, external otalgia, trauma,* and *myringitis.*

Pain in the Neck and Back

Neck pain is frequently caused by *arthritis,* which may show several joints painful and swollen in rheumatoid arthritis, painful joints but little swelling in degenerative arthritis, and also the pain and stiffness of hypertrophic spondylitis, which usually starts in patients over 50 years of age. Another frequent cause of pain in the neck is *torticollis* or wry neck, affecting one side and noted when forced movements are induced. *Suboccipital neuralgia* centers in the back of the neck, and a sensitive point may be detected midline from the mastoid to the first cervical apophysis.

Back Pain. Back pain, in the majority of cases of *arthritis,* is a result of hypertrophic spondylitis, with aching and stiffness on motion; it is less frequently found in rheumatoid arthritis, which usually affects younger patients. *Osteoporosis* causes bone pain, most frequently in postmenopausal women, but also as a senile condition. In *myelitis* there is also nervous symptomatology, such as paresthesias or paraplegia. Severe pain in the back is the first symptom of *spinal epidural abscess,* followed by other neurological symptoms like paresis or paralysis, and fever. Other pains along the spine come from *suboccipital neuralgia* starting at the back of the neck, *muscle strain* following excessive muscular effort, *fibrositis* (mainly noted on the neck and low back, with stiffness of the regional muscles), *tumors* of the posterior mediastinum (interscapular bothersome aching), *aneurism of the aorta* (if the tumor injures the spine), and the well-known *low back pain,* which may be due to infective disease, arthritis, metabolic bone diseases, deformities of the spine or the spinal cord, muscle diseases or reactions, acute sprain, disk lesions, or trauma. The symptom of back pain is also frequently related to general infections. *Variola,* currently rare, shows a typically diagnostic backache, and patients appear very ill. The rash determines the diagnosis. In *meningitis* a stiff neck points to cerebral congestion, and backed by other neurological signs and symptoms, indicates central nervous system involvement. In *encephalitis* the symptoms are more centered in the brain itself and may present varied combinations; in these two illnesses, meningitis and encephalitis, the diagnosis depends largely on examination of the spinal fluid. *Influenza* and *para-influenza* present an acute respiratory or abdominal condition accompanied by varying pain of many muscles and extreme weakness. In *myelitis* the dominant symptoms are paresthesia, tingling, hesitation in walking, and finally paralysis. *Rickettsial diseases (typhus, Rocky Mountain spotted fever, Q fever, and trench fever)* presents pains along the spine and in the legs, but headache is frequently the most prominent complaint (see section on headache for more information). *Spinal epidural abscess* is heralded by pain in the back (aggravated by motion), fever, paresthesia, or paresis. *Tuberculosis* of the mediastinum is suggested by the "mediastinal syndrome"—rachialgia (worse on lying in bed), dysphagia, and Horner's syndrome, plus other evidence of tuberculosis, such as fever and auscultatory chest signs. In *pancreatitis* the agonizing pain will be largely centered at the left side of the epigastrium.

Pain in the Extremities

Limb pain is a very frequent complaint. *Cramps* are involuntary, extremely painful muscle contractions, which occur because of ischemia or are due to unknown causes, usually appearing during bed rest. *Osteomalacia* is not rare among the elderly, with bone pain nocturnally or after exertion. There is articular pain, of a rheumatoid type or referred to other structures, such as muscles, blood vessels, or bones. There is also a tendency to spontaneous fractures. *Rheumatic fever* usually presents pain in the large joints and possibly cardiac murmurs. *Rheumatic pains* may be due to arthritis, with swollen, tender joints, or stiffness, or to rheumatoid arthritis, in which fever is a minor symptom or does not exist.

Coccidioidomycosis, or desert rheumatism, starts with an acute pneumonic picture followed by arthritis, conjunctivitis, and erythema nodosum. *Influenza* and *para-influenza* present the acute picture of a respiratory or abdominal infection, with general muscle aches. In *dengue* (the popular name of which, "breakbone fever," gives a good indication of the painful symptomatology) the picture is headache, muscle and joint pains, fever, and rash. *Trichinosis* also presents pain over all muscles, but with edema of the eyelids, diarrhea, fever, and marked eosinophilia as well. *Osteomyelitis* starts with fever and localized pain, tenderness, and swelling. *Tuberculosis* of bones follows other infections (lungs), and starts with limitation of motion. *Phlebitis* presents signs of venous obstruction, edema, local hyperthermia, fever, tachycardia, and local tenderness along the vein; with leukocytosis and more severe symptomatology in thrombophlebitis than in phlebothrombosis. In *gangrene,* dry or moist, there are necrossed tissues and a picture of severe infection. In *gout* the great toe is most often affected, with extremely intense pain, local swelling, and redness and shining of the skin. *Colorado tick fever* patients come from the West (March to August) and show a relatively severe clinical picture of a general infection, with muscle pains. They will have a remission and then a relapse of all symptoms. In *brucellosis* the pains occur together with gastrointestinal symptoms, sweating, enlargement of lymph nodes, and a characteristically undulant fever. *Relapsing fever* also occurs in patients from the West, who have been bitten by lice or ticks, presenting pains and a rash, and also showing a remission followed by relapse. *Leptospirosis* presents a similar infective picture together with a conjunctival effusion, remission, and relapse.

Bursitis presents pain when the corresponding muscle is in motion, of sudden onset and with local exquisite tenderness over the affected bursa. *Stress myalgia* follows unaccustomed exercise. In the rare cases of *polyarteritis nodosa* there are attacks of pain in the limbs, with arthralgia, fever, and moderate hypertension. Both *acrodynia* and *erythromelalgia* show painful red hands, of a more marked chronicity in the first instance. Only the tips of the fingers, which become cyanotic or blanched, will hurt for a few minutes in *Raynaud's disease*. Necrotic tissues show *gangrene,* humid and grayish in wet gangrene, and black in the dry type. Two main types of *osteosis* (Paget's and Recklinghausen) present only mild pain and are mainly diagnosed radiologically. In *brachial neuralgia* there are pain, numbness, and weakness variably distributed along the arm; in *sciatica* the neuralgic pain extends along the posterior aspect of the leg. Other neuralgic pains follow the distribution of the affected nerves, such as the *scalenus anticus syndrome* (felt in the arm during the night and accompanied by edema), *glomus tumor* (beneath the fingernails), *crural neuralgia* (along the anterior aspect of the leg), *meralgia paresthetica* (on the outer anterior aspect of the thigh), *causalgia* (with pain and paresthesias, usually following a trauma), *polyneuritis* (as implied by the name, with pain on the area of multiple nerves), and *radiculitis* (with typical violent pains mainly in the lower limbs and lasting only a few seconds). *Tumors* of all varieties usually cause pain in the limbs. *Gout* causes typical attacks, mainly on the great toe. And, finally, abnormalities of the feet, warts, painful heel, and so on, will also cause pain.

Other Pains

The following conditions will also cause pain. *Hemorrhoids* present swollen veins in the margin of the anus. *Periarteritis nodosa* may present a clinical picture similar to that of hemorrhoids, evaluated by rectoscopy. *Perianal abscess* is diagnosed by direct examination. *Anal fistula* adds pus discharge to the local pain, which becomes more intense during defecation. *Rectal prolapse* is diagnosed when the everted mucosa is seen. *Trauma* and *foreign bodies* in the anal area are evident. *Proctitis* presents colicky or continous pain, discomfort, and rectal tenesmus, and is diagnosed by rectoscopy. *Cryptitis* and *papillitis* cause pain during and after defecation, usually accompanied by pus discharge. *Cancer* usually presents symptoms similar to those of proctitis, and is diagnosed by rectoscopic examination. *Vulvitis* and *vaginitis* present symptoms of local inflammation, usually with leukorrhea (itching more marked in the case of *atrophic* or *senile* vaginitis). *Bartholinitis* presents a painful tumor in one of the labia. *Balantis* causes pain in the glans penis or the prepuce and shows the characteristic inflammation. *Hydrocele* and *hematocele* present a mass on one side of the scrotum. In *epididymitis, orchitis,* and *orchiepidydimitis* there is an enlarged epidydimus or testicle, usually painful. In *cancer* and *other tumors* of the testes, the enlarged lump suggests the diagnosis, which is confirmed by biopsy. *Varicocele* shows the characteristic "bag of worms" in the external genitalia. In *thromboangiitis* of the spermatic vessels the symptomatology resembles an acute epidydimitis. Finally, *torsion of the pedicle of the testis* causes intense pain with a swollen and tender testis.

CHEST PAIN

Pain in the chest is a common complaint of aging people. A distinction is frequently made relative to retrosternal pain, precordial pain, or pain in the side, but a strict delimitation of each topographic location of pain is not so easy. Precordial pain (located at the area of the apex of the heart) and retrosternal pain (located somewhat to the right of the foregoing location, exactly behind the sternum) are ordinarily not distinguished from each other by the layman, and even physicians are not careful to separate the two, since both may lead to the same diagnosis.

Angina Pectoris

Pain is the principal symptom, localized substernally and possibly radiating to the left shoulder, the left arm, or the jaw. Discomfort may be felt on the right shoulder and right arm, and may also exist with little or no substernal pain. The pain lasts for only a few minutes, rarely as long as half an hour or 1 hour, but it may be felt only as retrosternal oppression. Do not forget that among the elderly the outstanding symptomatology may be only weakness and/or dyspnea, either spontaneous or after exertion. There are no signs on auscultation or evidence of abnormal pulsations. A relation might be found to previous exertion, emotion, or gastrointestinal upsets (overeating, indigestion, meteorism). Patients may or may not complain of palpitation or digestive symptoms. A diagnosed anginal episode may be the first, or one in a series. The sequence of (a) provocation, (b) angina, (c) rest or nitroglycerin administration, and (d) relief is of diagnostic importance. During the anginal attack (not after it subsides!) there is a deflexion of the isoelectric line of the electrocardiogram (EKG) at the RS-T junction, or an inversion of the T wave. Signs of previous myocardial infarctions may help to establish the diagnosis of angina. During the intervals between attacks, we repeat, there are no EKG abnormalities, in pure anginal crisis, and diagnosis may be extremely difficult. Try to rule out a hiatal hernia, aortic valve disease, or even anemia or obesity.

The acute attack will be checked first by the patient's standing still or lying down from the beginning of the attack to its end, and by the classic use of nitroglycerin, which affords relief in less than two minutes, at times accompanied by headache caused by the medication.

> Nitroglycerin, 0.5 mg, or less, sublingual tablet, to be repeated as needed.

Relief is of such a specificity that when it fails, suspicion of myocardial infarction will arise. Also, the abuse of repeated administration of nitroglycerin will lead to tolerance of the medication; and large doses can cause nitrite poisoning, with flushed face, intense headache, dizziness, initial violent heart action which diminishes shortly, faintness and muscle relaxation, irregular respiration, mydriasis, diarrhea, and final syncope and cardiorespiratory failure.

Amyl nitrite pearls are a good substitute for nitroglycerin; the amount of the gas inhaled is varied according to tolerance and activity.

> Amyl nitrite, pearls, one pearl crushed and the gas inhaled.

General measures: Patient may engage in physical activity, but at a good tolerance level, and should follow a diet poor in fats, control body weight, avoid emotional or physical stress of any kind, observe bed rest whenever necessary, and avoid toxic habits (smoking, drinking alcohol, or caffeine) and any other error in hygiene.

Other vasodilators possessing slower and longer activity may be used, though not too much is to be expected from them.

> Pentaerythrityl tetranitrate, 10 or 20 mg tablets, one every 6 hours.

> Papaverine, 150 mg slow-release capsules, one every 12 hours.

> Mannitol hexanitrate, 15 or 30 mg by mouth, every 6 to 8 hours.

> Isosorbide dinitrate, 10 mg tablets, one every 6 hours.

> Erythrityl tetranitrate, 10 or 15 mg, sublingually, every 8 hours.

> Propranolol, 10 to 30 mg, by mouth, every 8 hours. Do not withdraw this drug at a rapid rate, since to do so may worsen angina.

The treatment of any coexisting disease should be pursued, particularly a cardiopathy, which should be at least supervised by a specialist.

Myocardial Infarction

Symptoms may range from practically none to the severe typical attack in its classic form with retrosternal pain together with an agonizing fearfulness. Fever, occasionally accompanied by chills, is rare, but it may occur, especially 1 or 2 days after the initial attack. Pain, also, may be absent, but the majority of older patients will complain of a sudden retrosternal discomfort or oppression, or will appear to be disoriented and confused.

It may strike either during bed rest or after exertion. The pain may be referred to the neck, shoulder, or mandible. The type of pain in infarction is the same as in angina, with the difference that anginal pain lasts a few minutes to less than an hour, with rapid relief obtainable on administration of nitroglycerin or amyl nitrate; whereas there is little, transient, or no pain relief in infarction.

Other frequent symptoms of infarction in the elderly are dyspnea, sweating, nausea, vomiting, weakness, and symptoms of congestive heart failure. There may be edema or hepatomegalia, a fall in blood pressure (more noticeable with a previous hypertension), weak rapid pulse or, at times, a slow pulse at the beginning, and arrhythmias. The diagnosis is based on the characteristic pain or discomfort, the electrocardiographic findings of initial elevation of the S-T segment and later inversion of the T wave, and the laboratory reports of leukocytosis and elevations of serum glutamic oxaloacetic transaminase (SGOT) and lactic acid dehydrogenase (LDH).

These patients are better referred to a cardiologist in a coronary care unit. Complete rest is needed, and may be achieved by narcotic analgesics, such as morphine or meperidine.

> Morphine, 10 mg by subcutaneous injection or 5 mg intravenously, if needed; and repeat in 30 minutes. When necessary, watch for induced bradycardia or hypotension. Use 5 mg more for stronger patients.

> Meperidine, 50 mg by intravenous injection, or 100 mg subcutaneously; repeat in 30 minutes if needed.

Treatment with anticoagulants can be started using heparin and warfarin, continuing with the latter if anticoagulants are later chosen. Oxygen is needed in most instances.

> Heparin (aqueous sodium), 7000 to 12,000 units, to start, by intravenous or subcutaneous injection; to be followed by 5000 to 9000 units, every 4 hours, until warfarin starts to work (check the clotting time).

> Warfarin, 30 to 40 mg by mouth, once the first day; 10 to 20 mg, once the second day; thereafter, 5 to 10 mg (more or less, as needed), every day (check the prothrombin time).

From the beginning watch for complications and treat them as soon as they arise. A drop in blood pressure may herald shock and calls for the administration of pressor drugs by carefully monitored intravenous infusions.

> Isoproterenol hydrochlorida, 1 : 200 solution (5 mg for each ml); put up to 10 mg (better *lesser* amounts) in 500 mg of 5% glucose, for intravenous infusion.

Bradycardia below 60 beats a minute requires atropine, larger doses if rate is too slow.

Atropine, 0.5 mg by intravenous injection.

Tachycardia is treated with lidocaine, and with quinidine when the former is discontinued or reduced in amount.

Lidocaine, 100 mg in 5 ml, 2.5 to 5 ml injected intravenously; followed by an intravenous infusion at a rate of 1, 2, or 4 mg per minute.

Quinidine, 200 mg tablets, four to six a day, in three or four installments.

Quinidine, as above, is also given for auricular flutter, fibrillation, and premature beats. Digoxin is also recommended for flutter, fibrillation, and tachycardia.

Digoxin, by intravenous injection, 0.75 to 1 mg in divided doses, during a 30-minute period, followed by quinidine by mouth.

If needed, to quiet the patient, tranquilizers should also be given, such as:

Phenobarbital, 30 mg or less every 6 hours, by mouth.

Diazepam, 5 mg tablets, one every 8 hours; rarely, 10 mg per dose.

In addition to complete bed rest, give a liquid diet the first few days; a bland diet will follow; resume normal activity at a slow pace—and avoid invalidism.

Pneumonia

The incidence of pneumonia notably increases with age, and it is a disease to be mindful of in dealing with patients suffering from chronic bronchitis. A number of forms of pneumonia are defined by cause and course: *pneumococcal, Klebsiella* (more frequent among the elderly), *Hemophilus influenzae, streptococcal, staphylococcal* (usually complicating influenza), *viral, Pneumocystis carinii,* and *aspiration* pneumonia (also of great interest in advanced age), as well as *pneumonitis.* The classification of pneumonia is based on the cause, which must be determined in all instances.

Tachypnea and tachycardia usually open the clinical picture, which presents an onset less acute for older patients than with younger ones; at times there is a slow start marked by general deterioration, or worsening of a previous disease by the sudden appearance of mental confusion or intense weakness. But there may also be the classic sudden shaking chill with pain in the diseased side of the thorax, worsened by effort or movement, and at times showing hctcrotopic referral to the shoulder, the flank, or the abdomen. There may be abdominal distention, dehydration, jaundice, symptoms similar to appendicitis, or cholecystitis; also painful tachypnea, tachycardia, delirium, and convulsions. The sputum shows a diagnostic, rusty aspect. The patient tries to lie on the affected side to restrain movements, the side where the auscultatory signs will appear. These will be: at first fine râles and diminished breath sounds; second, evidence of consolidation with bronchial breathing and often a pleural friction rub. Crepitant râles on bases are common in advanced age. Coughing is extremely annoying. At a third stage, resolution, evidence of consolidation fades, and the initial fine râles reappear. Leukocytosis is a common, but not constant, finding. The X-ray picture is characteristic when fully complete. Some cases require several films before the picture is diagnostic.

Aspiration pneumonia is very frequent among elderly persons with a chronic disease (bronchitis or cardiovascular, cerebral, or renal disease) or those suffering from dysphagia, shock, immobilization, oversedation, and the like. (Do not mistake for cancer the aspiration pneumonia due to oil drops.) In pneumococcal pneumonia the sputum is first pinkish, then becomes rusty, and finally turns yellowish purulent. In *Klebsiella* pneumonia the sputum is reddish, sticky (difficult to expectorate), and mucoid in nature. In staphylococcal pneumonia the sputum is copious, purulent, or blood-streaked, with a general salmon tinge. In *Hemophilus influenzae* pneumonia, it is also bloody, with an apple-green color, and also sticky. In viral pneumonia there is a muco-purulent sputum, scanty and rarely tinged with blood. The culture (and sensitivity) obtained from examination of the sputum is frequently diagnostic and should be done in all instances early in the attack. Patients under treatment with immunosuppressive agents may present an infection with *Pneumocystis carinii*. Terminal pneumonia is frequently due to infection with *S. aureus* or *E. coli*.

The basic routine treatment for all types of pneumonia is as follows: The patient will be confined to bed, at least for the time of fever plus 2 or 3 days after defervescence, or longer for those with more severe disease. Thereafter, start a gradual return to regular activity. Proper hygiene should be maintained at all times, with good sleep. Dehydration will not be allowed; give enough fluid to maintain 1000 to 2500 ml of urine, with special care for those who perspire profusely. At the start, a liquid diet is preferable, but a normal diet will be given as soon as possible, even with some increase in calories and vitamins. A free airway must be maintained at all times, even, if needed, with suction, endotracheal tube, or tracheostomy. Bronchospasm, frequent in patients with chronic bronchitis, is relieved with aminophylline. Oxygen, preferably humidified, will be administered with a nasal tube or a tent to those with dyspnea or cyanosis, but caution will be taken not to increase hypoventilation if a previous emphysema or chronic bronchitis is present; then stimulate respiration. Be sure that there is no constipation, and there are no bedsores. Watch for thrombosis, and give anticoagulants to those with a history of such ailment. Codeine is a great help for coughing and pleuritic pain.

Codeine, 30 mg, by mouth or subcutaneous injection, every 4 to 6 hours, as needed and tolerated.

Determine the type of pneumonia, since treatment depends on proper therapy against the cause of the disease. The most common types are viral and pneumococcal. For *pneumococcal pneumonia* the starting antibiotic of choice is penicillin, but the best is the one to which the germs are sensitive. Material for sensitivity, smear, and culture should be taken first, and changes made, if necessary, to the preferable antibiotic as soon as the report is obtained. Always watch for allergic reactions to antibiotics.

Crystalline penicillin G, 300,000 to 600,000 units, every 6 hours, by intramuscular injection; also 10 million units in 24 hours by continuous intravenous infusion. After improvement, give by mouth, 300,000 to 600,000 units every 4 to 6 hours.

Alternatives for those patients sensitive to penicillin, or those who do not respond to it, may be a cephalosporin in a serious illness and sulfisoxazole, erythromycin, lincomycin, or even a tetracycline for the less severe. Try to find the specific infective agent in all instances.

Cephalothin, 500 mg to 1, by intramuscular or intravenous injection, every 4 to 6 hours.

Cephaloridine (less painful intramuscularly), same dosage and timing as for cephalothin, but do not exceed 4g a day (nephrotoxicity).

Sulfisoxazole, 4 g as initial oral dosage, followed by 1 g every 4 to 6 hours. May be given intravenously, using a 5% solution, to start with 100 mg per each kilo of body weight followed by half the amount every 3 or 4 hours.

Erythromycin, 500 mg to 1 g, every 6 hours, by mouth. In severe cases, should be given intravenously (500 mg to 1 g, every 6 hours).

Lincomycin, 500 mg, every 6 to 8 hours, by mouth; or 600 mg, intramuscularly, once or twice a day, for more severe cases.

For *Klebsiella pneumoniae* (Friedlander's bacillus) the starting antibiotic of choice is kanamycin, given alone or with cephalothin. Gentamycin can be administered in resistant infections, if the specific one is not known. A tetracycline or chloramphenicol could also be tried, when necessary.

Kanamycin, by intramuscular injection, at a dosage of 15 mg for each kilo of body weight in 24 hours, given in divided doses two or three times a day (not to exceed 1.5 g a day, and in lower amounts in patients with renal insufficiency).

Cephalothin, 500 mg to 1 g, by intramuscular or intravenous injection, every 4 to 6 hours.

Gentamycin, by intramuscular injection, at a dosage of 1 to 3 mg for each kilo of body weight in 24 hours, in three or four installments. In some instances, 5 mg per kilo of body weight a day could be given. Use lower amounts for patients with renal insufficiency.

Chloramphenicol, 50 mg for each kilo of body weight in 24 hours, in divided doses every 6 hours. Can be given either by mouth or intravenously.

Doxycycline, 100 mg by mouth, once a day, the first three doses only 12 hours apart. May also be given by injection.

For *Hemophilus influenzae pneumonia* start with ampicillin or chloramphenicol.

Ampicillin, either orally, intramuscularly, or intravenously, at a dosage of 250 to 500 mg, every 4 to 6 hours.

Chloramphenicol (see above paragraph).

For *streptococcal pneumonia* start with penicillin G, or either erythromycin or a tetracycline. Follow with the specific antibiotic according to sensitivity, as soon as possible.

Penicillin G, 300,000 to 600,000 units, by intramuscular injection, every 6 hours, or 10 million units in 24 hours by infusion (for details see above).

Erythromycin, 500 mg to 1 g, every 6 hours, by mouth (for details see above).

Doxycycline, 100 mg by mouth, starting every 12 hours the first day, and then continuing once a day.

Staphylococcal pneumonia, particularly if it follows influenza, is a serious disease which requires the specific antibiotic; but to start, use a penicillase-resistant penicillin, a cephalosporin, or nafcillin.

Oxacillin, 50 to 1500 mg, every 4 to 6 hours, by intravenous injection; or 1 g by mouth, every 6 hours. (*Note:* Reactions may occur.)

Nafcillin, 500 to 1500 mg by intravenous injection, every 4 to 6 hours.

Cephalothin, 500 mg to 1 g, every 4 to 6 hours, by intramuscular or intravenous injection.

Viral pneumonia is treated like pneumococcal pneumonia. Tetracyclines could also be used.

Doxycycline, 100 mg by mouth, starting every 12 hours the first day, and then continuing once a day.

For *P. carinii pneumonia* use pentamidine isethionate or, perhaps preferably, a mixture of trimethoprim with sulfamethoxazole.

Pentamidine isethionate, 4 mg per kilo of body weight in 24 hours, in divided doses, by intramuscular injection.

Trimethoprim, 160 mg, plus sulfamethoxazole, 100 mg in tablets, every 12 hours, for 14 days.

In *aspiration pneumonia* ampicillin is a good antibiotic for initial therapy, though a corticoid should also be given.

Ampicillin, by parenteral administration, intramuscularly or intravenously, 250 to 500 mg, every 4 to 6 hours.

Hydrocortisone, 200 mg by intramuscular injection; repeating 50 mg, also by intramuscular injection, every 6 hours, for a total of 48 hours; and then 25 mg, intramuscularly, every 6 hours for the next 48 hours.

In *terminal pneumonia,* be it a gram-negative germ, *E. coli, S. aureus,* or even a virus, treat the infection aggressively and specifically.

Special procedures are also indicated in certain forms of pneumonia. In *Klebsiella* pneumonia treatment is urgent, since the mortality of untreated patients is very high (about 80%). In *staphylococcal* pneumonia it is extremely important to use an antibiotic to which the germs are sensitive. In *aspiration* pneumonia bronchoscopic treatment by a specialist should be considered for early removal of the causative irritant. Shock and pulmonary edema are treated by adequate parenteral fluid therapy with saline or dextrose, or as indicated by the blood electrolyte findings. Additional care should be taken as symptoms appear.

50% dextrose in saline, 500 to 2000 mg, timing according to condition.

If there is an accompanying *loss of blood,* preferably whole blood or at least dextran can be given.

Compatible blood, 500 mg to start, and the same amount every 30 minutes up to a total of 2 liters, or more if needed.

Abdominal distention (usually due to swallowing air) is treated with oxygen administration and a rectal tube. Gastric dilation may require continuous suction. Neostigmine might also help.

Neostigmine methylsulfate, 1:2000 solution, inject 1 ml subcutaneously.

When aspiration pneumonia is due to oily medications (*lipoid pneumonia*) the offending substance must be immediately discontinued. The general treatment is purely symptomatic, and when large masses are formed, surgery is often required.

Legionnaires' Disease

This disease may start with an acute flu- or pneumonic-like symptomatology: elevated fever, chills, chest pain, cough, and the corresponding râles or other sounds common with lung inflammation; but the onset may be not so dramatic. X-ray films show different pictures consistent with pulmonary involvement. In some instances the bacterium-like causative germ has been isolated from pleural fluid cultures; otherwise, no cause is usually found. Death is a frequent outcome.

Lately, erythromycin has been recommended for use by these patients.

Erythromycin, 250 to 500 mg tablets, to take 250 mg every 6 hours; or 500 mg every 12 hours. Larger doses could be used for severe cases.

Lung Cancer

The clinical course of bronchogenic carcinoma in the elderly is even slower than with younger patients; and coughing is usually the main symptom. Cough is nonproductive and annoyingly persistent; but most patients will attribute it to a chronic bronchitis or to cigarette smoking; so, be extremely careful when evaluating it. Pain is a late occurrence; or it may be due to complications, such as pneumonitis, abscess, or pleurisy. Whenever unresolved clinical pictures of this kind are present, think of a bronchogenic carcinoma; particularly if there has been an episode of hemoptysis, or localized wheezes are heard in one side of the chest. Particularly among the elderly, it is not rare that the first symptom is due to a metastasis, first in the bones, or in the pleura or the brain, with local evidence in each instance. Bronchiolar carcinoma, which is not a frequent cancer, gives bilateral signs and symptoms; when a profuse watery or mucoid sputum is present, physicians should think of this disease. Cytological and radiological studies are decisive in diagnosing lung cancer. Bronchoscopy, mediastinoscopy, and needle aspiration are excellent aids, also.

Surgery presents the only possibility for a cure, if performed early enough. Palliation is obtainable with radiation and chemotherapy—which should be performed by specialists.

Lung Abscess

Most abscesses of the lung are due to a previous aspiration pneumonia, or to some form of bronchial obstruction. After 10 to 14 days of induction there are chills with fever, chest pain, and coughing, dry at first then followed by expectoration of foul-smelling purulent sputum. Sweating, pulmonary consolidation, and hemoptysis may occur with periodic outbursts. X-ray may show an initial dense shadow and thereafter a central radiolucency, perhaps with a fluid level. Other less frequent symptoms are: anemia, weight loss, and malaise. Examination of the sputum is needed, preferably obtained by suction from the trachea, for tubercle bacilli and pyogenic aerobes and anaerobes. Bronchoscopy is advised in all instances, since cancer is a frequent cause of abscess.

Treat early and vigorously to avoid the development of a chronic condition which might require surgery. Both acute and chronic conditions may respond to antibiotic therapy. Give specific and intensive therapy for 1 or 2 months. Surgery is mandatory if resolution is not obtained. Drainage of secretions will be obtained by either the adequate position in bed or by bronchoscopic aspiration. A specialist should be consulted in these cases.

Any germ may be causative, but the ones most frequently found are staphylococci, aerobic pyogens, or anaerobes. The specific antibiotic will be given in adequate amounts. In the meantime, give penicillin or erythromycin in full amounts.

> Penicillin, 600,000 units every 6 hours, by injection. Treatment is to be continued for 1 or 2 months.

> Erythromycin, 500 mg every 6 hours, for those who cannot tolerate penicillin.

Atelectasis

Following sudden obstruction of lower air passages with a foreign body or thick secretion, side pain will be the first symptom, and then dyspnea, cyanosis, fever, and shock. Objective findings will be reduced expansion of respiratory movements, and diminution of respiratory sounds. In slowly developing atelectasis, due to tumors, symptoms are minimal except for coughing. Once the obstruction is completely established, the symptoms are the same as for acute atelectasis. X-ray and bronchoscopic examination findings are essential for diagnosis: retraction of ribs and diaphragm, narrowing of intercostal spaces, airless shadow, visualization of the obstruction, and retraction of the mediastinum toward the affected side. Best results are obtained by relieving obstruction and infection, the procedure carried out by a specialist. Symptomatic treatment will be also given.

Pleurodynia and Pleuritis

In pleurodynia sudden chest pain extends over the entire lower anterior chest, even to the epigastrium, and is accompanied by fever, symptoms of upper respiratory infection (sore throat, headache, and malaise), and aches over other muscles of the body. Painful muscles may appear swollen, and they are tender on palpation.

Fibrinous pleurisy also presents a sudden side pain with fever and malaise. The pain may be mild or very intense, related to respiration and coughing. It may radiate to the neck, shoulder, or abdomen, according to the location of the pleurisy. There is a shallow tachypnea as well as a friction rub heard on auscultation (do not take for pleuritic friction rub, the one heard on auscultation of dehydrated patients). When it is secondary to tuberculosis, pneumonia, pleurodynia, pericarditis, mediastinal diseases, rheumatic fever, uremia, polyarteritis, systemic lupus erythematosus, and so on, the symptoms of the underlying disease will enrich the clinical picture. If a pleural effusion is present (serofibrinous pleurisy), the clinical picture may be either abrupt or develop gradually with pleuritic pain. Depending on the amount of fluid, the symptoms will be from mild to severe dyspnea and circulatory embarrassment with the physical findings perhaps interfering with the normal sounds heard on auscultation. The best aids to diagnosis are X-ray and collection of pleural fluid for examination when it is present.

Pain will respond in most instances to:

> Codeine, 30 mg by mouth, every 4 hours, or by intramuscular injection, every 4 hours; shift to the oral route as soon as possible. Give 60 mg by mouth when needed and tolerated.

> Meperidine, 50 mg by intramuscular injection, four to six times a day. Give 100 mg if needed and tolerated.

> Morphine, 10 mg, by subcutaneous injection, repeated and increased as needed and tolerated.

If all these measures fail to control pain, use:

> Procaine, 10% solution, up to 5 ml, by injection,

for paravertebral infiltration to block intercostal nerves.

Pneumothorax

In traumatic or secondary pneumothorax the diagnosis is easy, but it is not so easy with a spontaneous pneumothorax occurring in an apparently healthy person. Most frequently, the onset is dramatic with sharp side pain, severe dyspnea with cyanosis, and dry cough. X-ray examination and the physical signs of diminished chest movements, diminished or absent respiratory sounds, hyperresonance, and hyperinflation confirm the diagnosis.

The elderly may present signs secondary to emphysema, lung abscess, cancer, or tuberculosis. Even though the pain may be considerable, its treatment is of little consequence while the intrapleural tension is present. The simplest measure to be taken is to give oxygen therapy; also a tracheal tube with suction to clear the bronchi and expand the lung. As a last resort, surgery may be needed. Take these patients to the hospital, under morphine sedation. For cough, give codeine.

Morphine sulfate, 10 mg by subcutaneous injection.

Codeine, 30 mg, by mouth or injection.

Pulmonary Infarction

Pulmonary infarction—very frequent among the elderly—starts abruptly with fever, substernal chest pain, dyspnea, and particularly anxiety. Other evidence of right heart failure and circulatory insufficiency may be present, such as edema, tender enlarged liver, and high venous pressure. Patients frequently have cough, and often varying amounts of hemoptysis. Auscultation reveals râles, sounds of consolidation, pleural rub, and gallop rhythm or accentuation of the second pulmonary valve sound. Cyanosis and pleural effusion may occur. Some cases show only hemoptysis. The SGOT and LDH values are significant when elevated. Radiologic or EKG studies help only in a few cases. A previous venous thrombosis or atrial fibrillation helps to evaluate the origin of the thrombus, particularly from legs or pelvic veins in the obese, or after surgery, fractures or lengthy bed rest.

Treatment is emergent: administer 100% oxygen by mask, heparin, meperidine or morphine for pain and sedation, and levarterenol for shock; request help of a chest surgeon for possible embolectomy; if needed, give cardiotonics.

The second phase of treatment consists of: continued bed rest, and heparinization while patient is confined to bed, thereafter changing to oral coumarin; also, antibiotics if there is an infection, removal of pleural effusions if they are present, and continuance of a close relationship with a chest surgeon for possible intervention. Prevent infarction by avoiding prolonged bed rest.

Heparin, 10,000 units, intravenously, every 4 to 6 hours, as indicated by continuous test of clotting time done before each injection; this will be continued for about 2 days, or while the patient is in bed; thereafter, change to:

Bishydrocoumarin, 200 to 300 mg by mouth, to start, followed by 50 to 100 mg, every 24 hours; for 3 to 6 weeks; check prothrombin activity frequently.

Morphine sulfate, 10 mg, by subcutaneous injection, repeated as needed and tolerated.

Levarterenol, 4 mg in each liter of 5% glucose, intravenously, to
maintain systolic pressure at 90 mm Hg.

Aortitis and Aortic Aneurism

Since most cases of aortitis are syphilitic in origin, the disease is declining in
frequency. Nevertheless, aneurismatic aortic dilation may result from arteriosclerosis. Only symptoms due to the enlarged vessel will be noticed,
depending on the involved sites: ascending aorta—visible pulsations, systolic murmur at the aortic area, and lower blood pressure in the right arm;
aortic arch—cough, hoarseness, distended veins in the neck, edema of the
face, dyspnea, and dysphagia; descending aorta—a paucity of symptoms,
with the condition only becoming noticeable when pressure erodes the spine
or ribs. Bulging of the artery as seen in X-ray films will help in the diagnosis,
at times needing the injection of radio-opaque material.

Treatment for cases of syphilitic origin will be as for syphilis, perhaps
better with repeated courses. Surgery may be advisable for selected patients. Watch for development of cardiac failure due to left ventricular
hypertrophy caused by aortic insufficiency; and for pulmonary diseases
which may be secondary to aortic aneurisms.

Herpes Zoster

Pain, at times a very severe neuralgia, may precede the skin lesions and
seriously interfere with sleep. The lesions are similar to varicella and herpes
simplex, but are limited to only one side of the body and correspond to the
cutaneous distribution of a nerve. In many instances, an intercostal nerve is
affected, and the lesions follow along its path, on one side of the chest. The
disease may start as an ordinary infection; and pain in the head may be
conspicuous in the cases of geniculate ganglion herpes corresponding to the
distribution of the ophthalmic branch of the fifth cranial nerve: head and
forehead, around the eyes, and the maxillary area. This is not a rare occurrence in advanced age.

When needed, smears from the floor of a vesicle will show the characteristic giant epithelial cells, after staining with Giemsa's solution. Pain can be
relieved, and the disease shortened by early use of corticoids; but it is
extremely important to differentiate herpes zoster from herpes simplex, particularly when located in the ocular area, because in herpes simplex corticoids are contraindicated.

Prednisone, to start with 40 to 60 mg a day, in divided doses;
decrease slowly to smaller amounts as soon as improvement is
noted; and after 7 or 10 days of therapy, discontinuance will be
started, also at a slow pace.

Triamcinolone acetonide, 40 mg suspension, for intramuscular injection in the gluteal area as the starting medication, to afford rapid relief; then continue with prednisone as stated above.

Give other analgesics when needed.

Acetylsalicylic acid, 300 or 600 mg, in tablets, every 4 hours, preferably with meals.

Codeine, 30 to 60 mg, by mouth, every 4 to 6 hours.

Acetophenetidin, 300 mg, by mouth, every 4 to 6 hours.

Propoxyphene hydrochloride, 65 mg, by mouth, every 4 to 6 hours.

Meperidine, 50 to 100 mg by mouth, every 4 to 6 hours.

Persisting neuralgia after disappearance of skin lesions is extremely frequent among the elderly. It might respond to infiltration of the affected area with triamcinolone acetonide, or with lidocaine or procaine solutions.

Lidocaine, 2% solution, 1 to 5 ml, for each specific painful area.

Procaine, 0.5% solution; inject a total of 200 ml in some 50 to 100 different points; the procedure may be repeated once a week for a few weeks.

Any of the above-mentioned analgesics may be of good use for postherpetic pain, including meperidine, which should not be denied to a suffering older person.

Pericarditis

In acute pericarditis, fever and chills are usually, but not always present. Pain is felt substernally or in the precordial area, radiating to the shoulders or the neck. It is more or less intense, increased by some positions—recumbent or prone—and relieved by others, such as leaning forward or sitting; it is also increased by movements of coughing or respiration. It may be mistaken for myocardial infarction because of its duration. There are: tachypnea, shallow respirations (particularly if the pleura is also involved), nonproductive cough, anxiety, and weakness. On auscultation the characteristic friction rub is heard during the complete heart cycle, except occasionally, only with the first or second sounds. Pain together with the friction rub will almost give the diagnosis, which is confirmed by EKG findings (elevated ST and flattened or inverted T waves) and laboratory reports of leukocytosis and elevated erythrosedimentation rate. If effusion occurs (more than 250 ml), X-ray findings will show an enlarged heart; also the auscultation sounds will change, diminishing or even disappearing. Large effusions cause cardiac tamponade, in which the veins of the neck are notably distended, dyspnea appears or increases, pulse amplitude decreases during inspiration, pulse pressure narrows, and after some time there are enlargement of the liver, ascites, and shock.

If a causative disease is known, it should be treated appropriately (infection, rheumatic fever, and the like). Analgesics are given for pain, and barbiturates for anxiety. Corticosteroids may help, not only in rheumatic fever, but for effusions, pain, and fever.

> Codeine, 30 mg, by injection or by mouth, repeated every 4 to 6 hours, as needed. Give 60 mg if needed and tolerated.

> Meperidine, 50 mg, by injection or by mouth, repeated as needed and tolerated. May increase to 100 mg, if allowed.

> Phenobarbital, 30 mg, by mouth, every 4 to 6 hours.

> Prednisolone, to 60 mg a day, in divided doses, by mouth, for 3 to 5 days; thereafter, decrease and discontinue the drug gradually, as is feasible.

Pericardiocentesis may be life-saving when the pressure of the effusion becomes dangerous. The help of a cardiologist is necessary, the work done in a well-equipped hospital. But if there is an emergency, infiltrate with procaine 2% solution after thorough sterilization of the area; sit the patient upright on a chair; use a 16- or 18-gauge needle with a short bevel and well fitting stylet (the needle connected to rubber tubing to prevent its excessive motion and also to a well-grounded electrocardiograph); puncture 1 cm within cardiac dullness, pushing slowly inward and slightly upward; withdraw liquid slowly and avoid touching the myocardium, as warned by the EKG machine (sudden elevation of ST5).

Rib Fracture

This is not a rare accident with the elderly. Following trauma, usually a fall, there is local pain, increased with respiratory movements, and particularly by pressure over the site of the fracture or bending the rib, thus forcing the normal arch to become shorter. X-ray films may be decisive in diagnosing the fracture, though linear fractures are not easily detected.

Firm strapping of the chest with adhesive, preferably of the antiallergic type, to immobilize the affected side, is suggested; or use a rib splint.

Heterotopic Pain

Heterotopic chest pain is pain referred to the thorax that originates in other regions of the body. Its principal sources are: (1) subdiaphragmatic abscess, (2) hepatic abscess, and (3) cholecystitis. Nevertheless, some purely abdom-

inal diseases may cause thoracic pain, even though the main symptomatology will be abdominal. The physician will always be on the alert for the
possibility of these occurrences (pancreatic diseases, for instance).

In *subdiaphragmatic abscess* there is pain, or at least discomfort, in the
lower part of the chest, radiating to the shoulder, and increased by pressure
beneath the ribs and directed inward. Radiologically, elevation and immobility of the diaphragm are important signs (usually on the right). Evidence of
previous pathology (perforation of a viscus, for instance), or a previous
surgical procedure, backs the diagnosis. The treatment is surgical (drainage),
together with the administration of the specific antibiotic and the soothing of
pain.

Hepatic abscesses are usually amebic, and other symptoms of amebiasis
can be found; gradual or sudden pain in the upper right quadrant appears, is
exaggerated by motion, and radiates to the lower chest or right shoulder. If
drainage is needed, it is better to aspirate. These abscesses usually respond
to emetine given with chloroquine or to metramidazole.

Cholecystitis, either acute or chronic, presents pain in the upper right
quadrant, which is increased by pressure, and radiates to the lower part of
the chest. There is usually a history of biliary colic. Always request the
advice of a surgeon; treat with analgesics, narcotics, antacids, anticholinergics, and sedatives.

ABDOMINAL PAIN

Prostatic Diseases and Cancer

A group of characteristic symptoms suggests prostatic lesions: abnormal
micturition (frequency, urgency, and an abnormal stream), hypogastric and
perineal pain together with a sensation of pressure, symptoms of cystitis,
and other general signs, depending on the extension of the lesions. In the
case of inflammatory changes (prostatitis) there may be fever. In prostatic
adenoma the symptoms are milder (dysuria, nocturnal erections, and so on).
In prostatic cancer the symptoms are not present for long periods, though
hematuria might be among the early symptoms. Adenoma and cancer are
very frequent among the elderly; so the physician has to be continuously
suspicious.

Prostatic diseases incite perineal heaviness associated with specific urinary symptoms, as pollakiuria, dysuria, urine retention, and perhaps painful
areas in the rectum and the hypogastrium. There may be an initial urethritis,
particularly gonococcic prostatitis. In the acute form there are systemic
symptoms such as fever. Both *acute* and *chronic prostatitis* present an enlarged prostate, felt on rectal examination, intensely painful in the acute, and
very painful in the chronic form. By pressure over the gland, some pus can
be obtained from the urethra, which will serve for diagnosis.

Prostatic adenomas (benign prostatic hypertrophy) are extremely frequent in men over 50 years of age: pollakiuria occurs mainly during the night; dysuria is manifested by a difficult onset of urine and a small, irregular flow. When the adenoma grows larger, symptoms are more marked, and others appear (retention of urine and systemic symptomatology).

Prostatic cancer shows a similar symptomatology, but an adenomatous tumor is smooth and uniformly enlarged, whereas prostatic cancer is irregular, harder, and without the central sulcus, as noted by rectal palpation. The serum acid phosphatase is elevated.

Treatment for acute prostatitis: Advise bed rest, force fluids, and give cool sitz baths, together with analgesics. The basic use of specific antibiotic therapy is required.

> Papaverine hydrochloride, 150 mg, in slow-release capsules, every 12 hours.

> Codeine, 30 mg, by mouth, every 4 hours. Give 60 mg, if needed and tolerated.

> Meperidine, 500 mg, by mouth, every 4 hours. Give 100 mg, if needed and tolerated.

> Belladonna tincture, 20 to 30 drops, in a little water, repeated as needed and tolerated (dosage could be decreased or increased).

In chronic prostatitis, if pain is severe, some of the above analgesics might be used, preferably in smaller amounts (not for the acute form). Hot sitz baths and long-term antibiotic therapy are for both types of prostatitis. Surgery might be indicated; so keep in touch with the urologist.

For prostatic hypertrophy (nonmalignant), any of the above maneuvers and analgesics could be tried. For malignancies, morphine and its analogues are needed, but surgery and other specialized techniques are to be decided on by the urologist.

> Morphine sulfate, 10 mg by subcutaneous injection, as needed and tolerated; 15 mg in some instances may be given.

> Meperidine, as stated above.

Cancer should be resected in toto, or at least to relieve obstruction. Orchiectomy and estrogens at a relatively high dosage, as well as radiotherapy, may give good palliation.

> Diethylstilbestrol, 5 mg a day. Any other equivalent estrogen may be used, such as stilbestrol, 20 mg a day, to increase to 1000 mg a day if there is not adequate response.

Bladder Diseases and Cystitis

Cystitis presents pain in the hypogastrium together with frequent and urgent urination. It may be either acute or chronic, and may be associated with fever. The next diagnostic step is to disclose the causative factor: gonococcus, *Escherichia coli*, tuberculosis, cancer, or others. Pus in the two glasses used for collecting urine is suggestive of cystitis; a more accurate diagnosis with specialized urologic techniques is needed. Terminal hematuria is also a sign of cystitis, while simple hematuria suggests cancer. Bladder irritability may be suggestive of hypertrophy of the prostate. Urinary retention is frequently accompanied by pain and tenderness in the hypogastrium. The dilated, hard, full bladder, which is felt on palpation, may be one of the first symptoms of prostatic enlargement.

Treatment for a bacterial cause may be by specific antibiotic therapy or chemotherapeutic agents (rapidly excreted sulfonamides, nitrofurantoin, methenamine mandelate, etc.). The following medications also have a particularly soothing effect.

Trimethoprim, 160 mg, plus sulfamethoxazole, 800 mg, by mouth, every 12 hours, for no more than 10 or 14 days.

Methylene blue, 65 to 130 mg, by mouth, every 8 hours (warn about discoloration of urine and staining of clothes).

Phenazopyridine hydrochloride, 200 mg, by mouth, every 8 hours (warn about discoloration of urine and staining of clothes).

Sulfisoxazole, 500 mg, tablets; six to eight tablets at once, then two to four tablets every 4 to 6 hours until temperature is normal for 48 hours.

Antispasmodics are helpful for the irritated mucosa of the bladder.

Tincture of belladonna, 10 to 20 drops, in water, every 4 to 6 hours.

Atropine, 0.5 mg tablets; half or one tablet every 4 to 6 hours.

Sedatives are frequently welcomed by patients (give only small doses).

Conditions due to "neurogenic bladder" or to infection may require analgesics and other drugs to allay pain or discomfort. The remaining treatment must be by a specialist.

For injuries to the bladder give codeine or meperidine, but the urologist will complete the examination and decide on further treatment.

Codeine, 30 or 60 mg, by subcutaneous injection.

Meperidine, 100 mg, by subcutaneous injection.

Pain occurs late in cancer of the bladder, but hematuria may warn of the presence of malignancy. As usual, morphine and its analogues will be given for help. Consult a urologist.

Morphine sulfate, 10 mg, by subcutaneous injection, repeated as needed and tolerated.

Meperidine, 50 mg, by subcutaneous injection, repeated every 4 to 6 hours. Give 100 mg if needed and tolerated.

Urethral Diseases

Pain may be perineal, but it may also be hypogastric. It is mainly local and increases during micturition. Purulent secretions are always present and are noted when the patient gets out of bed in the morning.

Urethral diseases are more frequently annoying in women: urethral caruncle may cause exquisite pain; it should be treated by a specialist (fulguration, etc.), but the use of methylene blue, phenazopyridine hydrochloride, belladonna tincture, and so on, may afford temporary relief. Infections should be treated accordingly.

Gastric Cancer

This type of cancer is among the most frequent malignancies, affecting more males than females, in many instances associated with atrophic gastritis, pernicious anemia, polyps, and ulcers. Cancer of the stomach will present pain of the same type as in peptic ulcer, but aggravated by the ingestion of food. Low gastric acidity is a differential sign (not always reliable) from the high acidity found in most cases of peptic ulcer. Other symptoms: anorexia (with a special dislike for meats), vomiting with coffee-grounds appearance from blood, weight loss, and characteristic findings on X-ray films. Epigastric pain is also felt in cancer of the ascending portion of the colon.

Morphine sulfate, 5 to 10 mg, intravenously, repeated in 15 to 30 minutes. Adjust dosage as needed and tolerated. Otherwise, morphine will be used subcutaneously, or alternate drugs will be administered, instead.

Morphine sulfate, 10 mg, by subcutaneous injection, repeated as needed and tolerated. Adjust dosage, and do not spare help.

Meperidine, 500 mg, by subcutaneous injection, repeated every 4 hours, or as needed and tolerated. Adjust dosage individually.

Codeine, 30 mg, by subcutaneous injection, repeated as needed and tolerated (average: every 4 hours). Give 60 mg if needed and tolerated.

Carcinoid syndrome with abdominal pain is treated with paregoric elixir or belladonna tincture whenever it is accompanied by diarrhea.

Paregoric elixir, up to 4 ml in water, repeated every 2 hours as needed and tolerated.

Laudanum (opium tincture), 20 to 30 drops in water, repeated as needed and tolerated.

Tincture of belladonna, 10 to 30 drops in water, repeated as needed and tolerated.

For this disease, corticoids might be of help, and serotonin antagonists are useful at times. But surgery is the best resort, whenever advisable. In all these instances, always be in touch with an experienced surgeon because resection is the only known cure, if done in time. Life may be prolonged with radiotherapy or chemotherapy supervised by a specialist.

Acute Dilation of the Stomach

Patients complain of fullness of the stomach, and, after a variable time, epigastric pain and vomiting of huge amounts of liquid will suggest acute gastric dilation. If it occurs in a bedridden patient after surgery, in pneumonia, heart insufficiency, or drug addiction, the condition leads to dehydration, loss of electrolyte balance, and shock.

A Levin tube will be the first measure to institute, to empty the stomach by continuous mild suction. In most instances, this will solve the problem within 1 or 2 days. Electrolyte balance and hydration will be checked and restored by means of intravenous fluids. Nothing should be given by mouth until dilation is controlled. An intravenous catheter is needed to pass glucose in saline solution and all electrolytes needed. When dilation is under control, stop the suction, and give fluids by mouth. If the fluid passes into the duodenum, the tube can be removed.

Chronic and Acute Gastritis

Chronic gastritis of the hypertrophic type may show symptoms suggestive of peptic ulcer. The diagnosis depends on gastroscopy, biopsy, and gastric analysis, which will be done for all patients to rule out cancer.

The atrophic type is due to iron deficiency anemia or pernicious anemia; the appropriate treatment will solve the problem. For hyperchlorhydria, antacids and anticholinergics are of some help in most instances. For hypochlorhydria, administer agents capable of liberating hydrochloric acid, and treat the basic cause as well. Patients will be advised to avoid gastric irritants (alcohol, spices, salicylates, coffee, and tea). Symptomatic relief, by the use of tranquilizers and anticholinergics, may be obtained.

Glutamic acid hydrochloride, 340 mg pulvules, one to three, before meals.

Phenobarbital, up to 50 mg, every 6 to 8 hours, by mouth. Adjust dosage.

Chlorpromazine, 50 mg, by mouth, every 6 to 8 hours. Adjust dosage.

Diazepam, 2 to 5 mg, by mouth, every 4 to 6 hours. Adjust dosage.

Acute gastritis may start with epigastric pain and cramps, like chronic gastritis, but with notably more marked symptoms, including nausea, vomiting, and anorexia. The final diagnosis depends on gastroscopy and adequate follow-up procedures. It may be phlegmonous, hemorrhagic, or corrosive.

Keep the patient in bed; give nothing by mouth; sedate the patient with drugs by the parenteral route. For phlegmonous gastritis, use broad-spectrum antibiotics until the specific one is known, and be in touch with a surgeon, since operative measures are usually required. Treat hemorrhagic gastritis similarly. In corrosive gastritis, treat the corrosive action aggressively, give infusions to avoid dehydration, and perform surgery whenever advisable.

Phenobarbital sodium, 75 mg ampoules, to inject 0.5 ml, intramuscularly; increase to 1 ml if needed and tolerated.

Hyperchlorhydria

This condition will rarely incite epigastric pain, but heartburn is the main symptom, at times very burdensome for the elderly. The diagnosis depends on adequate laboratory and X-ray studies. The drug market is glutted with over-the-counter medications for hyperchlorhydria (''heartburn''), none better than the other. Some may provoke untoward effects in certain individuals. Since the essential treatment of hyperchlorhydria does not differ too much from that for peptic ulcer, we refer the reader to the corresponding paragraph.

Peptic Esophagitis and Diaphragmatic (Hiatal) Hernia

Epigastric discomfort, pain, and heartburn are the main symptoms. In esophagitis there may be only superficial ulcerative lesions, or the lesions may be locally penetrating, accompanied by bleeding. The diagnosis is made by esophagoscopy and X-ray studies (barium meal). In diaphragmatic or hiatal hernia symptoms are similar, but at times there are no symptoms at all—which is something to keep in mind because the disease increases in frequency with advancing age. Hernia symptoms are dull, postprandial retrosternal pain together with hiccough, belching with acid reflux, dysphagia, and a pain that may disappear spontaneously in a short time. Anemia may result from "occult bleeding." Ordinarily these hernias are small (few or no symptoms), but they may be large (with dyspnea, cough, and so on). This diagnosis also is made by esophagoscopy and X-ray studies (barium meal).

Treatment is practically the same in both instances: weight reduction for the obese; avoidance of tight belts or tight clothing of any kind; sleeping with the head of the bed elevated about 22 cm (10 inches); avoidance of stooping, bending, lifting heavy weights, or use of anticholinergics (which may cause gastric retention); and administration of antacids (bismuth or bicarbonate in small amounts for short treatments, or magnesium oxide with calcium carbonate for long-term therapy).

Bismuth subgallate, 500 mg or more, by mouth, every 4 to 6 hours.

Bismuth subcarbonate, 500 mg or 1 g in capsules; 300 or 600 mg, in tablets; take from 500 mg up to 4 g a day.

Sodium bicarbonate, less than half a teaspoonful, every 4 to 6 hours.

Magnesium oxide, 15 to 60 g (according to individual reaction to avoid constipation), plus calcium carbonate, the amount needed to complete 120 g; give half or one level teaspoonful in half a glass of water, every 4, 6, or 8 hours.

Peptic Ulcer (Gastric or Duodenal)

Among the elderly, symptomatology is poor in peptic ulcer; either gastric or duodenal pain is mostly of moderate degree, and only occasionally may be acute. Acuteness, together with tenderness on palpation, suggests peritoneal irritation, mainly due to a penetrating lesion. The site of the pain is extremely variable: right side, left side, retrosternal, or in the chest. Symptoms of duodenal ulcer are usually more typical. Diagnosis is based on the exacerbation of symptoms from a chronic lesion; plus heartburn, abdominal distention, salivation, anorexia, nausea, vomiting, and weight loss. Bleeding or perforation is a frequent complication in advanced age. In all instances, the diagnosis depends on X-ray examination, gastroscopy, and gastric analysis. Cancer has to be ruled out. The fibroscope is a very good diagnostic tool.

During the acute stage, bed rest (avoid sores!) is imperative for 1 to 3 weeks, and a special diet should be followed, without any sort of irritants to the gastric mucosa (alcohol, spices, and so on), or those which the patient usually does not tolerate well. The diet has to be semibland, poor in fats (including milk and cream), not too bulky, and given on a rigid, regular schedule. It is best to add preparations of vitamins and minerals to this diet. At the beginning, the diet should be almost liquid (or with small amounts of milk). Analgesics are not the best help, but some relief is afforded by judicious use of antacids and anticholinergics (parasympatholytic drugs). A mixture of magnesium oxide and calcium carbonate may be of good use.

> Magnesium oxide, 15 to 60 g, balancing the dosage individually, to avoid constipation, plus calcium carbonate (to complete a total of 120 g), to give a half or one level teaspoonful in half a glass of water, every 1 or 2 hours until resolution of the ulcer.

Calcium may induce hypercalcemia; check blood calcium regularly, every 2 to 4 weeks, particularly at the beginning of therapy. Several of the pharmaceutical specialties, and even OTC preparations, may be used by these patients.

The number one anticholinergic drug is belladonna, given alternately with its active principle, atropine. When these drugs are used keep a constant watch for glaucoma or urinary retention.

> Belladonna tincture, 10, 20, or 30 drops in water, half an hour before meals and at bedtime. The dosage will be scheduled according to effect and individual tolerance.

Other parasympatholytic (anticholinergic agents) can also be used, such as dicyclomine hydrochloride or propantheline bromide.

When surgery is required, it seems best to do a simple gastroenterostomy, if dealing with frail elderly persons.

Intestinal Colic (Gastroenteritis)

Intestinal colic, the main manifestation of acute gastroenteritis or food poisoning, follows the ingestion of a noxious substance (food, alcohol, drugs, poisons), extensive burns, uremia, or an infective disease such as dysentery or typhoid fever. Pain is intermittent, of a colicky type, accompanied by nausea or vomiting, borborygmi, flatus, and diarrhea. Malaise, prostration, distended abdomen, and muscular rigidity are usual findings. Tenderness is elicited on palpation of the lower abdomen. The patient will adopt and continuously change bizarre positions seeking alleviation. Persistent vomiting leads to alkalosis; persistent diarrhea, to acidosis. Hypokalemia (muscular weakness, leading to muscular paralysis) may occur. Symptoms should subside in 2 days in pure intestinal colic; otherwise, efforts should be made to establish a correct and complete etiologic diagnosis. There will be no leukocytosis and constipation as in surgical abdomen and infective diseases, and no signs elicited on sigmoidoscopy, like dysentery and ulcerative colitis; nor will there be accompanying symptoms of intestinal obstruction, pancreatitis, appendicitis, and others.

These frequent intestinal symptoms may be due to several different causes and will be treated according to the etiology. Paregoric elixir or the camphorated tincture of opium is a classic remedy for the intestinal irritation and diarrhea, and is given to adults in doses of from 4 to 20 cc. Doses may be repeated every 4 to 6 hours. Give sulfas or an appropriate antibiotic if a bacterial infection is involved.

> Paregoric elixir, 4 ml in water; may be repeated every 4 hours; may increase up to 10 ml if needed and tolerated.

Opium together with belladonna may even give better results. Sedation will be induced by intramuscular barbiturates.

> Paregoric elixir and belladonna tincture, equal parts or double amount of paregoric (perhaps better), 1 to 1.5 ml, every 4 to 6 hours. Adjust dosage.

> Opium, 65 mg, and belladonna, 8 mg, for one suppository; insert one every 4 hours. Adjust dosage.

> Phenobarbital sodium, 1-ml ampoules containing 75 mg; to give 0.5 or 1 ml as needed and tolerated, by intramuscular injection.

Also, anticholinergic drugs (parasympatholytics) can be useful, particularly if there is diarrhea.

> Belladonna tincture, 10 to 30 drops, every 8 hours, according to need and tolerance.

> Atropine, 0.5 mg tablets; half a tablet, every 8 hours, according to need and tolerance.

> Dicyclomine hydrochloride, 20 mg, tablets, every 6 to 8 hours. Adjust dosage.

> Isopropamide iodide, 5 mg, tablets, every 12 hours. Adjust dosage.

> Propantheline bromide, 7.5 mg, tablets, every 6 or 8 hours. Increase to 15 mg if needed and tolerated.

Keep patients on bed rest and give nothing by mouth until nausea disappears; thereafter a light diet will be allowed. Protect carefully against dehydration (5% glucose in saline or a more adequate electrolyte protection). Use the appropriate antibiotic or sulfa if there is a known infectious component.

Colitis

Recently there has been a tendency to underestimate colitis as an independent clinical entity; nevertheless, among the elderly a chronic disorder of the colonic mucosa which presents evidence of inflammation is not a rare entity.

It may be due to atheromatosis, showing the traits of an ischemic colitis; or it may have a good vascularization, with sclerotic lesions—this happens more frequently. Many of these patients will react with intense fear of foods; they also may have sudden abdominal pain and loose stools with clots of blood, with vomiting, fever, and leukocytosis. A bruit over the superior mesenteric artery is not rare. For diagnosis, rule out Crohn's disease, ulcerative colitis, or any other form of colon pathology. X-ray findings will be very helpful in the diagnosis. There may be an extensive series of indentations and pseudo-diverticulae. Since gangrene may occur, a surgeon should always be at hand.

Bed rest will be advised during acute episodes. A bland diet is given at all times, avoiding food that may stimulate peristalsis. Sedatives and anticholinergics may decrease discomfort.

> Phenobarbital, 15 to 30 mg, two or three times a day, by mouth, as needed and tolerated.

> Belladonna tincture, 10 to 15 drops, in water, three times a day.

> Paregoric, 4 ml, three or four times a day, adjusting the dose to individual needs and reactions, to control severe diarrhea.

Ulcerative Colitis

Most frequently affected are young adults, 20 to 40 years of age, who complain of attacks of bloody diarrhea accompanied by abdominal cramps of increasing severity, which become intolerable with no pause at all, including the possibility of a serious toxemia—all the above supported by evidence obtained from proctosigmoidoscopic and X-ray examination. Rarely will the disease be seen in older age groups.

Hospitalize patients in bed, and give psychotherapy together with sedatives and tranquilizers. Apply heat to the abdomen; give antispasmodics and antidiarrheals, a bland diet, vitamins, and hematinics. Intravenous infusions are needed in almost all instances. Anemia should be treated if there is severe loss of blood. Also, corticoids are to be prescribed for all patients, to be gradually decreased when symptoms subside. Chemotherapy may be carried out with salicylazosulfapyridine, a sulfa, or a parenteral antibiotic.

Surgery is frequently advisable; so keep in touch with an experienced surgeon.

> Prednisone, 5 to 10 mg, every 6 hours.

> Salicylazosulfapyridine, 500 mg, tablets; take two to three every 6 hours, in individualized dosage, which may be given more frequently.

Crohn's Disease (Regional Enteritis)

Suggestive of Crohn's disease are fever, crampy pain, and diarrhea, the discomfort starting mainly in the right iliac fossa; also malnutrition with weight loss and a frequent (one in each four patients) mass formed by the inflamed bowel. Other complications include arthritis, dermic manifestations (erythema nodosum or others), fistulae in the anorectal area, or evidence of incomplete intestinal obstruction. Tenderness and muscle rigidity, of a voluntary type, are noted on palpation. In the *diffuse* form, signs and symptoms of malnutrition predominate; in the *inflammatory* form, fever and appendicitis-like symptoms; and in the *obstructive* form, symptoms and signs of incomplete intestinal obstruction. There is also the possibility of patients with abscesses and fistulae, which increase their deterioration. X-ray examination will confirm the diagnosis.

Treatment: bed rest; good nutrition, high in calories and low in residue; mucilaginous diet to increase intestinal bulk, to prevent irritation; antidiarrheals and anticholinergics to diminish abdominal cramps; corticoids during the acute stages; antibacterials when there is abscess formation or other infective complication; and surgery in selected cases, to be discussed with a skilled surgeon. Azathioprine has been recommended for these patients.

Psyllium hydrophillic mucilloid, powder, 1 teaspoonful (about 7 g) in water; from one to three doses a day is advised. Be sure to follow each dose by a second glass of water.

Aluminum hydroxide, 300, 450, or 600 mg tablets; or in liquid form, to provide an adequate dosage every 3 or more hours.

Tincture of belladonna, 10 to 30 drops, in water, before meals and at bedtime, as tolerated.

Paregoric, 4 ml in water, every 4 hours; adjust dosage.

Prednisone, to start with 60 to 80 mg a day, in divided doses; and decrease the amount as soon as there is improvement; after 1 month the dose should be less than 10 mg a day.

Gentamycin or kanamycin, as stated for peritonitis, q.v.

Azathioprine, 50 mg, tablets, to reach a daily dose of 3 to 5 mg per kilo of body weight in 24 hours; but the dosage has to be adjusted individually, carefully watching for adverse reactions, for which reason the drug should be handled only by experts.

Typhoid Fever

Pain is not always present in typhoid fever, but may eventually reach great intensity, suggestive of peritonitis but due to acidosis. In cases of typhic perforation of the intestines, it is really alarming.

The onset is gradual; symptoms worsen day after day until a peak is reached the second week; then they recede gradually during the third week. Fever rises from 38°C (100°F) to about 39.5°C (103°F) or over; there are malaise, headache and other pains, gastrointestinal discomfort, and the characteristic stupor. Many will present bradycardia, related to temperature, with a dicrotic pulse. At the beginning there may be constipation or diarrhea, but as the disease progresses there is always an intense diarrhea ("pea-soup"). The well-known rose spots appear at about the end of the first stage of the disease (seventh to tenth day), on abdomen and chest (small macules of a pink color, which fade on pressure). Unfortunately, a large number of patients will fail to show this rash. Coincident with the rash, splenomegaly develops.

Laboratory examination will reveal leukopenia (leukocytosis in complicated cases). *Salmonella typhosa* appears in the blood during the first week or in feces or urine at the end of the third week, and the agglutination reaction (Widal) is positive during the second week. Watch always for the onset of intestinal hemorrhage, signaled by a fall of fever, rapid pulse, hypotension, and sweating; and for intestinal perforation, suggested by abrupt onset of abdominal pain and other symptoms as with hemorrhage. Also, watch for the atypical clinical picture with predominantly respiratory symptoms (pneumotyphus), urinary symptoms (resembling nephritis), or neurological symptoms (psychotic or meningitis-like syndrome). The atypical signs are not rare among the elderly.

The patient has to be isolated and kept in bed, with the urine and feces well-disinfected. Keep the patient thoroughly clean, with dehydration avoided and nutrition and electrolyte balance well-maintained. Exercise the legs to avoid thrombosis and bed sores. In cases of severe constipation use only mild laxatives; for diarrhea, use paregoric or other antidiarrheal drugs. Transfusions may be needed. Corticoids will be given to the severely ill patient, particularly one in stupor. The infection will be treated first with chloramphenicol, and ampicillin will be used as a second choice. Start antibiotics as soon as possible, to improve the prognosis. In other countries the combination of trimethoprim with sulfamethoxazole has been highly recommended.

> Chloramphenicol, 100 mg or less (according to needs and tolerance) for each kilo of body weight in 24 hours, in divided doses, every 6 hours; by mouth or intravenously. Decrease and discontinue as soon as possible.

Ampicillin, 500 mg every 4 to 6 hours; start intravenously or intramuscularly; thereafter may be given by mouth.

Peritonitis

Peritonitis is always secondary to an infection located elsewhere in the body, mainly in the adjacent organs. Symptomatology depends on the causative factor. In most instances patients will appear acutely ill, and complain of an agonizing, constant pain in the abdomen, increased with motion, which makes them stay motionless with shallow respiration to avoid moving the diaphragm. During intestinal colics the patients freely move the abdomen when breathing. To obtain diaphragmatic immobilization, the patients adopt peculiar positions with flexed legs, so as to use only thoracic respiration. This is also helped by muscle rigidity (guarding) of the abdominal wall, which is a continuous rigidity in contrast with relaxation in other colicky pains. Pain and tenderness noted on palpation may be somewhat diffuse at the beginning; thereafter they are localized at the area of the underlying infective focus (appendix, stomach, etc.). Tenderness by rebound (pressing and suddenly relieving pressure over a distant abdominal point) is frequently noted. Rectal and vaginal examinations may also reveal painful spots, or painful masses. Unless the patient goes into shock, elevated temperature is the rule, tachycardia with weak pulse is present, and chills are almost the rule. Check the pulse every 10 minutes, since it progressively increases in rate, so helping the diagnosis.

The hippocratic facies, drawn, pinched, and livid, is a characteristic of this diagnosis. The general condition seems very poor, though less severe in localized peritonitis; but the less acute or even absent pain of peritonitis with large effusion does not exclude the extreme severity of the condition. Unfortunately, elderly patients may not complain much of their symptoms, regardless of the seriousness of the disease. All pain and related symptomatology may subside if paralytic ileus ensues as a complication.

Polymorphonuclear leukocytosis is an important laboratory sign but may be less conspicuous in the elderly and in cases with severe infections, thus indicating a poorer prognosis.

The search for the underlying causative factor is fundamental to adequate treatment; at the same time it provides a good indication of the extent and character of the peritonitis.

Because peritonitis is almost always secondary to a previous disease, symptoms of the original sickness precede and accompany it. Diseases of the gastrointestinal tract are of primary importance, particularly perforations from peptic ulcers, appendicitis, cancer, and diverticulitis; diseases of the female pelvic organs are important among women, particularly infections following salpingitis, abortions, or the puerperal state.

Post-surgery and *traumatic peritonitis* are easily diagnosed, since each case follows the causative incident, although these conditions are less often seen because of the use of adequate anti-infective therapy.

Peritonitis due to infective diseases is also easily diagnosed when the corresponding symptoms are superimposed on those of pneumonia, bacteremia, typhoid fever, influenza, or other acute infection.

Peritonitis due to local diseases of the pelvis or the abdomen—abscesses (perigastric, periduodenal, subdiaphragmatic), or diseases of the gall bladder, kidney, or appendix—is another type. Infections of the lymph glands, veins, uterus, or tubes are included. The diagnosis depends on the findings in the previous condition.

Peritonitis due to abdominal diseases is perhaps the most frequently seen, and usually follows an acute abdomen. The diseases of the digestive system to be considered are: peptic ulcer (gastric or duodenal), acute cholecystitis, pancreatitis, acute appendicitis, and in the first place perforation of a viscus by peptic ulcer, acute erosive gastritis, or cholecystitis. Diseases of the urinary system are: pyelonephritis (rare occurrence), perirenal abscess, or renal carbuncle. Other diseases to be considered are: acute salpingitis, rupture of ectopic pregnancy, occlusion of the mesenteric vessels, diseases of the spleen (mainly rupture or infarction), mesenteric adenitis (rare), and torsion of cysts, organs, or pedunculated tumors.

A surgeon must be called as soon as the diagnosis is established, since no treatment but surgery is likely to check the progress of the infection. Prepare the patient with intravenous fluids and continuous gastric suction; give analgesics for pain and antibiotics against fecal flora (the specific one will be used as soon as it is known), and send him to the hospital with no delay.

Meperidine, 100 mg, by intramuscular injection, every 4 to 6 hours.

Kanamycin, 15 mg per kilo of body weight in 24 hours, in divided doses, intramuscularly, every 8 to 12 hours, not to exceed 1.5 g a day. Watch for toxic reactions.

Gentamycin, 1 to 5 mg per kilo of body weight in 24 hours, in divided doses, intramuscularly, every 8 hours. Watch for toxic reactions.

Perigastritis

Perigastritis, a sort of localized peritonitis, is usually secondary to a preceding peptic or duodenal ulcer (q.v.). A painful mass is noted in the epigastrium or a little to the right. At times a wasted patient, almost cachectic, may give the erroneous impression of cancer. Pain is continuous or may be alleviated by a change of position, and the fever is of the febricula type. The final diagnosis is made by X-ray examination.

This is a surgical problem, and should be referred to a surgeon. To allay pain an analgesic can be given. Treat the source of the intra-abdominal infection.

Codeine, 30 or 60 mg, by injection, every 4 to 6 hours.

Meperidine, 100 mg, every 4 to 6 hours, by mouth or subcutaneously.

Gentamycin or kanamycin to start; see above paragraph.

Acute Suppurative Gastritis

On the occurrence of an abrupt elevation of temperature, chills, very intense epigastric pain, dry tongue, vomiting, severe diarrhea, rigid distended abdomen painful on pressure, weak, rapid pulse, and prostration there will arise the suspicion of acute suppurative gastritis. Other forms do not show such a fulminating onset, and their symptoms are not as severe as in acute suppurative or phlegmonous gastritis. A great number of cases are diagnosed only at autopsy because of difficulties in diagnosing the disease.

An aggressive treatment with kanamycin or gentamycin will start the antibiotic regimen; the specific drug will be substituted as soon as known. The patient will be sent for surgical treatment as indicated.

Kanamycin, 15 mg per kilo of body weight in 24 hours, in divided doses, by intramuscular injection, every 8 to 12 hours, not to exceed 1.5 g daily.

Gentamycin, 5 mg per kilo of body weight in 24 hours, in divided doses by intramuscular injection, every 8 hours.

Acute Cholecystitis

This is a frequent disease among the elderly, occurring most often when there are also gall stones. Patients will present fever, chills, and very intense pain, in the right hypocondrium or the nearby epigastrium, or as heterotopic pain referred to the shoulder, particularly the right, but at times the left—and also to the right infrascapular area. Nausea, abdominal distention, and jaundice may occur. Murphy's sign becomes positive (pressure on the right hypocondrium elicits pain on deep inhalation). Muscle rigidity and splinting of respiration might be noted. X-ray examination might show the presence of stones or the obstructed duct of the gall bladder. Differentiate cholecystitis very carefully from pneumonia, peptic ulcer (particularly perforated), pancreatitis, appendicitis (particularly retrocecal), and especially myocardial infarction.

Treatment: Order bed rest and give parenteral fluids while the acute phase is active, and nasogastric suction if abdominal distention is a disturbing factor. Pain is usually relieved by papaverine and atropine; meperidine may be required, at times, but morphine should not be given. Antibiotic therapy will serve to treat the infection or an infective complication.

Papaverine, 30 mg per 10-ml ampoule, by intramuscular injection; give 1 ampoule every 3 to 4 hours, as needed and tolerated.

Atropine, 0.4 mg per ml, by intramuscular or intravenous injection, 1 or 1.5 ml, every 6 to 8 hours, as needed and tolerated.

Meperidine, 50 mg, by subcutaneous or intramuscular injection, every 4 to 6 hours; may increase to 100 mg, if needed and tolerated.

Ampicillin, 250 mg, by intravenous injection or by mouth, every 8 hours.

Doxycycline, 100 mg, daily (the first day, every 12 hours), by mouth or by injection.

At times, surgery is advisable.

Chronic Cholecystitis and Biliary Colic

Chronic cholecystitis with lithiasis is a very frequent disease of the elderly. It is possible, particularly when previous attacks have occurred, for the diagnosis to be made by the patient himself because of the location of a sudden, acute sharp pain at the right side of the upper abdomen, radiating to the back or the right shoulder or arm, or, very rarely, to the left shoulder. The pain is intermittent and possibly accompanied by nausea, vomiting, sweating, and extreme hyperactivity, ordinarily following a heavy meal. A pure biliary colic runs its course with or without moderate fever; a notable elevation of temperature, with chills, occurs only when there is some sort of infection (cholecystitis). On palpation, there is tenderness, and possibly a sensation of an enlarged tender mass in the region of the gall bladder. This tenderness is found even without a typical location of pain (heterotopic or diffuse pain, without radiation). Reflex spasm of the abdominal muscle may occur. Following the attack, jaundice and dark urine may appear. There are no urinary symptoms (dysuria and hematuria), as in renal colic; no red urine, as in porphyria; no cardiovascular symptoms, as in myocardial infarction; no increased abdominal borborygmi, as in intestinal obstruction.

Many patients will present very little symptomatology. Complications may occur as liver abscess, sclerosing cholangitis, or cancer. The symptoms that chronic cholecystitis presents are of insidious onset, but are almost always the same: namely vomiting, dyspepsia, or pain. Attacks are to be differentiated from hiatal hernia, renal ulcer, urinary infections, and colonic disorders. Do radiologic examinations.

The very severe pain of biliary colic should be controlled as soon as possible because it is really excruciating. Papaverine may suppress the spasmodic contractions of the biliary duct muscles, and thus the colic.

> Papaverine hydrochloride, 60 to 100 mg, by intramuscular injection; repeat if needed and tolerated.

Avoid morphine, as it may increase biliary spasm. In case of papaverine failure, the second choice will be meperidine.

> Meperidine, 50 mg, by intramuscular injection.

Meperidine also may increase biliary spasm. Only after the failure of both papaverine and meperidine can we use morphine (with caution because of possible increase of spasm). If no antibiotic has been chosen and in the absence of a sensitivity test, ampicillin or tetracillin can be started.

> Morphine sulfate, 10 mg, by subcutaneous injection, or intramuscularly, if preferred; repeat if needed and tolerated.

Use a nasogastric tube for suction when there is abdominal distention; provide hydration by the venous route when it seems necessary. After the colic is over, the advisability of surgery will be discussed with a specialist, particularly when dealing with patients over 70 years of age, for whom it is not always indicated. In most instances of biliary colic the disease of the ducts has an infective component; so for the prevention of later septic complications use antibiotics: the specific one is best, otherwise, a broad-spectrum drug will be used instead.

> Ampicillin, 250 mg, every 8 hours, by mouth or intravenously.

> Tetracycline, up to 500 mg every 6 hours, by mouth, or 250 mg every 6 hours, intravenously.

Most patients will require weight reduction and a diet with as little fat as possible.

Cancer of the Liver

Waiting for pain warnings will delay the diagnosis of cancer of the liver because it will occur in a deteriorating cirrhotic patient who also presents masses, or ascites, or is in a pre-comatose state. These weak, underweight, cachectic persons will show a tender enlargement of the liver, or the hard mass may be scattered, nodular, and irregular. Usually this happens with metastatic carcinomas, and an arterial murmur may be heard on auscultation of the region. Other tumors may also be detected in other areas. Arteriography and liver scanning will help in diagnosis. A liver biopsy will be decisive. Some ascitic patients will have malignant cells in the fluid.

Treatment is purely symptomatic, since chemotherapy and surgery are of little help at this time. Liver transplants are under study.

Gall Bladder and Bile Duct Carcinomas

These occur above 60 years of age, more frequently in women past 70, but are rare. Symptoms are of a nonfunctional gall bladder, and the diagnosis is made by intravenous cholangiography.

Surgery is the only treatment, though many cases are inoperable.

Subphrenic (Subdiaphragmatic) Abscess

This condition will present pain in the right flank (or low chest) with radiation to the right shoulder. Symptoms include fever with spikes and elevation and immobility of the right diaphragm with or without gas in the intestinal spaces. It is a condition mostly due to a previous surgical procedure or perforation of a neighboring organ.

Drainage of the abscess performed by a surgeon is the best choice. Analgesics will be given to allay pain, and antibiotics or sulfas to resist infection.

Codeine, 30 to 60 mg by mouth, every 4 hours.

Kanamycin, 50 mg for each kilo of body weight every 24 hours, in four installments. Watch for toxic reactions.

Gentamycin, 1 to 3 mg for each kilo of body weight every 24 hours, in three or four installments. Watch for toxic reactions.

Pancreatic Colic and Acute Pancreatitis

In both *acute* and *chronic pancreatitis,* pain is not exactly of a colicky nature; it is constant and widespread, with a principal left epigastric location. Other symptoms include weakness (because of hypokalemia), constipation with steatorrhea (rarely diarrhea), dramatic mental changes, shock, and possibly peritonitis. The pain is very severe, agonizing, constantly accompanied by shock in acute hemorrhagic pancreatitis, and without shock but with the appearance of a very ill patient in acute and chronic pancreatitis. The sudden, severe pain is exaggerated in certain positions, such as lying supine, and it may radiate to the chest (substernal), the flanks, or the back. Tenderness is elicited on pressure on the epigastrium, where some muscular rigidity is also found. Only rarely will there be no pain. Consequences of pancreatic juice spreading into the chest cavities are: pneumonia, pleural effusion, and pulmonary atelectasis, the symptoms of which diseases may play an outstanding role in the overall clinical picture. Laboratory findings may help to diagnose a pancreatic condition by elevated serum amylase (over 300 Somogyi units), leukocytosis, and roentgenographic examination.

In *pancreatic colic* there is no hard rigidity of abdominal musculature like that in peritonitis from viscus perforation, as from peptic ulcer or gall bladder. There is no radiation to the shoulder, but there is a relatively good general condition, as in biliary colic; there is no early elevation of serum glutamic oxaloacetic transaminase, as in myocardial infarction; there are no urinary symptoms (hematuria, dysuria), as in renal colic of the left kidney; there is no fecal vomiting and visible peristalsis, as in intestinal obstruction; nor is there bloody diarrhea, as in mesenteric thrombosis.

Since severe pain is the principal symptom, its treatment should be the first aim. Start with papaverine hydrochloride, which may suppress the spasm of the duct and allay pain. Meperidine will be given next, if papaverine cannot control it. If both fail, atropine will be given; only as a last resort will morphine be used, but very cautiously, since the risk of increasing the muscle spasm is greater with morphine than with meperidine. Pentazocine is also advised as a first choice.

> Papaverine hydrochloride, 60 mg, by intramuscular injection; to be increased to 100 mg and repeated if needed and tolerated.

> Pentazocine, 30 mg in each ml; inject every 4 hours, or as needed and tolerated.

> Meperidine, 50 mg, by intramuscular injection; may use 100 mg if needed and tolerated.

> Atropine, 0.4 to 0.6 mg, by subcutaneous injection.

> Morphine sulfate, 10 mg, by subcutaneous injection.

These drugs may be repeated judiciously. A nasogastric tube for continuous duodenal aspiration will counteract gastrointestinal distention. Intravenous fluids and blood, in cases of hemorrhagic pancreatitis, are a must. Peritoneal dialysis will be considered for selected cases. As complications arise, they should be treated adequately. Check for hypocalcemia and hypokalemia, and, if there is a deficiency, monitor the electrolytes; treat with calcium and potassium salts if they are needed.

> Calcium gluconate, 10% solution; inject 10 ml, every 4 hours.

> Potassium gluconate, elixir containing 20 mEq in 15 ml; give this amount two or three times a day.

In case of infection, use antibiotics: the specific one, a broad-spectrum antibiotic, or those against fecal flora.

> Tetracycline, up to 500 mg, every 6 hours, by mouth; or 250 mg, every 6 hours, by intramuscular injection.

> Ampicillin, 250 mg, every 8 hours, by mouth or intravenously.

> Kanamycin, 50 mg for each kg of body weight in 24 hours, in four installments, taking care to note any toxic reactions.

Gentamycin, 1 to 3 mg for each kg of body weight in 24 hours, in three or four installments.

Chronic Pancreatitis and Cancer of the Pancreas

There is a very similar clinical picture in both instances: pain as in acute pancreatitis, but much less severe (relieved by bending forward) and with less radiation; anorexia, weight loss, and weakness; with steatorrhea in pancreatitis and jaundice in cancer. Most patients will vomit. In pancreatitis there is usually a history of abusing alcohol. In the cases of cancer, the peak incidence occurs above 80 years of age. Both diseases must be differentiated from biliary pain and gastric ulcer; and the jaundice, from that induced by drugs, particularly tranquilizers and psychotropics. The laboratory will correlate fecal fat estimation with the size and number of fat globules in the stools as revealed microscopically. The serum amylase is not always elevated. Radiologic studies will be of some help for the diagnosis of pancreatic cancer, in which instance thrombosis, emboli, and liver enlargement may occur.

For treatment give pancreatic extracts and vitamins. Propantheline is advocated for pain, but other antispasmodics may also be used. In all instances the advisability of surgery will be discussed with an experienced surgeon.

Pancreatic extracts, several brands available.

Vitamins, several multivitamin preparations available.

Propantheline, 15 mg tablets; take one after each meal and one at bedtime.

Diverticulitis

Diverticulosis is very frequent over 60 years of age. The acute attack of diverticulitis is almost identical with an acute attack of appendicitis, but located at the left side. There may be fever, chills, nausea, vomiting, abdominal distention, constipation, or, more rarely, diarrhea, and, above all, acute pain, located at the left iliac fossa, increased by pressure and frequently accompanied by muscular rigidity. The pain may be similar to colic pains. There may be a history of diarrhea alternating with constipation. When the attack of diverticulitis is followed by abscess formation, all symptoms increase notably, and evidence of intestinal obstruction or even peritonitis is added. The location of the physical findings depends on the site of the diverticulae. The final diagnosis is made by a barium enema.

Treatment: For the acute stage prescribe bed rest, fluids and electrolytes by intravenous drip, nasogastric suction if there is vomiting or abdominal distention, antispasmodics for diarrhea and cramps, opiates for bleeding or imminent perforation, analgesics for pain, and antibiotics for the infection (try to determine and use the specific one). Always be in touch with a surgeon, since almost any complication will require surgical care (abscess, hemorrhage, perforation, obstruction).

Papaverine, 30 mg in each ml; give by intramuscular or intravenous injection, from 1 to 4 ml every 3 to 4 hours, as needed and tolerated.

Atropine, 0.4 mg, by intramuscular or intravenous injection, every 6 to 8 hours, or as needed and tolerated.

Morphine sulfate, 10 mg by subcutaneous injection, every 4 to 6 hours, or as needed and tolerated.

Meperidine, 50 mg, by subcutaneous or intramuscular injection, every 4 to 6 hours; or 100 mg if needed and tolerated.

Kanamycin, 15 mg per kilo of body weight in 24 hours, in divided doses, intramuscularly, every 8 to 12 hours, not to exceed 1.5 g a day.

Gentamycin, 2 or 3 mg per kilo of body weight in 24 hours, intramuscularly, in divided doses, every 8 hours.

Appendicitis

Many elderly patients will start appendicitis with little or no symptomatology, but the course is sometimes very severe and rapid. Other cases usually begin with acute pain, of a colicky nature, first noted in the epigastric area and aggravated by pressure over the right iliac fossa, where it locates thereafter. The skin of that area is hypersensitive; and the local muscles tend to be rigid. Fever rises slowly or not at all; nevertheless, there are tachycardia and leukocytosis. The appendicular points (McBurney, etc.) are very sensitive and may provoke a rebound pain when the pressure is exerted over a distant point, as the left iliac fossa, and suddenly released. Nausea, vomiting, anorexia, or constipation may be present. Symptoms may vary according to the anatomical location of the appendix: retrocecally or retroperitoneally, muscle rigidity will be less marked; if the appendix is in the pelvis, tenderness will be elicited almost only by rectal or vaginal examination. Good diagnostic points are the location of the pain, the increasing leukocytosis, and a moderate fever.

Consult a surgeon to remove the appendix at the earliest possible time. Maintain continuous suction through a nasogastric tube, good hydration, and electrolyte balance, and use specific antibiotics, if known, at a high dosage. Meperidine or codeine may help to control pain.

Chloramphenicol, 100 mg, or somewhat less, per kilo of body
weight in 24 hours, in divided doses, every 6 hours; dosage to be
decreased and discontinued as soon as possible, either by mouth or
intravenously.

Ampicillin, 500 mg, every 4 to 6 hours; intravenously or intramuscularly; may use oral route afterward.

Cephalothin, 500 mg to 1 g, every 6 hours; by intravenous injection
(injection into the muscle is painful, but may be done).

Meperidine, 50 mg, by intramuscular injection, repeated or increased to 100 mg as needed and tolerated.

Codeine, 30 mg, by subcutaneous injection, every 4 to 6 hours; give
60 mg if needed and tolerated.

Perforation of the Stomach

A patient with a known, or an unknown, peptic ulcer suddenly suffers an
extremely violent pain in the abdomen, exactly of the type described for
peritonitis. It happens spontaneously without any preceding effort, trauma,
or known condition that would suggest a cause for the perforation. It is
accompanied by profuse sweating, immobility, rigidity of the abdominal
wall, and a change of an initial relatively slow and full pulse into a rapid,
weak one introducing other symptoms of shock, such as low blood pressure,
collapse of veins, increased thirst, and decreased renal output. Blood-tinged
vomit is diagnostic. If there is no history of a previous ulcer, the diagnosis
becomes extremely difficult. An acute erosive gastritis will give the same
clinical picture after the total erosion of the stomach wall. A finding of air
within the abdominal cavity upon roentgenographic exploration is almost
pathognomonic.

Surgical repair must follow this diagnosis immediately. Since the pain is
extremely severe, meperidine should be given, a nasogastric tube placed for
continuous suction, and shock watched for and prevented or treated if
necessary.

Meperidine, 50 to 100 mg, by intramuscular injection, as needed
and tolerated.

In the case of erosive gastritis, efforts will be directed toward finding an
offending cause, mainly toxins, or alcohol or drugs (acetylsalicylic acid). If
there is such a causative factor, it should be totally eliminated. If pain is
intense enough, give meperidine; otherwise, give antacids by mouth. The
disease should be terminated in less than 2 days.

Sodium bicarbonate, powder, half a level teaspoonful or less, with water.

Any of the OTC preparations—without aspirin!

Intestinal Perforation

Most cases are due to typhoid fever or appendicitis. It may occur during the course of any intestinal erosive disease, when a sudden clinical picture resembling an acute peritonitis will take place, with a drop in temperature and the onset of pain, especially marked in the lower right abdomen. Perforation can also occur in cases of intestinal diverticulosis, cancer, and tuberculosis. Roentgenological examinations will disclose the presence of air in the abdominal cavity.

Once there is no doubt as to the need for an urgent operation, a surgeon will be immediately consulted. Help the patient to allay pain and apprehension; and prevent the almost inevitable infection of the peritoneum with the intestinal flora: pass a tube to protect against distention, start the administration of intravenous fluids to avoid shock, give meperidine, and begin antibacillary therapy.

Meperidine, 50 mg, by subcutaneous or intramuscular injection. There is no need to repeat.

Gentamycin, 1 to 3 mg for each kg of body weight and period of 24 hours, in divided doses. Watch for toxic reactions.

Kanamycin, 50 mg for each kg of body weight and period of 24 hours, in four installments. Watch for toxic reactions.

Perforation of the Gall Bladder

The sudden onset of the peritonitic syndrome in a patient with acute cholecystitis, particularly if symptoms of obstruction are present (jaundice), will point to the diagnosis of perforation of the gall bladder. If the perforation occurs toward a neighboring organ (liver, diaphragm, stomach), the clinical picture will be that of localized peritonitis, pancreatitis, subphrenic abscess, etc.

In general, the procedures to follow are similar to those outlined above. The help of a surgeon will be required immediately.

Gastric and Intestinal Obstruction

The clinical syndrome of acute intestinal obstruction centers around severe abdominal pain and vomiting. The syndrome varies: it is more severe with obstruction of higher portions, of an agonizing colicky type; but if the obstruction is in the colon, pain will be intermittent, of a crampy character. Vomiting of food is rapidly followed by biliary emesis; to wait for fecaloid vomiting to establish the diagnosis is an error, because of the late occurrence of this symptom. Small amounts of feces can be passed out in very low colonic obstructions; but a total suppression is the rule. Unfortunately, feces suppression is not an early symptom and not reliable as a basis for diagnosis. It occurs late in the case of high obstruction, and is not complete in the case of lower colonic obstruction. Abdominal rigidity opens the clinical picture, which changes soon, little by little, to the distended abdomen of meteorism. Pronounced epigastric distention corresponds to gastric dilatation; distention of the middle part of the abdomen points to a small intestine obstruction; obstruction of the colon produces a peripheral, horseshoe-like distention. Later, the dilatation becomes generalized. Visible peristaltic contractions may occur. Late in the course of the disease there are dehydration and an abnormal electrolytic balance.

The diagnosis of the cause of the obstruction is the second step: stricture, intussusception, volvulus, compression, impaction, etc. An early laparotomy is both diagnostic and therapeutic.

In many cases of gastric obstruction there is severe pain (and vomiting). Start giving antacids.

Sodium bicarbonate, half a level teaspoonful of powder, or less.

Any of the OTC preparations; before feedings.

A bland diet (not to be given while pain persists) together with vitamins and minerals is advisable. If it fails, a nasogastric tube for continuous suction will be placed. Watch the electrolyte concentration, and correct deficits, when present. The tube should be used as soon as the formal diagnosis of gastric obstruction is made. Surgery will be considered when the obstruction is due to an underlying peptic ulcer.

In cases of intestinal obstruction the patient will be confined to bed; surgery will be considered from the beginning, and performed as soon as the patient is ready, particularly in cases of strangulation or infarction. Pain has to be controlled immediately, since it may reach intolerable proportions.

Meperidine, 50 to 100 mg, by intramuscular injection.

Codeine, 60 mg, by intramuscular injection.

Papaverine hydrochloride, 60 to 100 mg, by intramuscular injection.

A Levin tube must be used for continuous suction, and parenteral fluids will be given, according to the electrolyte profile, particularly following vomiting. Sedatives and tranquilizers may help for tension and restlessness. Shock will be watched for, and treated from the beginning.

Rupture of the Spleen

Rupture of the spleen usually follows a traumatic injury of the organ (accident, or forceful palpation of an enlarged spleen) and will present a very intense pain at the left flank with radiation to the shoulder. There are also: symptoms of internal hemorrhage, such as hypotension and tachycardia, with or without shock; muscle rigidity; and peritonitic symptoms. These symptoms may be delayed if the capsule ruptures somewhat later after the accident.

Immediate splenectomy is mandatory. If pain is severe, meperidine may be given.

> Meperidine, 50 mg, by intramuscular injection. An additional 50 mg may be given if needed and tolerated.

Mesenteric Vascular Occlusion

Sudden, very severe pain in the abdomen, frequently accompanied by bloody stools and vomiting, suggests mesenteric occlusion due to arteriosclerosis or polyarteritis. In most instances there are a tender abdomen, vomiting, signs of internal hemorrhage, and rapidly progressive shock, and death may occur. Elderly patients who are known arteriosclerotics and show other vascular symptoms would suggest mesenteric occlusion. It also may occur following abdominal surgery.

For mesenteric vascular diseases (ischemia or occlusion), the only logical approach is surgery. Help with analgesia and anticoagulants.

> Morphine sulfate, 10 mg, by subcutaneous injection.

> Papaverine hydrochloride, 10 to 30 mg, intravenously.

> Procaine, 1.5% solution, to inject 25 ml epidurally.

> Heparin, 10,000 units parenterally, every 6 hours, the coagulation time checked to be no less than 20 minutes. At the same time start with a coumarin.

> Bishydroxycoumarin, tablets, containing 25, 50, or 100 mg; give 300 mg the first day, 200 the second, and 50 to 100 mg thereafter— prothrombin time checked to be 15 to 30% of normal (then discontinue heparin).

Aneurism of the Abdominal Aorta

This is a disease almost exclusively of the elderly. A pulsating mass may be the only symptom of aneurism; but it is not rare that there is pain in the medial segment of the abdomen, radiating to or referred to the back or the groin and pudendal parts. Also, the pulsating mass may or may not be tender on palpation; when tender, ordinarily it is fixed. Because most of these aneurisms are atherosclerotic, they are easily visualized by X-ray.

Pain is felt by many patients with aortic aneurism, particularly if it is of the dissecting type. Surgical treatment is the most rewarding therapeutic approach, and with the facilities available in some highly specialized centers, results are good. Cases with normal blood pressure may benefit from the use of propranolol.

> Propranolol hydrochloride, 20 mg, by mouth, every 6 hours; or 1 to 2 mg, by intramuscular injection, every 6 hours.

Patients with elevated blood pressure will be treated to reduce the hypertension if after study of the various factors involved, that seems likely to be of benefit.

Aneurism of the Iliac Arteries

There is a pulsating mass in either the right or the left iliac fossa, which does not suggest relationship with the digestive system. There is an intense pain radiating to the corresponding muscle.

Treatment is as for aortic aneurism.

Occlusion of the Pelvic Arteries

This starts with severe pain, numbness of the lower limbs, and lack of pulsations with changes of color of the sites, depending on the obstructed blood vessel. In case of doubt, the help of a specialist will be required.

Treatment is largely surgical. For prevention and amelioration of effects, vasodilators may be given.

> Papaverine hydrochloride, 60 to 100 mg, by intramuscular injection, every 6 hours.

> Nylidrin hydrochloride, 6 mg, tablets; one or two every 6 hours (or 8 hours).

> Nicotinic acid, 50 mg, tablets; one, two or three every 8, 12, or 24 hours.

> Isoxsuprine hydrochloride, 10 or 20 mg, tablets; one or two every 6 to 8 hours.

Cyclandelate, 200 mg, tablets, every 6 hours, before meals and at bedtime.

Pyelitis and Pyelonephritis

A differentiation between pyelitis and pyelonephritis is rarely accepted. In what could be considered a pure pyelitis there is almost always involvement of the renal tissue. Many cases are secondary to a previous infection, and only rarely is a primary infective focus known. This is the most frequent kidney disease of the aged, and in many instances it is asymptomatic. The main symptoms are: dysuria, frequent urination, turbid urine with pus, chills and fever, hypertension, and abdominal pain in the corresponding flank, with or without radiation to the pudendal parts. Pain may be dull or show acute crises; also the general symptoms may be more or less marked or even absent (in these last cases, pyuria is the only symptom). Tenderness is found in the corresponding costovertebral area. Some abdominal rigidity may be present in more acute cases, and an enlarged renal mass may be felt. Chronic cases may run prolonged courses, even for years, with occasional recrudescence of more acute symptoms with practically an asymptomatic interval between the crises. Elevated BUN is a frequent finding; pyuria is characteristic in all instances, but is not always present, in spite of the frequent bacteriuria found in elderly persons. X-ray pictures are revealing only when dilatation of the renal pelvis occurs. The disease is frequently due to urinary obstruction.

Specific antimicrobial therapy will be carried out in each case. To alleviate pain, advise bed rest, force ingestion of fluids (even give intravenous infusions whenever needed), and prescribe any of the following drugs:

Acetylsalicylic acid, 600 mg, in tablets, every 4 to 6 hours, preferably with meals.

Acetaminophen, 600 mg, by mouth, every 6 hours.

Acetophenetidin, 300 mg, by mouth, every 4 to 6 hours.

The patient should be sent to a urologist for evaluation, since surgical procedures are needed at times. Antibiotics or sulfas are needed in most instances.

Hydronephrosis

Almost always a tumor is felt on palpation, which may or may not cause discomfort, noted as dull abdominal pain; and may or may not be constantly present, since it may disappear between the pain crises (Dietl's crises). Fever and pyuria may be concomitant symptoms, particularly the latter. The diagnosis depends on the recurrence of Dietl's crises or the persistent tumor with discomfort in the corresponding flank. Radiologic studies and other urologic examinations (ureteral reflux, rapid drip from a ureteral catheter) may help in diagnosis.

Treatment of pain in cases of hydronephrosis is a very minor matter.

Codeine, 30 or 60 mg, by mouth, every 6 to 8 hours.

Papaverine hydrochloride, 150 mg, in slow-release capsules, one every 12 hours.

The patient must be referred immediately to a urologist for treatment.

Perirenal Abscess

In most instances there is dull pain in the corresponding flank; however, the pain may be either acute or absent. In the costovertebral region there is also pain, and tenderness. Muscle rigidity may be present. Fever may be present, and a mass may be palpated. When the abscess irritates the psoas muscle, there is some flexion of the leg upon the body. X-ray examination adds more diagnostic evidence (the kidney shows less mobility, and its shadow is obliterated).

Pain will be treated with analgesics of the type of codeine and with methylene blue, phenazopyridine hydrochloride, or anticholinergics.

Codeine, 60 mg, by mouth, every 4 hours.

Methylene blue, 65 or 130 mg, by mouth, every 8 hours (inform about discoloration of urine and staining of clothes).

Phenazopyridine hydrochloride, 200 mg, by mouth, every 8 hours (inform about discoloration of urine and staining of clothes).

Tincture of belladonna, 15 to 30 drops in water, every 4 to 8 hours, according to tolerance.

Atropine sulfate, 0.5 mg, tablets; half or one tablet every 8 hours, according to tolerance.

These patients should be referred immediately to a urologist. The basic treatment depends on adequate selection of the antimicrobial therapy and the indicated surgical procedures.

Kidney Abscess

This disease is also known as renal carbuncle or cortical abscess. The symptoms are identical to those of perinephritic abscess. The diagnosis is made by pyelography, showing distortion of the calyces.

Patients should be referred to the urologist at the earliest possible moment because the basic treatment here depends on adequate selection of drugs to combat the infection or to protect surgical procedures. To allay pain, on a temporary basis, use the drugs advised above for perirenal abscess.

Movable Kidney

A movable kidney will produce intermittent hydronephrotic crisis (q.v.) and the possible palpation of the movable organ. Some patients refer to dull, vague abdominal pain.

Viscerae that can be easily displaced from their normal position do need surgical fixation. At times, pain may be felt and help needed. Before injecting analgesics give a placebo. If it does not work, give the following medication:

> Meperidine, 50 mg, by subcutaneous injection; follow with same dose by mouth every 4 hours. May increase to 100 mg, if needed and tolerated.

> Morphine sulfate, 10 mg, by subcutaneous injection; or half the dose by the intravenous route, if so needed; follow with meperidine by mouth, as stated above.

Tuberculosis of the Kidney

Dull pain is very frequently felt in the corresponding flank and costovertebral region. The outstanding symptom is frequency with terminal painful dysuria. The diagnosis depends on urine cultures (should be repeated, if negative) and the X-ray film (characteristic moth-eaten areas together with irregularly narrowed and dilated ureters).

The basic care for tuberculosis of the kidney depends on a long-standing antituberculosis drug administration and performance of any form of needed surgery.

> Isoniazid, 300 mg a day, in one dose; plus

> Rifampin, 15 mg for each kilo of body weight (600 mg) a day, in one dose; plus

> Ethambutol, 15 mg for each kilo of body weight, in one dose a day; plus

> Pyridoxine, 30 mg, three times a day.

Treatment of pain is a serious problem for the patient. Use any of the following for this purpose.

Codeine, 30 to 60 mg, by mouth, as needed and tolerated, every 6 to 8 hours.

Meperidine, 50 (or 100) mg, by mouth, every 4 to 6 hours.

Propoxyphene hydrochloride, 65 mg, by mouth, every 6 hours.

Cancer of the Kidney

This cancer affects mainly males and soon metastasizes (lungs, bones, and liver). Symptoms are: dull pain in the corresponding flank, a palpable mass, hematuria (the most important symptom) that on occasion may provoke colicky pain (clot formation), and fever. Radiologic studies are essential for diagnosis (irregular shape, distortion, displacement). Surgery may be both diagnostic and curative or, at least, palliative.

As usual, chemotherapy (which is of not too much help) and surgery are the essentials of the treatment. Allaying pain is only a palliative measure.

Morphine sulfate, 10 mg, by subcutaneous injection, increased and repeated as needed and tolerated.

Meperidine, 50 mg, by subcutaneous injection, every 4 to 6 hours, increased and repeated as needed and tolerated.

Codeine, 60 mg, by subcutaneous injection, every 4 to 6 hours, as needed and tolerated.

Polycystic Kidneys

Suggestive symptoms are: pain in one or both flanks and costovertebral areas, dull and constant or of an intermittent colicky character; palpation of a tumor, sometimes giving the impression of a bunch of grapes; and hematuria. When the findings are bilateral, the diagnosis of polycystic kidneys is easier; otherwise pyelograms are needed for better accuracy. Check patients with hypertension or pyelonephritis for polycystic kidneys.

There is very little to do for polycystic kidneys, except to protect against infection, or to treat it, and to treat hypertension whenever it appears. Pain in the flanks is only episodic and not always intense enough to command special care.

Renal Lithiasis and Colic

A constant, dull pain in the corresponding flank is suggestive of lithiasis. The diagnosis depends on radiography because not all patients with renal stones suffer agonizing colic. However, they may complain of backaches, which are due to impacted stones or infection, so that the treatment has to be surgical or dependent on antimicrobial drugs.

A renal colic frequently begins with vague low back pain that soon turns into an excruciating pain felt from the corresponding costovertebral area and flank down to the corresponding side of the external genitourinary organs (penis and testis, in the male; labia majora, in the female) or even the thigh. Precordial pain is not a rarity. Sweating, vomiting, and syncopal symptoms accompany the intense pain, which appears intermittently, and remains as a less severe discomfort between attacks of colic. If the physician does not examine the patient at the beginning of the crisis, it will be prudent to determine the exact nature of the pain, since further in the course it becomes more generalized, suggesting an abdominal crisis, particularly intestinal obstruction. Typical signs and symptoms are: dysuria or anuria; hematuria, with or without small clots; chills and fever; and the expulsion of solid sediment (sand, calculus)—but, unfortunately, not all patients present these typical features. Pain is elicited on pressure over the renal area or over the ureter. Ordinarily, the clinical picture will suggest the diagnosis, which is confirmed by laboratory tests: the urinalysis shows micro- or macrohematuria and large quantities of urates or other salts; a radiologic examination might reveal a calculus, either directly or using contrast media. The diagnosis of renal colic must be completed by identifying the cause of the obstruction: lithiasis provoked by an excess of uric acid, phosphates, calcium, alkaptonuria, hypovitaminosis A, oxalates, cystine, and so on; or pyelitis, hydronephrosis, kinks or strictures of the ureter, cancer, and renal tuberculosis.

Pain is the main symptom; it is among the worst pains one can suffer, and must be controlled as soon as possible.

> Morphine sulfate, 10 mg, by intravenous or intramuscular injection; to be repeated in 10 to 15 minutes; and then every 3 to 4 hours, as needed, by subcutaneous injection.

> Meperidine, 100 mg, by intramuscular injection, repeated in 1 or 2 hours; and then every 3 or 4 hours, as needed.

The patient will be referred to a urologist for further evaluation and treatment.

Diabetic Acidosis

The patient presents a gradual onset, but as soon as symptoms of acidosis become obvious, he looks extremely ill. Symptoms of an acute abdomen may become apparent, and more than one patient has been erroneously sent to the operating room with violent abdominal pain, vomiting, meteorism, fever, and leukocytosis. A genuine "acute abdomen" may develop in a diabetic patient, but the first thought whenever this situation occurs is that a diabetic acidosis is present. Symptoms of diabetic acidosis can be detected by dry and flushed skin, dry mouth and intense thirst, hyperventilation (air hunger) with acetone odor to breath, tachycardia, weak pulse and the characteristic laboratory findings of hyperglycemia, glycosuria, and decreased CO_2 combining power of the blood plasma.

Start the specific treatment and refer the patient to a specialist in diabetes for further care. Insulin is to be given from the outset, and an intravenous infusion will be started immediately with hypotonic saline with sodium bicarbonate. The remainder of the treatment requires specialized antidiabetic techniques.

> Regular insulin, 200 to 700 units, or even somewhat more, during the first 24 hours; starting with 50 units by subcutaneous injection together with 50 units by the intravenous route, particularly if there is any sort of circulatory collapse; repeating with 75 to 100 units every hour until some benefit is obtained, and then decreasing the frequency.

Hypoglycemia

Acute abdominal pain may also be due to a hypoglycemic syndrome, generally developing after excessive injection of insulin (more rarely, spontaneously). Symptoms are moist and pale skin, hunger, shallow respirations, full and bounding pulse, tremors, and possibly convulsions. Hypoglycemia, below 60 mg per 100 cc of blood, is pathognomonic. Appendicitis or cholecystitis may be taken for hypoglycemia.

The objective of the treatment is to restore immediately the lost balance of blood sugar concentration. A patient still alert, or semialert, will take any form of sugar by mouth: a few teaspoonfuls of sugar (sucrose) or glucose (dextrose), fruit juices (better with sugar), honey, candies, and so on. Patients potentially subject to hypoglycemia (insulin users, patients with hyperinsulinism, and so forth) must always carry lumps of sugar with them. If the patient is not able to swallow, use:

> Dextrose, 23% solution, to inject intravenously, 40 to 80 ml—equivalent to 10 to 20 g of glucose.

The patient should be referred to a diabetes specialist for further treatment.

Adrenal Crisis

Acute adrenal insufficiency showing the characteristic helpless asthenia with, possibly, severe acute abdominal pain radiating to the back and/or legs, vascular collapse, and renal shutdown, might suggest gastric or intestinal perforation; but these symptoms may occur in acute overwhelming infective conditions or follow surgery, trauma, or dehydration.

As soon as the diagnosis is made, the patient will receive hydrocortisone (sodium succinate or phosphate), followed by 1000 ml of 5% glucose in isotonic saline with an additional 100 mg of hydrocortisone, given in a 2-hour period. The total 24-hour dose of hydrocortisone should reach 300 mg or more, and additional saline will be given to normalize hydration and natremia. At times, vasopressor drugs are needed; but at this point the patient will be referred to an endocrinologist for further treatment. Antiinfective agents should also be given.

Hydrocortisone, 100 mg, by rapid (30 seconds) intravenous injection.

Glucose, 5% in isotonic saline, with 100 mg hydrocortisone added, to be given within a 2-hour period.

Porphyria

Most cases of porphyria will present chronic abdominal pain. Painful abdominal crises may be of a diffuse character. Other symptoms of the disease will be also present (constipation, skin eruption, change of color of the urine, and so on).

A diet high in proteins and carbohydrates will help to control all symptoms, including pain. If it is really necessary, give codeine, meperidine, propoxyphene hydrochloride, or chlorpromazine, which may help to control pain as well as possible mental symptoms.

Heterotopic Pain

Diseases not arising directly from abdominal organs may refer pain to this section of the body. The following are the most important ones.

Pneumonia in the right inferior lobe may cause abdominal pain located at the right iliac fossa. Avoid an erroneous diagnosis of appendicitis.

Pleurisy and *pleurodynia* may act like pneumonia, but pleural symptoms are evident.

Pulmonary infarction may resemble biliary colic or occlusion of the mesenteric vessels; but intense dyspnea and bloody sputum may direct attention to the respiratory system.

Myocardial infarction may cause more abdominal than thoracic or epigastric pain. A history of anginal attacks may be helpful.

Though it is not exactly heterotopic pain, *poisoning* may cause abdominal pain when due to gas, ammonia, bismuth, caffeine, cantharides, carbon tetrachloride, colchicin, digitalis, formaldehyde, benzene, phosphorus, thallium salts, or turpentine oil.

HEAD AND FACE PAIN

Pain in the head is the most common of all pains, and is one frequently suffered and complained of by the elderly. In many instances there will be a hazy distinction between headache and confusion because the latter may be directly derived from the pain; nor will there be a clear delimitation from the site of origin, since there are patients with glaucoma who complain of headache rather than the excruciating pain in the eye. Thus headache is not a reliable symptom to construct a diagnosis on, particularly among frail and deteriorated patients of advanced age. Nevertheless, in all instances pain serves as an important clue to the onset of a disease, whether it be headache or any other pain.

Common Cold

Headache is a frequent complaint, together with rhinitis, coughing, and general malaise. Care should be taken not to mistake a common cold for other disease also accompanied by rhinitis, particularly if sore throat is present, or if other symptoms appear; it is important to rule out influenza among the elderly because of the frequent and serious pneumonic complication.

Rest is important, liquids should be taken in strict balance with the liquids lost, and drugs are to be given only when needed. When headache becomes intolerable, acetylsalicylic acid may be tried; give codeine if coughing increases the headache. A combination of codeine and acetylsalicylic acid gives better results than either drug used alone.

> Codeine, 15, 30, or 60 mg, by mouth, every 4 to 6 hours, as needed and tolerated.

> Acetylsalicylic acid, 500 or 600 mg, in tablets, every 4 to 6 hours, preferably with meals.

Influenza (Grippe) and Similar Diseases

Sudden elevation of temperature, chills (may be absent), headache or confusion, muscular pains, intense malaise, and weakness (very important) are characteristic. Respiratory involvement is usual. During an epidemic outburst, there is little diagnostic doubt: a common cold will show few or no constitutional symptoms; bacterial diseases will present leukocytosis instead of the influenza leukopenia. A final diagnosis is made by isolation of the virus from garglings (early stages) or serum tests (acute phase and convalescence).

The parainfluenza viruses provoke a disease clinically identical to influenza, differentiated only by laboratory tests (complement-fixation, hemagglutination-inhibition, and so on). The adenoviruses also cause syndromes with a similar clinical picture.

There is no specific therapy, but the severity of most of the symptoms requires help. Patients will be kept in bed, carefully watched for complication (pneumonia), and treated symptomatically. Because of the presence of fever and headache, acetylsalicylic acid should be given first. When patients start to cough, codeine should be added to the above medication, but preferably at a low dosage. Nasal obstruction may help to increase, or at least maintain, the headache: give ephedrine or phenylephrine. For type A influenza, amantadine is recommended by some physicians; when there is nervous involvement, use dexamethasone with mannitol by intravenous injection (or peritoneal dialysis).

Acetylsalicylic acid, 600 mg, in tablets, every 4 hours, preferably with meals. If needed, give the medication more frequently, to obtain effective analgesic and antithermic results.

Codeine, 15 to 30 mg, by mouth, every 4 or 6 hours.

Ephedrine, 1, 2, or 3% solution; instill a few drops (or use a spray) into each nostril, repeating every 4 or 5 hours.

Phenylephrine, 0.1 or 0.5% solution; instill a few drops (or use a spray) into each nostril, every 4 or 5 hours.

Amantadine, 100 mg capsules, to take one every 12 hours during 10 days; when used as a preventive measure, to be taken for up to 90 days, if so needed. Watch for central nervous system reactions.

Dengue

Dengue presents a sudden onset, with severe pain in the joints and muscles ("breakbone fever"), frequently mistaken for influenza. In the first stage of the disease, there is a transient flushing or frank eruption of a pale pink macular rash in the face, followed by a remission of symptoms, lasting for 3 or 4 days; then there is a second stage, when the eruption is more marked and similar to measles or scarlet fever. Superficial lymph nodes may be enlarged, and splenomegaly noted. Laboratory tests are made for leukopenia, mouse antibody neutralization, hemagglutination, and virus isolation. Also, avoid confusion with yellow fever, typhus, malaria, or pappataci (sandfly) fever.

There is no specific therapy. For the headache, an ice cap is always helpful. The most important drugs to consider here are codeine and acetylsalicylic acid; but in some instances other salicylates might also be effective. If the patient falls into shock, expand blood volume with dextran or an infusion correcting electrolyte imbalance, when present.

Colorado Tick Fever

Patients are found in, or have come from, the western part of the United States. The disease occurs mainly from March to August. Onset is with sudden fever, chills, and severe pain in the head and muscles. Accompanying symptoms are photophobia, nausea (with or without vomiting), anorexia, and a possible mild nonspecific rash. Diagnosis is reinforced when these symptoms reappear following a remission of 2 or 3 days. There is leukopenia with a shift to the left. The virus may be inoculated into laboratory animals and identified.

There is no specific therapy. Acetylsalicylic acid ordinarily controls pains, and perhaps other symptoms of the disease. Other salicylates and coal-tar derivatives may also be effective.

Septicemia (Bacteremia)

Symptoms are fever, commonly of the hectic type (septic fever), mostly with chills and headache, skin rashes (often purpuric or petechial), and a previous known infection. The disease is suspected when there is no improvement in due time from such an infection, or if, instead, there is an exacerbation of septic symptoms (the site of origin may be unknown). It usually follows erysipelas, tonsillitis, otitis, urinary sepsis, tooth abscess, and so forth. In turn, bacteremia may produce new focal sites of infection, particularly in the heart (check continuously for early endocarditis); watch for signs from the central nervous system (mainly meningitis), vascular system (thrombophlebitis), lungs (abscess, pneumonia, infarct), skeletal system (osteomyelitis), and so on. In most instances blood cultures will establish the diagnosis. Gram-negative infections may lead to severe clinical pictures ending in shock.

The basic treatment depends on the offending infecting organism and its sensitivity to antibiotics, which will be administered accordingly. It will not be forgotten that control of the infection will result in control of the symptoms. Codeine is the first choice for aches and pains. Other analgesics, or combinations of analgesics, can be used whenever needed. When the offending organism is not known, start with a broad-spectrum antibiotic or give nafcillin, oxacyllin, lincomycin, or any other similar drug. Gram-negative infections are treated with gentamycin, either alone or with penicillin or ampicillin (also a cephalosporin). In case of shock use blood expanders and correct acidosis.

> Doxycycline, 100 mg by injection, every 12 hours the first day; once a day thereafter. May use 200 mg for very severe infections.

> Nafcillin, 6 to 8 g in 24 hours, in divided doses, every 4 to 6 hours, by intramuscular injection.

Lincomycin, 600 mg by intramuscular injection, every 12 to 24 hours.

Gentamycin, at a dosage of 5 mg for each kilo of body weight in 24 hours, by intramuscular injection divided into three installments.

Penicillin, 600,000 units or more, by injection, repeating as needed.

Ampicillin, 200 to 300 mg for each kilo of body weight, by intravenous injection, in four installments.

Dextran or electrolyte solutions, by intravenous infusion.

Scarlet Fever (Scarlatina)

This disease starts with fever, headache, vomiting, sore throat, malaise, flushing of the face (with a pale area around the mouth), and the so-called strawberry tongue. The red exanthem starts on the neck and the chest, disappears under pressure (digital or with a glass slide), presents dark red lines (Pastia's lines) in the skin creases, and covers the whole body in 2 or 3 days. The red rash may be slight or even absent; then rely on other symptoms to make the diagnosis. Desquamation (even without detected exanthem) starts during convalescence, is more marked in the palms and soles, and may serve for a retrospective diagnosis. The detection of a group A streptococcus with erythrogenic toxin will solve the problem in doubtful cases.

Antibiotic therapy, with penicillin, is specific for scarlet fever. Other symptoms will be treated as they arise.

Crystalline penicillin G, 600,000 units every 6 hours by intramuscular injection; or 10 million units in 24 hours by continuous infusion. After improvement, give 600,000 units every 6 hours, by mouth. Adjust dosage to the severity of the disease. If there is intolerance to penicillin, use equivalent antibiotics.

Typhoid Fever and Other Salmonelloses

All salmonelloses, including typhoid fever, may show such a mild symptomatology that they might run their course as a mild gastrointestinal upset or be totally unrecognized. When fever is present, showing toxemia, headache becomes a part of the clinical picture. Either diarrhea or constipation may be present, as well as a relatively slow dicrotic pulse. If severity of the symptoms (particularly fever) steadily increases, the diagnosis will be suspected. The fever reaches a peak in about 1 week, is sustained for 1 or 2 weeks, and gradually decreases in about 1 week (but any type of fever may occur!); the typical typhoid roseola (rose spots), which disappears under pressure, is found on the abdomen and chest at about the second week. The diagnosis is confirmed by finding typhoid bacilli or positive laboratory tests.

Antibiotic treatment is specific, particularly with chloramphenicol or ampicillin. For headache, use codeine injections. Acetylsalicylic acid and similar drugs should not be given because of gastrointestinal irritation. Analgesics with narcotic properties should be avoided or given guardedly because of the danger of increasing the stuporous condition of many of these patients.

> Chloramphenicol, 1 g by mouth, every 6 hours during the febrile stage; thereafter, half the amount for 2 weeks.

> Ampicillin, 100 mg for each kilo of body weight in 24 hours, divided into six doses (every 4 hours). Can be given orally.

> Codeine, 30 to 60 mg, by subcutaneous injection, every 4 or 6 hours, as needed and tolerated.

Other salmonelloses will be detected only by laboratory procedures, since the clinical pictures are identical with typhoid fever. The therapeutic advice will be similar to that for typhoid fever, with less emphasis on antibiotic therapy, which may prolong the carrier state.

Shigellosis

Dysentery was a very common occurrence years ago, but now is rarer, though it still can affect patients with no respect to age. With debilitated and frail elderly persons, it usually starts abruptly, with cramps in the lower abdomen, diarrhea frequently tinged with blood and filled with mucus, more or less elevated temperature, headache, progressive cloudiness of the sensorium, lethargy, convulsions, and other symptoms indicating debilitating dehydration. On palpation, the abdomen is tender and irritated with some areas of ulceration when checked by sigmoidoscopy. Diagnosis is achieved by identification of the *Shigella* in stool cultures. Differentiate it from amebic dysentery, salmonellosis, and ulcerative colitis. A large number of cases will show only a milder symptomatology, warranting a favorable prognosis.

Whenever possible, avoid the use of antibiotic therapy; nevertheless, if needed, ampicillin is the drug of choice.

> Ampicillin, 100 mg for each kilo of body weight in 24 hours, divided into four doses, given for about 1 week, terminated as soon as the symptoms abate.

The main care with these patients is to avoid dehydration, preferably with continued infusions, monitoring electrolytes. Keep them isolated in bed; give a light, fluid diet, but only after a few hours of absolute rest to the bowel. For cramps, give paregoric or belladonna. Disinfect stools carefully.

Paregoric, 4 or 5 ml in water, every 4 hours.

Tincture of belladonna, 10 to 20 drops in water, as tolerated and needed.

Brucellosis (Malta Fever, Undulant Fever)

Headache occurs during the acute stage of the disease; the phases of elevated temperature are heralded by cephalalgia. Sweating, generalized aches, weakness, anorexia, lymphadenopathy, splenomegaly, and chilly sensations might suggest the diagnosis. Orchitis is not prevalent in the United States as in other countries.

A tetracycline, either alone or, for seriously ill patients, in combination with streptomycin, is a wise choice. For the treatment of headache, codeine, acetylsalicylic acid, or a combination of both can be administered. In patients with severe toxemia, the adjunctive use of a corticoid might be of help, but never given for more than 3 or 4 days.

Tetracycline, 500 mg, every 6 hours, by mouth, avoiding milk and antacids.

Streptomycin, 500 to 1000 mg, every 12 hours, by injection. Watch for injury to the 8th cranial nerve.

Codeine, 30 or 60 mg, by subcutaneous injection to start, followed by the same dosage and timing after some effect is obtained. Give every 4 to 6 hours, according to results and tolerance.

Acetylsalicylic acid, 300 mg, plus codeine, 30 mg, in capsules or tablets, one or two every 4 to 6 hours, according to response.

Prednisone, 20 mg, every 8 hours, by mouth.

Hydrocortisone, 50 to 100 mg, every 8 hours, by mouth.

Meningitis

A meningitic reaction is suggested by a complex of fever, headache, possibly with backache, confusion, seizures, and stiff neck, which calls for an immediate examination of the spinal fluid, usually following a known infection (otitis, mastoiditis, sinusitis, brain abscess, generalized infections). In bacterial meningitis the course is very rapid, to lethargy and coma. Tuberculous meningitis is less acute, with the initial focus almost always known. In viral meningitis the course is also rapid. Diagnosis depends on the examination of the spinal fluid: bacterial meningitis with increased pressure, increased number of cells and elevated proteins, decreased glucose, and possibly identifiable bacteria; viral meningitis with fewer cells, the amount of glucose normal, and isolation of the virus possible. A fully developed clinical picture of meningitis will also include contracture of other muscles besides those of the neck, such as opisthotonos, strabismus, and flexion of the legs; paralysis of the pupils, limbs, and face; itching of the nose, vomiting, constipation, generalized hypersensitivity, hyperacusis and photophobia, bradycardia, and delirium. Unfortunately, this clear-cut picture is not always present. The well-known meningitic reflexes will be looked for: Babinski's (extension of toe on plantar irritation), Brudzinski's (legs are flexed when the neck is forced to flexion), Kernig's (the above-flexed patients resist attempts to restore them to extension). The elderly frequently react with seizures, cerebral edema, and shock.

Isolate patients on bed rest, and observe all regular hospital measures for acute cases, as hydration, electrolyte balance, elimination, and nutrition. The specific antibiotic will be promptly given, in full amounts. For meningococcus, pneumococcus, streptococcus, *Proteus,* or *H. influenzae* infections, give ampicillin; for staphylococcus, methicillin; for *E. coli,* kanamycin; for *Pseudomonas,* polymyxin B. For pain use corticoids as soon as possible; analgesics will be only a second choice. For seizures give diazepam; for cerebral edema, mannitol. Treat shock as usual (blood expander, electrolyte infusions, and so forth).

> Ampicillin, 200 mg for each kilo of body weight in 24 hours, by intravenous injection of fractional doses, every 3 or 4 hours.

> Methicillin, 100 to 200 mg for each kilo of body weight in 24 hours, by intramuscular injection of fractional doses, every 4 hours.

> Kanamycin, 15 mg per kilo in 24 hours, intramuscularly, in two or three installments (not to surpass 1.5 g per day).

> Polymyxin B, not to surpass 200 mg per day; 1.5 to 2.5 mg per kilo in 24 hours, in three intramuscular injections (additional 2.5 mg a day intrathecally, for no more than 3 days, could be a useful boost).

> Cortisone, 24 mg, by mouth, four or five times a day, according to needs and tolerance.

> Diazepam, 5 mg, every 4 to 6 hours.

> Mannitol solution, to inject 2.5 g for each kilo of body weight, by intravenous infusion.

Encephalitis

Symptoms may begin suddenly or in steps, with cephalalgia, malaise, insomnia, chills, fever, and others, depending on the area most affected. Convulsions, myoclonus, hemiplegia, ocular paralysis, and medullar or cerebellar symptoms may occur when the cortex is affected; backache is commonly due to muscle spasm or irritation of the spine. The general picture may be one so mild as to be unrecognized (as is found in most cases of St. Louis encephalitis) or be extremely severe (as in Eastern encephalitis, with hyperpyrexia, convulsions, and coma). Among the diagnostic possibilities are also the Japanese B, the Murray Valley, and the arthropod-borne encephalitides. Other intracranial complications to be looked for are due to systemic infections, such as brucellosis, measles, influenza, mumps, poliomyelitis, vaccinia, and varicella; or to parkinsonism, hemorrhage, drug therapy, or perhaps other causes.

When the infectious agent is known, etiological treatment can be carried out in many instances. Independent of this attack on the cause, relief of the burdensome headache is imperative. Corticoids may be of help, particularly when given early in the disease, and especially if it is of viral origin. Excessive intracranial pressure causing headache may be lowered with mannitol or urea–invert sugar preparation given by infusion. The first analgesics to be used should be either acetylsalicylic acid, codeine, or a combination of the two. If insufficient relief is obtained by the above medication, meperidine could be tried, but not for too long a time.

> Prednisone, 5 to 20 mg, every 6 hours, according to needs and results.

> Acetylsalicylic acid, 300 mg, plus codeine, 30 mg, in capsules or tablets, two every 4 hours.

> Meperidine, 50 to 100 mg, by intramuscular injection or by mouth, every 4 hours.

> Mannitol solution, by intravenous infusion, giving 2.5 g for each kilo of body weight.

Glanders (Farcy)

Glanders has an abrupt and violent beginning: high fever, chills, headache, and prostration, which follow exposure to horses. Often a painful ulcer is the point of initial infection. The diagnosis is established by laboratory procedures. There is also a chronic form with painful ulcers and repetitious fulminating recurrences.

Specific therapy is to be prescribed whenever possible: the soluble sulfonamides (sulfadiazine) continued for at least 20 days; or chloramphenicol or chlortetracycline for at least 2 weeks. In severe cases the association of two antibiotics or an antibiotic and a sulfa is better. The disease does not respond to penicillin or streptomycin. When cephalalgia is troublesome, use acetylsalicylic acid.

Sulfadiazine, tablets, 0.5 g, four to twelve tablets daily.

Chlortetracycline, tablets, 250 mg, four tablets daily, between meals.

Chloramphenicol, tablets, 250 mg, four tablets daily, between meals.

Tularemia

Tularemia in all its forms is characterized by a febrile attack, with headache, other symptoms of infection, extreme weakness, chills, and sweating. At the site of inoculation, a papule appears; it rapidly ulcerates, and lymphedema develops (which may suppurate and drain). An atypical pneumonia follows. Identification of the causative *Pasteurella* gives the diagnosis.

Streptomycin is the first choice; a tetracycline or chloramphenicol, the second. Headache may become burdensome, at times, even to the point of requiring injections of codeine.

Streptomycin, 500 to 1000 mg every 12 hours, by injection. Watch for injury to the 8th cranial nerve.

Tetracycline, not to excede 500 mg every 6 hours, by slow intravenous injection; but it will be given orally as soon as possible, 500 mg every 6 hours (avoid milk and antacids).

Codeine, 30 or 60 mg, subcutaneously, every 3 or 4 hours, as needed and tolerated. Same dosage could be given by the oral route, either from the beginning of therapy or after obtaining some relief from the use of injections.

Relapsing Fever (Recurrent Fever)

After the first attack of fever and sweating, an intense headache will occur. The clinical picture subsides by crisis, and after a period of remission reappears. Additional relapses may occur, at longer intervals. The diagnosis depends on the finding of *Borrelia* in peripheral blood.

A tetracycline or chloramphenicol has to be given only during the attacks, *never* at the end of any relapsing attack or during the intervals, because of the possibility of provoking a serious Herxheimer reaction. The attacks are accompanied by a characteristic severe headache, which fortunately responds very well to the administration of codeine.

Tetracycline, 500 mg, every 6 hours, by mouth. Avoid milk and antacids.

Codeine, 30 or 60 mg, preferably by mouth, every 4 to 6 hours. If needed, subcutaneous injections may be given, with the same amount of medication and timing.

The Leptospiroses (Weil's Disease and Others)

Symptoms are headache, photophobia, fever, and generalized algias, particularly in arms and calves. Conjunctival hemorrhage is almost characteristic.

Penicillin or a tetracycline is recommended, but not always effective. The headache usually responds to the administration of acetylsalicylic acid, codeine, or similar analgesics.

Rickettsial Diseases (Typhus, Rocky Mountain Spotted Fever, Q Fever, Trench Fever)

Headache of a severe character is a paramount symptom in all rickettsial diseases. Elevated temperature and a rash are also common to most of them. Diagnosis depends on laboratory tests. The rash of the typhus group begins on the back and chest; that of Rocky Mountain spotted fever, on the flexor surfaces of wrists, ankles, and back; that of trench fever, on chest and abdomen. In Q fever, a rash may be present or, possibly, respiratory symptoms.

Chloramphenicol and the tetracyclines are the first choice. For the treatment of cephalalgia do not give acetylsalicylic acid, since it increases the already profuse sweating of these patients, thus risking dehydration. Meperidine can be tried, but with caution, because in severe cases it may depress the respiratory centers. The first choice is codeine.

> Chloramphenicol, 50 mg for each kilo of body weight in 24 hours, divided into four installments; start by intravenous injection; as soon as possible decrease dosage and resort to oral administration. Higher dosages may be given if needed.
>
> Codeine, 30 to 60 mg, by subcutaneous injection or by mouth, every 4 to 6 hours, as needed and tolerated.

Syphilis

All clinical forms of syphilis may present headache: in cerebral syphilis it may be excruciating; its intense pain may also be found in gummata, osteitis, arteritis, and meningitis, as well as in tabes and general paresis. Headache may be present during the secondary or the late stages of the disease; or may be a symptom heralding an otherwise ignored syphilitic infection. The clinical history and laboratory tests will give the final diagnosis.

Antibiotic therapy is mandatory. Symptomatic treatment for cephalalgia will be carried out, whenever needed, with acetylsalicylic acid, codeine, or any other acceptable analgesic.

Lymphogranuloma Venereum

The disease is suggested by the presence of a shallow ulceration and the development of a well-marked regional lymphadenopathy, particularly in the inguinal area. A complicating meningitis should be considered: in this rare complication cephalalgia is an indicative sign.

Chemotherapy, with a sulfa drug, alone or with tetracycline, is effective treatment. Headache is rarely severe, and should respond satisfactorily to any antalgic.

Sulfadiazine, tablets, 0.5 g, two at once, then one four times a day.

Malaria

Headache, usually severe, accompanies the hot stage of malaria, when flushing of the face and elevation of temperature take place. The sequence "chilling, heating, and sweating" is almost pathognomonic. Other details and the detection of the parasite in blood smears will indicate the type involved.

Chloroquine and chlorguanide are usually considered the first choice. Quinine is still an important drug, not only as an antimalarial, but also as an analgesic and antipyretic. When the preferred antimalarials are not effective or available, quinine might be used instead.

Chloroquine, 1 g, to start, followed by 500 mg after 8 hours, and then 500 mg daily, for 4 days (for all plasmodia).

Amodiaquine, 600 mg, or even up to 1 g, to start, followed by 400 mg daily, for 2 days (for *P. vivax* and *P. malariae*).

Quinine, 1 g every 8 hours, during the first day of treatment, followed by 600 mg every 8 hours for about 1 week (for *P. falciparum*).

Plague (Bubonic Plague)

Headache is not constantly found or characteristic of this serious disease. Diagnosis is given by enlarged lymph nodes, or the syndromic complex of pneumonia, pharyngitis, or meningitis, confirmed by the recovery of the infective germ.

Antibiotic therapy must start immediately with streptomycin, the tetracyclines, or chloramphenicol. The use of narcotic analgesics is to be discouraged; codeine, acetylsalicylic acid, or both are usually effective.

Streptomycin, 500 to 1000 mg every 12 hours, by injection. Watch for injury to the 8th cranial nerve.

Chloramphenicol, 50 mg for each kilo of body weight in 24 hours, divided into four installments, starting by intravenous injection; to decrease dosage and start oral administration as soon as possible. Higher dosage may be given.

Tetracycline, not to exceed 500 mg every 6 hours, by slow intravenous injection in severe cases; resort to oral administration as soon as possible, at a rate of 500 mg every 6 hours (avoiding milk and antacids).

Yellow Fever (Black Vomit)

Symptoms are elevated temperature, albuminuria, jaundice, and hematemesis (black vomit), beginning abruptly with headache, generalized pains, flushed face, and a rise in pulse rate. Diagnosis is made by specialized laboratories. The disease will be found only in endemic areas, or in persons coming from these places.

No specific treatment is known. Severe headaches should be relieved. Because of the impairment of the gastric mucosa, salicylates should be avoided. Instead, codeine or meperidine can be given. Avoid dehydration, and give all symptomatic help.

Hypertension

Hypertensive bouts may be accompanied by a revealing headache, and occur together with dizziness, asthenia, palpitations, and insomnia. The diagnosis is made by blood pressure evaluation. The headache may occur during the morning hours, be located in the occipital area, and increase with effort.

Treat hypertension adequately; and, if needed, give mild analgesics. For the relief of nocturnal headache, sleep with the head on a higher position than the rest of the body (block under the bed, extra pillows, elevation of the mattress, and so on).

Hypotension

Hypotension headache (most frequently in the occipital area) is modified by the position of the body and effort. These patients feel weak and faint easily, some when getting up from bed. Any debilitating disease may cause hypotension.

Headache may be relieved with mild analgesics. If syncope occurs, it will be treated according to the regular procedures.

Heart Failure

Congestion because of poor circulation will interfere with oxygenation of tissues. Respiratory symptoms (dyspnea, coughing, and râles heard on auscultation) are conspicuous in left heart failure. Prominent in right heart failure are edema, epigastric distress due to enlargement of the liver, and congestion of the abdominal viscerae causing anorexia and constipation. Headache of nonspecific nature may accompany either type of heart failure.

This headache sometimes requires drastic measures, such as the use of morphine, hydromorphone, meperidine, or anileridine. On occasions codeine may be sufficient to control the situation. Some patients may respond to milder analgesics.

> Morphine, 10 mg, by subcutaneous injection, every 4 hours, as needed and tolerated (may increase to 15 mg).

> Hydromorphone, 1 or 2 mg, by subcutaneous injection, every 4 hours; as needed and tolerated.

> Meperidine, 50 mg, by intramuscular injection or orally, every 4 hours; or 100 mg, as needed and tolerated.

> Anileridine, 25 mg, by intramuscular injection or by mouth, every 6 hours, as tolerated.

Arteritis

Inflammation of the temporal arteries provokes headache, tenderness, and local pain, which exacerbates on pressure and during mastication. Fever and loss of weight are also noted.

Arteritis affecting the temporal artery requires immediate and active treatment for the prevention of blindness, as intracranial arteries might also be involved. Corticoids are mandatory; salicylates are of good help.

> Cortisone acetate, 50 mg in each ml of the suspension; inject 100 mg every 8 hours, intramuscularly until symptoms begin to subside; immediately, start decreasing the injected amount, to 200 mg a day, and then to 100 mg a day (always in divided doses); and as soon as the situation is under control, discontinue it gradually. Keep the reduced dosage at a level sufficient to ensure continuing action.

> Hydrocortisone, to start with 300 to 500 mg in 24 hours, the schedule being similar to the one above.

> Prednisone, to start with 80 mg a day, in divided doses, the schedule being similar to the one developed for cortisone, above.

Dexamethasone, to start with 4 to 5 mg a day, in divided doses, the schedule as above.

With such an elevated dosage, sodium retention is a possibility to keep in mind; salt ingestion should be drastically reduced, additional potassium given, and frequent determination of electrolytes performed.

Sodium salicylate, 600 mg (if tolerated) by mouth, every 4 hours.
To increase tolerance, thyroid extract (30 mg a day) may be tried.

Brain Tumors and Cysts

Symptoms depend on cranial hypertension and the localization of the new mass: intense cephalalgia together with projectile vomiting and papilledema (characteristic of cranial hypertension), bradycardia, epileptic seizures, ophthalmoplegia, and behavioral disorders. This cephalalgia interferes with sleep, and may be more severe at the site of the lesion, is resistant to ordinary analgesics, and may mimic migraine; if the tumor localizes in the pituitary gland, the headache is mostly frontal, and the patient complains of extreme weakness.

Hydatid cyst of the brain is frequent in Europe but relatively rare in the United States. Ordinarily, a previous cyst is found elsewhere in the body (liver). Diagnosis is made by X-ray examination and laboratory tests (eosinophilia, Carson's test, complement fixation).

Surgery is the only approach to these problems, except for some tumors sensitive to radiation. For the relief of headache, prior to surgery, the best measure to be taken is the intravenous administration of a 50% glucose solution. Avoid lumbar puncture.

Glucose 50% solution; inject intravenously 25 ml (most cases will respond well to this amount) or up to 50 ml.

Subdural Hematoma

Headaches following an injury to the head, immediately or after the first few days, particularly if accompanied by irritability and mental confusion, may be indicative of subdural hematoma. A spastic hemiplegia is a later confirmation of the intracranial bleeding. The cerebrospinal fluid will appear tinged with blood.

The condition requires surgery, particularly when progressing symptoms reveal increasing pressure within the skull due to an increase in the size of the lesion. Narcotic drugs should not be given when increased intracranial pressure is one of the causative factors of pain.

Subarachnoid Hemorrhage

The bleeding is frequently preceded by a sudden and very intense cephalalgia, frontal or occipital to start, then becoming generalized, possibly following previous exertion of some kind. Loss of consciousness may last for a few moments or hours in smaller hemorrhages, or until death in severe ones. Neck stiffness is constant; convulsions and fever are common. The spinal fluid pressure is elevated, as well as its content of red blood cells.

As usual with these intracranial problems, narcotics are to be considered contraindicated. If the diagnostic tapping is followed by alleviation of the headache and the other symptoms, lumbar puncture will be considered the best help for these patients, repeated until the bleeding stops. Consider the use of antihypertensive drugs, diazepam, corticoids, and correction of the electrolyte imbalance. Codeine and acetylsalicylic acid should be tried for help.

Intracranial Abscess

Headache ranges from mild to severe, and convulsions usually are the first indication of an abscess, together with other signs of increased intracranial pressure (vomiting and papilledema). A previous septic lesion developing neurological symptoms may suggest the formation of an intracranial abscess.

Each case requires individualized therapy: surgery, antibiotics, or analgesics.

Epilepsy

The diagnosis of epilepsy is very difficult when the first seizure occurs after 60 years of age. Headache may be a part of the aura complex, and follows most attacks; but there are also headaches similar to migraine that appear between the principal epileptic seizures. Electroencephalograms are not always informative.

When epilepsy is due to a known cause, the treatment should be addressed to this underlying factor, and measures against cephalalgia itself taken only when needed. The mild analgesics may be given. Treatment with diphenylhydantoin, phenobarbital, or diazepam will be evaluated in each instance.

Neuroses and Emotions

When due to neuroses and emotions, headache is often of a bizarre type, lacking features from which a diagnosis could be made. For this reason care must be observed not to take a neurotic or an emotional cephalalgia for an organic disease, or vice versa.

The basic neurotic problem will respond better to psychotherapy, preferably by a specialist; however, under the skillful management of any understanding doctor the neurotic symptoms are likely to improve. When the headache follows a more or less intense emotional shock (an accident, a distressing situation), the first attempt made will be to quiet the patient.

Migraine

Headache is the dominant symptom affecting the whole head or the right or the left side alone (hemicrania). During the attack, nausea and photophobia are important symptoms. Often photophobia, visual aura, scintillating scotoma, nervous irritability, and nausea precede the attack. The recurrent pattern of these symptoms may warn some patients of the coming of a typical attack.

In cases due to allergic diseases, desensitization or avoidance of the allergen will be a necessary treatment (there has been considerable question about allergy being the sole cause of migraine). If the symptoms are slight, acetylsalicylic acid, codeine, or a similar analgesic will help. If no effect is noted following the first or second dosage, ergot derivatives will be used instead. In really severe cases, the ergot derivatives should be the first drug given by injection, particularly when vomiting does not allow oral medication. Ergotamine, by the intravenous route, may increase vomiting, at times. Dihydroergotamine is a good, effective alternative. Administration of ergot derivatives can be repeated after 1 or 2 hours, whenever necessary, and the therapy can be complemented with the same drugs given orally. The addition of caffeine may be of help for some of these patients.

> Ergotamine tartrate, 0.5 mg in solution, by subcutaneous injection; or, for more active and rapid effect, 0.25 mg in solution by intravenous injection. This will terminate the attack in most instances.

> Dihydroergotamine, 1 mg in each ml solution, to be given by intramuscular or subcutaneous injection. Inject only 1 ml. It may also be given by vein.

> Ergotamine tartrate, 1 mg, by mouth, every 4 hours the first day; every 8 hours, thereafter, as needed.

> Caffeine, 100 mg, by mouth, every 6 to 8 hours.

Histamine Headache

This headache shows some similarities to migraine. It affects one side of the head and the corresponding eye, temple, face, and neck. Other symptoms are localized vasodilation, edema, watery eyes, and running nose.

Treatment will follow the same rules: to start with a regular analgesic drug (acetylsalicylic acid, codeine, pentazocine, propoxyphene hydrochloride) or resort to ergot derivatives (ergotamine tartrate, dihydroergotamine) whenever the first trial fails or the attack is severe. Antihistaminics should be used.

Ergotamine tartrate, 0.25 mg, by intravenous injection; or 0.5 mg in solution, by the subcutaneous route.

Dihydroergotamine, 1 mg in each ml of solution, by intramuscular or subcutaneous injection. Also, in emergent situations dihydroergotamine in the same amount of 1 mg can be injected intravenously.

Chlorpheniramine maleate, 8 mg, by mouth, every 8 or 12 hours.

Cyproheptadine, 4 mg, by mouth, every 6 to 8 hours.

Hay Fever

A frontal headache accompanies the classic symptoms of itching nose, eyes, and pharynx, watery nasal discharge, and sneezing.

Pollinosis requires complete and continuous treatment, which will be carried out according to the rules given by allergists. Additional treatment with antihistaminic drugs is helpful. The treatment of headache, per se, is of little importance, since it usually responds well to antihistamine therapy, either alone or together with a sympathomimetic drug of the type of ephedrine.

Chlorpheniramine or cyproheptadine, as above.

Ephedrine, 25 mg, by mouth, every 6 or 8 hours.

Pseudoephedrine hydrochloride, 60 mg, by mouth every 6 to 8 hours.

Anaphylactic Shock

A pounding headache with throbbing in the ears accompanies a sensation of extreme anxiety and uneasiness, following the injection of an offending allergen. Intense peripheral vascular collapse and other allergic symptoms may appear. Fatal cases are not rare.

All efforts will be directed to saving the patient from this threatening reaction by immediately giving epinephrine by intravenous infusion.

Epinephrine, 0.5 mg in 10 ml of saline solution; inject slowly into the vein.

The remainder of the treatment depends on the occurrence, or not, of respiratory difficulties and hypotension, which conditions will be treated accordingly, including the use of resuscitation, if necessary.

Gastrointestinal Diseases

Dyspepsia or *indigestion* may present as nausea, frequently with vomiting, weakness, sweating, vertigo, and headache. Other forms of *gastroenteritis* or *colitis* may add fever, with or without chills, diarrhea, constipation, or anorexia. Of the divergent causes producing these symptoms, those involving a simple chemical malfunction of the upper digestive tract (dyspepsia or indigestion) are recognized by their evanescence and ready response to spontaneous efforts at their correction. The irritants should be eliminated or neutralized; established infection should be treated with antitoxin or antibiotics and rest. Therefore, for nausea and vomiting give copious fluids, followed (when irritant is eliminated) by opium and belladonna for diarrhea; maintain hydration; treat intestinal infection; advise a liquid diet, gradually adding solid elements.

Codeine sulfate, 30 to 60 mg, by mouth or by subcutaneous injection, every 6 hours.

Acetaminophen, 600 mg, by mouth, every 8 hours.

Tincture of opium (laudanum), 20 to 30 drops in water, repeated as needed.

Tincture of belladonna, 10 to 30 drops in water, repeated as needed and tolerated.

Ampicillin, or preferably kanamycin or gentamycin, at accepted dosages.

Hepatic Headache

Intense cephalalgia is part of the symptom complex of acute yellow atrophy. Also complained of are abdominal pain in the right upper quadrant, vomiting, jaundice, or convulsions. Often, there is a preceding or chronic liver disease with headache. If hepatic function is under great stress, it is better not to give analgesics; instead, the use of corticoids is advisable. Consider hepatitis, fulminant, submassive, and prolonged, resulting in cirrhosis, portal or postnecrotic, and chronic intoxication that produces alcoholic liver.

Prednisone, 5 to 15 mg, by mouth, every 6 to 8 hours, for a few days, decreasing the dosage when improvement is noted, and starting discontinuance gradually after a few days of treatment.

Triamcinolone acetonide, 40 mg, suspension, for intramuscular injection in the gluteal area, to start medication, and then continuing by the oral route.

Paget's Disease

Pain in the skull and other bones is a symptom of the disease, manifested by early decalcification of bones, which produces softening and bowing. The changes occurring in the head lead to a triangular appearance of the face. The diagnosis is made by X-rays.

Most of the symptoms will have to be treated as they become apparent. Initial bouts of headache will respond well to common analgesics. In advanced cases, when pressure may be a contributing factor, X-ray therapy should be tried. Estrogens or androgens (according to sex) have been recommended. Calcitonin is now highly praised.

Intracranial Calcifications

X-ray examinations may show intracranial calcifications in patients with neurological disturbances who also complain of headache. Cranial hypertension may be present in some instances. Epilepsy and vertigo may accompany the calcifications.

The basic treatment belongs to the neurologist and the neurosurgeon. When pain is distressing, use meperidine or codeine, and for less marked pain acetylsalicylic acid or propoxyphene hydrochloride.

Muscle Strain

An occipital headache will be present when the muscles of the back of the head are tense and tender in cases of anxiety, or of cervical spondyloarthrosis. A characteristic gesture is pressing the neck muscles with one or both hands while moving the head backward.

The headache is relieved as soon as the neck strain subsides under treatment. An adjuvant dose of an analgesic is of additional help. Muscle relaxants should be considered for this purpose. Relaxation of muscles may be helped by medication of the type of meprobamate or carisoprodol.

Codeine, 60 mg, by mouth, every 4 to 6 hours.

Meprobamate, 400 mg, every 4 to 6 hours, by mouth.

Trauma to the Head

Pain will follow any injury to the head. A very close surveillance, or an initial surgical approach, is mandatory.

Drugs for the relief of pain may be needed: common analgesics or even narcotics. All cases should be transferred to the hospital, particularly if the patient has been found unconscious, a fracture is disclosed, convulsions are present, or shock develops.

Meperidine, 50 mg, by mouth or by injection; or 100 mg, as needed and tolerated. Either meperidine, morphine, or any other narcotic, if given, will be observed very closely for its effects upon the respiratory centers, to avoid dangerous depression.

Heat and Heatstroke

Excessive heating may provoke headache, heat cramps, or heat prostration. In the last condition, circulatory collapse is manifested, starting with headache, irritability, cramps, and weakness. In heatstroke (sunstroke) the symptoms are similar (headache, irritability, collapse), with elevated body temperature over 40.5°C (105°F). When excessive heat threatens collapse of the patient, headache is one of the premonitory symptoms.

The administration of analgesics capable of inducing diaphoresis is contraindicated; and in order not to depress respiratory centers, narcotics are also to be avoided. In both instances, heat and heatstroke, the first attempt will be to decrease body temperature (particularly in the case of sunstroke), by using an ice cap and blankets cooled with water or by placing the patient in an ice-water bath. Rectal temperature will be checked frequently and not allowed to fall below 38°C (about 101°F). The complete treatment will follow well-established rules.

High Altitude

Persons not accustomed to high altitudes may develop anoxic symptoms when they come to these elevations. If they are rapidly transported, symptoms appear suddenly: dyspnea after light effort, dizziness, weakness, cyanosis, palpitation (tachycardia), possibly hemorrhages, and headache. The chronic state is revealed by dyspnea, dizziness, and headache, although as a rule there is no discomfort or disability after a sojourn of 2 to 4 weeks. Psychic aberrations may occur, particularly in the acute form.

Narcotic analgesics are positively contraindicated because of depression of the respiratory centers. The first approach is to decrease physical activity until the body accommodates to the new environment of an atmosphere poor in oxygen. When symptoms become annoying or dangerous, oxygen can be given by mask.

Hypoventilation

This condition occurs in pneumonia, chronic emphysema, pneumothorax, or any other form of obstruction to ventilation. Anoxemic symptoms include disturbance of electrolyte balance, headache, and symptoms of each of these diseases. Toxemias producing a depression of the respiratory centers (opium and related drugs) will induce hypoventilation. Toxic gases will impair the oxygenation of blood and tissues: carbon monoxide intoxication ordinarily begins with headache, and then other nervous symptoms are added, such as vertigo and loss of consciousness. Carbon monoxide–hemoglobin replacing oxyhemoglobin causes the characteristic redness of the skin. Inert gases of all sorts may substitute for oxygen in some situations, thus interfering with respiration.

In acute poisoning by gases, particularly carbon monoxide, immediate administration of 100% oxygen by inhalation is mandatory. Rest is required to decrease the oxygen requirement, and will be maintained until respiration and oxygenation become normal. Oxygen will be given by mask when symptoms become noticeable or severe. Do not give narcotic analgesics because they will depress the respiratory center, and use all other analgesics sparingly. In cases of CO_2 retention, with hypoventilation and hypoxemia, oxygen may *increase* the inhibition of the respiratory center, thus making necessary the use of analeptics or respiratory stimulants.

> Ethamivan, by intravenous infusion, at a dosage of about 0.1 mg for each kilo of body weight per minute, as required.

> Caffeine sodium benzoate, U.S.P., 500 mg; inject intramuscularly.

Cerebral Anoxia from Hematic Conditions

Acute posthemorrhagic anemia: there is direct or indirect evidence or history of blood loss, dizziness, faintness, more or less marked pallor, sweating and thirst, tachycardia, and progression into shock. *Chronic blood loss:* evidence of bleeding is not always clear; fatigability, weakness, and perhaps other symptoms of depleted vitality are observed (a blood count will give the final clue to diagnosis). Causative factors must be found. *Arteriovenous shunts and some forms of anemias* will also interfere with the adequate oxygenation of tissues. Among the symptoms of anemia—pallor, dyspnea, asthenia, and psychic changes—cephalalgia also has a place. Some *toxic substances* will interfere with respiration because of their power to transform hemoglobin into different compounds. Toxic drugs are the nitrites, chlorates, and sulfas, among others.

For acute posthemorrhagic anemia the treatment is that of shock. For chronic posthemorrhagic or iron deficiency anemia treatment will be directed toward the blood deficiency. Other anemias are to be treated following the same principles. In the case of headache due to cerebral anoxia caused by congenital heart disease or shunt, if the patient is of an advanced age, the symptomatic treatment, as stated above, will be of some help; but the basic treatment is that applying to the underlying cause. If the cephalalgia is a consequence of a toxic reaction to a drug (sulfas, chlorates, and so on) first discontinue that drug; second, try to eliminate it from the body; and last of all, try a mild analgesic, if it is really needed.

Toxic Headache

Tobacco in large amounts will provoke headache together with other neurological symptoms (confusion, weakness, twitchings, convulsions), symptoms from the gastrointestinal tract (painful abdominal cramps, vomiting, diarrhea), and even collapse and coma if absorption has been excessive. Death may occur (respiratory paralysis).

Intoxication by *lobelia* may cause similar symptoms.

Caffeine (coffee and tea) intoxication may also begin with headache and other neurological symptoms. Pain of a burning nature is felt in the throat; there is ringing in the ears; tachycardia and thirst may be dominant symptoms. As in the case of tobacco intoxication, anamnesis will reveal an inordinate use of these beverages.

Poisonings by *CO and other gases* must be considered occupational poisonings. Persistent headaches not due to evident causes should be investigated from the industrial risk point of view, as in the case of laborers who work in locales with an excess of carbon monoxide or any other toxic gas. Additional symptoms due to each particular toxic gas should be sought.

In *uremia* due to chronic nephritis headache is a very important symptom, but the usual clinical picture is that of a formerly known progressive renal insufficiency, with or without edema. A previous acute glomerulonephritis occurs in the great majority of patients. Neurological, respiratory, gastrointestinal, and circulatory symptoms reveal the serious nature of the intoxication, due to nitrogen accumulating in the blood. It is a terminal phase of chronic kidney disease; it may also occur as a result of acute kidney diseases, and regress when the basic condition improves. Laboratory tests will give an accurate diagnosis.

At the beginning of *diabetes,* when hyperglycemia is not yet controlled, or whenever hyperglycemic bouts occur, headache is common, as it also is whenever acidosis develops during the course of the disease. Headache may be present at the preclinical stage, when prediabetes may be suspected if minimal changes in glucose tolerance occur in patients with relatives suffering from the disease. When polydypsia, polyuria, polyphagia, and itching accompany the headache, there will probably be sugar in the urine, confirming the diagnosis.

Hypoglycemia results from an overdose of insulin or from going many hours without taking food; it presents headache, sweating, trembling, weakness, palpitation, psychological changes (similar to drunkenness, with which it has been confounded), and finally syncope, which may occur early. Psychological symptoms predominate when hypoglycemia develops slowly after use of long-acting insulins or oral drugs. Also, symptoms may appear at higher blood sugar levels when the hyperglycemia of a diabetic patient is lowered too rapidly.

Treatment. Anoxic toxins will induce anoxemia, which is to be treated with oxygen inhalation plus the basic therapy for each particular toxin. A severe tobacco intoxication may paralyze respiration; oxygen is also to be given in this instance, frequently together with artificial respiration. For the resulting headache, an ice cap is the best aid. In case of headaches due to coffee or tea intoxication, morphine is the drug of choice because it will also help to decrease caffeine hyperexcitability.

> Morphine, 10 (or 15) mg, by subcutaneous injection.

Carbon dioxide and other gases may also interfere with proper oxygen absorption, thus provoking a syndrome similar to any other hypoxic or anoxic condition. The administration of oxygen, frequently together with respiratory stimulants, is the correct therapeutic approach.

> Ethamivan, by intravenous infusion, at a dosage of about 0.1 mg for each kilo and minute.

> Caffeine sodium benzoate, U.S.P., 500 mg; inject intramuscularly.

Carbon monoxide intoxication requires immediate removal of the patient from the place of contamination; complete avoidance of any effort; artificial respiration (with oxygen inhalation); administration of mannitol or hypertonic urea, to combat cerebral edema whenever present. If needed, because of the severity of symptoms, an exchange transfusion can be given. Analgesics are of very little help in these cases.

> Mannitol solution; inject 2.5 g for each kilo of body weight, by intravenous infusion.

> Hypertonic urea solution; inject 1 g for each kilo of body weight, by intravenous infusion.

Uremia, diabetes, and hypoglycemia, as noted above, are frequently accompanied by headache. The basic treatment of each condition is paramount. In some instances, the use of a mild analgesic can be considered a good adjuvant therapy.

Ovaric Headache

Many headaches are intimately related to the ovarian function, such as menstruation, menopause, and so on. On the other hand, headache of all types (particularly migraine) is by far a disease of women. At the menopause headache is a bothersome and frequent symptom.

Hormones (estrogens, or a combination of estrogens and a progesterone) are the basic treatment. Any analgesic drug can be given as adjuvant, emergency treatment. It is to be noted that ovarian headache can be of a cerebrovascular nature (migraine), and in these cases it should be treated accordingly.

Acidosis

In metabolic acidosis (following excessive absorption of chloride, loss of bicarbonate, renal disease, diabetes), there are pain (do not mistake it for an acute abdomen!), hyperpnea, nausea with or without vomiting, and other signs of dehydration (inelastic skin, dry mouth, sunken eyes). Laboratory tests will make the diagnosis clear.

Treatment is to be addressed to the cause (diabetes, renal failure, diarrhea, as the most frequent etiologic factors), and the metabolic imbalance corrected by intravenous infusions of bicarbonate whenever indicated. In respiratory acidosis due to depressed respiratory centers, impaired mechanical respiration, or carbon dioxide intoxication, the treatment is the same as for hyperventilation: rest, oxygen therapy, and avoidance of narcotic analgesics.

Alkalosis

Symptoms include irritability, particularly tetany. Correct the deficit of water, sodium, chloride, and potassium by giving these substances either by mouth or by intravenous infusion.

Respiratory alkalosis may be due to neurotic hyperventilation or toxemia (lesions of the central nervous system, hepatic coma, salicylate poisoning, fever, and so on). Give oxygen, or simply, as in the case of neurotic hyperventilation, ask the patient to breathe into a paper bag (do not use a plastic bag). Sedatives may be helpful.

Phenobarbital, 15 or 30 mg, by mouth, every 6 to 8 hours.

Diabetic Acidosis

Diabetic acidosis shows abdominal pain (sometimes leading to the erroneous diagnosis of "acute abdomen") in a known diabetic patient (rarely an unknown one), who slowly deteriorates and then appears extremely ill, with dry and flushed skin (important symptom), an acetone odor to the breath (also, an important symptom), and exaggerated hyperglycemia and decreased CO_2 combining power of the plasma (which are diagnostic).

No direct treatment for pain is advisable; but antidiabetic therapy should be started and a diabetologist called immediately. First make a thorough test of the urine (sugar, albumin, diacetic acid, acetone), draw blood for laboratory procedures (glucose, cholesterol, SGOT, BUN, electrolytes), and inject into the vein 50 units of regular insulin, particularly if there is any suspicion of circulatory collapse. With an additional 50 units injected subcutaneously, the initial 100 units required will be complete. Thereafter, repeat 75 to 100 units subcutaneously every hour until the symptoms and the blood and urine chemistry have improved; then, decrease the amount of insulin, to reach a 24-hour amount of 200 to 700 units. At times, larger amounts are needed! Also, start intravenous infusions promptly with hypotonic saline and sodium bicarbonate. The rest is up to the specialist.

Hypoglycemia

Symptoms of hypoglycemia, which are confirmed by the findings of low levels of blood glucose, include: sweating, tremor, weakness, behavioral changes, dizziness, convulsions (even coma), and occasional epigastralgia.

The objective of treatment is rapid restoration of blood sugar concentration, which is easily achieved with sugar. Most persons who fall into this category are still alert enough to swallow a few spoonfuls or lumps of sucrose (plain sugar), honey, or candy, or to drink fruit juices and sweet beverages. It must always be remembered that all persons subject to hypoglycemic attacks (insulin users, patients with hyperinsulinism) must carry lumps of sugar with them at all times, to be taken at the first warning. If the patient is not able to drink or swallow, give an intravenous injection of dextrose. Refer the patient to an endocrinologist or a diabetologist.

Dextrose, 25% solution (1 g = 4 ml); inject intravenously 40 ml (10 g) or 80 ml (20 g).

Trigeminal Neuralgia

A very severe pain, frequent in the elderly and presented in the form of relatively brief attacks involving one half of the face (in relation to the affected branch of the trigeminal nerve), is suggestive of the name "tic douloureux," otherwise known as trigeminal neuralgia. There are trigger areas, which are hypersensitive and may excite an attack of pain when irritated or merely touched. The condition will not be confounded with migraine or with other forms of neuritis (tumoral, post-herpetic, and so on). A good clue will be given by precipitation of attacks by washing the face, exposure to cold, eating, drinking, or even talking. *Suicide* is a threat among the elderly, because of suffering from the severe pain.

The first treatment trial can be made with cyanocobalamine (vitamin B_{12}), in large amounts by the intramuscular route. This treatment could be repeated, even without pain, after a 1- or 2-month interval, a few times. The second trial can be with carbamazepine, which is very effective. Also, anticonvulsants of the type of diphenylhydantoin may be used and expected to be effective in many cases. Surgery is the final resource: first, the injection of alcohol into the ganglion or into the affected branches of the trigeminus, which may allay pain for months and even years; and second, neurosurgery.

Cyanocobalamine, 1 mg (1000 μg) by intramuscular injection, daily for 10 days.

Carbamazepine, 200 mg, tablets, half a tablet twice daily; increasing dosage according to results and tolerance.

Diphenylhydantoin, 100 mg, tablets; one every 6 hours.

Herpes Zoster

Patients over 50 years of age are the ones most frequently affected by herpes virus, and develop characteristic lesions of zoster. The clinical picture usually opens with fever and chills, the vesicular rash rapidly following. There are tense vesicles upon an erythematous base, the base generally less inflamed than in cases of herpes simplex. The outstanding differential clue is that in herpes zoster the vesicles always follow the path of distribution of a nerve. In the head it may be the ophthalmic, otic, or pharyngeal nerve. The corresponding area usually presents intense pain, which may precede the rash, persists during its acme, and in about 10% of affected elderly persons may even increase and continue after disappearance of the skin lesions. Interference with sleep is extremely budensome. On rare occasions the eruption may become generalized, but there is a clear-cut setting on the path of the nerve initially affected. For diagnosis, if needed, take smears from the floor of a vesicle for detection of giant epithelial cells stained with Giemsa's solution.

Ophthalmic herpes zoster is found over the cutaneous distribution of the nasociliary nerve or other branches of the ophthalmic; thus the vesicles erupt around the eyes, from forehead to nose on one side of the face. There may be, in addition to pain, edema and inflammation of tissues, causing serious ocular lesions in many cases (conjunctiva, ciliary body, and other locations).

Otic herpes zoster provokes a sudden onset of pain and fullness in the ear, tinnitus, and some sort of hearing impairment. Pain may reach extremely acute proportions. There is also swelling of the area and a corresponding adenopathy. Vesicles are noted in auricles or the ear canal.

Pharyngeal herpes zoster presents the characteristic vesicles within the mouth on the pharyngo-tonsillar area, only on one side. There may also be pain, occasional paresis on the affected side (differentiated from Bell's palsy because in the latter there are no vesicles), and other symptoms of otic herpes zoster.

Corticoids are positively contraindicated in herpes simplex (!), but their use is advised and usually very rewarding in herpes zoster. Persisting neuralgia after disappearance of skin lesion might respond to infiltration of the affected area with triamcinolone acetonide and lidocaine solution.

Prednisone, to start with, at 40 mg a day, to rapidly decrease the dosage; but discontinuance has to be slow.

Triamcinolone acetonide, 40 mg in suspension; inject into gluteus muscle (or affected area), in starting corticoid therapy, for rapid relief.

Lidocaine, 2% solution; use 1 to 3 ml.

Codeine, 30 (to 60) mg, by mouth, every 4 hours; may also be given by subcutaneous injection. This medication, and vitamin B_{12}, are recommended for otic zoster.

Sinus Pain

Acute sinusitis begins abruptly or gradually with pain which increases or appears under pressure in the area corresponding to the affected sinus or sinuses. Heterotopic pains, radiating to the head, teeth, and ears, and fever, periorbital edema, photophobia, general malaise, and even vertigo make up the syndrome.

Chronic sinusitis is less conspicuous. Pain might be the only symptom, either headache, toothache, or simply local pain or tenderness over the sinuses.

Local pain varies in accordance with the affected sinus: supraorbital in frontal sinusitis; teeth, cheek, and forehead in maxillary sinusitis; occipital, parietal, root of the nose, or neck pain in ethmoid or sphenoid sinusitis. The final diagnosis is made by noting purulent discharge from the affected sinus and by the use of transillumination or X-rays, or direct irrigation by catheter or puncture.

For the treatment of acute sinusitis, advise bed rest, light diet, moderate intake of fluids, local heating, local decongestants, adequate antibiotic therapy, and the use of analgesics. Local decongestants help to control pain, either when given by mouth or instilled into the nose. Broad-spectrum antibiotics are fundamental in the treatment of sinusitis, both acute or chronic, together with surgical procedures to be initiated by a specialist. Chronic sinusitis requires more specialized care, with irrigations, removal of polyps (if present), antrotomy, and so on, and adequate antibiotic therapy.

Papaverine hydrochloride, 150 mg, in slow-release capsules, one every 12 hours.

Meperidine, 50 (to 100) mg: starting by subcutaneous injection and continuing by mouth every 4 to 6 hours.

Pseudoephedrine hydrochloride, 60 mg, tablets, every 6 to 8 hours.

Phenylephrine, 5% solution, three or four drops into the nostril of the affected side.

Broad-spectrum antibiotics; to choose an adequate one and use it in full dosage.

Erysipelas

Not too frequent with the elderly, this acute disease begins with pain, fever, chills, and a localized red rash (around the nose or mouth, most frequently) with a distinctly demarcated margin, which is firm to the touch and swollen, particularly at the periphery. Malaise, nausea, and vomiting are not rare occurrences; redness spreads peripherally, and in severe cases there are vesicles or bullae. A frequent starting point is the angle of the mouth. It is caused by a streptococcus.

Since beta-hemolytic streptococci are mostly sensitive to penicillin, give this antibiotic. The patient will observe bed rest, with the head elevated. Hot packs on the lesion help to control pain. Acetylsalicylic acid will serve for both pain and fever.

Procaine penicillin, 600,000 units solution by injection, every 8 or 12 hours.

Injuries to the Face

These injuries may be: contusions, bruises, wounds, fractures, burns, and so on. The diagnosis is easily made from the clinical history and physical appearance. For fractures, particular symptoms and X-ray evidence will assure the diagnosis.

Except for contusions and bruises, all injuries to the face should be referred to a surgeon, either general or plastic. After a thorough cleansing of the lesion, some analgesic will be given, according to the intensity of the pain. The pain of contusions will be treated with cool compresses as well as salicylates and similar drugs. Bruises may receive similar care, or will be treated with local anesthetic solutions—of course, after thorough cleansing and good protection with local antibiotics and covering.

Benzocaine, 5 or 20% ointment; apply locally, once or twice a day.

Bone Pain

This facial pain may be due to an injury, an infection, arthritis, or a tumor, and is treated accordingly. In all instances, if pain is severe enough, a narcotic analgesic will be used. Otherwise, a salicylate or similar drug will be given. The basic condition provoking pain will receive adequate care, be it arthritic, rheumatic, infective, or tumoral.

Codeine, 30 (to 60) mg, by subcutaneous injection, every 4 hours.

Meperidine, 50 (to 100) mg, by subcutaneous injection, every 4 to 6 hours.

Glaucoma

There is always some sort of pain, ranging from mild to excruciating, related to the eye. When the cause of glaucoma is unknown, it is a primary glaucoma; if known, secondary glaucoma. Suspicious cases will be promptly referred to an opthalmologist.

Chronic open-angle glaucoma shows a frequent need for change of glasses, and there are minor visual disturbances (halos around lights, mild pain, and so forth); the diagnosis depends on the finding of increased intraocular pressure, at times following provocative tests (water ingestion). At times it is asymptomatic, and has to be searched for and diagnosed to avoid loss of vision.

Acute angle-closure glaucoma presents attacks of increasing symptomatology of a relatively chronic nature (halos around lights, pain, and so forth), which last for a short time and recur frequently until the characteristic brutal attack takes place (severe pain, loss of vision, nausea and vomiting, chemosis, lacrimation, dilated pupil, turbid aqueous fluid, and highly increased ocular tension—even perceptible to touch).

Chronic angle-closure glaucoma consists of repeated attacks which are characteristic, similar to those in acute angle-closure glaucoma, but less marked.

Secondary glaucomas follow the clinical course of the causative disease, namely: uveitis, a space-occupying lesion (tumors) or cataracts, and the use of corticoids for the treatment of any disease. Under these circumstances, an attack of ophthalmodynia with increased ocular tension is diagnostic of secondary glaucoma.

The excruciating pain suffered by a great number of patients, seriously interfering with adequate rest, frequently requires emergent treatment to decrease intraocular tension. But since the selection of therapies depends on whether it is a primary or secondary glaucoma, an open-angle glaucoma, and so on, it will be better carried out by an experienced ophthalmologist.

The acute attack of glaucoma requires immediate treatment, and must be referred to the ophthalmologist at the earliest possible moment. For the acute-closure glaucoma, start interim treatment with pilocarpine:

Pilocarpine, 2% solution; instill one drop every second (five times); thereafter one drop every minute (five times) and finally one drop every half hour.

Pilocarpine should be instilled, also, in the other eye, as follows:

> Pilocarpine, 0.5% solution; instill one drop every 3 hours.

Effectiveness is noted when myosis occurs. If the treatment fails, give acetazolamide:

> Acetazolamide, 500 mg by intramuscular injection.

Surgery is the last and usually curative measure, which will be decided upon by the ophthalmologist. Nevertheless, if the patient has aphakic eyes, this lack of a lens in both eyes makes it preferable to use isoflurophate.

> Isoflurophate, 0.1% ophthalmic solution, to instill two drops every 8 hours, for 3 days; during nighttime isoflurophate, 0.025% ophthalmic ointment, will be used.

For open-angle glaucoma pilocarpine is still the drug of choice, though acute attacks may be prevented with glycerin given by mouth, acetazolamide by injection (intramuscular or intravenous), or intravenous urea if the former drugs fail.

> Pilocarpine, 1 to 4% solution, to instill one drop every 4 hours, or as decided by the specialist.

> Glycerin, 1 or 2 g for each kilo of body weight, in a mixture with equal parts of water.

> Acetazolamide, 500 mg by intravenous injection (or intramuscularly); or 250 mg in tablets, not more frequently than every 6 hours.

> Urea, 30% solution, give 1 to 5 g for each kilo of body weight by the intravenous route, making sure that there is adequate kidney function.

Secondary glaucoma can be treated with corticoids and acetazolamide, or as decided by the specialist.

> Prednisone, 5 mg repeated every 4 hours, until symptoms abate (10 mg can be given in special cases); then, reduce dosage and discontinue it very slowly after 8 to 10 days of treatment.

> Acetazolamide; see above lines.

Conjunctivitis

The first symptom noted is a painful sensation, as if a foreign body were in the eye, followed by lacrimation, photophobia, a more or less marked discharge of pus, and the characteristic redness of the conjunctiva, which confirms the diagnosis. Care must be taken to differentiate the various types of conjunctivitis: chronic or acute catarrhal inflammation, gonococcal, and the different types of viral conjunctivitis and trachoma. In trichinosis, there are pain, subconjunctival hemorrhage, and edema of the lids. Take material from the secretion for culture, and sensitivity to antibiotics. Refer patient to an ophthalmologist for diagnosis, if necessary.

To treat, remove foreign bodies, if any, whenever the procedure is within one's capabilities. Rarely, pain will require local anesthesia, which can be achieved with holocaine or pontocaine, for example. Most frequently, as soon as the specific treatment with antibiotic suspensions or solutions is started, pain subsides. These antibiotics can be given alone or with corticoids, which are a must in the case of allergic conjuctivitis.

> Holocaine, 1% solution; instill one or two drops into the conjunctival sac.

> Pontocaine, 0.5% solution; instill one or two drops into the conjunctival sac.

> Cortisone, 15 mg for each g of an ophthalmic ointment, to be applied every 6 to 8 hours.

Keratoconjunctivitis

Symptoms are: pain (severe), other symptoms of conjunctivitis (lacrimation, photophobia, purulent discharge), and, on examination, small yellow-gray phlyctenulae found on the conjunctiva or the limbus. The *sicca-syndrome* (Sjögren's) presents an absolute lack of tears, and usually is accompanied by arthritic symptoms.

The patient should be sent to an ophthalmologist for treatment. Cases of regular keratoconjunctivitis are treated with a combination of antibiotics and corticoids. Seldom will the pain be so annoying as to require the use of local anesthetics. For the sicca-syndrome use artificial tears and try corticoids at low dosages, skipping days for better tolerance.

> Neomycin sulfate, 5 mg, plus hydrocortisone acetate, 10 mg, for each ml of ophthalmic suspension; instill two or three drops every 4 to 6 hours.

> Neomycin sulfate, 5 mg, plus polymyxin B sulfate, 10,000 units, and hydrocortisone acetate, 10 mg, for each ml of ophthalmic suspension; instill two or three drops into the conjunctival sac every 4 to 6 hours.

> Tetracaine, 0.5% solution; instill two or three drops into the conjunctival sac every 4 to 6 hours.

Cocaine, 4% solution; instill two or three drops into the conjunctival sac every 4 to 6 hours.

Prednisone, tablets containing 1, 2.5, or 5 mg each; take no more than 5 or 10 mg a day, to start; reduce dosage as soon as possible, taking 1 or 2.5 mg every other day or leaving longer lapses between the days of medication.

Interstitial Keratitis

Symptoms are: pain, lacrimation, photophobia, a grayish infiltration of the cornea (deep layers), new growth of vessels around the limbus, and a progressive loss of vision. Other forms of keratitis always cause pain, lacrimation, photophobia, and, in some instances, loss of vision. Scattered punctate infiltration of the superficial layers characterizes *superficial punctate keratitis;* ulceration forming branched lesions that resemble the veins of a leaf (with knoblike ends) is called *dendritic keratitis;* a disc-shaped deep inflammation is *disciform keratitis*.

A combination of antibiotics and corticoids will be advised, specially if syphilis is a factor. The patient will be referred immediately to an ophthalmologist for further treatment.

See above formulations.

Ulcers of the Cornea

Symptoms are: pain, lacrimation, photophobia, a localized point of necrosis in the cornea (grayish superficial lesion), and possible perforation at a later stage.

Obtain material for germ culture and sensitivity; give, immediately, adequate and specific local and general antibiotic therapy. If pain is very annoying, local anesthetics can be prescribed. For deep ulcerations, atropine will be mandatory. In all instances refer the patient to an ophthalmologist.

Pontocaine, 0.5% solution; instill two or three drops into the conjunctival sac every 4 to 6 hours.

Cocaine, 4% solution; instill two or three drops into the conjunctival sac every 4 to 6 hours.

Atropine, 1% solution; instill one drop into the conjunctival sac, no more than three times a day (every 8 hours).

Iritis and Iridocyclitis

Symptoms of *iritis* are pain (radiating to the temple), edema of the upper eyelid, lacrimation, photophobia, swelling, color changes of the iris, a miotic pupil irregular from synechiae, and marked congestion of blood vessels around the cornea. *Iridocyclitis* shows the same symptoms, but they are more severe, and the injection of the blood vessels of the conjunctiva is more marked.

Dilate the pupils with atropine; give local corticoids, of the type of cortisone, dexamethasone, and so on; and analgesics, if needed. Refer the patient to a specialist.

Atropine, 1% solution; instill one drop into the conjunctival sac every 8 hours.

Cortisone, 15 mg for each g of the ophthalmic ointment; apply every 4 to 6 hours.

Codeine, 30 (to 60) mg, by mouth, every 4 hours; inject, if needed.

Endophthalmitis and Panophthalmitis

Intense pain in the eye, with marked congestion of the blood vessels and chemosis, rapid loss of vision, and production of pus, indicates the onset of an *endophthalmitis* (suppuration is limited to the retina and the uveal tract) or a *panophthalmitis* (suppuration involves the whole eye). An early diagnosis is imperative, and treatment requires an ophthalmologist from the beginning.

The severe pain that always accompanies the condition has to be relieved immediately, with codeine, meperidine, or even morphine. It is desirable that secretion be taken for culture and sensitivity to antibiotics, since antibiotic therapy is to be started as soon as possible, with the specific antibiotic or at least with a broad-spectrum one. Antibiotic therapy, of course, has to be given systemically.

Codeine, 60 mg, by subcutaneous injection or by mouth, every four hours.

Meperidine, 100 mg by subcutaneous injection or by mouth, every 4 or 6 hours, as needed, but only for a short time.

Morphine, 10 to 15 mg by subcutaneous injection, every 4 hours, as needed and tolerated; also not for a prolonged period of time.

Optic Neuritis and Retrobulbar Neuritis

Optic neuritis provokes pain on eye motion and some sort of disturbance of vision, from enlargement of the blind spot to complete blindness of the affected eye. *Retrobulbar neuritis* also presents pain, constant and aggravated by eye motion, and rapid loss of vision, with only a little hyperemia of the retina.

The patient will be referred to a specialist. Meanwhile, analgesics can be given for the relief of pain, as well as corticoids—which will serve a double mission: to allay pain and to avoid reactive irritation.

> Codeine, 30 (to 60) mg, by mouth, every 4 hours; or by subcutaneous injection, if needed, particularly at the start of treatment.

> Prednisone, 5 mg, one or two tablets every 6 hours; decrease the dose when pain subsides, and discontinue therapy very slowly after some 10 days of treatment.

Dacryocystitis

Diseases causing obstruction of the lacrimal ducts are frequent in old age. In the acute form, there is pain at the medial canthus of the eye, with redness and edema over the region of the lacrimal sac, with lacrimation and other symptoms.

Pain may be relieved by common analgesics. Hot compresses, applied over the affected area for 10 minutes, three or four times a day, are also helpful. The rest of the treatment depends on an ophthalmologist for antibiotic therapy and drainage, if needed.

Hordeolum (Sty) and Blepharitis

Hordeolum is characterized by pain, redness, and swelling of the eyelid (the inflammation more localized at the site of the infection), restricted to the superficial layers of the eyelid. In *blepharitis* there is no actual pain but a sensation of discomfort (burning, itching) of the eyelid, which appears inflamed and excretes some pus.

Local treatment can be given with ophthalmic antibiotic ointments, either alone or with corticoids. In the case of hordeolum the mixture of corticoids and antibiotics may abort the sty; also, the sty may mature more rapidly if hot compresses are used, applied for 10 minutes, three or four times a day. Drain pus by incising the sty.

> Neomycin sulfate, 5 mg, plus polymyxin B sulfate, 10,000 units, and hydrocortisone acetate, 10 mg, for each ml of ophthalmic suspension; instill two or three drops into the conjunctival sac every 4 or 6 hours.

Orbital Cellulitis

Symptoms are: very severe pain in the orbit, exophthalmos, restricted mobility of the eye, edema of lids and conjunctiva, and frequently a history of infection elsewhere in the body (paranasal sinuses, mouth, and so on).

A help to the general treatment of orbital cellulitis (rest, hot application, and *antibiotics*) will be to minimize pain with analgesics of the type of codeine, acetylsalicylic acid, and so forth. Rarely, stronger analgesia will be needed, provided that emesis will not be a complication which might cause eye damage.

Errors of Refraction

These conditions usually cause caphalalgia, the sensation of strained eyes, headache, and at times local pain.

The patient will be referred to an ophthalmologist for corrective eyeglasses.

Traumatic Lesions to the Eye

The obvious nature of traumatic lesions, all accompanied by pain, makes any discussion of this subject unnecessary.

Besides the surgical management urgently needed in most of these cases, the patient has to be relieved of the pain he is suffering. Morphine should not be used, because of the frequency with which it induces vomiting, endangering a damaged eye. In most instances codeine will control the pain.

Furunculosis and External Otitis

Frequent sites of furunculosis are the canal of the ear and the auricle itself. Pain is the dominant symptom, and the presence of the furuncle is disclosed together with diffuse inflammation of the canal.

Pain has to be relieved with analgesics, and local heat applications started as soon as possible. A thorough cleansing of the ear canal is imperative, and will be done immediately, gently using an irrigator or syringe, with sodium bicarbonate, 3% solution. After irrigation of the area, it will be dried with a cotton applicator. Thereafter, local treatment with antibiotic preparations will follow, by applying the solution to a loose cotton pledget in the canal, or, if preferred, applying an antibiotic ointment. To control the swelling of the canal, in acute external otitis and in furunculosis, the use of aluminum acetate (Burow's solution) may be very helpful. Put a loose gauze strip or a piece of cotton into the canal, and keep it wet with the aluminum acetate solution by adding a few drops every 3 or 4 hours; but this procedure is not to be done for more than 2 days. This will allow a better application of local antibiotics. Furuncles are to be incised after pus is well localized; but incision is not always advisable, and should be left to the specialist. Systemic antibiotics must be started at the outset, and continued 2 days after the infection is cleared up. It is best to use the specific antibiotic; but, in any case, use a broad-spectrum one.

Traumatic Lesions to the Auricles and External Canal

These lesions are always obvious, and the diagnosis is easily made. Most are due to foreign bodies inserted into the canal.

These foreign bodies have to be removed at the earliest possible time; but since it is very easy to damage the eardrum during the removal, it is advised that the procedure be done by a specialist or at least someone expert in the technic. Residual pain may be treated with local anesthetic solutions. Contusions, wounds, frostbite, and so on, will be treated as elsewhere in the body: by cold compresses, local disinfection, stitches, and so forth. In the case of wounds, it is best to follow the advice of an expert on how to preserve the normal shape of the auricle. In case of large hematomas, remove blood, apply pressure, and avoid infection by a sterile procedure. For residual pain either use local anesthetics, as stated above, or give analgesics.

Myringitis

There is a severe local pain in the ear, with more or less marked deafness and systemic symptoms (fever). Otoscopy will show the eardrum red and often covered with vesicles.

Give an analgesic to control pain, control the infection with adequate antibiotic therapy, and add corticoids that may help for a more rapid improvement; but do not delay in referring the patient to an otologist.

Otitis Media

This is a common complication of infective diseases involving the nasopharynx: pain within the ear, varying degrees of deafness, fullness inside the ear, tinnitus, and more or less marked constitutional symptoms (fever, malaise, and so forth). Otoscopy will reveal an inflamed eardrum with possible bulging. In chronic otitis media there is also pain, but it may recede after a time.

Ordinarily otitis media requires surgery, which should be done by a specialist. Pain may be relieved by means of analgesics when it is due to acute serous otitis, acute purulent otitis, chronic secretory otitis, and chronic purulent otitis. In the case of complicating eustachian tube inflammation, in acute serous otitis, in chronic secretory otitis, and in chronic congestive otitis, the use of a vasoconstrictor by the nasal route is advisable.

Inflation of the eustachian tube is a procedure that should be left to the specialist. Antihistamines, systemic descongestants, and antibiotics can be of great help.

Ephedrine, 1% solution, to instill in the nose two or three drops, two or three times a day.

Chlorpheniramine maleate, 8 mg, by mouth, every 6 to 8 hours.

Pseudoephedrine hydrochloride, 60 mg, tablets, every 6 or 8 hours.

Mastoiditis

Pain on the mastoid area, with or without edema at the same site, which follows a chronic or even a recent infection in the ear or a treatment of the area by antibiotics, suggests mastoiditis. Take cultures of secretions from any infection in the ear before starting antibacterial medication. Since this is a problem to be solved by a specialist, the patient will be referred to an otologist after receiving an injection of codeine to allay pain. Chronic cases will also be scheduled to receive specialized care because complications are manifold and prone to occur, including severe ones such as brain abscess, lateral sinus phlebitis, and meningitis.

Codeine, 60 mg, by subcutaneous injection.

Buccal Dysphagia

This disability occurs in all painful inflammatory diseases of the mouth. Only a brief summary will be given here of the treatment for this pain when it makes eating difficult. (More details will follow immediately.)

Caries and *pulpitis*: cleanse the affected area and put a cotton plug with clove oil on the sensitive spot.

Dento-alveolar abscess: treat with analgesics of the salicylate type, and similar drugs; if fever is also present, with antibiotics. As soon as pus is localized, the abscess must be incised.

Xerostomia or dryness of the mouth: this condition is frequent in later years, owing to reduced fluid intake, mouth breathing, or sicca-syndrome. Persons with sicca-syndrome comprise about 25% of patients with xerostomia; they may respond to small amounts of corticoids, on alternate days for better tolerance. Also, wet the mouth with saline or water.

Buccal aphthae: local anesthetic medication will be given before each meal. Mouthwashes and vitamin therapy are also advisable.

Gingivitis and *stomatitis:* treat according to the causative factor, namely, diabetes, leukemia, pernicious anemia, or toxic agents, including drugs. Local irritants (calculus, infection, redundant gingiva, and so forth) will be removed. Use frequently a plain water mouthwash, cleansing solutions, and, if necessary, local anesthetics.

Vincent's angina: use analgesics of the type of salicylates and the like, and wash the mouth with hydrogen peroxide (in equal amounts of water). Clean the infected area and follow the mouthwash of hydrogen peroxide with a mouthwash of a dilution of Fowler's solution of arsenic, meticulously prepared and reliably supervised.

Glossitis: treat with anesthetic solutions and very careful oral hygiene.

Injuries to the mouth: refer to an oral surgeon, but pain has to be controlled with analgesics, mostly of the narcotic type, together with local applications of cold (ice bags), starting at the first visit of the patient.

Postextraction pain: treat with warm saline to cleanse the socket and a few drops of an anesthetic solution, repacking after cleansing every other day, and give analgesics by mouth.

Pulpitis

There is a sharp pain, intermittent and not always well localized by the patient. The diagnosis is made by X-ray and electric examination.

Pain may be relieved by cleansing the cavity very carefully, removing all food debris, and applying oil of cloves. Further treatment is entirely in the dentist's domain; but meanwhile efforts will be made to avoid accumulation of food in the cavity.

> Oil of cloves; soak a cotton applicator, and put it in the cavity.

> Clove oil plus zinc oxide powder; mix to make a semisolid mixture, and apply it to the cavity.

Dento-Alveolar Abscess

This condition, which is secondary to suppurative pulpitis, is characterized by local inflammation of the gingiva and extended edematous reaction to the nearby facial structures. It may appear without previous pulpitis.

The use of analgesics is of help. Codeine may be given by injection. If there is fever, an antibiotic should be added, and the antibiotic therapy maintained until some sort of surgery is performed. The specific antibiotic should be used; otherwise, penicillin is advised. In the case of fluctuant swelling at the site of the root of the affected tooth, an incision should be made to drain the pus, and the pus collected and sent to the laboratory for culture and sensitivity to antibiotics. Also, hot saline mouth rinses may help.

> Codeine, 30 (to 60) mg, by mouth, every 4 hours; or by intramuscular or subcutaneous injection.

Penicillin (procaine), 600,000 units every 6 or 8 hours, by injection. Also, could be given by mouth in appropriate dosage.

Gingivitis and Stomatitis

In *gingivitis* there are pain, swelling, redness, and bleeding of the gingivae. It is a syndromic complex that may reveal other diseases: diabetes, leukemia, scurvy, pellagra, or intoxication by diphenylhydantoin (Dilantin) or heavy metals. Pain is not rare, particularly in secondary forms or forms characterized by their severity.

Stomatitis or inflammation of the oral mucosae may constitute a painful condition independent of or secondary to other diseases. Symptoms vary from a relatively mild inflammation with little pain, to extremely painful necrotizing or gangrenous lesions. Direct smears or cultures from the lesions will help to diagnose the etiological factor. A general examination of the patient will help to disclose any underlying disease (scurvy, pellagra, agranulocytosis, leukemia, bacterial or fungal diseases, syphilis, or scarlet fever). (See also the following paragraphs.)

Gangrenous Stomatitis

Noma or gangrenous stomatitis is characterized by a grayish slough of all the buccal mucosae, which swell, and turn red and, finally, black, all this accompanied by only moderate pain.

Treatment depends on the cause: diabetes, pellagra, toxic agents (including drugs), pernicious anemia, or leukemia. Any irritating cause must be removed, such as calculus, local infection, or redundant gingiva. Local treatment will include mouthwashes with hydrogen peroxide, sodium borate, or perborate. The application of a local anesthetic to painful areas is also helpful, in the form of mouthwashes or ointment.

Hydrogen peroxide, diluted in equal parts of water.

Sodium perborate, 1 teaspoonful in a glass of water.

Lidocaine, 2% solution, a few drops in a tablespoonful of water.

Benzocaine, 5% ointment, applied locally.

Vincent's Angina

This necrotizing gingivostomatitis presents a sudden onset with fever and painful bleeding of the gingival area, the oral mucosa, and the pharynx, including the tonsils.

Advise rest, a bland diet, multivitamins, and strict avoidance of smoking. Any analgesic may be given to relieve pain, but it will almost completely

subside in the great majority of cases following the use of frequently repeated mouthwashes with hydrogen peroxide, followed by specially supervised mouthwashes of diluted potassium arsenite solution.

Hydrogen peroxide, mixed with equal parts of water, to be used as
mouthwash, after each meal and at bedtime.

Fowler's solutions (potassium arsenite solution), 0.2 ml, (three
drops) diluted with one-fourth glass (60 ml) of water. Hold in mouth
for 2 minutes and spit out. Do not swallow.

Aphthae

Aphthae are very painful small, shallow ulcers, round or ovoid in shape.
Most commonly only one ulcer appears during each attack, occurring anywhere within the mouth.

No specific treatment is known. Mouthwashes are good: hydrogen
peroxide, sodium perborate, sodium borate. Some physicians advise the use
of multivitamins to prevent recurrences, but they have not been proved
effective. The best measure is good oral hygiene. Anesthetic medication
applied locally may be a minor help.

Glossitis

The inflammation of the tongue may be either chronic or acute, primary or
secondary, and may manifest itself under several different types, as follows:

Systemic infections: the condition is not always painful, but on some
occasions its intense inflammation may provoke discomfort. Pain may occur
when fissures are formed.

Traumatic: lesions are due to irritation from teeth or orthodontic devices
in the mouth. Pain is the main manifestation. Heavy smokers and drinkers
often show glossitis, not always painful.

Pellagra: glossitis may reach important proportions, but is not the principal symptom of the disease. Its manifestations vary from an inflammation
occupying only the borders and tip of the tongue, to a massive ulcerative
stomatitis.

Ulcers: they are always painful, particularly when touched, and may be
provoked by a neighboring irritating tooth, coughing (if located in the fre-
num), self-biting (epilepsy), or a generalized stomatitis. Cancer of the tongue
begins with a painful ulcer, which bleeds easily. Tuberculosis ulcers are
relatively large and very painful. Treat according to the cause. Locally,
relieve pain by the use of some anesthetic before eating. Advise a nutritious
diet, multivitamins, and careful oral hygiene. All sorts of toxins and irritants
have to be avoided (spices, strong beverages, and tobacco). In the case of
glossodynia, local anesthesia must be obtained by local injection, better if

accompanied by corticoids orally. Also, antihistamines, sedatives, tranquilizers, and vitamins may be used with benefit; and estrogens in the menopausal woman. Glossodynia with xerostomia will force the use of pilocarpine.

See formulas for anesthesia, above.

Pilocarpine, 20 mg a day, in divided doses.

Dysgeusia

A disturbed sense of taste may force the patient to dislike food, thus leading to malnutrition and weight loss, a situation not too rare among the elderly.
Keep the mouth clean, and instill 2 or 3 drops of zinc sulfate solution.

Zinc sulfate, 0.2% solution, two or three drops, two or three times a day.

Neoplasms

Ulcers or tumors located anywhere in the mouth will suggest the possibility of cancer as soon as they are indolent, or painful with a burning sensation, most frequently, or bleed easily. Tumors do not become painful until their healing is delayed.
Malignancies in the mouth are treated by either radiation or surgery. For the treatment of pain, regular analgesics should be used first, and narcotics given when necessary.

Postextraction Pain

Pain follows most extractions of teeth, because of the traumatism and also because of the previous infection. Delayed pain indicates socket reinfection.
Irrigate the socket with warm saline, either alone or with a few drops of an anesthetic. Pack loosely with gauze strips soaked with a mixture of guaiacol and glycerin. Repack, every other day, after cleansing. Give oral analgesics also.

Lidocaine, 2% solution.

Cocaine, 5% solution.

Arthritis of the Temporomandibular Joint

Symptoms are severe arthralgia and limitation of movement of the mandible, ordinarily affecting only one side.
Treatment includes resting the joint, soft diet, analgesics, relaxants, and,

if needed, tranquilizers. When this treatment fails, it will be better to consult a specialist, particularly if local injection of corticoids also fails.

Trauma to the Mouth

Localized pain and perhaps abnormal mobilization of the effected parts may indicate a fracture of the bones of the mouth. These fractures are frequently compound.

All severe injuries to the mouth are to be treated by an oral surgeon. In the meantime, efforts to alleviate pain will be welcome. Apply an ice bag, externally.

Meperidine, 100 mg, by mouth, every 4 hours.

Codeine, 30 (to 60) mg, by mouth, every 4 hours; may be injected.

The *lack of teeth* constitutes some sort of traumatism which should be avoided by the use of an adequate prosthesis.

Pharyngeal Dysphagia

Dysphagia occurs in all inflammatory diseases of the pharynx. A symptomatology similar to that of retropharyngeal abscess may be noted in cases with caries of the cervical vertebrae; but in this instance, pain may be absent. Diagnosis depends on X-ray examination. There are also a few forms of dysphagia caused by spasms of the pharyngeal muscles, which may or may not be painful: rabies, tetanus, tetany, encephalitis, strychnine intoxication, and others. Pharyngitis and tonsillitis are, perhaps, the most frequent causes of pharyngeal dysphagia.

The first step will be to identify the causative germ, determine its sensitivity to antibiotics, and give the indicated one. To treat pain, swab the pharynx with anesthetic solutions and prescribe an anesthetic gargle containing phenol, 0.5%, particularly before meals.

Tonsillitis and Pharyngitis

The prevalent symptomatology is that of pharyngitis, but in most instances the tonsils are also involved: the pharynx will be red and swollen and show mild or marked exudates, together with the tonsils, which may appear enlarged and show some purulent secretions in true tonsillitis; and there is pain which increases on swallowing. If the disease is merely confined to this area, general symptoms will be absent, except, at times, for fever. In other instances the underlying diagnosis must be established. In adenoiditis there is also nasal obstruction, but this condition will be rare in the elderly.

Influenza: presents upper respiratory symptoms, fever, generalized aches, and marked weakness.

Scarlet fever: shows a rather severe angina followed by the erythematous rash.

Rheumatic fever: presents a relatively complex picture of angina and one or more of the following: articular pains, cardiac or neurologic involvement (murmurs or chorea), or skin reactions (nodules, erythema marginatum or nodosum).

Diphtheria: covers the tonsils and pharynx with a grayish membrane, which leaves a bleeding surface when detached.

Agranulocytosis: starts abruptly with angina, local ulcers, septic fever, and regional adenopathy, mostly in patients under treatment with certain drugs.

Acute leukemia: presents a picture similar to the former one, with dermic symptoms, as petechiae or other forms of bleeding.

Vincent's angina: shows extensive buccal reactions, mainly bleeding gums and ulceration.

Herpangina: gives a picture of common angina together with herpetic vesicles.

Zoster angina: is like herpangina but occurs only in one side of the pharynx.

Detection of the causative infective agent and its sensitivity to antibiotics will permit effective radical treatment. If the pain requires special measures, it will help to swab the pharynx with an anesthetic solution. Also, it will help to put an ice collar around the neck or to take analgesics by mouth. If an abscess develops, it should be opened for drainage, if necessary. A specialist should be consulted in many instances.

Peritonsillar Abscess

Symptoms are: severe pain at one side of the throat, swelling and tenderness of the corresponding jaw and adjacent tissues, edema of the uvula, which appears displaced on examination, as well as symptoms of systemic infection.

For peritonsillar abscess the effective treatment is surgical drainage when fluctuation is evident. The incision is made at the point of localized swelling or softening. Often these cases require the surgical skill and judgment of a specialist. Since this area is extremely sensitive, some sort of anesthesia can be given, but its effectiveness is impaired by the presence of violent inflammation. Wash the mouth with antiseptics after a thorough cleansing following evacuation of pus. After incision, injection of codeine is helpful.

Cocaine, 10% solution; apply with an applicator to the surface to be incised.

Procaine, 2% solution; inject locally.

Laryngitis

Hoarseness is the main symptom of either acute or chronic laryngitis. Pain on swallowing may be more or less marked, as well as a constant ache located in the lower oropharynx. Diphtheric and tuberculous laryngitis must be ruled out in all instances. Also a thorough search must be made for neoplasms of the larynx and pharynx, particularly in chronic conditions. The causative factor may be primary or a complication of respiratory or systemic infections; it must be basically treated and eliminated whenever possible.

Advise rest of the voice, a humid atmosphere, steam inhalations at frequent intervals (either water alone or with eucalyptol: 1 teaspoonful added to each quart of water), and anesthetic lozenges (dibucaine, 1%). For cough, codeine and expectorants can be given if necessary. A specialist should be consulted in most cases.

> Potassium iodide, saturated solution (1g for each ml of water), 300 to 600 mg (5 to 10 drops) in water every 2 hours, to help expectoration.

> Glyceryl guaiacolate, 100 mg for each 5 ml of water or syrup; 5 to 10 ml every 2 to 4 hours.

PAIN IN THE NECK AND SPINE

Torticollis (Wry Neck)

There is pain on the side of the spasm, exaggerated when the patient tries to move the head to a normal position from the forced torsion against the affected muscle, which appears tense and painful to the touch. Torticollis might be an independent clinical entity (torticollis "a frigore"), but it is mostly secondary to other causes (rheumatism, injuries, inflammatory lesions of the spine, neuritis, or even diseases of the central nervous system).

In treating torticollis, massage and heat applications are effective. Anticholinergics may give more encouraging results. Also, tranquilizers may help, as well as muscle relaxants, the latter preferred in most instances.

> Belladonna tincture, five, ten, or more drops, in a little water, every 4 to 8 hours, according to effects and tolerance.

> Meprobamate, 400 mg, by mouth, every 6 hours.

> Carisoprodol, 350 mg, by mouth, every 6 to 8 hours.

Severe cases need a head halter to apply traction; some will need a collar. These cases will be better under the care of a specialist.

Deformities of the Cervical Spine

Fusion of vertebrae may be due to infections, injuries to the spine, or abnormal congenital development. There is limitation of movements; and the diagnosis will depend on the clinical history and X-ray findings.

Cervical ribs cause pain or paresthesias in the shoulder and arm (scalenus anticus syndrome). The elongated rib may be detected on palpation (rarely on inspection). For more details see below, the paragraph on "Scalenus Anticus Syndrome," in the section "Pain in the Extremities."

Curvatures of the spine: there will be pain in the neck and the back from the various curvatures of the spine, such as kyphosis, scoliosis, lordosis, or a combination of them. The diagnosis is made by simple inspection and palpation.

Treat the fusion of vertebrae resulting from infective processes with special emphasis on the infection; but physical measures are important in almost all cases, even though pain is not always too distressing and surgery is available. The advice of a specialist is desirable.

For cervical ribs, physical therapy is advised, with surgery as required, and analgesics for pain.

Curvatures of the spine cause pain mostly because of muscle strain. The logical treatment, therefore, is to give cholinergics or muscle relaxants, but it is better under the direction of a specialist.

Suboccipital Neuralgia

Symptoms include pain in the back of the neck, at times more marked on one side, and occasional muscle spasm. A sensitive point might be detected by pressing at the center of a line traced from the mastoid to the first cervical apophysis.

This type of neuritis responds very well to infiltration with anesthetic solution into the tissues on the occipital area, at the level of the hairline. Also, traction or a neck collar might help many patients, particularly if analgesics are added. When the above measures fail, surgery might be the best approach, if advised by a specialist.

> Procaine, 1% solution; inject up to 10 ml diffusely into the occipital area.

> Lidocaine, 1% solution; inject 5 to 10 ml diffusely into the occipital area.

Infectious Diseases Causing Spinal Pain

Smallpox (variola) is characterized by fever together with a painful rachialgia and headache, myalgias, chills, and tachycardia. The typical eruption establishes the diagnosis (macules, papules, umbilicated vesicles that turn into pustules, all of them appearing in only one crop of eruptions, first on the face). Symptomatic therapy is the method of treatment. Pain may be relieved with acetylsalicylic acid or codeine. Because of their effects upon the central nervous system, particularly the respiratory centers, do not give narcotic analgesics in these cases.

Meningitis and *meningismus* cause pain in the back accompanying the characteristic agonizing headache. There are fever, stiff neck, and positive Kernig's and Brudzinski's signs. Laboratory tests establish the diagnosis. Meningism will induce the same symptomatology but without the evidence of meningeal infection. As soon as the diagnosis is completed, specific therapy will be started immediately, together with measures for dehydration and for electrolytic changes. Corticoids may help.

Influenza provokes a mild rachialgia, myalgias, other pains, and the common and revealing respiratory symptoms. These discomforts ordinarily respond well to the use of analgesics.

Pleuritis, if located at the central portion of the diaphragmatic pleura, causes pain referred to the neck and shoulder, the thorax, and the back. Hearing a pleural friction rub is characteristic. Common analgesics are usually effective in relieving these complaints. Adhesive strapping can also give relief. At times there is need for stronger drugs, either morphine or paravertebral procaine infiltration. Codeine should be tried before resorting to stronger drugs, since it helps mitigate the pain and allay cough reflexes.

Spondylitis: Infections in the spine cause symptoms of rheumatic pain and limitation of motion, or even more important complaints. Tuberculosis provokes severe pain that may awaken the patient from his sleep; X-ray plates will give a clue to the problem, but the diagnosis depends on the demonstration of bacilli by laboratory tests. Gonococcal spondylitis is frequent among patients infected with the gonococcus. In brucellosis there is a clinical picture similar to tuberculosis, though pain occurs earlier and suppuration is not so prevalent. Streptococcal infections may locate at the spine and provoke a spondylitic syndrome. In all these cases, the X-ray examination is very important. Each individual case of spondylitis will require individual basic care; but nearly all require the help of analgesics for the relief of pain.

Rheumatoid Spondylitis

This is mostly a disease of young people, rarely seen in elderly patients. Pain is the first symptom, starting at the lower portion of the spine and spreading upward progressively. It is accompanied by stiffness of the column. The condition of the patient is worse when he leaves his bed in the morning. Outbursts of pain and stiffness last only for days or weeks, and then subside for a time. The vertabrae are tender on pressure. X-ray examination and laboratory tests are essential for diagnosis.

In rheumatoid (ankylosing) spondylitis, in addition to physical care, the patient will receive analgesic and anti-inflammatory drugs. The basic drugs to be tried are indomethacin, phenylbutazone, and oxyphenbutazone, but always with due precautions because of untoward effects, particularly hematologic ones (aplastic anemia, agranulocytosis, leukopenia, and so on).

> Sodium salicylate, 600 mg, by mouth, every 4 hours, with meals or antacids; the addition of small amounts of thyroid extracts, 30 to 60 mg a day, may help for tolerance.

> Prednisone, 5 to 20 mg a day, to be decreased slowly and discontinued when effects are noted.

> Indomethacin, 25 mg, by mouth, every 8 to 12 hours.

> Phenylbutazone, 100 to 200 mg, by mouth, every 8 hours.

Hypertrophic Spondylitis

Osteoarthritis of the spine is a disease of the elderly, since most healthy people will show some osteoarthritic changes of their vertebrae after 50 years of age. Pain is of little interest, though aching and stiffness on motion can be detected in most cases.

Physical treatment is needed, as a firm pillow and mattress, neck collar or brace with traction. Analgesics are always of help for relief of pain, but narcotics are not recommended for these patients.

Climacteric Vertebral Osteoporosis

Pain is the main symptom of this condition, with a decrease of bone mass; the diagnosis is made after an X-ray examination, and should be completed before more severe symptoms arise (collapse of vertebrae).

This reaction is much rarer with the administration of estrogen and progesterone (with due precautions because of recent warnings about induction of cancer), but requires some help with analgesics to alleviate the symptomatic pain. Salicylates and the like are desirable.

Senile Vertebral Osteoporosis

Senile osteoporosis starts after the climacterium. Pain is relieved by rest. Spontaneous fractures may occur when the disease is advanced.

In women, the treatment should be as for climacteric osteoporosis. Androgens and also other anabolic steroids will be tried on men. Analgesics will be of some help.

Vertebral Osteomalacia

This condition is due to deficient calcification of bones and may occur in patients losing calcium in the urine or with other impairment of bone calcium deposition. Pain in the spine is a prominent symptom (not always present), and collapse of the vertebrae may occur later in the disease. Symptoms of tetany will be present when blood calcium is low.

Besides the specific treatment with vitamin D, a high calcium diet will be of positive help. In many instances the physician will have to resort to analgesics.

Curvature of the Spine

Lordosis, kyphosis, and scoliosis may provoke pain in the back. The diagnosis is obvious.

Since pain is mostly due to muscle strain, the logical approach is to use papaverine, belladonna, atropine, meprobamate, carisoprodil, and so forth. But the basic treatment should be directed by an orthopedist.

Papaverine hydrochloride, 150 mg, in slow-release capsules, one every 12 hours.

Tincture of belladonna, five to ten drops, three to six times a day, or more; according to needs and tolerance.

Meprobamate, 400 mg, by mouth, every 6 hours.

Carisoprodol, 350 mg, by mouth, every 6 to 8 hours.

Spinal Myelitis

Pain in the back may accompany some cases, and its nervous pathology should be traced to a possible cause by syphilis, tuberculosis, or bacterial infections.

The help of a neurologist may be needed. Maintain good nursing care, care of the bladder (including catheterization in most cases), care of the bowels (enemas, at least every other day), and use of an air mattress, and turn the patient every 2 hours, at the same time giving thorough care to the skin. Since paraplegics are protein losers, this element in the blood must be kept at normal levels. Antibiotics will be given according to each individual infection.

Spinal Epidural Abscess

Severe pain in the back, aggravated by motion of the spine, is symptomatic. Paresis, paralysis, or paresthesias, and septic symptoms complete the syndrome.

Surgery and antibiotic therapy are the essentials of the treatment.

Diseases of the Mediastinum

Diseases of the posterior mediastinum may account for spinal pain—interscapular, not intense but bothersome. It is exaggerated in bed. Dysphagia or the Horner syndrome may be present.

Esophageal dysphagia may be due to esophagitis, or may be extraesophageal. *Esophagitis* is the main cause of this form of dysphagia, which has been described before (see under "Abdominal Pain"). Differentiate it from cardiac pain (there is also dyspnea) and from pain related to posture and meals. *Extraesophageal dysphagia* will differentiate lodging of food in the lower esophagus (usually following a history of choking), spasms (usually accompanied by spasms of other muscles and relieved by drinking tepid water), achalasia of the esophagus (uncoordinated propulsion of contents, leading to strictures and dilatation), intrathoracic diseases due to tumor (cancer, lymphoadenopathies) or aneurismatic changes of the great vessels, pseudobulbar palsy due to cerebro-vascular disease, and moniliasis. Most of these conditions are to be treated by the specialist.

Tumors are the main source of mediastinal symptoms. They may be benign or malignant; radiography is the best diagnostic procedure. Esophagoscopy or broncoscopy can be used. The management is surgery whenever indicated for both benign and malignant growths, and chemotherapy or radiotherapy as indicated. Pain requires the use of narcotics.

> Morphine sulfate, 10 to 15 mg or more, by subcutaneous injection, repeated as needed and tolerated. Meperidine or codeine may be injected, instead.

Tuberculosis of the fibrotic type may stimulate the mediastinal syndrome. Symptoms due to tuberculosis are also present. Pain along the spine in cases of tuberculosis of the mediastinum may be due to pleural reaction if not to direct infection of the surrounding structures. Regular analgesics will be tried first—perhaps with some emphasis on codeine because it may also alleviate coughing. Narcotics are the last resource. The treatment of tuberculosis is essential.

Aneurism of the aorta: circulatory or respiratory symptoms may appear first. Pain will be present when the aneurism injures the spine. The basic treatment depends on the judgment of the specialist in cardiovascular conditions.

Referred Spinal Pain (Heterotopic Pain)

Abdominal symptomatology is the focal point of the clinical picture of the three following diseases, which may also present heterotopic spinal pain.

Biliary lithiasis may provoke pain radiating to the spine and the right shoulder (in rare instances, the left shoulder). The treatment includes the care of an acute attack (colic), for which it is advised to give, first, an injection of papaverine; as the second choice, an injection of meperidine, or better, meperidine with papaverine; and only as a last resort, morphine. Bed rest, hydration, gastric suction for the relief of abdominal distention, and antibiotics are needed. In cholecystitis, antacids as well as antispasmodics and sedatives give good results.

Peptic ulcer may cause spinal pain in a few patients. Peptic ulcers respond to antacids and anticholinergics.

Pancreatitis may cause pain in the spine in some cases. The best drug to treat this pain is codeine.

Low Back Pain

Infective Diseases. Low back pain may be more prominent than the pain in the upper spine in infections like smallpox, meningitis, or some cases of influenza.

Rheumatic Diseases. Except for the location of the pain, there is no difference between aches provoked by rheumatoid and hypertrophic spondylitis.

Metabolic Bone Diseases. Pain may be located low in the spine in climacteric osteoporosis, senile osteoporosis, and osteomalacia.

Deformities of the Spine. Curvatures such as scoliosis, kyphosis, and lordosis (particularly the last) may initiate low back pain.

Diseases of the Spinal Cord. In these diseases, pain may be low when caused by myelitis.

Muscle Diseases and Toxic Reactions. These diseases may also cause low back pain.

Injuries. The main complaint in this group of patients is the strain of an unusual effort, particuarly in lifting heavy objects, violent movements of the trunk, jumping, or falling on the feet. Often, the protrusion of an intervertebral disk is the cause of the pain. Each individual case will require its own physical therapy or surgical procedure, but the adjuvant use of analgesics is to be advised to alleviate suffering.

Acute Sprain. Acute sprain starts suddenly with pain in the lumbar spine following either an unusually heavy effort or even a movement that is performed every day. The patient cannot straighten up or move, and the pain increases for the following 1 or 2 hours. Rarely, the symptoms develop later on. The muscles are tense and tender to pressure. In general, the symptomatology corresponds to that of fibrositis (q.v.). Bed rest, local heat, and massage are important parts of the treatment; but the help of analgesics and muscle relaxants is valuable.

Fractures. Pain and muscle spasm are important symptoms. On examination there is local tenderness, and perhaps a deformity. The diagnosis is made by X-rays. Absolute immobilization and surgical care are essential for these cases, but analgesics are needed, starting with codeine or meperidine, and thereafter salicylates or similar analgesics.

Codeine, 30 to 60 mg, by subcutaneous injection, every 3 to 4 hours during the first 2 days; thereafter, by mouth, every 4 hours.

Meperidine, 100 mg, by mouth, every 4 hours, for 1 or 2 days; then to be followed by any other analgesic.

Disk Lesions. These lesions may be either traumatic or degenerative. Except for acute injuries (see above), forces acting constantly upon the last two vertebrae and their articulations will provoke low back pain. X-ray examination is imperative.

Protusion of the Intervertebral Disk. This condition often produces low back pain radiating to the thighs and aggravated by effort. There are spasms, local tenderness, and limitation of motion. Neurological symptoms may develop (depression of reflexes, paresthesias, and so on). An X-ray picture ordinarily establishes the diagnosis. In both the acute and the chronic stages of the disease, analgesics will help, as will muscle relaxants. Physical therapy is always needed, and surgical procedures are frequently a necessity.

Chronic Low Back Pain. Besides sources already indicated, the condition may also be due to sacralization of the 5th lumbar vertebra or lumbarization of the 1st sacral vertebra, spondylolyis, or spondylolisthesis. The pain may be continuous or intermittent, ordinarily aggravated by motion and mitigated by rest, heat, or massage. On examination, no abnormal signs or structures are usually found. Patients do not complain of sharp pains, but of annoying dull aches that do not interfere too much with daily activities. Besides the general measures necessary to handle these patients, the use of analgesics, particularly salicylates, is to be encouraged. At times, surgery is needed for the total relief of some patients.

Psoitis. Psoitis may be due to an infection of the spine, and so will present rachialgia; but the main symptoms are found in the legs.

Heterotopic Low Back Pain. There are a few diseases that may cause referred pain to the low spine. We shall mention some of them: biliary lithiasis, pancreatitis, kidney diseases (acute nephritis, renal colic, pyelonephritis, hydronephrosis), diseases of the uterus, prostatic diseases, and others. *Hernia in Petit's triangle* is a rare occurrence, found among elderly people with habitual constipation or who do unusual strenuous exercise. The swelling in the lumbar region may be very small. Other symptoms of herniation may be found. Surgery is the best approach, if feasible.

PAIN IN THE EXTREMITIES

Arthritis

Symptoms similar to rheumatism will be caused by the invasion of a joint by gonococci or tubercle bacilli, which are frequent offenders, along with staphylococci, streptococci, or pneumococci. Symptoms include limitation of movements, pain, and stiffness. In *acute arthritis* a joint becomes hot, red, and swollen. In *tuberculous arthritis* the symptoms are confined to one joint and show a chronic course. In *gonococcal arthritis* there is a previous urethritis, and the local symptoms are intense, occurring with fever and malaise. Other infective agents also cause acute and systemic symptoms. The diagnosis is made by isolation of the causative germ from the synovial fluid. In *gouty arthritis* the local symptoms will refer to the great toe, but tophi may be found in any tendon, joint, or bursa. Discharge of urates may take place, particularly in the hands and feet, from longstanding, prominent tophi. Symptomatology may show an acute or chronic course. The acute attack usually involves one joint; the pain reaches excruciating intensity (with shiny, red, hot, and tender skin), and may last a few days, at the beginning, but recur in a chronic form. Gout brings on limitation of movements and distortion of the joint. The diagnosis is made by detection of high levels of uric acid in the blood (over 8 mg/100 ml) and response to the use of colchicine internally.

Acute septic arthritis will be treated with adequate antibiotic therapy, aspiration and irrigation of the infected joint, and drainage whenever indicated. These measures will allay pain; but it can be helped with immobilization (using splints, if necessary) and elevation of the joint, the application of hot compresses, and the use of analgesics. In chronic septic arthritis, surgery and antibiotic therapy are the most important measures to be taken. Analgesics may be of some help.

Other forms of arthritis, as Reiter's syndrome, sarcoidosis, neurogenic, and chondrocalcinosis, should be treated for the basic cause, or at least symptomatically.

Gout treatment requires a well-planned way of living: keeping within normal weight limits, avoiding foods or beverages known to cause individual attacks, avoiding long fasting periods, not allowing dehydration or acidosis, and using colchicine together with probenecid or sulfinpyrazone as the basic medication. Probenecid and sulfinpyrazone will not be given to those with acute attacks. When these drugs fail to work, give allopurinol, provided this drug is well tolerated (itching is an early sign of intolerance). For acute gout, colchicine is the drug of choice. As alternates, indomethacin, or phenylbutazone, and corticoids are very effective medications. If the pain is very severe before the anti-gout agents produce their effect, give codeine or meperidine by subcutaneous injection.

> Colchicine, 0.5 mg, by mouth, every hour until the relief of pain or the appearance of nausea or diarrhea; 1 mg may be given every 2 hours; 4 to 8 mg are needed, in total, to control an attack. For chronic use, start with 0.5 mg, by mouth, every 8 hours, and decrease to 0.5 mg once a day after a few days.

Probenecid, 500 mg, tablets; start with half a tablet every 12 hours, for 7 days, and then one tablet a day or as needed and tolerated.

Sulfinpyrazone, 100 mg, by mouth, every 12 hours; increase gradually to 200 mg every 12 hours, as needed and tolerated.

Allopurinol, 100 mg, by mouth, every 12 hours, according to blood uric acid response, or, in severe cases, increase to 300 mg every 12 hours. Do not give this in acute gout.

Indomethacin, 25 mg, by mouth, every 8 hours; increase to a total of 200 mg a day, in divided doses, but for no more than 3 days.

Phenylbutazone, 100 mg, by mouth, give 400 mg a day at the start, in divided doses; follow with 200 mg a day, in two installments, until the attack is controlled, but not for more than 3 or 4 days.

Prednisone, 5 mg a day, by mouth, together with colchicine. Decrease and discontinue administration as soon as possible.

Codeine, 60 mg, by subcutaneous injection.

Meperidine, 100 mg, by subcutaneous injection.

Rheumatic Fever

Symptoms are almost identical with those of rheumatoid arthritis: they commonly follow a bout of pharyngitis, and are associated with heart murmurs, precordial pain, arrhythmia, pericardial friction rub, and even heart failure. Some patients also show skin rashes or chorea. The detection of beta-hemolytic streptococci is diagnostic.

Salicylates are almost specific for rheumatic fever, and will be given from the very beginning in large amounts in severe cases. These patients will also receive antibiotics (penicillin) and corticoids (prednisone), the latter to be replaced by salicylates if they prove ineffective after a trial of about 5 days. By this time, the patient should be treated by a specialist; but if care is needed, start corticoids immediately. Additional treatment, particularly in case of complications, will be advised by the specialist.

Acetylsalicylic acid, 600 mg, in tablets, every 4 hours, preferably with meals.

Acetylsalicylic acid, when larger doses are needed: to start with 60 mg for each kg of body weight, in four or six doses given during the 24-hour period; to increase to 90, 120, and 180 mg for each kg of body weight, also in six divided doses during the day. The medication will be given with meals, whenever possible, or accompanied by sodium bicarbonate, 300-mg tablets or the amount of powder taken with the point of a knife. Try thyroid extract (30 mg a day) to increase tolerance, but only small amounts.

Prednisone, 5 to 10 mg, by mouth, every 6 hours. After 3 weeks the dosage should be gradually decreased, to give a total treatment time of about 6 weeks. At times, higher doses are needed, up to 20 or even 40 mg every 6 hours; withdrawal will take a longer time. For prolonged treatments use the lowest effective dosage and skip days, at least every other day.

Rheumatoid Arthritis

This is a disease of younger people, but it may become abruptly apparent after 60 years of age, with pain in several joints, all of them swollen and tender on palpation. In the adult type, smaller joints (fingers, wrist, feet) are affected more frequently than the larger joints (hips, shoulders, knees, elbows), the reverse of the juvenile type; but the actual prevalent frequency is: fingers, knee, shoulders, toes, and elbows. Pain is worse after periods of inactivity. The muscles corresponding to the diseased joints are stiff, and the stronger flexors produce the typical cramped position of the affected parts. In the adult type, muscles become atrophied and give a noticeable fusiform shape to the fingers. Watch for the development of malignancies.

Advise bed rest, but only within certain limits, alternating with well-planned physical activity including progressive increase of exercises, to a reasonable working ability below the tolerance of the joints. There will be 4 to 8 additional hours to the regular 8-hour night rest; and also articular rest, with the use of splints, and so on, whenever advisable. Moist or radiant heat will help to allay pain and relax muscles. The use of salicylates will be the basic therapy, before resorting to corticoid or chrysotherapy, or other drugs.

Acetylsalicylic acid, 600 mg, tablets, every 4 hours; preferably after meals, and accompanied by a small daily dose of thyroid extract (15 to 30 mg a day, by mouth).

Sodium salicylate, 600 mg, by mouth, as above.

Sodium salicylate in larger doses; 1200 mg by mouth, every 4 to 6 hours, to increase to 2 g every 4 hours. Those who do not tolerate salicylates well should receive the help of antacids, to protect against local irriation (sodium bicarbonate, 300-mg tablets or the amount of powder taken by the point of a knife); also, the use of small amounts of thyroid extract (15 to 30 mg a day) will increase the tolerance in many cases.

Prednisone, 5 to 10 mg every 6 hours. As soon as the patient improves, but by 3 weeks at the latest, the dosage should be decreased, so that the complete treatment lasts for about 6 weeks, or less. Intra-articular injections (hydrocortisone, 25 to 50 mg) may be given. For more prolonged treatments, give the smallest effective dosage, skipping days, at least every other day.

Gold sodium thiomalate, in increasing dosages of 10, 25, 50, and 100 mg for each ml. Use 10 mg once the first week; 25 mg once the second week; thereafter, 50 mg once a week, to reach a total administration of 1 g (19 injections of 50 mg). If the response is good, decrease the dosage to 50 mg every 2 weeks; then, every 3 weeks; and finally maintain, tolerance permitting, 50 mg once a month for a long time.

Gold thioglucose (aurothioglucose), 10, 50, and 100 mg for each ml. To be used as above.

Degenerative Arthritis

This disease causes painful joints, but there is no involvement of muscles or swelling of the joints. This form of arthritis ordinarily begins after 40 years of age; the patients are mostly obese and do not compain of systemic changes.

Obese and hyperactive patients should avoid unnecessary stress on the affected joints, or even have the aid of supportive devices. The obese must regain normal weight. Apply heat locally. Orthopedic measures are needed, at times. The rest of the treatment will follow the same steps as for rheumatoid arthritis (see above paragraph).

Bursitis

This ailment brings on very intense pain when the corresponding muscle is in motion and its tendon presses over its bursa. In *acute bursitis* the symptoms appear suddenly, with pain, local tenderness, and limitation of movement. In *chronic bursitis* the symptoms are similar, and the muscle becomes atrophic because of lack of exercise. The most frequently involved bursa is the subdeltoid, and the pain is referred to the shoulder. Pressure on the bursa causes pain.

Within the first few hours of the onset of symptoms, radiotherapy usually gives very good results. Also, the early administration of corticoids will control symptoms rapidly in many cases. For well-established cases, rest, immobilization, applications of local heat, and the use of analgesics are needed. Some patients may also need the intra-articular injection of corticoids.

Prednisone, 5 mg, every 8 hours; decrease the dosage as soon as the effects are noted, and discontinue it gradually over a period of 15 or 20 days.

Hydrocortisone acetate, 25 mg in 1 ml suspension; inject from 1 to 5 ml into the bursa.

Stress Myalgia

Normal, healthy elderly persons will complain of stress myalgia some hours (next day) after any strenuous or prolonged unaccustomed use of muscles. Pain will occur in the muscles used for that exercise.

Rest, massage, heat applications, analgesics, and muscle relaxants will help to improve the situation.

Meprobamate, 400 mg, by mouth, every 6 hours, for a total of 2 or 3 days.

Myositis

Muscle pain and inflammation are the common symptoms of *trichinosis*. There are initial gastrointestinal symptoms followed by fever and edema of the eyelids. All muscles may be involved, especially the abdominal muscles. Suggestive for diagnostic purposes are an early eosinophilia and the ingestion of poorly cooked pork. Pain may be relieved with codeine, but a more specific treatment of the disease may include corticoids, thiabendazole, and pyrvinium pamoate.

Thiabendazole, 25 mg for each kilo of body weight in 24 hours, in divided doses (preferably, every 12 hours), to be given for 4 to 10 days.

Pyrvinium pamoate, 5 mg for each kilo of body weight, by mouth in one single dose (which may be repeated after 2 weeks).

Polymyositis presents inflammatory and degenerative changes of muscles and skin, the latter with edema and the former swollen. During the acute episodes of pain, corticoids and analgesics may help. Physical therapy may also be useful.

Prednisone, up to 60 or 80 mg a day for as long as needed, or until symptoms of hyperdosage appear.

Fibromyositis is noted by pain, tenderness, and stiffness of muscles and joints, usually following infection, trauma, extreme weather, or other causes. It may respond to rest, heat, massage, splints, hard mattress, salicylates, and local injection of anesthetics.

Procaine, 1% solution; inject 0.5 or 1 ml into the nodules.

Stiff-man syndrome shows a tonic muscle rigidity with episodic aching and tightness lasting for weeks or months. Avoid any stimulation likely to provoke spasms; give myoneural blocking agents (succinylcholine), or diazepam, or use lidocaine for peripheral nerve blocking.

Succinylcholine, 20 mg in 1 ml solution; inject intravenously 10 to 30 ml.

Diazepam, 5 (to 10) mg, by mouth, every 8 hours.

Lidocaine, 1 or 2% solution; inject in affected areas, up to 1 to 4 ml each.

Cramps

The extremely painful involuntary muscle contraction is characteristic. Cramps may be due to an unknown cause: nocturnal cramps; or they may be due to insufficient blood flow to a muscle. Common causes are dehydration, neurologic etiology, *tetany,* or *tetanus,* in which cramps are the outstanding symptom.

In tetanus, treatment of the infection comes first: give tetanus immune globulin and penicillin; and thereafter chlorpromazine and meprobamate. Cramps due to hypocalcemia (tetany) are treated with calcium salts, together with vitamin D, dihydrotachysterol, or parathyroid hormone (check calcemia to adjust dosage).

Calcium gluconate, 10% solution; inject 10 to 20 ml.

Dihydrotachysterol, 0.125 mg in capsules; give 0.75 to 2.5 mg a day, in divided doses.

Parathyroid hormone, 50 to 100 units by subcutaneous or intramuscular injection, repeating every 6 to 8 hours, but to no more than 1 week.

Cramps due to poor vascular supply may be improved by massage, hot applications, and the use of vasodilators.

Papaverine hydrochloride, 150 mg in slow-release capsules, every 12 hours. If necessary, it could be injected.

Polyarteritis Nodosa

Not a frequent disease, it is characterized by attacks in which muscular pain in the extremities (or in the abdomen) and arthralgias are associated with fever, malaise, a moderate hypertension, and an elevated eosinophilia. The symptomatology is extremely variable and may refer to the heart (cardialgia or any other heart disease), kidneys (glomerulonephritis), gall bladder (hepatic colic), or gastrointestinal tract (appendicitis, proctitis, and so forth). The diagnosis is established by biopsy.

Fever and pain may respond well to salicylates. The basic treatment will be carried out with corticoids.

> Prednisone, 5 to 10 mg, two or three times a day; to decrease dosage, but not stop its use.

Erythromelalgia

The attack may follow heating, and also a dependent position of the arms, arm swinging, or exercise; the hands become painful and red. It is relieved by cooling or elevation of the limbs.

If erythromelalgia accompanies organic neurologic diseases, hypertension, gout, or polycythemia vera, any of these diseases must be treated. If not (primary erythromelalgia), acetylsalicylic acid should be tried first, which drug should also be used as pain reliever for secondary erythromelalgia. It is beneficial to cool and elevate the affected limb. Severe, unresponsive cases have to be treated surgically, crushing or sectioning the nerve.

> Acetylsalicylic acid, 600 mg, tablets, every 4 hours; to continue two or three doses after the attack is over.

Acrodynia

Symptoms are similar to erythromelalgia—hands are painful and red; the difference consists of chronicity and the occurrence of sweating and bothersome paresthesias. Most cases are due to mercury poisoning, which condition is the one to be remedied.

Avoid further contamination with mercury, a step that may be enough for recovery; give pyridoxine, and detoxify with dimercaprol (BAL) or penicillamine.

> Pyridoxine, 50-mg tablets, two a day.

> Dimercaprol (BAL), 100 mg for each ml solution: give 3 (to 5) mg for each kg of body weight; every 4 hours the first 2 days, every 6 hours the following day, and every 12 hours thereafter, for a total of 10 to 15 days. Check carefully for tolerance.

> Penicillamine, 250 mg in capsules, to start taking this dosage every 6 hours on an empty stomach. The dosage may be increased up to a total of 4 or 5 g a day, in divided doses.

Raynaud's Disease

Pain in the tip of the fingers is associated with blanching or cyanosis. Attacks last a few minutes, rarely more than 1 hour. When repeated, they give origin to a local, painful ulceration that may end in gangrene. Women are more frequently affected than men. Typical attacks may also occur in toes, nose, and ears.

Smokers have to give up the habit; the hands and the body must be kept warm at all times. Recommended medications are vasodilators, tranquilizers, reserpine, and methyldopa. Surgery is the last resort, when the use of vasodilators fails.

> Papaverine hydrochloride, 150 mg, slow-release capsules, one every 12 hours. May also be injected.

> Nicotinic acid, 50- or 100-mg tablets; take 50 to 150 mg, one to three times a day.

> Reserpine, 0.25-mg tablets: start with one dose a day; increase up to four or eight tablets a day (in divided doses), as needed; to establish a maintenance therapy of one tablet a day.

> Methyldopa, 125- or 250-mg tablets; take about 500 mg in three or four installments (adjust dosage).

Gangrene

Dry gangrene: necrotic tissues show a black appearance. *Wet gangrene:* the color is grayish and the tissues show edema, blisters, and necrosis. Necrosis occurs more frequently in the fingers and toes, but other parts of the body can be affected.

Any of the diseases that are prone to cause gangrene (diabetes, etc.) must be aggressively treated. The patient must be on bed rest, the limb placed horizontally or slightly elevated, the lesion covered with wet dressing (sterile saline), and antibiotics used either locally or systemically whenever indicated. Once gangrene is established, pain must be relieved by means of analgesics and the patient referred immediately to a surgeon for further evaluation.

> Meperidine, 100 mg, by subcutaneous injection.

Traumatic Lesions

The diagnosis is obvious in the great majority of cases. There may also be accompanying skin lesions. A *contusion* can produce a subperiosteal hematoma. *Luxations* and *fractures* give origin to characteristic signs and symptoms. Contusions, dislocations, and fractures are the common injuries to the upper limbs.

Contusions, with or without hematoma, are treated at the start with ice packs for 20 minutes. Thereafter, hot compresses could be used; and very rarely analgesics will be needed. Fractures and luxations will be sent to an orthopedic surgeon, but the first aid will include relief of pain and apprehension. Dislocations are also treated with ice packs at the start, applied to the site for 20 minutes, every 6 to 8 hours; hot packs or compresses would be useful only after the second day, but with care not to cause a burn. If the pain is severe enough for more drastic measures, infiltrate the painful area.

Osteomyelitis

Symptoms are pain, fever, and restricted motion. The bone is tender on palpation, and may show some swelling and fluctuation. The diagnostic evidence might appear late, depending on X-ray examinations.

Treatment is designed to manage properly the bone (or generalized) infection, bascially with adequate specific antibiotics and surgery. Soothing pain is only a minor part in the treatment of osteomyelitis, either acute or chronic. Pain shall be relieved, but not abolished, by means of analgesics.

Tuberculosis of the Bones and Joints

Limitation of movement may be the first symptom (might be caused by muscle spasm). Mild pain may also be noted at the early stages. Any bone may be affected, particularly the spine and legs, and the clinical course is usually intermittent. Diagnosis depends on the finding of tuberculosis elsewhere in the body (lungs), the X-ray picture, or the finding of the tubercle bacillus in exudate or sputum.

Total therapy includes rest, diet, chemotherapy, and surgery.

Osteosis

In Paget's and von Recklinghausen's diseases pain is not intense. The diagnosis depends on X-ray examinations and the bone deformities.

Parathyroid hyperfunction requires surgery. Following parathyroidectomy there is frequently a need to give vitamin D. Analgesics will afford symptomatic relief of pain.

Bone Cysts

These cysts may be mildly painful, and the deformity poorly marked. There are X-ray findings, which may give the diagnosis.

Curettage is the only good approach to therapy of bone cysts, whenever it is possible. If there is pain, some relief may be obtained with analgesics.

Osteomalacia

Intense bone pain, more intense at night and during exercise, ushers in the clinical picture of osteomalacia. Spontaneous fractures and deformities of the bone suggest the diagnosis, which is confirmed radiographically.

Pain should be relieved with analgesics; but the basic treatment depends on the specific cause. Osteomalacia of the adult responds, almost specifically, to large doses of vitamin D. When it is due to pancreatic insufficiency, it requires not only higher calcium intake, but also vitamin K, and, more important, pancreatic enzymes. In cases of sprue, a special diet, vitamin B_{12}, and folic acid are essential for recovery. All patients with osteomalacia will receive calcium therapy by mouth, and will be checked for blood calcium levels periodically.

> Vitamin D, 100,000 units, once a day. If larger doses are needed, check blood calcium.
>
> Calcium lactate, powder, 1 level teaspoonful, three times a day.
>
> Calcium gluconate, 10% solution; inject 10 to 20 ml, intravenously; or calcium gluconate, 1-g tablets, two to five tablets, 1 hour after each meal.
>
> Pancreatin, 250 to 500 mg, with meals.

Milkman's disease may cause pain in the arms, but the main symptomatology is found in the legs. It is a special form of osteomalacia, and should be treated as such.

Pernicious Anemia

Bone pains are usually present, and should be noticed; but the important symptoms on which diagnosis depends are lingual, gastrointestinal, and, most important, degenerative changes in the nervous system. The blood picture will show a macrocytic anemia, the stomach contents will be achlorhydric, and the therapeutic trial with vitamin B_{12} or radioactive vitamin B_{12} will be positively effective.

Relief of pain, on a temporary basis, will be achieved by means of analgesics; but the treatment of the disease depends on the use of cyanocobalamin injections.

> Cyanocobalamin (vitamin B_{12}), 100 or 1000 mcg ampoules; to use regularly 100 μg one or three times a week, until blood returns to normal levels; thereafter, only one injection a month.

Myeloma

Multiple myeloma causes scattered skeletal lesions; pain in the bones, limbs, or trunk; headache; malaise; and weight loss. The diagnosis is made by radiography and biopsy of a lesion.

Radiotherapy, surgery, and chemotherapy may ameliorate the disease. For pain, radiotherapy is the best approach. Analgesics may be used, including narcotics. Also use splints, dietetic supplements, and, if needed and tolerated, chemotherapeutic alkylating agents managed by a specialist.

Neoplasms of Bones

Pain is the most important symptom in the great majority of bone tumors, particularly malignant ones. In *osteoid-osteoma,* pain increases during the night hours. In *osteogenic sarcoma,* pain is followed by swelling, as also happens in *Ewing's tumor. Metastasis* from the breast, prostate, lungs, thyroid, and kidney also begins with pain. The diagnosis depends on X-ray examination and biopsy.

The essentials of treatment depend on surgery, chemotherapy, and radiotherapy, the latter being capable of allaying pain to a great extent. Whenever necessary, the use of analgesics will be considered, either regular or narcotic analgesics.

Brachial Neuralgia (Cervical Root Syndrome)

Brachial neuralgia shows numbness and weakness variably distributed along the arm, from shoulders to fingers. It may be preceded by a crisis of wryneck, or pain in the arm may be the first symptom to appear. Also, there are paresthesias, hyperesthesia, and an increase of pain when one is stretching the nerve. As a result of pain, a change in posture may result ("leading chin"). On palpation, pain is elicited by pressure over the involved roots, in the cervical region, or over the nerves in the arm.

Pure brachial neuralgia is rare. Most cases are due to disk diseases in the spine, heart troubles, arthritis, neoplasms, and cervical rib. Each of these conditions will receive adequate treatment, and the use of analgesics will be common to all.

Scalenus Anticus Syndrome

A neuralgia is felt in the arm, at times together with edema, worse during the night and better after the arm is moved. The scalenus anticus syndrome seems to be due to anomalies of the cervical column, and is more frequent among women.

Surgery applied to the cervical ribs, fibrous bands, or the muscle itself is the only means to a complete cure. Otherwise, order bed rest, with traction on the neck; a sling to support the arm; and pillows to support the shoulders. Analgesics may afford temporary relief.

Polyneuritis

This disease is characterized by the involvement of multiple nerves, with pain scattered over all involved areas, symmetrically distributed, and affecting mainly the limbs. In the arms, pain is noted in the portion closer to the shoulder, the forearm, or the hand. Muscular atrophy, particularly of the hand, may be another symptom.

The patient will stay in bed and receive analgesics for pain. As soon as pain is relieved, massage and passive motion will start. Slings and stretching will be used. Prevent contractures. The basic cause will be treated accordingly, such as poisoning, infections, nutritional and metabolic causes, and cancer. Give a high caloric diet and vitamins of the B complex.

Causalgia

This syndrome frequently follows injury of a nerve. Pain is excruciating, and associated parethesias worsen the situation, particularly cutaneous hyperesthesia. The slightest touch to the skin triggers an attack of pain. Patients try to keep the limb motionless, and a secondary muscle atropy may supervene, vasospasm may be severe, and dystrophies may be a consequence.

In mild cases, keep the extremity cool and well-protected against any sort of stimulus. With this protection and the use of analgesics, the disease may subside in a few months. Severe cases, or those which do not improve from the above care, will be treated by sympathectomy.

Glomus Tumor

Most of these tumors, over 30% of all the cases, originate beneath the fingernails. There is a bluish mark in the skin or nail, over the tumor. Pain radiates to the arm, and increases with the slightest stimulation.

The only hope for cure is surgical removal.

Heterotopic Pain in the Shoulder

Pain in the shoulder may reflect several different diseases with no interrelationship among them, such as diseases of the ribs and the sternum, pleuritis, pleurodynia, pneumonia and other lung diseases, mediastinal diseases, and biliary lithiasis and colic; and there is also the heterotopic pain that follows the ingestion of large amounts of food. The referred pain is but a small part of each particular clinical picture, but in rare instances it may be the only symptom, as may happen in chronic calculous cholecystitis. Also, the pain provoked by diseases of the mediastinum and of the aorta, and particularly angina pectoris, may radiate to the shoulders and even the whole arm.

Tennis Elbow

This radiohumeral bursitis causes a very intense pain at the slightest movement of the involved muscles. It occurs more frequently among tennis players, but may be brought on by other motions, such as using a screwdriver or some motion in a manufacturing routine. The pain centers over the lateral epicondyle of the humerus, which is tender on pressure. Violent dorsiflexion of the hand aggravates the pain, and the local injection of an anesthetic will abolish it—the correct diagnosis can be based on this information.

At the beginning, pain may be relieved, if the patient is a tennis player, by the use of a racket with a heavier frame, massage of the painful area, application of heat, and the administration of analgesics. Nonplayers will observe the same routine, including any change in procedure that could be equivalent to the change in the handle of the racket. Chronic established pain will be relieved with analgesics and avoidance of the offending movements or even having the arm immobilized in a brace or a splint. The so-called trigger points may be infiltrated by using corticoids or corticoids with local anesthetics.

> Hydrocortisone acetate, 25 mg in 1 ml, suspension; inject about 1 ml, or less, into each point.

> Procaine, 1% solution; inject 1 ml into each point.

Climacterium

At the cessation of gonadal activity different symptoms may appear. Pain in the bones, particularly in the limbs, may suggest the erroneous diagnosis of rheumatism. Even actual bone lesions may accompany these climacterium pains.

Since rheumatism-like pains are frequent during the climacterium, they should be treated as such, in addition to the common treatment of this stage of human life. Estrogens and progesterone are to be given to balance the endocrine deficiency. Males will use androgens. The rest of the therapy will be similar to that for osteoporosis. Regular analgesics will help.

Cushing's Disease

In both Cushing's disease and Cushing's syndrome, bone pains are felt in the areas where osteoporosis is found in the X-ray films. The diagnosis cannot be based on these pains alone.

In most instances, pain affects the head or the back; but it may also involve the limbs. Nevertheless, it is of a minor degree, and treatment can be carried out with acetylsalicylic acid or similar drugs.

Coxalgia

This disease may be a form of tuberculous arthritis in the coxal joint, not too frequent among the elderly. The initial symptom is pain and limping (pain referred either to the hip or the knee). There is a limitation of movement, and patients tend to stand on the healthy leg, the affected leg placed in a typical position, flexed, abducted, and with external rotation. This results in muscle atrophy and, finally, fistulization of an abscess. An early diagnosis is difficult: a patient begins to limp and shows the foregoing symptoms; the X-ray examination is of little help, as only some decalcification is seen, and only later on the cartilage lesions appear.

The treatment of coxalgia due to arthritic tuberculosis is that of tuberculosis itself, with streptomycin, isoniazid, and paraaminosalicylic acid, all three given initially for 6 months, then followed by isoniazid and paraaminosalicylic acid for 18 additional months. Secondary drugs will be used in resistant cases. For the symptomatic treatment of pain resort to papaverine, codeine, or meperidine.

Bursitis of the Leg

Most frequently women may complain during the climacterium of intense pain in the medial aspect of the tibia, particularly distressing when using stairs. Other forms of bursitis will show the typical symptoms of the disease.

If it is treated at the outset with either radiotherapy or corticoids, the results are almost always gratifying. When the disease is well established, it will require rest, immobilization, application of local heat, and intrabursal injection of corticoids. The pain can be helped with the usual analgesics.

> Prednisone, 5 mg, every 8 hours; decrease the dosage when effects are noted, and discontinue it slowly, for a total treatment period of up to 15 to 20 days.

> Hydrocortisone acetate, 25 mg in each ml, suspension; inject from 1 to 5 ml into the bursae.

Psoitis

Either spontaneous pain or pain induced on deep palpation is noted in one or both iliac fossae. This pain is usually accompanied by muscle rigidity, which causes a typical position of the leg, namely, flexed and abducted; the patient bending forward when walking. Psoitis is rarely an independent problem, and a cause must be sought, as tuberculous spondylitis, perinephritic abscess, appendicitis, or adrenal tuberculosis.

Treat the cause with antituberculous drugs or antibiotics; and perform surgical procedures whenever needed. Analgesics will give only minor relief.

Contracture of the Achilles' Tendon

The peculiar restricted dorsiflexion of the ankle occurs with pain along the metatarsal arch. Pain referred to the calf is increased by walking barefooted or by using flat shoes or slippers.

The administration of analgesics helps to allow better manipulation, with massage, exercise, and gradual stretching of the tendon. Contracture not responding to this therapy will be treated surgically, for lengthening of the tendon.

Varices

Frequent among the elderly, varices in the legs may cause some pain and paresthesia, some ankle edema, and even trophic changes in the skin, sclerosis or ulcers, when circulation has been disturbed for long periods. The diagnosis is evident because of the varicosities visible under the skin.

The regular treatment of varicositis, mainly located in the legs, is to use elastic protective stockings (which are to be replaced appropriately), intermittent elevation of the affected legs, injection of sclerosing agents, and surgery whenever advisable.

Phlebitis

Phlebothrombosis: pain is minimal, elicited often in the calf by dorsiflexion of the foot. *Thrombophlebitis:* there is intense pain, with tenderness on palpation and swelling of the leg; also systemic symptoms are usually present, such as fever and malaise. The femoral and popliteal veins are the ones most frequently affected by phlebitis.

In superficial phlebitis, order rest, elevation of the affected limb, application of heat, and surgery if necessary (ligation in extensive or progressive cases; or stripping). Use anticoalgulants only in rapidly progressive cases. Phenylbutazone is useful in many instances. The involvement of deep veins requires bed rest, elevation of the affected limb, elastic bandage, anticoagulant therapy, surgery in many cases, and gradual walking after 5 to 10 days of absolute rest. The advice of a specialist will be requested.

> Heparin (aqueous sodium), 7,000 to 12,000 units initially, by intravenous or subcutaneous injection; to be followed by three-fourths of this dosage every 4 hours, until warfarin or bihydroxycoumarin starts to work. Check for clotting time.

> Warfarin, 30 to 40 mg, by mouth; once a day the first day; 10 to 20 mg, the second day; 5 to 10 mg, as needed, thereafter. Start at the same time as heparin, and control with the prothrombin time, checked often.

> Phenylbutazone, 100 mg, every 8 hours, for at least 5 days; but do not give it to patients with peptic ulcer.

Intermittent Claudication

Pain with paresthesia, muscular weakness, and/or cramps, forces a person walking in the street to stop suddenly; after a few moments he is able to resume walking, until the next attack. Oscillometry gives low readings.

Since this pain lasts only seconds or minutes, there is no need to use analgesics. Prevent pain by advising the patient to walk slowly, with short steps, to avoid stairs and hills as much as possible, or to stop frequently, more often than he ordinarily would, for a few seconds before continuing walking. Exercising, by walking until pain starts, will be done every 4 or 5 hours during the day to increase the number of new collateral vessels. Surgery (sympathectomy) is a final procedure, when conservative measures fail.

Thromboangiitis Obliterans

Pain of the type of intermittent claudication may be the first sign of Buerger's disease. Gradually or suddenly, more severe pain becomes persistent, and an area of gangrene is delineated in the toes or the metatarsal region. Diagnostic signs of arterial insufficiency are the changes in color of the feet and toes: red (rubor) when dependent, and pale (pallor) when elevated above the level of the heart. Trophic changes of the affected area (nails and skin) may develop. Ulceration and gangrene could be the final outcome.

Stop smoking, and take very good care of the feet by cleansing them with oil, if dry, or alcohol, if soft; try to keep the nails soft and corns in good shape; keep the extremities warm but not hot, avoid garters, prevent mycotic infections and infections of abrasions; finally, exercise the limbs judiciously. Vasodilators may be used, but they are of little help and may cause some harm. Treat any infection vigorously with antibiotics; and treat gangrene, if it is present. Sympathectomy is considered a practical remedy. Diphenylydantoin may control pain.

> Diphenylhydantoin, 100 mg, by mouth, every 8 hours; in emergent situations give the first 100 mg by intramuscular injection.

Gangrene

Treat diabetes vigorously, or any other condition capable of causing gangrene. If gangrene develops, the limb should be placed horizontally or slightly lowered. Cover the lesion with wet dressing (sterile saline or antibiotics, if infected), give analgesics, and refer the patient for further evaluation and action to a surgeon.

Pain in the Bones

Traumatic pain. Fractures and dislocations are diagnosed by inspection, manipulation, and the finding of loss of function; and are confirmed by X-ray examination. Sprains and strains are noted in the joints and tendons; the immediate pain is caused by distention or pressure of tissues by extravasated blood; and the late pain, which is accompanied by further swelling, by an outpouring of lymph around the injured tissues. Ankle sprain is a very frequent occurrence. Relieve its pain with ice packs applied to the site of the injury, for 20 minutes every 6 to 8 hours; and the next days with hot packs or soaks, but avoiding burns. Exercise and start using the sprained ankle as soon as possible; and in case of suffering infiltrate the painful area with procaine hydrochloride, 1% solution, injecting up to 10 ml. Dislocations are treated as sprains, but more time will be given for recovery, with more attention to the healing of muscles and tendons; and since surgical repair is needed at times, the cases should be evaluated by a surgeon. Fractures require the skill of an orthopedic surgeon, but there is almost always the emergent need of relief of pain, with analgesics, or even narcotics, according to effects and tolerance. Contusions, with or without hematoma, only need the help of ice packs.

Osteosis, of the type of osteosis parathyroidea cystica, presents the problem of parathyroid hypersecretion, which has to be controlled surgically by removal of the hyperfunctioning gland. At times, it is necessary to give vitamin D after surgery.

Bone cysts. Whenever necessary, curettage is the only treatment for bone cysts; but if they are painful, some relief may be given with analgesics.

Osteomalacia responds, almost specifically, to large doses of vitamin D. If it is due to insufficiency of the pancreas, also give pancreatic enzymes, calcium, and vitamin K. Most patients with osteomalacia should receive a prolonged calcium therapy, for which reason they have to be periodically checked for calcium blood levels. In cases of sprue, vitamin B_{12}, folic acid, and a special diet will be given. Analgesics are good for pain.

Milkman's disease may cause bone pain so severe that walking is impossible. There are occasional fractures of a spontaneous character; and the disease runs a chronic course. The typical bands or striae in the shaft of the long bones, as seen in X-ray films, will confirm the diagnosis. Treat as for osteomalacia.

Polycythemia vera is a disease that very frequently presents pain in the legs; but this is only a minor symptom, mentioned here as a brief reminder of the fact.

Sciatica

There is a neuralgic pain, either continuous or by crises, accompanied by numbness, which extends along the posterior aspect of the leg, from the hip to the ankle. Tenderness is elicited on palpation of the nerve, all along its course. Also, pain increases when stretching the nerve (Lasegue's sign). Eventual changes are muscle atrophy, diminished reflexes (Achilles), limitation of motion, deformities, trophic changes, and so on. Sciatica may be secondary to other diseases or lesions that injure the nerve, and which must be diagnosed adequately.

Pain along the nerve is mostly due to herniated disks or tumors (including prostate tumors), which will be treated accordingly, in most instances by surgical means. Palliative treatment will be given by analgesics, narcotics, when needed, and possibly vitamins of the B complex. This neuralgia may also be due to general infections, syphilis, poisoning, or metabolic causes, which will be treated with the adequate antibiotic or the corresponding therapy for the causative factor. In most of these cases analgesics, including narcotics, may be of help.

Crural Neuralgia

There is pain along the anterior aspect of the leg, with paresthesias frequently associated, quadriceps atrophy, and diminished or absent patellar reflex. Crural neuralgia is secondary to infection or tumor of the abdominal organs.

The basic treatment will be with antibiotics or surgery. Pain may be relieved with analgesics, and some help may be obtained by the use of vitamins of the B complex.

Meralgia Paresthetica

There are paresthesias (burning, tingling, numbness) or actual pain noted on the outer surface of the thigh.

Decompression of the fascial canal of the nervus cutaneus femoris lateralis may be required; but a trial will be given to avoidance of external pressure or constriction, the use of vitamins of the B complex, and analgesics.

Radiculitis

The typical tabetic violent pains mainly affect the lower limbs. They are sudden in onset and persist for only a few seconds. Very frequently, these fulgurant attacks are the first and only evident symptoms of tabes dorsalis. Other tabetic symptoms and signs are suggestive of the diagnosis: locomotor ataxia is the most characteristic, with its associated derangements of pupillary and tendinous reflexes, and visceral crises. Examination of the spinal fluid is diagnostic. Vertebral diseases may also provoke radiculitis.

Tabes dorsalis is treated with penicillin G (large doses) for 10 to 20 days; with a second course usually needed, as evaluated from spinal fluid examinations performed every 3 months. Other cases need the advice of a specialist to manage herniated disk and to decide on traction and massage, the use of a firm, flat bed, and possible surgery according to age and emotional status. In addition to these measures, analgesics and muscle relaxants are reliable for the relief of pain.

Multiple Sclerosis

The extremely varied symptomatology of multiple sclerosis and its characteristic bouts and remissions may indicate the diagnosis. Pains are noted in legs and other parts of the body.

Multiple sclerlosis has no specific therapy; only symptomatic and general care can be offered, including reasonable activity, massage, psychotherapy, a good nutritious diet, vitamins, avoidance of early treatment of complications, and so on.

Tarsitis

Pain and diffuse inflammation of the foot are noted, with diffuse pictures of the tarsal bones obtained in X-ray films. Find the etiologic factor (tuberculosis, gonococcus, and so forth).

Treat the cause using the specific antibiotic. For pain, temporary relief will be given by analgesics.

Metatarsalgia

Pain beneath the three middle metatarsal bones, most frequently associated with tender calluses in the same area, is symptomatic.

Place a rubber support behind the heads of the metatarsal bones; alternatively, a transverse bar on the outside of the shoe or adhesive strapping applied to a pad cut in the form of a triangle could be used. Exercise the affected muscles, picking up marbles with the toes. Codeine or papaverine may help.

Neuralgia of the Feet

Pain in one or both feet, in the heel, in the sole, or in the metatarsal area, may be noted.

Treat a local or general cause, if known. Block the nerve, if necessary. Use vitamin B_{12} by injection if there is impairment to its gastrointestinal absorption. Since carbamazepine has proved effective in a number of patients suffering from other types of neuralgia, it could be tried in these cases.

Carbamazepine, 200 mg, by mouth, every 6 to 8 hours.

Painful Heel

Pain in the heel may be due to plantar periostitis or bursitis of the Achilles' tendon. Calcaneous spurs may be seen in X-ray films.

Check shoes for proper size and shape; correct abnormalities such as flat foot, spurs, or strain in the Achilles' tendon; advise the patient to keep within the normal weight range, to use massage, to apply warm soaks, and to use a rubber ring to protect the painful heel. Use analgesics, or inject cortisone locally.

Codeine, 30 (to 60) mg, by mouth, every 6 hours.

Papaverine hydrochloride, 150 mg, in slow-release capsules, one every 12 hours.

Hydrocortisone, 25 mg, solution, to inject into the painful area; may repeat three times a week.

Plantar Neuroma

Severe pain is felt and elicited on palpation, in the web between the third and fourth toes. In the early stages, instead of a severe pain there may be paresthesias in the adjacent toes. The lesion is usually unilateral.

Physical devices may help, such as a rubber support behind the metatarsal heads. The best choice is radical surgery for excision of the involved nerves.

Plantar Wart

A wart is found beneath the metatarsal heads, tender to pressure and causing limping.

Since plantar warts may be very painful and are almost always very difficult to treat, it is best to send the patient to an experienced dermatologist or podiatrist. For temporary relief use a rubber ring, metatarsal pad, or bar, etc., for protection. Give analgesics, if needed.

Fracture of the Humerus

Elderly persons who fall on the shoulder or upon the outstretched hand may incur a fracture of the upper extremity of the bone. Unfortunately, the fracture frequently becomes impacted, and there is no deviation. For this reason, when the accident occurs, X-ray studies have to be made in two planes to disclose the injury, since a fracture with dislocation of the head of the humerus requires surgery.

Immobilize the shoulder with a pad placed between the arm and the chest, a sling holding the flexed forearm fastened by a circular bandage going around the arm and the thorax. After 48 hours, apply heat and start a gentle mobilization of the segment. Of course, it is better to request the help of an orthopedic surgeon.

Fracture of the Radius

Colles' fracture of the distal portion of the radius is a common result of a fall upon the outstretched hand, with the typical silver-fork displacement because the distal fragment is brought upward and backward.

Reduce the fracture and keep the segments immobilized in a cast or plaster splint for about 1 month; however, the splint will not be used with the frail and debilitated patient, who will exercise the shoulder and elbow every day to avoid stiffness ("frozen shoulder").

Dislocation of the Shoulder

If following the accident the hand can be put on the opposite shoulder and the elbow brought toward the thorax, dislocation may be ruled out; but it is better to do a radiologic examination in case of doubt.

Heat, a sling, and early exercises are advisable for elderly persons suffering this kind of injury.

Fracture of the Pelvis

This accident is frequent with the elderly, the injury carrying a very serious prognosis. Displacement is minimal or totally absent; nevertheless, the site of the fracture is exquisitely sensitive to pressure exerted on the iliac crests or the femoral trochanters. X-ray films will disclose the extent of the injury. Check in all instances for secondary injury to soft tissues, such as the urethra, the bladder, and so forth.

Fracture of the pelvis is a very serious accident, for which reason the patient will be promptly transferred to a hospital and be put under the care of an orthopedic surgeon. Watch for complications.

Fracture of the Femur

This is another serious and frequent injury among the elderly, usually the fracture of the neck of the femur, which shows some shortness of the limb with outward rotation when the patient lies on his back. X-ray films will give the final diagnosis.

Transfer the injured person promptly to a hospital, to be kept under the care of an orthopedic surgeon. Watch for complications.

Fracture of the Patella

Neither frequent nor rare, this injury may occur with or without separation of fragments. Radiological studies are always needed for the diagnosis, and for evaluation of the procedure to follow.

Linear fractures are of relatively little importance and can be treated with a plaster cast; but more serious lesions require surgery, which will be done by a specialist.

OTHER PAINS

Injuries to the Neck

Violent wrenches of the head may give rise to *strain of the neck* when only muscles are overstretched, or *sprain of the neck* when muscles and ligaments are involved together. The so-called *whiplash injury* occurs when a car is hit from behind by another car, the lesions ranging from sprains to dislocations or fractures. Except in car accidents, these lesions are not too frequent among the elderly. In all instances, an X-ray film should be made for an adequate evaluation of lesions.

Treat with bed rest, and use traction if the injury is of some importance. Use analgesics and muscle relaxants, and massage the area when soreness subsides. At the slightest suspicion request the help of a surgeon.

Dislocation of a Vertebra

This condition causes pain and stiffness, with motion limitation. X-ray studies are needed to rule out fractures.

As usual, reduce the dislocation and maintain traction. A plaster jacket will be used for about 1 month.

Fracture of a Vertebra

Vertebral fractures result from car accidents or falls, and elderly persons are more sensitive than youngsters to these injuries. Severe pain starts immediately, and the muscles become stiff, showing some spasm. Jerks or wrenching of the neck, with paresis or paralysis below the injury, reveal spinal cord involvement. X-ray films will diagnose the fracture.

Handle these cases with extreme care, to avoid further injury to the spinal cord. Grasp the head, keeping it in a straight line with the body while the patient is moved to a stretcher and thereafter until he is placed on a bed, maintaining traction with a head halter (use 2 to 3 kg—5 to 6 lb). Immediately call a surgeon for help.

Hemorrhoids

Hemorrhoidal crises are usually painful; the external hemorrhoids distend suddenly and hurt during defecation, and the distended veins, which are easily seen in the margin of the anus, may bleed; internal hemorrhoids may protrude from inside, and then are painful and also may bleed. Pain is worst with coincident anal fissure. Thrombosed hemorrhoids are extremely painful: the average hemorrhoidal volume increases and becomes irreducible. When there is a clinical picture of rectal involvement (pain of either a colicky or a continuous nature in the rectal area, sensation of presence of a foreign body, constipation alternating with bloody or mucopurulent diarrhea, and systemic symptoms, particularly of a mental nature), the first disease to consider is internal hemorrhoids.

Consult a proctologist. Prolapsed hemorrhoids will be gently replaced with the help of a wet piece of toilet paper or paper towel, since the use of lubricated gloves will easily allow further prolapse. Thrombosed hemorrhoids will be treated with cold or hot sitz baths, as preferred by the patient, and analgesics; but the final steps will be taken by the proctologist, who will evacuate the thrombus or excise the whole tumor. For local pain, when there are no other accompanying symptoms, the use of antihemorrhoidal suppositories is advisable.

Polyarteritis

Rectal pain will occur with polyarteritis when the rare rectal location of the lesions occurs. There may also be other symptoms of the disease; but the diagnosis is always very difficult, depending on the evaluation of the rectal symptoms and exploratory findings (arterial nodosities seen by rectoscopy), which are associated with a febrile reaction apparently of an uncertain nature.

Therapy will give mostly poor results. Corticoids are an acceptable medication, though not much hope should be held for their overall success. Meperidine or codeine may be given as emergent medications.

Prednisone, starting with a high dosage; 20 to 40 mg a day in divided doses; this to be decreased and then discontinued as soon as possible.

Perianal Abscess

Symptoms include piercing anal pain, frequently associated with fever and urine retention. The diagnosis is made by direct examination of the area, which shows localized tenderness, swelling, and redness.

Treatment depends on the use of antibiotics and incision when the pus has collected. Analgesics will only give some temporary relief.

Anal Fistula

This fistula generally follows a perianal abscess, and the first symptom is pain, together with an intermittent pus discharge. The diagnosis is made by finding an opening in the skin adjacent to the anus.

Surgery is the rational treatment for the problem. Papaverine, codeine, meperidine, and suppositories will only afford palliative respite.

Anal Fissure

Fissures are among the most common causes of anal pain, as well as hemorrhoids. A sharp pain makes defecation very difficult, which pain then persists and becomes increasingly severe. A careful examination will disclose the fissure.

Anesthetic ointments applied before and after defecation will help to allay pain. Antispasmodic drugs will also be of help. But surgery is the only positive solution.

Lidocaine, 5% ointment; apply locally whenever needed, particularly before and after defecation.

Belladonna tincture, 15 to 30 drops, in water, every 4 to 6 hours, as needed and tolerated.

Rectal Prolapse

Pain is minimal or even absent, except in cases of associated hemorrhoids, inflammation, or fissure in ano. The everted mucosa will assure the diagnosis.

The replacement of the prolapsed rectal mucosa in its proper location is to be done immediately. Put the patient in a genupectoral position (or merely a lateral position) and with a wet gauze or cotton gently, but firmly, push the mass through the anal opening. After that is done, attach a cotton ball firmly to the anoperineal area, to prevent further prolapsing. Give mineral oil, and instruct the patient to defecate without any straining on the rectum. If it is present, treat proctitis; and if they seem to be needed, use sclerosing agents. Refer the patient to a surgeon.

Trauma to Anus and Rectum

It is not difficult to evaluate the causative injury and the resultant pain. A severe injury may perforate the rectal walls and provoke peritonitis and shock.

Treatment is surgical, and important injuries need immediate repair. Minor injuries only need a thorough cleansing and disinfection. Cold compresses will help, and anesthetic solutions will afford temporary relief.

Cocaine, 5 to 10% solution; instill a few drops on lacerated tissues.

Foreign Bodies

The condition is not too frequently found in older persons. Pain and bleeding are the most notable symptoms, and there may be a history of the insertion of a foreign body; but this may also be denied. It will be noted by rectal palpation, in most instances; and finally the fact will be confirmed by X-ray examination, or by rectoscopy.

Remove the foreign object in all instances. First try natural removal, through the anus; if that is not feasible, it is a matter of surgery. Give meperidine, methadone, or morphine to allay pain and nervousness during the procedure.

Proctitis

Pain may be colicky or continuous, accompanied by discomfort and tenesmus; efforts to defecate are fruitless, passing nothing or only mucus and gas; constipation alternates with bloody and/or mucus diarrhea; and there are dyspeptic and mental symptoms. The diagnosis is made by rectoscopy: a red, edematous, and even purpuric mucosa is found. Proctitis may be bacteriologically diagnosed: due to dysentery, tuberculosis, syphilis, or gonorrhea; or it may be nonspecific.

The basic treatment depends on the underlying cause. To allay pain, at least defecation pain, make the stools softer; to protect against ano-rectal spasm, give belladonna; and if there is diarrhea, which may increase the pain, add opium derivatives.

Dioctyl sodium sulfosuccinate, 50 to 250 mg, in capsules; take up to 250 mg, as needed to soften stools, without provoking unpleasant side effects.

Belladonna tincture, 10 to 30 drops, in water; three or more times a day, as needed and tolerated.

Paregoric elixir, up to 4 ml in water, repeated as needed and tolerated.

Cryptitis and Papillitis

Symptoms include pain during and after defecation, generally accompanied by blood or pus discharge. The diagnosis is made by local examination: tenderness, thickness of the crypts of Morgagni, and spasm of the sphincter. In *papillitis* there is a constant urge to defecate, pain being only mild. An enlarged papilla (not a hemorrhoid!) may protrude or can be seen by rectoscopy (not a polyp!).

Consult a proctologist for the best way to treat any of these situations. There is a basic need to eradicate the causal infection. Increase the bulk of the stool with medication and high-residue diet, and use a stool softener to allay pain. Crypts may benefit from local application of phenol or carbolfuchsin solutions.

> Methylcellulose, or sodium carboxymethylcellulose, 500 mg, tablets; one to three tablets every 6 to 12 hours, according to effect and tolerance, accompanied by a glass of water.

> Dioctyl sodium succinate, 50 to 250 mg, in capsules; give up to 250 mg in a day, according to effects and tolerance.

> Phenol, 5% oil solution.

> Carbolfuchsin compound (Castellani's paint), solution.

Lymphogranulomatosis

Symptoms are: pain, constipation alternating with diarrhea, and sensation of a foreign body, together with other symptoms of stricture. The feces may be thin and irregularly shaped. Tenesmus and mucosanguineous diarrhea are not too rare, as well as complicating perianal fistula and abscess.

Treat with sulfadiazine or a tetracycline. The enlarged and possibly ulcerated lymph nodes may require rest, warm compresses, and analgesics.

Polyps and Benign Tumors

These polyps and tumors may be accompanied by mild or no pain. Hemorrhage is the most important symptom. Rectoscopy will provide the final diagnosis.

Surgery is the logical approach. If needed, codeine or papaverine will be given.

Cancer

Symptoms may be any of those corresponding to proctitis; pain may occur late in the disease. In all cases suggesting rectal involvement, a rectoscopic examination is mandatory to rule out cancer.

Removal in due time is the only hope for cure. In other cases, radiotherapy or chemotherapy will be helpful. For palliative treatment for pain, start with analgesics, thereafter to resort to narcotics as needed.

Rectal Spasm

This spasm occurs as a cramplike unpleasant feeling located above the anus. It starts in a mild fashion and increases rapidly. It may associate with abdominal cramps, or may follow sexual intercourse. No lesions are discovered by rectoscopy, or at most some vascular congestion is found by sigmoidoscopy.

Eating or drinking something (gastro-colic reflex) may terminate the spasm; if it fails, give a small enema or dilate the anus in a gentle maneuver. Meperidine may be needed on some occasions.

Vulvitis and Vaginitis

Acute vulvitis: there are pain and local imflammation, usually diagnosed on inspection of the area. *Chronic vulvitis:* symptoms include pruritus, purulent discharge, and pain. *Vaginitis:* the pain is more deeply centered, usually with leukorrhea or purulent discharge where the causative germ may be found. *Atrophic* or *senile vaginitis:* itching is more worrisome than true pain; the condition of the mucosa will disclose the diagnosis.

When there is not too marked an inflammation, cold compresses of aluminum acetate will give good results. With inflammation, sitz baths or hot compresses are better. Antihistaminics and corticoids may help. For vulvitis and vaginitis keep the area clean, avoid dryness caused by soaps or the like, advise the use of absorbent and loose clothes, and give specific antibiotic therapy. Temporary relief will be obtained with warm douches, not too frequently repeated.

Aluminum acetate, 5% solution, to soak compresses.

Dyphenhydramine, 25 or 50 mg, every 6 to 8 hours.

Prednisone, 5 mg, once or twice a day; to decrease and discontinue as soon as possible.

Saline solution, for vaginal douches, prepared with sodium chloride, 1½ level teaspoonfuls in a liter of water.

Bartholinitis

Pain is located at one side of the vulva, accompanied by local inflammation and the presence of an extremely painful tumor in the corresponding labia, with or without fluctuation. Diagnosis is made by inspection and palpation.

Refer patient to a gynecologist for surgical drainage. Apply hot compresses to hasten collection of pus or abortion of the abscess. Give antibiotics and analgesics.

Balanitis

Patients refer pain to the glans penis or the prepuce, and the diagnosis is made by inspection.

Cleanse the area with hydrogen peroxide, zephiran, potassium permanganate, or boric acid with talcum.

Hydrocele

The main symptom is the mass of fluid in one side of the scrotum; pain is minimal. Fluctuation and positive transillumination will give the diagnosis.

Treatment will consist of aspiration of fluid or hydrocelectomy.

Hematocele

Pain is minimal; there is a sensation of heaviness; the tumor in the scrotum is hard on palpation, does not transilluminate, and does not admit any differentiation of the involved structures, namely, testis, epididymus, tunica vaginalis, and so on.

Aspiration or other form of surgery will be needed.

Epididymitis

Infection of the epididymus centers on the superoposterior side of the testis and forms a tender lump, with pain, except in the case of tuberculosis. Check for the causative factor.

Advise rest, cold compresses (or hot, if so preferred by the patient), sedation, and antibiotherapy, specific when known.

Orchitis

There is an enlarged testis, tender on palpation, painful at all times, which follows an infectious disease or other etiological factors such as surgery, trauma, stress, and so forth. In *orchiepididymitis* the inflammation of both the testis and the epididymus is evident. A good number of cases of orchitis are true orchiepididymitis, and the symptoms of both diseases are noted in the same patient.

The urologist will evaluate surgery and antibiotic therapy; but the patient will be helped with rest, support of the bursae, cold compresses, and analgesics.

Cancer and Other Tumors

Pain is not an important symptom because it appears late. The tumor is evident, and has to be identified by biopsy.

Surgery is the best solution, whenever possible, and will be evaluated by a urologist.

Varicocele

The mass of varicose veins is felt like a bag of worms in the external genitalia of both men and women, with little or no pain.

During acute exacerbation put the patient to rest in bed, with cold compresses and elevated genital area. If treatment starts early, it may arrest the process; but generally surgery is needed.

Thromboangiitis of the Spermatic Vessels

Symptomatically this condition resembles an acute epididymitis (determine exactly the site of the inflammation in the corresponding blood vessels).

Treat like thromboangiitis of the legs, use diphenylhydantoin, and discuss sympathectomy if there is a worsening of the disease. Stop smoking.

Diphenylhydantoin, 100 mg, by mouth, every 8 hours; first dose intramuscularly in emergent situations.

Torsion of the Pedicle of the Testis

There is extremely intense pain, with a tender and swollen testis. Contraction of the cremaster muscle makes the testis stay high in the scrotum, which becomes edematous. There are systemic symptoms, such as fever, nausea, with vomiting, following necrosis of the gland.

Refer the patient immediately to a urologist or a surgeon, since surgery is the only way to save the testicle from gangrene, unless a manual reversal of the torsion can be performed. If it occurs in the right testicle, the torsion takes place clockwise, so it has to be reversed counterclockwise; if it occurs in the left testicle, it takes place counterclockwise and has to be reversed clockwise. For the very acute local pain an injection of morphine or meperidine will be recommended.

Morphine sulfate, 15 mg, by subcutaneous injection.

Meperidine, 100 mg, by subcutaneous injection.

III. UNCONSCIOUSNESS

HANDLING THE UNCONSCIOUS PATIENT

Rules for handling unconscious patients have been well established by emergency services in hospitals all around the country. This paragraph mainly relates to resuscitation procedures to start immediately, when needed, because of a diagnosis of *cardiac arrest* in which there are no pulse, no heart sounds, and no respiratory movements. Under these circumstances, first try elevation of the legs (only for 30 seconds); if that is not effective, do not persist, but thump the precordial area of the chest forcefully in an attempt to end asystole. But do not delay beginning cardiac compression (also called cardiac massage) and mouth-to-mouth pulmonary ventilation (also called artificial respiration), provided there is a free airway. If there is not, make it patent, carefully avoiding aspiration of secretions. Put the patient on a firm surface-floor, or a hard board on the bed, tilt the head back so the tongue lifts from the back of the throat, and breathe forcefully into the lungs of the patient, to have him inhale, repeating inflation of the lungs four times, then compressing the chest, also forcefully, against the back, repeating 15 times, at a rate of 75–80 each minute. Then, follow a ratio of 15 compressions to two quick inflations, if you are alone giving help. If you have help, give five compressions while the other person gives one inflation. There will be rapid transportation of the patient to the hospital; as soon as this is done, cardiac activation will be restored by electrical means supervised by a cardiac specialist.

Most patients will be unconscious, but with no emergency need for care, as no cardiac arrest will be present. There is time for a more detailed examination, beginning with a *clinical history* given by relatives or witnesses to the incident. Do not trust too much—but do not totally discard—data provided by the same patient during lucid periods. The physician may infer or approach a correct diagnosis from this information: use of drugs (for instance, insulin), poisoning, an accident, or a previous sickness. This examination will be completed as sketched here, by any skilled practitioner.

1) History—if available, given by relatives, witnesses, or the patient.
2) Eye examination
   a) Pupils—size, reaction to light
   b) Corneal reflex
   c) Fundi (papilledema, sclerosis, retinitis)
3) Neurological examination (level of consciousness)
   a) Neck (stiffness)
   b) Movements of limbs (hemiplegia)
   c) Reflexes (tendons, skin surface)
   d) Convulsions, paresis, tremors
4) Electrocardiogram, blood pressure, pulse, heart auscultation

   5) X-ray studies of skull and lungs
   6) Laboratory procedures
        a) Blood—glucose, BUN, Na, K, CO_2, Cl, CBS, coagulation time, culture, and sensitivity of infecting bacteria
        b) Urine—glucose, protein, ketones, culture, and sensitivity
        c) Spinal puncture—including culture and sensitivity of bacteria
        d) Blood in feces
        e) Toxic substances—stomach, blood
   7) Temperature
   8) Skin—injuries, congestion
   9) Nose—cerebrospinal fluid or blood
   10) Ears
   11) Mouth—bitten tongue
   12) Lungs—type of respiration, odor, auscultation
   13) Cardiovascular to complete blood pressure in both arms, peripheral vessels
   14) Abdomen—walls, masses, pain (if sensitive enough)
   15) Electroencephalogram, if indicated.

Further examination could show more diagnositc signs and symptoms:

Anisocoria or different pupillary size is seen as an index of fracture of the base of the skull or other form of cerebral compression, the moderately dilated pupil pointing to the side of initial injury (when the pupil is widely dilated it denotes a more severe compression, and when both are totally midriatic a severe midbrain disturbance has been sustained—Hutchinson's pupils). Also, it may reveal a meningeal infection, encephalitis, cerebral tumor, or some intoxication, such as alcohol, or uremia. In injuries its real value is to disclose cerebral damage in cases of trauma.

Midriasis may also indicate an intoxication, as from atropine, cocaine, or food, or meningoencephalitis, epilepsy, cranial tumors, or advanced states of cerebral trauma.

Miosis also may indicate intoxication from opium and derivatives, particularly morphine; as well as alcohol, uremia, and, particularly, tabes dorsalis.

Light reflex is lost in tabes dorsalis, encephalitis, meningitis, chronic alcoholism, cerebral arteriosclerosis, cerebral tumor, lesions of the cervical medulla, and some special cases of diabetes.

Corneal reflex speaks for life if present.

Papilledema is a very important sign of brain tumors, appearing earliest in cerebellar, mesencephalic, and parietoccipital tumors. It is also of significance in traumatic lesions with hemorrhage, alcoholic intoxication, arterial hypertension, and chronic nephritis. Usually, when an unconscious patient shows evidence of papilledema, a diagnostic lumbar puncture should be considered, since it generally means increased intracranial pressure requiring emergency measures.

Sclerosis and *retinitis* are evidence of vascular disease, particularly indicating arterial hypertension, and are found in diabetic and albuminuric retinitis.

Neurological examination will start with assessing level of consciousness, according to response to increasing force of stimuli, symmetrically performed, as in this series: loud voice, shaking, slapping, stroking soles of feet, pinching, or pressing supraorbital nerve. Patient may be totally or partially aroused, at least for a while; or the response may be solely to move some muscles as if avoiding excitation. Should the latter occur unilaterally, it will indicate paralysis of the opposite side; anesthesia is indicated by the lack of response from a particular site of stimulation.

Neck rigidity indicates meningeal involvement, cerebellar pathology, tetanus, and/or toxoplasmosis.

Impaired movement of limbs and loss of tone may be indicative of hemiplegia (hypotonus on the paralyzed side; but hypertonus on the same side when the reflexes return). This is a good sign in traumatic and hemorrhagic cases. The simplest method is to raise and let fall one limb after another; paralyzed limbs fall more rapidly.

Tendon reflexes are usually hyperactive in alcoholism and other intoxications: strichnine, atropine, tetanus, rabies, pneumonia, and typhoid fever, pyramidal lesions, etc. In this last instance unilateral hyperreflexia may indicate hemiplegia, the meningeal reaction to hemorrhage, encephalitis, and so on. Diminished reflexes may also indicate increasing intracranial pressure. For evaluation of diminished reflexes, it will be necessary to consider the natural regression of reflexes noted with some frail, debilitated, or deteriorated elderly persons.

Plantar reflexes with extension of toes (positive Babinski) will indicate a lesion of the pyramidal tract due to hemorrhage, meningitis, tumors, or some chronic condition.

Convulsions, paresis, or *tremors* will be noted and will complement the foregoing findings.

An *electrocardiogram* will show whether the problem is a myocardial infarction, or there is a basic arrhythmic condition, such as fibrillation. *Radiologic* studies are needed to determine the extent and quality of injuries to skull, bones, and joints, and the extent of lung changes, since pneumonia is not only a primary but very frequently a complicating disease at advanced age.

Laboratory findings are among the essential requirements for an accurate diagnosis. Draw *blood* for glucose, urea nitrogen, sodium, potassium, carbon dioxide, chlorine, coagulation time, and complete blood counts, together with culture and sensitivity tests. *Culture* and *sensitivity* studies are also to be performed with urine, feces, spinal fluid, and sputum. Save *urine* for glucose, protein, ketone bodies, or any evidence of kidney involvement; and *feces*, to detect blood or any other suspected abnormality. *Gastric juice* (blood, also, for some) serves to determine the nature of toxic agents that have been swallowed.

Cerebrospinal fluid will provide extremely useful information. It will appear turbid or frankly purulent in cases of meningitis and of brain abscess if draining into subarachnoid spaces. It will be bloody in cerebral hemorrhage or accidental injury of recent occurrence. In old hemorrhages, the fluid appears yellowish. The pressure is increased in cases of meningitis, hemorrhages, and brain tumors, and in some severe cases of arterial hypertension; it is decreased if there is obstruction, such as with tumors, fractures, or abscesses. Glucose is increased in encephalitis and decreased in meningitis; protein is increased in cases of meningitis, obstruction within the spinal canal, or brain tumor, and when there is encephalic edema. The cell content is increased in all instances of meningitis and encephalitis, the polymorphonuclear neutrophiles predominating in meningitis. The outstanding features of the fluid are summarized as follows:

> Hemorrhage—Increased pressure, bloody or xanthochromic.
> Meningitis—Increased pressure, polymorphonuclear neutrophiles, and protein; and decreased glucose.
> Encephalitis—Increased pressure, protein, and glucose (all moderately), and a mild lymphocytosis.
> Brain tumor—May be normal or show increased pressure, usually with moderate increase of lymphocytes and protein.
> Brain abscess—Increased pressure, protein, and cells.

Temperature, if elevated, suggests infection. Nevertheless, this is not a very reliable indicator among the elderly, who may react with little intensity, particularly in the presence of an overwhelming infective disease.

Skin changes from injuries or injections are always indicative of a trauma, a reaction to a drug, or some other problem.

If *nose* and *ears* show signs of injury along with the skull, it will be assumed to be serious if blood or clear spinal fluid is noted exuding.

Mouth: check the tongue, which will appear bitten in cases of epilepsy.

Lungs are to be checked in cases of pneumonia, infarction, aspiration of irritants, pneumothorax, or any other aggression to the respiratory organs. Check for the type of respiration, odor of breath, and auscultatory signs.

Cardiovascular system: check blood pressure in both arms, the rhythm and quality of the pulse, the heart sounds, and the condition of the peripheral blood vessels. Pressure is elevated in stroke, low in shock.

Abdomen: check for localized pain, tenseness of muscles, bowel activity, meteorism, and the presence of masses.

Finally, an *electroencephalogram* may help to disclose epilepsy, and other brain lesions.

It seems appropriate to give the reader a short summary of how to check abnormalities found in the patient with a *brain injury:*

1 Weigh the patient's problems at once, and concentrate on those that appear life-threatening.
2 Check for adequate heart action.
3 Be sure there is a patent airway, and ensure proper oxygenation immediately.
4 In falls or car accidents look for cervical spine fractures, an important matter when attempting trachea intubation.
5 Describe the patient's reactions exactly in a simple checklist.
6 Check pupils, since unilateral dilation or fixation will require immediate surgical care. These patients may also present hypertension and/or bradycardia—in case of hypotension look for another cause than injury.
7 Bleeding from the ear canal or behind the drum indicates fracture of the base of the skull.
8 In case of car accident or fall, suspect neck injury in the unconscious patient with muscle hypotonia, diaphragmatic breathing, flexed forearms, and hypotension. Priapism is suggestive of spinal cord injury.
9 Check neck injury by additional radiological studies of all seven cervical vertebrae. A widening of soft tissue shadow of the posterior pharynx suggests local blood extravasation and spine injury.
10 Check all scalp wounds, to look for bone lesions.
11 In addition to a good radiologic study for cranial injuries, computed tomography, cerebral angiography, and an echoencephalogram might be done, as well as a lumbar puncture and an electroencephalogram.
12 Find out how the incident happened, if there is a previous history of any disease; put the patient in a side position if necessary, to avoid aspiration until intubation is done. If the patient is in shock, check for ruptured viscus, aspiration, or obstruction; find out if there are associated injuries (chest, abdomen, spine); and end with a complete examination and the needed remedies.

STROKE

General Considerations and Diagnosis

A stroke can be defined as a sudden, vascular, enduring loss of neurological functions characterized by unconsciousness followed by paralysis. Before the attack there may be headache, dizziness, nausea or vomiting, and transient weakness or paresthesis on one side of the body. Frequently the attack strikes the patient by surprise, and he is unaware of the impending danger. Usually the onset is sudden with complete loss of consciousness, as in a very deep sleep, with a fall, if the subject is out of bed. Symptoms include: stertorous respirations, or breathing following the Cheyne-Stokes rhythm, a flushed face, a bradycardic full pulse, usually an elevated blood pressure, complete muscular relaxation but characteristically without any tone on one side of the body, thus indicating a paralyzed area; at times the head and eyes are turned toward the injured side of the brain, or one of the cheeks inflates rhythmically with respiration (showing paralysis). These symptoms plus lack of reflexes with a positive Babinski's sign all point to the diagnosis of stroke. Some patients are not unconscious, but they will present most of the reviewed symptoms and signs of stroke. Clinically, at times the pattern of the paralysis makes it possible to incriminate the diseased artery.

The lumbar puncture may have blood in the liquid, which will show elevated pressure. Radiographic studies done by specialists will be one aid to the final diagnosis.

Strokes are due to:

> Cerebral hemorrhage
> Cerebral thrombosis
> Cerebral embolism
> Cerebrovascular insufficiency
> Brain tumor or abscess
> Cardiac diseases
> Hemopathies
> Cerebral infections

In the following pages we shall deal with the most important diseases, in order of frequency, affecting people over 50 years of age and capable of provoking strokes.

General Treatment of Stroke

The acute attack requires complete bed rest, carefully avoiding injuries (pressure ulcers, but mainly trauma to the agitated patient). Parenteral infusions are needed to give nutrients and medication, since no attempt will be made to give anything by mouth to the unconscious patient. Some sedation is usually needed for the agitated patient. Lumbar puncture will be used if it lowers elevated intracranial pressure; otherwise, it will be performed very carefully, only for diagnostic purposes. Catheterization of the bladder is also needed.

Great controversy exists about the use of anticoagulant therapy, which may help some and hurt others.

It is best to call a neurosurgeon immediately, who will evaluate the possibility of some sort of successful surgery for each individual patient.

Intracranial Hemorrhage

Any form of intracranial bleeding may cause a stroke whenever the bulk of extravasated blood is capable of damaging brain structures, either following an injury or because of vascular deficiency.

Subdural hematomas cause symptoms to appear immediately after an injury to the head; but in some instances these symptoms will not occur until a few days later, in which case the subdural hematoma presents irritability and mental confusion. There may be headache, and not rarely other symptoms of stroke, among them spastic hemiplegia, which confirms the intracranial bleeding. Other symptoms of stroke may appear in different combinations and intensity. The cerebrospinal fluid will appear tinged with blood. The diagnosis depends on radiologic findings (plain films, angiogram, pneumogram) and at times is helped by reading focal slow waves of low amplitude in the electroencephalogram.

Surgery is the best approach, particularly when progressing symptoms reveal increasing pressure within the skull. A neurosurgeon will be consulted immediately, since evacuation of the hematoma is the best procedure. Narcotic drugs should never be given when increased intracranial pressure is suspected.

Subarachnoid hemorrhage. A frank clinical picture of stroke may start its symptomatic complex; or a sudden and very intense headache appears, possibly following a previous exertion of some kind. The headache may be frontal or occipital to start, then becoming generalized; and the loss of consciousness may last for only a few minutes or hours, in smaller hemorrhages, or until death, in more severe ones. Stiffness of the neck is constant; convulsions and fever are common. The spinal fluid will be under elevated pressure and will show large amounts of red cells. A good number of older patients with subarachnoid hemorrhage may present a history of recurrent attacks, with cephalalgia, stiffness of the neck, and hypertension. Kernig, Brudzinski, and Marañon's signs are positive. Paresis of the limbs is not infrequent. Radiologic studies are not very informative but may show aneurismatic calcifications or an aneurismatic pattern of the circle of Willis.

The help of a neurosurgeon is needed to evaluate the advisability of surgical treatment. Medically, aminocaproic acid may be given as an antifibrinolytic agent while there is active bleeding. If the diagnostic tapping is followed by alleviation of the headache and other symptoms, lumbar puncture will be considered the best help, repeated until the bleeding stops. Do not use narcotics.

> Aminocaproic acid, 250 mg in each ml (20-ml vials), to start with 20 ml intravenously, followed by 4 or 5 ml every hour until a plasma concentration of 13 mg% is reached. Do not exceed six vials (120 ml) in 24 hours. Always use infusions with 5% glucose or saline.

Intracerebral hemorrhage will rapidly provoke headache and hemiplegia, leading immediately to loss of consciousness. The clinical findings will be rich in neurological manifestations together with elevated blood pressure, and other evidence of cardiovascular disease. The paralysis will occur according to the bleeding vessels. The accident may happen during exertion of some kind, mostly in patients with a previous tendency to bleed, who suffer from liver cirrhosis or a hemopathy. The spinal fluid is bloody, and the radiologic studies are of help in diagnosis.

The advice of a neurosurgeon is essential in order to decide what steps to follow.

Arterial involvement will be evidenced not only by radiologic and other diagnostic procedures, but also by the appearance of focal signs and symptoms, as summarized in the following list:

Vertebral and basilar arteries: loss of consciousness and memory; confusion, hemiplegia (or other forms of paralysis), dysarthria, blindness, deafness, dysphagia; and when the patient may become ambulatory, ataxia.

Middle cerebral artery: monoplegia or hemiplegia and hemianopsia of the same side; scintillating scotoma or numbness.

Posterior cerebral artery: symptoms similar to the above, plus blindness not too rarely.

Anterior cerebral artery: weakness or numbness of the leg opposite to the lesion.

Internal carotid: confusion and personality changes, transient blindness or dimness of vision; and weakness or numbness on the opposite side to the lesion.

Cerebrovascular Insufficiency

Cerebrovascular insufficiency, with transient or permanent injury to the nerve cells resulting in a stroke syndrome (more frequently only a transient syncope or focal neurological impairment), can occur as a consequence of the occlusion of extracranial arteries (carotid or basilar artery), small emboli, or sudden changes in systemic pressure. The symptoms will be identical with those of a stroke due to embolism or hemorrhage; but some distinctions are to be found in the case of occlusion of the arteries mentioned above.

Internal carotid occlusion. The final hemiplegic features are generally preceded by hemiparesis on the side opposite the lesion, blindness of the eye on the affected side, episodes of incoordinated speech or frank aphasia, emotional behavior changes, and lowering of intelligence. The terminal hemiplegia usually comes with aphasia. Should the patient develop a good collateral circulation, no symptoms will be present. Arteriography is decisive in diagnosing this condition; but ocular tonometry will indicate carotid occlusion if the pressure in the eye of the affected side is less than one half that of the normal eye.

Anticoagulant therapy is of help in internal carotid occlusion, but not to be carried out with the severely hypertensive patient (may cause bleeding). Many cases will greatly benefit from surgery (replacement, thromboendarterectomy), for which a neurosurgeon will be consulted.

> Heparin, 10,000 units, given intramuscularly or intravenously, every 6 hours, checking clotting time, to be no less than 20 minutes.

> Bishydroxycoumarin (25, 50, 100 mg tablets), give 300 mg during the first day, 200 mg the second, to follow with 50 to 100 mg to bring prothrombin time to 15 to 30% of the normal, discontinuing heparin when this medication becomes effective.

Cerebral Thrombosis

Usually, the accident is totally unrelated to trauma or exertion, and progresses gradually to show the entire symptomatology, the loss of consciousness occurring relatively late. Previous attacks of aphasia, dizziness, paresis, or other neurological symptoms almost always have occurred, with rapid improvement becoming apparent between them. The great majority of the patients will present marked evidence of arteriosclerosis (coronary vessels, aorta, cardiovascular diseases, and so on), and most will show symptoms and signs of the involved arteries, which may be as in the cases summarized above, or any of the following, all of which symptoms also occur in cerebral embolism.

> Vessels of the aortic arch: intermittent claudication, difference of blood pressure taken in both arms, absent or almost absent pulsation in the common carotid.

> Subclavian steal syndrome: occurs because of occlusion of the subclavian and the innominate arteries, causing dizzy spells.

The established clinical picture is similar to that for intracranial hemorrhage or embolism, but with a slower onset; there is an almost identical symptomatology. Radiologic studies with arteriography will help in determining the injured vessels.

Anticoagulant therapy may help only a few patients, and presents a real risk of bleeding in many others. The surgical management of the stenosed vessels will be left for specialists to decide. Other measures will be taken for rehabilitation of the patient, which holds true also for patients suffering different forms of stroke. Exercising will start the second or third day after the accident, or when the patient regains consciousness. Adequate training of the active hand for personal care will also start soon. The first phase will be in bed; the second, on standing, which will take place after 4 or 5 days. In each phase gradual movements, according to the capabilities of each individual patient, will be ordered, from easier ones to those more complicated or requiring more strength. The final goal is to put the patient as close as possible to complete self-care and even a relatively normal life. Use of medication is of relatively little help; perhaps some improvement will be given to the confused or depressed patient with dextroamphetamine.

Dextroamphetamine, 10 mg once a day of a long-acting preparation.

Cerebral Embolism

Usually a fulminant onset occurs in these cases, with development of a full clinical picture of massive stroke; but in many instances there is a rapid improvement. The neurological symptoms depend on the involved vessel, as shown in the previous paragraphs, q.v. A substantial number of the elderly with cerebral embolism are known patients, suffering from coronary thrombosis, myocardial infarction, atrial fibrillation of longstanding duration, endocarditis, thrombosis of the carotid, infections causing clots of blood or pus, drops of fat from bone fractures, and perhaps lesions in the abdomen or lower limbs. Radiologic studies will be helpful in determining the site of the embolus.

Since there is no known therapy for this contingency, the surgical approach is the only solution when advisable and possible.

Basilar artery occlusion. The occlusion of the vertebral or basilar arteries, usually partial, causes intermittent neurological symptoms: confusion, dizziness, impairment of speech or vision, weakness, and numbness of the limbs. When occlusion becomes complete, there are: behavioral and emotional changes, dysarthria, dysphagia, ophthalmoplegia, pupillary abnormalities, and a lethal outcome.

Since surgery is practically inaccessible for most cases, anticoagulation is the only hope, whenever it is possible to carry it out (see above).

Arteriosclerosis and Atherosclerosis

Arteriosclerosis (a generic term, but not synonymous with the types included) presents itself as hyperplastic sclerosis of the small arteries (related to arterial hypertension), Mönckeberg sclerosis of the medial layer of the arterial muscle, and atherosclerosis of the intima of the aorta and other large arteries.

Symptoms depend on the site where atheromatose lesions occur, namely, cerebral, coronary, aorta, or peripheral arteries. The most important are:

1. *Cerebral deficit,* starting with forgetfulness of recent events, followed by confusion, behavior changes, and finally thrombosis or hemorrhage.
2. *Coronary deficit,* causing different arrhythmias, cardiac failure, angina, and finally myocardial infarction.
3. *Deficit in extremities,* notably the legs, with intermittent claudication ending in gangrene.
4. *Kidney deficit,* characterized by impaired urinary concentration ability and consequent hypertension.
5. *Deficit of the terminal aorta,* with intermittent claudication extended to the muscles of the calf, the thighs, and the buttocks; mostly bilateral and progressive; men may also complain of impotence.

Arteriosclerosis and atherosclerosis are mostly found in advanced age, although not all older persons will show these changes in their arteries. Persons likely to have arteriosclerosis are patients over 45–50 years of age (particularly men) who are subject to any of the predisposing factors: diabetes or any other carbohydrate dismetabolism which may affect the metabolism of lipids; diseases of the elderly mainly characterized by elevated blood cholesterol or triglycerides; ecologic factors, such as diet, smoking, personal behavior, and local arterial structure caused by hypertension or involvement of arterial walls; and also heredity or infections.

The general trend in handling arteriosclerosis will follow these steps: (1) prophylaxis against the disease; (2) early pre-lesional treatment; (3) treatment of the established disease to stop the progress of atherogenesis, to avoid thrombosis, and to deal with the possible accidents of thrombosis, infarcts, and sequels in the brain, the heart, or another site. For prophylaxis advise your patient to stay on a low-fat diet, with fats constituting no more than 20% of the total caloric intake and mostly using polyunsaturated fats; to maintain adequate physical activity; and to take some antilipemic drug, such as clofibrate, estrogens (only for women), thyroid extracts, treatment of diabetes (it is unfortunate that phenformin has been banned from the market, since it used to help in these cases).

Clofibrate, 500 mg capsules; take one four times a day.

Conjugated estrogens, 0.625 or 0.3 mg tablets; take one a day for 21 days, with pauses of 7 to 10 days.

Thyroid extract (thyroglobulin); tablets containing about 15 to 30 mg, according to tolerance.

The basic drugs for the early treatment of the disease are the vasodilators, which will be selected according to the most affected vessels. Peripheral-acting vasodilators will help in the brain, the limbs, the internal ear, and the eye. There are many on the market, most of them with similar activity (nylidrin, cyclandelate, isoxsuprine). For dilation of coronary arteries, there are also several brands to choose from (pentaerythritol tetranitrate, isosorbide, and nitroglycerin for acute attacks). Dilators of the skin vessels, useful in superficial trophic lesions, are also numerous (tolazoline hydrochloride, nicotinic acid, nicotinyl alcohol).

Nylidrin, tablets containing 6 mg; take one every 8 hours.

Pentaerythritol tetranitrate, 10 mg tablets; take one every 6 hours (may increase to 20 mg tablets, if so needed and tolerated).

Tolazoline hydrochloride, 25 mg tablets, four times a day, or a higher dosage if needed and tolerated.

Nitroglycerin, 0.3 to 0.6 mg sublingual tablets, to place under the tongue (effects noted in less than 2 minutes, lasting less than 40 minutes). For prolonged effect long-acting preparations have been advised, but their usefulness has not yet been well substantiated.

Further treatment will be that of each established disease, according to the accepted trends in each instance.

Temporal Arteritis

Inflammation of the temporal arteries may precede a stroke, to which it might be linked, which is not too rare an event among the elderly. There is a clinical symptomatology of headache, other pains, and local tenderness; eye impairment may be revealed by visual symptoms, a more important ischemic optic neuritis, or blindness. Frequent complications are diffuse polyarteritis (characterized by multisystemic manifestations with fever, weight loss, hypertension, diarrhea, and dermic symptoms) and polymyalgia rheumatica. The final diagnosis is made by biopsy of the artery, and strongly suggested by an elevated sedimentation rate.

The early diagnosis of temporal arteritis is of great importance because the disease usually responds well to corticoid therapy.

Prednisone, 60 to 80 mg to start, to decrease to low dosages as soon as symptoms are under control; for chronic treatment, give medication every other day.

Arterial Hypertension

Either patients with known hypertension or those still without that diagnosis may reach the advanced stage, when neurological conditions will induce a state of unconsciousness. This will be a stroke in the great majority of instances, but it may also be a shock or simply a syncope. In the case of stroke, the diagnosis will be easy to make: all pertinent symptoms will be present, including the elevated blood pressure, but naturally varying according to the lesions present in each case. Of course, the diagnosis depends heavily on the past history of the patient, with evidence of a known hypertensive condition. During these hypertensive crises when the diastolic blood pressure runs over 150 mm Hg, other symptoms are present, such as those corresponding to acute hypertensive encephalopathy (very intense cephalalgia, convulsions, nausea and vomiting, drowsiness, cramps or twitching of the muscles, papilledema, and retinal hemorrhages), leading to a more or less complete stroke; or those corresponding to pulmonary edema; or acute dissecting aneurism of the aorta.

Emergency hospitalization is required, preferably in an intensive care department under supervision of specialized personnel, to maintain a continuous monitoring of vital signs and variations in blood components. The severe cases will be treated with sodium nitroprusside or with diazoxide, rapidly acting antihypertensive drugs (but special care will be maintained to avoid or check an excessive drop of blood pressure). If there is no imminent risk to be feared, use either reserpine, hydralazine or methyldopa. Once the blood pressure is under control, the regular antihypertensive method suitable for that particular patient will be followed.

> Sodium nitroprusside; 50 mg vial will give 100 μg in each ml when added to 500 ml of 5% glucose, to give 0.5 to a maximum of 8 μg each minute in a continuous intravenous infusion. Higher dosage might be given if needed and tolerated. Keep a continuous watch for an excessive fall of blood pressure.

> Diazoxide, 300 mg in a 20-ml vial, to be injected intravenously, rapidly and undiluted into a peripheral vein; a second injection may be given if the first one does not accomplish reduction in a lapse of no more than 30 minutes; further injections should be given as needed and tolerated at intervals of 4 to 24 hours, but not for more than 4 or 5 days.

> Reserpine, to give a daily dose of 0.1 mg, or to continue the dosage established by previous treatment.

> Methyldopa, to give a daily dose of 500 mg or to continue the previously established regimen (to a regular dose of 2000 mg a day; rarely 3000 mg a day).

> Hydralazine hydrochloride, to give 50 mg a day or to continue the preestablished dosage (maximum of 250 mg a day).

Brain Tumors and Cysts

The main symptoms are a result of cranial hypertension and the localization of the new mass, but older people frequently start symptoms with a strokelike hemiplegic outburst. An intense cephalalgia together with projectile vomiting and papilledema are characteristic of cranial hypertension. Also there may be behavioral disorders, bradycardia, epileptic seizures (these occur primarily with infarction), and ophthalmoplegy. The intense cephalalgia interferes with sleep, increases with effort, may be more severe at the site of the lesion, and is resistant to ordinary analgesics. It may mimic migraine. If the tumor localizes in the pituitary gland, the headache is mostly frontal, and the patient may complain of extreme weakness.

Hydatid cyst of the brain, frequent in Europe, rare in the United States, affects children more often than adults. A previous cyst is ordinarily found elsewhere in the body (liver). Headache may be the first manifestation of an expanding mass within the skull, even when it occurs in a patient in general good health. Very rarely it will cause strokelike symptoms. Diagnosis is made by X-ray examination and laboratory tests (eosiniphilia, Carson's test, complement fixation).

Surgery is the only logical approach to these problems, except for some tumors sensitive to radiation, or in persons over 80 years of age, particularly when they are in deep coma, with unequal pupils or stertorous breathing. For the relief of headache, prior to surgery, the best measure to be taken is the intravenous administration of a 50% glucose solution.

> Glucose, 50% solution; inject intravenously 25 ml—most cases will respond well to this amount—up to 50 ml.

Narcotic analgesics are not indicated for these patients. The risks of lumbar puncture (mobilization of the tumor to obstruct cerebrospinal pathways) make this procedure inadvisable.

Intracranial Abscess

Stroke symptoms are variable, ranging from mild to severe, convulsions being the first indication of an abscess, in many instances. Other signs of increased intracranial pressure, such as vomiting and papilledema, are usually present. Sometimes a previous septic lesion developing neurological symptoms will suggest the formation of an intracranial abscess.

Each case requires individualized therapy with surgery, antibiotics, and analgesics.

Epilepsy

Epilepsy is the first disease to suspect when a patient lying unconscious on the floor (or the bed) also presents generalized and severe clonic convulsive movements of the body, frothing at the mouth, most frequently tinged with blood because of tongue biting, and fecal and urinary incontinency. Since in most instances epilepsy starts early in life, the patient will be a known epileptic. It is not exceptional, however, for the first attack to occur late in life. After the attack, the patient is disoriented and then falls into a deep sleep. This clinical picture corresponds to the grand mal seizure. Other forms of epilepsy may also occur: petit mal, psychomotor seizures, and

Jacksonian epilepsy. The last type may correspond to local or focal irritation of the brain by tumors or other lesions. In this instance, the seizure starts as a local clonic spasm in the limbs or face, usually with no loss of consciousness, except when the seizure becomes generalized. The diagnosis depends on finding typical waves in the electroencephalogram and an increase of glucose and calcium in the blood. The pneumogram, the angiogram, and scanning are very useful in detecting new formations or other lesions in the brain. Usually, the clinical diagnosis is easy. Always check for injuries that may occur during the fall, particularly fractures.

When epileptic seizures occur, they are not treated per se—but care will be exerted to avoid further injuries. After the seizure, a schedule for treatment will be planned, accordingly: either to reinforce a previous one, or to start a new regimen. When the seizure is due to a known cause (symptomatic epilepsy), the treatment will be addressed to this underlying factor. Phenobarbital and diphenylhydantoin are the drugs commonly used for the treatment of grand mal seizures. Other drugs may also be employed. In status epilepticus, when seizures follow seizures without a pause, useful drugs are diazepam, phenobarbital, and paraldehyde.

> Phenobarbital; give 25 or 100 mg four times a day, according to needs and tolerance.

> Diphenylhydantoin, 100 mg three times a day, or a double dose if needed and tolerated—watch for hypertrophy of gums and neurologic side effects.

> Phenobarbital, injectable, 400 mg given slowly by vein—may increase to 800 mg if needed and tolerated.

> Diazepam, 2-ml ampoules containing 10 mg of the drug; inject intravenously at a very slow rate for the elderly; better to start with 5 mg, repeating at 10- to 15-minute intervals, not to exceed a total of 30 mg a day.

> Paraldehyde; inject 4 to 5 ml intramuscularly, repeating the same amount after a reasonable interval if needed; 1 or 2 ml mixed with a triple volume of saline can also be injected intravenously, but at a very slow rate—the intramuscular route is always preferred.

Migraine

In migraine a throbbing cephalalgia is the dominant symptom, either spread over the whole head or affecting only one side (hemicrania). During the attack nausea and photophobia are important symptoms. It is not common for migraine to start at an advanced age—on the contrary, it frequently disappears after the climacterium. There are patients, mainly women, who are the principal subjects of migraine, who may develop ocular symptoms with scotomata, blurred vision, transient hemianopsia or amaurosis, aphasia, and a convulsive state similar to a *stroke*. The attacks last for a few hours or even days, if untreated; they are frequently preceded by symptoms similar to an aura; and they are repeated at intervals.

If an allergen is found to be the cause of migraine, desensitization or avoidance of the allergen will cure or improve the disease. In other instances give regular analgesics if the symptoms are only of a mild nature (acetylsalicylic acid, codeine, or equivalent drugs). For more severe cases or those which do not respond to the initial treatment, give an ergot derivative.

> Acetylsalicylic acid, 600 mg, in tablets, every 4 hours while the attack lasts.

> Codeine, 30 (to 60) mg, by mouth or by subcutaneous injection if the case seems to be more severe, repeated every 4 hours.

> Ergotamine tartrate, 0.5 mg in solution, by subcutaneous injection, or 0.25 mg, by the intravenous route (this route may cause or increase vomiting).

> Dihydroergotamine, 1 mg in each ml; inject as needed subcutaneously, intramuscularly, or intravenously, instead of the ergotamine tartrate.

Mitral Stenosis

When symptoms of stroke develop in patients with known mitral stenosis, it may be assumed that a thrombus coming from the left atrium has reached cerebral arteries. These thrombotic accidents may also occur in other vascular areas (visceral or peripheral arteries). Rarely, the diagnosis of mitral stenosis must be made in other instances when an elderly person has a stroke. At the apex of the heart a loud snapping of the first mitral sound is heard followed by a low-pitched rumble, usually accompanied by a "thrill," but the rumble may possibly be absent when there is a large thrombus in the left atrium. The blood pressure is about normal, but it may be elevated for some of those in stroke. Hepatomegaly, peripheral edema, and pleural effusion together with electrocardiographic signs (broad or tall peaked P waves) will point out right ventricle involvement (hypertrophy and failure). Most cases will present dyspnea (exertional or nocturnal), relatively frequent hemotysis, and pulmonary infections. The X-ray picture will depict a straight left border of the heart with a large left atrium (also a large right ventricle and pulmonary artery if there is pulmonary hypertension).

The treatment of the stroke accident will follow standard procedure; that for the valvular stenosis will be surgical whenever possible. Discuss with a heart surgeon the pros and cons for each individual patient, since age is not a contraindication for these prosthetic corrections.

Polycythemia

Bleeding and thrombosis are common complications of polycythemic conditions. When hemorrhage or the thrombus occurs in the brain, a stroke leads the clinical picture. The symptoms are those already well known: headache, vomiting, loss of consciousness, and paralysis of one side of the body. When polycythemia is a basic component, there are other symptoms also present to complete the diagnosis. The patient shows a dusky redness of the skin, prominent in the lips, the fingernails, and the mouth and conjunctiva. There is complaint of weakness, malaise, headache, itching after bathing, acral pain, and inability to concentrate and to work. The ophthalmoscope shows tortuous, black retinal veins. If there is neither bleeding nor an increased plasma volume, there will be a confirmatory increase of red cells in the blood count, well over the 6.5 million level. The hemoglobin is over 18 per 100 ml, and the hematocrit over 55% (for women these limits are somewhat lower). Symptoms of gout may appear.

Treat polycythemia by venesection, removing about 1 liter—more or less, as needed—every week, until the hematocrit falls to no more than 45%, repeating treatment whenever it approaches 50%. Radiophosphorus and chemotherapy with chlorambucil or melphalan may be tried. These procedures are better handled by a specialist.

Thrombocytopenic Purpura

A stroke due to thrombocytopenic purpura or thrombotic thrombocytopenic purpura is usually fatal. The attack is preceded by a sudden appearance of petechiae and other bleeding spots (gastrointestinal bleeding, gums, nose, hematuria, vaginal bleeding). In the chronic form patients commonly present easy bruising and petechiae on pressure areas. The diagnosis is made by the low platelet count, below 100,000 per cubic ml, and the prolonged bleeding time.

The cerebral hemorrhage is very difficult to stop, owing to the low coagulability of the blood. A surgical trial may be given in some selected cases. The best treatment is to avoid the causes provoking hemorrhage (trauma, great effort, offending drugs). Splenectomy will be considered for selected cases.

Leukemia

Leukemia is usually a disease of younger people, but it may occur at any age. In both the acute and the chronic form, hemorrhages may infiltrate the central nervous system and give the clinical appearance of a stroke, usually seen in patients with white cell counts over 300,000 in each cubic mm. Common symptoms are: hepatosplenomegaly, generalized adenopathy, sudden onset of fever, sore throat, joint pains, petechiae or any other form of bleeding from the mouth or the lungs, thrombocytopenia, anemia, and the revealing hemocytogram with immature and abnormal white cells (myelocytes with peroxidase-staining cytoplasmatic granules: lymphocytes, without them). The diagnostic approach will evaluate a previous clinical picture with malaise, weakness, anorexia, pallor, fever, bone and joint pains, hepatosplenomegaly, and some instances of bleeding. The hemogram is mandatory.

There are several different schedules of treatment designed for each variety of leukemia, but because of the complexities involved the help of a specialist should be requested. The treatment of stroke will follow the regular pattern.

> Acute lymphocytic leukemia: start treatment with vincristine and prednisone.

> Acute myelocytic leukemia: use the COAP or the VAMP schedules (Cytoxan, Oncovin, Ara-C, and prednisone, in the first instance; and vincristine, amethopterin, mercaptopurine, and prednisone, in the second).

> Chronic lymphocytic leukemia: do not treat the asymptomatic patient; for hemorrhages due to the leukemic condition give the adequate chemotherapy (chlorambucil or cyclophosphamine), or if due to chemotherapy, discontinue it and give corticosteroids.

> Chronic myelocytic leukemia: use X-ray therapy, radiophosphorus, or busulfan, which is considered the drug of choice.

Meningitis

Following a period of vague symptomatology, the elderly may give the first evidence of a serious condition when they develop paralysis of limbs and face, contracted pupils, and a very rapid course, to lethargy and loss of consciousness. Suggestive of a meningitic reaction is a complex of fever, headache, possibly with backache, and stiff neck, which calls for an immediate examination of the spinal fluid. A full clinical picture of meningitis will also include: contracture of other muscles besides those of the neck, such as opisthotonos, strabismus, and flexion of the legs; itching of the nose; vomiting; constipation; generalized hypersensitivity, hyperacusis, and photophobia; bradycardia and delirium. Unfortunately, this clear-cut picture is not always present. The well-known meningitic reflexes will be looked for: Babinski's (extension of the toe on plantar irritation), Brudzinski's (legs are flexed when the neck is forced to flexion), and Kernig's (the above-flexed legs resist attempts to restore them to extension). In all instances the final diagnosis depends on the examination of the spinal fluid: in bacterial meningitis there are increased pressure, increased numbers of cells and elevated protein, decreased glucose, and possibly identifiable bacteria; in viral meningitis, there are fewer cells, the amount of glucose is normal, and the isolation of the virus is possible.

Isolate patients in bed and carefully observe all regular hospital measures for acute cases (hydration, electrolyte balance, elimination, and nutrition). The specific antibiotic will be promptly given, in full amounts. For infections with meningococcus, pneumococcus, streptococcus, *Proteus,* or *H. influenzae,* give ampicillin; for staphylococcus, methicillin; for *E. coli,* kenamycin; for *Pseudomonas,* polymyxin B. For pain use corticoids as soon as possible. Also try to normalize blood volume and pressure with electrolyte solutions and perhaps isoproterenol.

> Ampicillin, 200 mg per kilo in 24 hours, by intravenous injection of fractional doses, every 3 or 4 hours.

> Methicillin, 100 to 200 mg per kilo in 24 hours, by intramuscular injection of fractional doses, every 4 hours.

> Kanamycin, 15 mg per kilo in 24 hours, intramuscularly, in two or three installments (not to surpass 1.5 g a day).

> Polymyxin B, not to surpass 200 mg a day; 1.5 to 2.5 mg per kilo in 24 hours, in three intramuscular injections (an additional 2.5 mg a day, intrathecally, for no more than 3 days, could be a useful boost).

> Cortisone, 25 mg, by mouth, four or five times a day.

> Prednisone, 5 mg, as above.

> Dexamethasone, 0.5 mg for each dose, for a total of 2 to 3 mg a day.

Encephalitis

Extremely acute attacks of encephalitis cause shock before the clinical picture is well established; otherwise, shock is a late occurrence. The patient may have had high fever (rarely, hypothermia) and will show the common neurological symptoms of the disease, with backache, headache, stiff neck, malaise, insomnia, vomiting, convulsions, myoclonus, tremors, ocular paralysis or other forms of palsies, hemiplegia, and a more or less marked loss of consciousness; all this in varied combinations, from very mild (as in St. Louis encephalitis) to very severe (Eastern encephalitis). The clinical examination of the patient will reveal exaggerated deep tendon or absent superficial reflexes; and the spinal tap shows elevated pressure, increased protein, and perhaps isolation of the causal virus, thus differentiating this condition from meningitis.

Put patients in bed, and carry out hospital care. Viral encephalitis has no etiologic treatment. When the infecting germ is known, give the *specific antibiotic.* Corticoids administered early in the disease will help headache and convulsions. Analgesics may be given. Excessive intracranial pressure usually responds to mannitol or urea-invert infusions. Phenobarbital may control convulsions.

Prednisone, 5 to 20 mg, every 6 hours, according to needs and results; to be reduced and discontinued gradually.

Mannitol, 10% solution, by intravenous infusion.

Phenobarbital, 65 mg, by mouth or by injection, according to needs and results.

Meningovascular Syphilis

When large vessels are involved in meningovascular syphilis, stroke symptoms are prone to occur. The previous symptomatology is that of a common case of syphilis followed by headaches, irritability, paralysis, and altered reflexes (particularly those for light and accommodation), with the regular laboratory reports. This condition is, of course, a manifestation of tertiary syphilis, which requires immediate and adequate treatment (including the treatment of stroke).

Penicillin is the drug of choice for these patients, and efforts will be made to use it during the latent stage if primary and secondary syphilis have not been detected and treated in due time. Large doses of short-acting penicillin are preferred; and all patients should be rechecked at relatively frequent intervals.

Penicillin G, 600,000 units daily, by intramuscular injection, for 15 to 20 days; in resistant cases even 24 million units could be given intravenously for 10 to 20 days.

SHOCK

General Considerations and Diagnosis

The definition and concept of shock is not the same for all authors. Nevertheless, it is generally agreed that in shock there is a profound depression of both the circulatory and the nervous systems, with the natural consequences of this situation. The clinical situation results in marked arterial hypotension, rapid and weak pulse, dyspnea due to deficient ventilation, a pale and clammy skin, more or less intense clouding of consciousness, decreased urinary output, acidosis, and a general condition of extremely serious depression of vital factors which follows a trauma or any other form of extreme aggression.

Causes of shock are: (1) *loss of fluid* due to hemorrhage, burns, vomiting, diarrhea, peritonitis, trauma, surgery, or nephrosis; and (2) *vascular low resistance* due to massive sepsis, a condition relatively frequent among the elderly suffering from gram-negative infections; also diabetes, cancer, pneumonia, meningitis, or other chronic depletion, and among those receiving radiation therapy, corticoids, or immunosuppressive drugs; as well as in those with intense pain, spinal injury, or who use vasodilating drugs or suffer anaphylactic shock, intoxication with hypnotics, or other drug reactions.

General Treatment of Shock

Each variety of shock will require its own specific treatment, but there are rules to be followed, which are summarized here.

To evaluate results properly, a continuous record of the state of consciousness, blood pressure, pulse, respiration, temperature, and skin condition will be maintained with utmost precision.

Patients will be placed in bed with the legs only slightly elevated and will be watched for patency of the airway. If necessary, cleanse the airway or intubate, and assist respiration as needed and possible. Oxygen therapy is always necessary if indicated by cyanosis, dyspnea, or blood values. An indwelling urinary catheter is advisable to assure elimination and also to promote organic perfusion. Keep the patient reasonably warm, the temperature checked at frequent intervals. Perform all required tests (laboratory, blood pressure, central venous pressure, cardiac function) as indicated.

Check pain as soon as possible, but avoid morphine, oral medication, and subcutaneous injections. Since intravenous infusions are rapid, use the tubing for infusing codeine, or meperidine at least.

> Codeine, 30 to 60 mg, intravenously, repeated as needed and tolerated.

> Meperidine, 50 (to 100) mg, by the intravenous route, repeated as needed and tolerated.

Blood volume must be replaced and maintained, starting with about 100 to 1500 ml of saline and following with plasma expanders or blood transfusions. The total amount to be given can be evaluated from the changing levels of central venous pressure or the clinical response. If dextran is given, a 10% solution in 5% glucose (or saline) will be infused in an initial amount of 100 to 150 ml during the first hour to be followed by less than 1000 ml in 24 hours (some 10 ml for each kilo of body weight a day). Nevertheless, dextran may cause pulmonary edema, renal shutdown, or heart failure, particularly in patients with known cardiac or renal diseases, or who are markedly dehydrated. In these cases, transfusions of well-matched blood are preferable.

> Dextran 40, 10% solution in saline.

Dopamine, either alone or with levarterenol, may help to increase blood pressure. These substances may be tried, carefully, avoiding anginal pain, ventricular arrhythmias, or local tissue necrosis due to extravasation.

Levarterenol, 4 to 6 mg added to 1000 ml of dextrose in water, to be infused in about 1 day.

Dopamine hydrochloride, 200 mg ampoules diluted in 500 ml of 5% dextrose in saline (there are 400 μg of dopamine in each ml); give 2 to 5 μg/kg/minute at the start, and increase gradually to a maximum of 30 to 40 μg/kg/minute, or as needed and tolerated.

In cases presenting oliguria or suspected of cerebral hypertension, mannitol can be given, added to the infusion used.

Mannitol, 10 to 25% solution, 200 ml to 1 liter, in 500 to 1000 ml of saline.

Corticoids are advised by some practitioners, to be used early in cases of suspected shock, but to be discontinued at the slightest suspicion of an adverse reaction.

Blood Loss

Hemorrhage is a relatively frequent cause of shock. The symptomatology is similar to that of common shock: vertigo or dizziness; weakness; faintness; profuse sweating followed by thirst; hypotension, not to be confused by a transient previous phase of moderately elevated blood pressure; tachycardia with feeble pulse; and a final stage of frank depletion. Laboratory reports will reveal marked anemia because of the decrease of red cells and hemoglobin; but it is very important to remember that during the first hours there is always the possibility of evidence of blood concentration, with elevated figures for cells and hemoglobin.

External hemorrhage is usually easy to detect: epistaxis, hematemesis, hemoptysis, or a severe injury. The blood is seen externally.

Epistaxis.   Hemorrhage from the nose is usually due to direct trauma to the mucosal vessels, such as cracking of mucosa from extreme dryness, infection, nose-picking, foreign body, fracture, or hemic diseases; but among the elderly important considerations will be hypertension and neoplastic ulceration. When the blood follows a retrograde path, it may suggest hemoptysis or hematemesis; in some of these cases even the rhinoscope may not show the bleeding spot. Fortunately, most cases of epistaxis are not severe enough to cause shock.

Hematemesis.   Blood expelled from the gastrointestinal tract through the mouth may come from esophageal varicosities or from gastric ulcerations. Blood from esophageal varicosities is of the venous type (darker in color), and is regurgitated rather than vomited; also there is usually a previous portal hypertension due to liver disease. Vomited blood from the stomach may also be of the dark hue, but in the case of massive hemorrhages it may be bright red. A known previous history may help in diagnosing the condition, namely, the existence of a peptic ulcer, the habitual ingestion of antacids, or the use of ulcerogenic drugs.

Hemoptysis.   Blood coming through the mouth from the lungs is neither vomited nor regurgitated—it is coughed. This blood is usually bright red and frequently frothy and mixed with mucus or with pus. It is profuse in benign bronchial adenoma, tuberculosis, aortic aneurism, and injuries.

Internal hemorrhages may demand the treatment of shock or the control of active bleeding.

Gastrointestinal Hemorrhage.   This hemorrhage may cause a mild syncopal attack that will be followed by vomiting of blood or by melena; soon, a hypovolemic shock will appear, with hypotension, weakness, dizziness, tachycardia, and feeble pulse. Other symptoms are related to the causative disease, namely, peptic ulcer, gastric cancer, or gastritis.

Ruptured Aneurisms.   The most important ones, for our consideration, are those of the thoracic and the abdominal aorta, and those arising from the arteries of the lower limbs. In the first instance, symptoms are similar to those of myocardial infarction, but the pain radiates to the back, abdomen, and hips; there is a previous hypertensive condition; and the event occurs more frequently among males. Depending on the site of rupture, there may be additional symptoms of cardiac tamponade, or a frank hemoptysis. A ruptured abdominal aortic aneurism may present initial mild symptomatology, but soon a sudden severe pain will appear, together with a mass in the abdomen or the flank, pulsating and expanding, and possibly subcutaneous ecchymotic bleeding in the flank or the groin. Ruptured aneurisms of the lower limbs are easy to diagnose because of the ischemic or gangrenous changes that occur distally.

Essentials for the treatment of shock due to blood loss are blood transfusion (plasma is an acceptable alternate, in many instances) and surgery when no improvement occurs after 12 to 24 hours of medical remedies. Other measures for the care of shock will be put into practice. Do not use morphine in the case of gastric lesions (may cause vomiting), and avoid oral and subcutaneous medications. Keep a good record of vital signs. Watch continuously for airway obstruction, and keep the patient in bed with the legs only slightly elevated. If needed, intubate and give oxygen. At all times maintain perfect hospital care. Place an intravenous catheter as soon as possible, not only for needed transfusions, but also for the administration of other needed drugs, particularly codeine or meperidine, for pain.

Codeine, 30 to 60 mg, intravenously, repeated as needed and tolerated.

Meperidine, 50 (to 100) mg, intravenously, repeated as needed and tolerated.

Blood for transfusion, well-matched, to be given at a reasonable speed to improve symptoms soon, and to control the situation in less than 24 hours (otherwise, resort to surgery).

Calcium gluconate, 10% solution, to give 10 ml for every liter of blood, always injected slowly intravenously. This is an advisable precaution.

For more details of treatment, see under "General Treatment of Shock," earlier in this section.

Dehydration

Strictly speaking, dehydration refers to deficit of water; but in most instances there is a concomitant deficit of electrolytes, particularly sodium. In severe cases, shock is a consequence. Symptoms are: decreased skin turgor (inelastic and wrinkled), dryness of mucosae (more apparent in the mouth and tongue, which becomes shrunken and corrugated), ashen hue of integuments, decreased intraocular pressure, cramps, hyperthermia, hypotension, and finally lethargy, confusion, and marked oliguria. Laboratory reports will show only modest decreases of natremia; renal compromise will show in increased BUN and creatinine. The common causes of dehydration are listed below.

Diarrhea, vomiting, or both; generally caused by gastrointestinal obstruction, such as pyloric stricture or intestinal obstruction; or by cholera, enterocolitis, hemorrhages from the digestive tract, or any other disease compromising the intake of water.

Gastric or any other form of gastrointestinal suction.

Deprived ingestion of liquids or excessive elimination because of sweating or urination (polyuria).

Hemorrhages of all sorts, which may also present dehydration.

Uremia.

Diabetes mellitus, and diabetes insipidus.

Severe liver diseases (cirrhosis, other causes of ascites).

Adrenal insufficiency.

Chronic renal diseases.

Burns, heatstroke, sunstroke.

Other forms of cachexia due to malnutrition.

When shock occurs under these circumstances, efforts will be made to correct the water deficit as soon as possible, and the first medication to be given should be isotonic saline, intravenously, which will be periodically readjusted as needed. Nevertheless, all patients knowingly suffering from any of the above-mentioned diseases will be protected from the occurrence of this dangerous event—as will, naturally, all those unable to drink adequate amounts of water, such as the unconscious, the psychotic, and the like.

> Isotonic saline, 1000-ml bottle, to be infused intravenously at due speed to correct symptoms at the earliest possible moment.

> Dextrose in water, 5%, to use as above.

> Isotonic saline, with potassium (40 mEq in 500 ml).

Peptic Ulcer

Bleeding and perforation are frequent complications of peptic ulcers (either duodenal or gastric) which will usually cause marked shock. *Bleeding ulcer* symptoms are: a mild syncopal attack followed by vomiting of blood or by melena, soon turning into a clinical picture of shock with hypotension, weakness, dizziness, tachycardia, feeble pulse, sweating, thirst, chilliness, and a desire to defecate. *Perforated ulcers* provoke a sudden, acute epigastric pain radiating to the shoulder or the lower right quadrant, which thereafter lessens for a while, and is accompanied or followed by nausea and vomiting, fever, prostration, tachycardia, rebound tenderness, strong rigidity of the abdominal muscles, absent bowel sounds, and the classic chamber of free air in the abdominal cavity as seen in X-ray films.

The great majority of these patients will show a previous history of peptic ulcer with epigastric pain, almost always related to feeding time and relieved by the ingestion of food or antacids, but recurring with emptying of the stomach (hunger pains). If the pain occurs at a higher location, it may indicate the presence of an esophageal ulcer. A tender spot is noted on palpation at the painful region. There are also nausea and vomiting (may be bloody), anemia, and heartburn. Laboratory tests will show elevated acidity of the gastric contents, but there are patients with lower secretion of acid. The final diagnosis depends on fluoroscopic and radiologic examination, and must rule out cancer.

Following the essential measures for the treatment of shock, patients will be promptly transferred to a hospital, where strict care will be maintained at all times, with careful recording of vital signs, and immediate placement of an intravenous catheter for transfusions and medication. Patients will be in bed, with the legs only slightly elevated, and if necessary, intubated and receiving oxygen. Basically, start with blood transfusions (plasma is an acceptable alternate); but if there is no improvement in 12 or 24 hours, surgery is inevitable. Codeine or meperidine will allay pain; dopamine (alone or with levarterenol), hypotension; mannitol, cerebral hypertension or oliguria. Do not give morphine or corticoids to these patients.

Blood for transfusion, given at a reasonable speed for improvement of symptoms, but for no more than 24 hours without improvement, at which time surgery becomes mandatory.

Calcium gluconate, 10% solution; administer 10 ml intravenously at a very slow rate for each liter of blood transfused, as an advisable precaution.

Codeine, 30 to 60 mg, intravenously, repeated as needed and tolerated.

Dopamine hydrochloride, 200 mg ampoules diluted in 500 ml of 5% dextrose in saline (there are 400 μg of dopamine in each ml); give 2 to 5 μg for each kilo of body weight every minute at the start, increasing gradually to a maximum of 30 to 40 μg , as needed and tolerated.

Mannitol, 10 to 20% solution, 200 ml to 1 liter, in 500 to 1000 ml of saline.

Once the situation is controlled, the patient will receive the regular treatment for peptic ulcer. First, plan an adequate diet. Since chronic epigastric dull pain is the most frequent manifestation, patients will receive antacids and parasympatholytics (anticholinergics), sodium bicarbonate being the one preferred by most patients; but this medication should not be given for long-term therapy, with a mixture of magnesium oxide and calcium carbonate preferred in this case (check at intervals for hypercalcemia). During acute stages order bed rest, bland diet deprived of any kind of irritant, and phenobarbital if there is marked anxiety. When surgery is required, a simple gastroenterostomy seems to be the best procedure for frail elderly persons.

Esophageal Varices

Hematemesis in which the blood coming from the mouth is regurgitated rather than vomited will suggest esophageal varicosities. In other words, if hematemesis is accompanied by vomiting efforts, the blood is suspected of coming from the stomach; if it is only regurgitated, without vomiting discomfort, it may be from the esophagus. Blood from the stomach is usually preceded by a history of peptic ulcer; blood from esophageal varicosities, by a previous liver disease. These patients are frequently alcoholics or may present clinical jaundice. Other symptoms include: hepatomegaly (may be associated with splenomegaly), fetor hepaticus, ascites (not a rare occurrence), spider angiomas on the skin, and liver palms. Laboratory reports will show increased bilirubin, transaminases, and alkaline phosphatase. The final diagnosis will be given by a fiberoptic esophagogastroduodenoscopy: X-ray films may also be informative. These varicosities will rarely cause shock because of bleeding, but it is a possibility. The symptoms will be those of shock, as described in the preceding paragraphs, q.v. for more details.

Shock will be treated, accordingly, with bed rest, the legs only slightly elevated, maintenance of a patent airway (oxygen if needed), placement of an intravenous catheter, and administration of blood (or plasma), dopamine, mannitol, or any other needed medication. The use of pituitrin frequently controls the bleeding. If it fails, use a triple-lumen tube (Sengstaken-Blakemore). Finally, discuss the possibility of surgical decompression for the causative portal hypertension.

> Pituitrin S, 20 units in 50 ml of 5% dextrose, given intravenously at a slow rate (20 to 30 minutes); may be repeated.

Acute Gastritis

Either the acute simple, or the acute corrosive gastritis may cause shock because of diarrhea or hemorrhage. In the first instance, there are anorexia, diarrhea, colicky pains, prostration, and dehydration following the use of chemical irritants (particularly, salicylates) or infections. The acute corrosive gastritis follows the ingestion of corrosive substances, usually in attempted suicide. The differential diagnosis is given by corrosion seen in the mouth and pharynx. Fiberoptic endoscopy will differentiate these two conditions, the second being more likely to cause symptoms of shock.

Whenever it is present, treat shock in the usual way (see above entries). In addition, in acute simple gastritis treat the accompanying infection and the water or electrolyte imbalance; sedatives and antidiarrheics may be of help. In acute corrosive gastritis the treatment of shock will require more active efforts, together with the use of antacids and the specific antidote, whenever known. Meperidine will be preferred for pain, but morphine will be strictly avoided. Lavage will be performed only if there is no risk of perforation, and not done when corrosion is severe. In this last instance, emergency surgery will be considered.

> *Corrosion caused by acids:* administer magnesium oxide, or use milk or egg albumin. Also, milk of magnesia is helpful.

> *Corrosion caused by alkalis:* make a mixture of equal parts of water and vinegar, and give about 500 ml; diluted citrus fruit juice can be given, or citric or tartaric acid (2 to 4 g, in water); melted margarine, melted butter, or milk may protect the mucosa. Do not treat pain with morphine; give meperidine instead (50 to 100 mg, by injection). Early corticoid therapy may help for strictures.

Gastric Cancer

Not rarely, aged males will present shock due to hemorrhage caused by gastric cancer because the disease may be totally asymptomatic for relatively long periods of time, or so vaguely disturbing that patients do not request medical help. Once the diagnosis of shock due to abdominal hemorrhage is established (see previous paragraphs in this section), the possibility of cancer will be suggested by a previous weight loss in a patient with some gastrointestinal discomfort, who is or has been considered anemic because of paleness, and who presents a palpable mass in the abdomen. The final diagnosis is made by X-ray examination or by endoscopy, which can also be of help in doing a biopsy or a cytologic examination.

Surgical resection will be the best resource, whenever applicable. Radio- and chemotherapy are good palliative methods and may prolong life. For more details see the chapter on tumors and ulcers.

Gastric Benign Tumors

The clinical situation is exactly the same as with gastric cancer, and the final diagnosis will be given only by X-ray and endoscopic procedures.

Surgery is the best approach for those bulky tumors prone to cause massive gastrointestinal hemorrhages.

Mesenteric Occlusion

Acute conditions usually start with generalized abdominal pain of either sudden or slow onset, always steady and severe. In some instances there are colicky intermissions. Other gastrointestinal symptoms are ordinarily present: nausea, vomiting, diarrhea, prostration, and other evidence of shock; all these together with abdominal distention, tenderness on palpation, and, finally, signs of peritoneal irritation. The clinical symptoms of an acute abdomen, together with hemoconcentration, marked leukocytosis with a shift to the left, melena, and X-ray examination showing some gaseous distention and peritoneal fluid, will help one to reach the final diagnosis, thus eliminating, mainly, pancreatitis (elevated amylase) and perforation (peritoneal air).

Because of an extremely serious prognosis, surgery is advisable in most instances to resect the gangrenous portion of the bowel or perform an embolectomy or thrombectomy. In addition, the regular treatment for shock will be put into effect immediately. Anticoagulants will not be given to these patients, who should be protected with antibiotics against infections caused by fecal flora.

Kanamycin, 50 mg for each kilo of body weight in 24 hours, in divided doses by intramuscular injection.

Gentamycin, 1 to 3 mg for each kilo of body weight in 24 hours, in divided doses by intramuscular injection.

Meperidine, 50 to 100 mg, by intramuscular injection, to allay pain; repeated as needed and tolerated.

Diarrhea and Vomiting

When either diarrhea or vomiting caused by an inductive disease reaches considerable proportions, the loss of water and electrolytes will easily induce shock. Listing all possible diseases here is unnecessary; the reader will find many references to them in these pages. The only additional instruction here is that one must put into practice the treatment for shock, as stated at the beginning of this section, along with the treatment for each specific disease.

Acute Pancreatitis

Acute pancreatitis always causes a very severe clinical picture, with shock occurring in many instances and always in the acute hemorrhagic type—with fever, which may follow pain and will reach 38° to 39°C (100° to 102°F). Pain, mainly located at the left side of the epigastrium, spreads to almost all of the abdomen; it is constant and very severe, exaggerated by certain positions (lying supine), elicited (actually increased) by pressure on the epigastric area, and accompanied by local muscle rigidity. Pancreatic juice spreading internally may provoke pneumonia, pleural effusion, or pulmonary atelectasis, with all the accompanying symptomatology. The laboratory will report leukocytosis and elevated serum amylase (over 600 Somogyi units). X-ray films will help the diagnosis. If the pancreatic condition refers only to a pancreatic colic, there will be no muscle rigidity. Acute pancreatitis must be differentiated from peptic ulcer, gall bladder disease or colic, myocardial infarction, renal colic of the left kidney, intestinal obstruction, and mesenteric thrombosis.

Keep patients in bed, and strictly follow the regular hospital care: nasogastric tube to combat gastrointestinal distention, intravenous fluids (nothing should be given by mouth), blood transfusions in cases of hemorrhagic pancreatitis, peritoneal dialysis for selected cases, antispasmodics or analgesics to allay pain (selected in this order: papaverine hydrochloride, meperidine, atropine, morphine sulfate), calcium salts for hypocalcemia, and antibiotics (the specific one, whenever known) to check infection. Treat other complications as they arise, including shock.

Papaverine hydrochloride, 60 to 100 mg, by intramuscular injection, repeated as needed and tolerated.

Meperidine, 100 mg, by intramuscular injection, repeated as needed and tolerated.

Atropine, 0.4 to 0.6 mg, by subcutaneous injection; watch for intolerance.

Calcium gluconate, 10% solution; inject 10 ml, every 4 hours (check calcemia).

Tetracycline, up to 500 mg, every 6 hours, by mouth; or 250 mg, every 6 hours, by intramuscular injection.

Ampicillin, 250 mg, every 8 hours, by intravenous injection or by mouth.

Kanamycin or gentamycin may also be considered for administration for infection.

Peritonitis

The outstanding symptom of peritonitis is abdominal pain, which may cause the older patient to lapse into shock. If due to a perforation, the pain will be excruciating, but it will be less marked when due to local infection or to infections carried by the blood. Characteristically, the peritonitic patient will lie on his back, immobile, legs flexed upon the abdomen (at times, straightened), with superficial respirations. Hiccup, together with shoulder pain, suggests diaphragmatic involvement. Diarrhea, nausea, and vomiting—occasionally of fecal character—may be present. Initially, the abdomen is somewhat distended and rigid, becoming more so thereafter, with borborygmi evident in the first stage and silent when paralytic ileus supervenes. Chills and fever are characteristic, and tachycardia increases gradually. In advanced stages, the drawn, pinched, and livid *facies hippocratica* is evident.

Post-surgery and traumatic peritonitis is diagnosed because each case follows the causative incident (now less often seen because of the use of adequate anti-infective therapy).

Peritonitis due to infective diseases is diagnosed when the corresponding symptoms are superimposed on those of pneumonia, bacteremia, typhoid fever, influenza, or other acute infection.

Peritonitis due to local diseases may be of the pelvis or the abdomen, such as abscesses (perigastric, periduodenal, subdiaphragmatic), or of the gall bladder, the kidney, or the appendix. Infections of the lymph glands, veins, uterus, or tubes are included. The diagnosis depends on the findings of the previous condition.

Peritonitis due to abdominal diseases, perhaps the most frequently seen, usually follows an acute abdomen. The causative diseases of the digestive system are: peptic ulcer (gastric or duodenal), acute cholecystitis, pancreatitis, acute appendicitis, and perforation of a viscus by peptic ulcer, acute erosive gastritis, or cholecystitis.

Diseases of the urinary system include: pyelonephritis (rare occurrence), perirenal abscess, or renal carbuncle.

Other diseases to be considered are: acute salpingitis, occlusion of the mesenteric vessels, diseases of the spleen (mainly rupture or infarction), mesenteric adenitis (rare), and torsion of cysts, organs, or pedunculated tumors.

A surgeon is to be called as soon as the diagnosis is established, since surgery is likely to check the progress of peritonitis. Prepare the patient with intravenous fluids, all efforts to combat shock, and continuous gastric suction; give analgesics for pain, and antibiotics against fecal flora (the specific one as soon as it is known).

Meperidine, 100 mg, by intramuscular injection, every 4 to 6 hours.

Kanamycin, 15 mg per kilo of body weight in 24 hours, in divided doses, intramuscularly, every 8 to 12 hours, not to exceed 1.5 g a day.

Gentamycin, 1 to 5 mg per kilo of body weight in 24 hours, in divided doses, intramuscularly, every 8 hours.

Injuries

Concussional results of any traumatic lesion may cause a more or less marked shock because of pain or the effects upon sensitive organs. Trauma to the head may lead to stroke due to brain hemorrhage (q.v., in the previous section). Following any accident such as a car accident or a fall, carefully check the patient.

Head: examine the scalp for wounds, lacerations, or contusions; the deeper bony structures, for depressions.

Eyes: note pupil size, particularly regarding equality and reflexes.

Ear and nose: check for escape of cerebrospinal fluid in cranial fractures; or a less suggestive local hemorrhage.

Cardiovascular: check blood pressure, heart rate, rhythm, quality of pulse.

Skin: hematomas, lacerations, or wounds may indicate lesion in the limbs, the thorax, the back, or other areas.

Neurological: check for abnormal reflexes or for paralyses.

Cranial injuries may provoke stroke or shock. In the case of stroke there will be a loss of consciousness followed by paralyses, stertorous respirations or respirations of the Cheyne-Stokes type, flushed face, bradycardia with full pulse, normal or relatively elevated blood pressure, head and eyes "looking" at the injured side of the brain or one of the cheeks inflating rhythmically with respiration, lack of reflexes, or a positive Babinski's sign. In the case of shock there will be marked arterial hypotension with tachycardia and weak pulse, dyspnea due to deficient ventilation, pale and clammy skin, all pointing to a profound depression of the circulatory and nervous systems.

Intracerebral hemorrhage: symptoms are as stated above; the diagnosis is made by angiography.

Extradural hemorrhage: there is usually a transient loss of consciousness, and signs of increased intracranial pressure develop gradually; X-ray pictures may show a fracture crossing the middle meningeal groove.

Subarachnoid hemorrhage: there is a painful stiff neck, and fresh blood in the cerebrospinal fluid.

Subdural hematoma: vague but typical symptoms are headache, slowly progressive weakness of one side of the body, vomiting, and other neurological symptoms and signs; there will be paralyses, papilledema, and mental changes; X-ray studies may help in diagnosing the condition (shift of the pineal gland and distortion of the ventricles).

These cranial injuries require an emergency treatment for shock, as stated earlier in this section, with hospitalized patients resting in bed, the legs only slightly elevated, with adequate means for respiration, urine excretion aided by an indwelling catheter, pain controlled with meperidine, blood loss replenished with transfusions of blood or plasma, dopamine to increase blood pressure, mannitol to check cerebral hypertension, and antibiotics to prevent an additional infection. Consider surgery.

Meperidine, 50 to 100 mg, intravenously, repeated as needed and tolerated.

Blood for transfusion, well-matched, to be given at a reasonable speed to improve symptoms soon, and to control shock in less than 24 hours.

Calcium gluconate, 10% solution, to give 10 ml for every liter of blood, slowly injected in the vein.

Dopamine hydrochloride, 200 mg ampoules diluted in 500 ml of 5% dextrose in saline (400 μg of dopamine in each ml); give from 2 to 5 μg for each kilo of body weight each minute at the start; increase gradually to a maximum of 30 to 40 μg for each kilo of body weight every minute, or as needed and tolerated.

Mannitol, 10 to 25% solution; give 200 to 1000 ml added to 500 to 1000 ml of saline.

Penicillin; give 600,000 units every 6 to 12 hours.

For more detailed information, see the corresponding paragraphs under the heading "Stroke," early in this section.

Other injuries are less prone to cause shock, but they may, mainly with the frail elderly. It will be well to give special and extra care to all injuries, especially in these patients with reduced vitality. If the patient is anxious, mitigate the condition with mild sedatives; if he is depressed, give caffeine in the form of a strong coffee infusion. Otherwise, follow the advice given in the preceding paragraph.

Burns

The diagnosis is obvious in the great majority of cases. There has been a close relationship with a very hot object, a flame, or corrosive or radiating substances. The results may be: *first degree* burns, with only erythema of the skin; *second degree* burns, when vesicles are added to the erythema; and *third degree* burns, when the damage extends beyond the dermis into the deeper layers of the skin. Shock will occur among the elderly whenever the burned surface reaches a little over 9% of the body surface. The classic "rule of nines" establishes that one whole arm or the head represents 9% of the total surface; also, each are the anterior and posterior surfaces of the legs, the upper trunk, and the lower trunk (11 segments multiplied by 9 is 99, plus 1% reserved for the genital area). When such a person seeks help with second or third degree burns covering more than 9% of the body surface, do not wait for the development of shock to start adequate treatment. Give it immediately. If he is more severely burned, send him to a specialized hospital. Watch in all instances for dehydration, which is a critical state. The ideal hydration level is shown by a urinary level of about 30 to 50 ml every hour (more than 100 ml indicates overhydration; less than 30 ml, underhydration); but these figures are valid only for the first 2 days and if there is no acute renal insufficiency. After that time, check turgor of the normal skin and moisture of the tongue. Edema may also indicate overhydration (we are not talking about the characteristic edematous reaction of the burn sites).

Treatment for minor burns requires only cleansing and protection. Codeine may be given for comfort. More severe burns may require some sort of minor surgery or debridement. Patients with severe burns over more than 9% of the body surface will go into shock in 2 to 3 hours; it is for that reason that an adequate treatment for shock must be started immediately. Blood (plasma or dextran) is to be given in all instances from the very beginning of treatment, together with equal amounts of electrolyte solution (lactated Ringer's) and 5% dextrose in water or the same electrolyte solution, to compensate for insensible loss. The accepted required amounts for the first 24 hours are 1 ml of each liquid for each kilo of body weight and for each 1% burn area, plus one half of these amounts for insensible perspiration, as shown in this example: 1 ml of blood (or plasma) × 25% burn area × 65 kg (about 140 lb.) = 1625 ml; 1 ml electrolyte solution × 25% burn area × 65 kg = 1625 ml; plus 5% dextrose or electrolyte for compensation: one half of 1625 = 812.5 ml; total amount of infused liquid is 4062.5 ml (half of it given during the first 8 hours, though not all authorities agree). The highest burn surface used in these calculations will be 50%; that is, for 80% burn surface the calculation will estimate only 50%. Also, no more than 200 kg of weight will be considered. The second day only half the total amount of infused liquid will be given. If blood or plasma is not available, electrolyte solutions can be given if the burn area is less than 40%. If there is acidosis, give bicarbonate solutions, included in the total estimate. The care of the skin is a matter of minor surgery, but requires grafts for extensive third degree burns. Use the open or the closed method, as feasible; and take the greatest precautions to avoid infections. Mafenide or butesin picrate is advised for this purpose, as a cream to be applied locally. Immunize against tetanus in all extensive burns. Established infections will be treated with the specific antibiotic.

Codeine, 30 to 60 mg, by intravenous injection.

Blood (well-matched for each patient), for transfusion.

Lactated Ringer's solution, 1000-ml flask; use following the above-mentioned indications.

Mafenide cream, one tube, apply locally.

Sunburn, Sunstroke

Sunburn occurring during the summer season will mostly show a mild discomfort from the resultant erythematous and vesicant reaction. But particularly among the aged, after a relatively prolonged exposure, there are some acute cases which will show fever, chills, and shock. The *dermic* symptoms appear as erythema and edema followed by vesiculation and oozing, and later on by exfoliation and tanning. Patients may complain of precordial distress and headache, and not rarely will present cramps. Even with relatively mild cases, watch for complication: renal failure, hyperkalemia, or, as stated above, cardiovascular collapse or marked shock. Usually, the diagnosis is easy because of the history. The laboratory will report hemoconcentration and proteinuria. It will be wise to check for diseases predisposing to photosensitivity, as porphyria. Avoid the use of light-sensitizing cosmetics and drugs (8-methoxysoralen, sulfonamides, phenothiazines).

Shock will be treated as usual, with efforts to decrease body temperature starting with a tub bath or iced sheets to decrease rectal temperature, but not below 38.5°C, checking every 10 minutes. Resultant hypothermia, which frequently occurs, will be treated with warm blankets, hot drinks, or heating pads. Locally, use wet, cool dressings; but not an oily preparation. General treatment is aimed at control of fever, pain, and collapse.

Sodium chloride, 1% solution; use ad libitum.

Sodium bicarbonate, 2 to 5% solution; use ad libitum.

Calamine lotion; apply locally after using any of the above, three or four times a day (do not allow excessive drying of the skin).

Starch lotion, use like the above calamine lotion, but only twice a day.

Acetylsalicylic acid, 600 mg, tablets; take every 4 to 6 hours, preferably with meals.

Prednisolone, 5 mg a day (or several times a day) in more severe cases.

Heatstroke

Those persons exposed for a time to some sort of elevated temperature by any form of heating will react with heatstroke when debilitated by age or any other cause. This condition will follow a course with two main stages: first, headache, dizziness, nausea, visual disturbances, and possibly convulsions; second, development of a shock state, with sudden loss of consciousness, very high fever, arrythmic tachycardia, dryness of the skin (from lack of sweating), flushed and hot skin, and hypotension. When a patient reacts in this manner to heat, he has to be watched in the future because of the almost certain repetition of the reaction when he is exposed, even if to lower temperatures than those that caused the first attack.

The treatment is that stated for shock, but in general will follow the same directions as for sunstroke, discussed in the preceding paragraph, q.v.

Pulmonary Infarction

Pulmonary infarction starts abruptly with fever, substernal chest pain, anxiety, dyspnea, and not rarely shock, which almost immediately follows the starting symptoms among the elderly. Other evidence of right heart failure and circulatory insufficiency may be present (edema; tender, enlarged liver; high venous pressure). Patients frequently have cough, and often various amounts of hemoptysis. Pain may vary according to location of the infarct: precordial or retrosternal if the left lower lobe is affected. Small infarcted areas are practically symptomless. Auscultation reveals râles, sounds of consolidation, pleural rub, and gallop rhythm, or accentuation of the second pulmonary sound of the heart. Cyanosis and pleural effusion may occur. SGOT and LDH are significant when elevated. X-ray films help only in a few cases. Electrocardiograms will only give evidence of cor pulmonale.

Initial treatment is emergent: 100% oxygen by mask; heparin, meperidine, or morphine for pain and sedation; levarterenol and other adequate measures for shock. Request the help of a chest surgeon for possible embolectomy. If needed, give cardiotonics. The second phase of treatment includes continued bed rest, and heparinization while confined in bed, thereafter changing to oral coumarin; use antibiotics if there is an infection, remove pleural effusions if they are present, and maintain a close relationship with the chest surgeon for possible intervention.

Heparin, 10,000 units, intravenously, every 4 to 6 hours, as indicated by continuous test of clotting time done before each injection; it will be continued for about 2 days, or while the patient is in bed; thereafter change to:

Bishydrocoumarin, 200 to 300 mg, by mouth, to start, followed by 50 to 100 mg, every 24 hours, checking prothrombin activity, for 3 to 6 weeks.

Morphine sulfate, 10 to 15 mg, by subcutaneous injection, repeated as needed and tolerated.

Levarterenol, 4 mg in each liter of 5% glucose, intravenously, to maintain systolic pressure at 90 mm Hg.

Metaraminol, 100 mg in 1000 ml of 5% glucose, for slow infusion. Isoproterenol, 2 (to 4) mg in 1000 ml of 5% glucose, for slow infusion capable of maintaining adequate blood pressure.

Atelectasis

In acute pulmonary atelectasis the main symptomatology consists of fever, dyspnea, cyanosis, tachycardia, some sort of chest pain, wheezing, cough, restricted chest expansion on respiration, and narrowing of the intercostal spaces. Extensive atelectasis may cause shock among elderly patients, but usually of short duration. X-ray findings show displacement of the mediastinum and "ground-glass" density of the collapsed lung. The disease has to be differentiated from pneumonia, or from pulmonary infarction.

Treatment should be carried out in the hospital, preferably by a specialized team. Shock will be treated as needed.

Septic Shock

Usually shock is prone to occur in the course of severe infective diseases, but it will also happen in milder forms when frail older people are involved. To the particular symptoms of the causative disease, at times those of *peripheral vasodilation* are added. The resulting hypotension brings on a very weak and rapid pulse, cadaveric pale face, sweating, superficial respirations with anoxia, hyposthenia, apathy, immobility, or restlessness, and may lead to disrupted consciousness from septic shock. The most frequent causes of this reaction are listed below.

Severe neutropenia in cancer, with or without chemotherapy.

Infections of the genitourinary tract or following urologic procedures.

Shock to the upper respiratory tract in tracheostomy, or the use of endotracheal tubes or respirators with aerosol.

Reaction following any surgical procedure, even of a very minor nature (such as the placement of catheters).

Anaerobic infections affecting the skin (necrotizing cellulitis), the brain (abscess, empyema), or the lungs (aspiration pneumonia, lung abscess), and septicemia.

Viral infections causing severe reactions, such as influenza, hemorrhagic dengue, yellow fever, rickettsioses.

Bacterial infections when there are poor defenses or great toxicity, particularly those affecting the central nervous system.

In most instances there will be a previous diagnosis of the causative disease, and probably such a disease will be under treatment. The occurrence of shock will indicate that either the personal defenses or the treatment itself is poor. Under the circumstances, more aggressive treatment will be started immediately; and a recheck of specific antibiotherapy will be requested from the laboratory, in order to proceed adequately. Usually, very large amounts of antibiotics will be needed in these cases. In addition to the specific anti-infective therapy, the treatment for shock will be carried out in all its details, paying special attention to the maintenance of good organ perfusion by giving adequate amounts of blood, plasma, or other suitable solutions. Most patients will also need to reinforce heart function with isoproterenol or dopamine; but it will be wise not to give vasoconstrictors (such as levarterenol), which may hamper perfusion. The electrolyte balance will be kept within appropriate levels at all times.

Blood for transfusion; give at a reasonable rate for prompt effect.

Calcium gluconate, 10% solution; give 10 ml for each liter of blood, slowly injected into the vein; as a good addition when blood is given.

Dopamine hydrochloride, 200 mg ampoules diluted in 500 ml of 5% dextrose in saline, supplying a concentration of $400\,\mu$g of dopamine in each ml; give 2 to $5\,\mu$g for each kilo of body weight to start, and then increasing gradually to a maximum of 30 to $40\,\mu$g for each kilo of body weight every minute, or as needed and tolerated.

Electrolyte solutions, as needed.

Influenza

Shock is a frequent outcome of influenza whenever fever and toxemia, or either one, is severe, or as a complication if pneumonia appears, or when the patient is old or debilitated. Prostration is marked, and all the usual symptoms are intense, as noted by the physician during the patient's lucid intervals. These symptoms are: sore throat, cough, headache, generalized pains, and extreme weakness. The face is frequently flushed, the eyes are congested, and the gastrointestinal functions are disturbed. Most cases with shock may also have pneumonia, which will be suspected if the fever does not subside in 4 or 5 days, or reappears following a frank remission. An accurate diagnosis of influenza depends on isolation of the causative virus by hemagglutination or complement fixation, which will differentiate the several para-influenza varieties, as well as some other organism possibly implicated. Leukopenia is the rule for pure influenza; leukocytosis may be noted when there are other infectious complications. Weakness, when prolonged after subsidence of the clinical picture, will confirm the diagnosis of influenza because it is usually more marked than the expected weakness most older persons experience after any debilitating disease.

Immunization against influenza should be done for all patients over 65 years of age before the usual epidemic season starts, in November. The Guillain Barré syndrome, affecting very few recipients, should not preclude the practice of immunization, particularly if the patient is feeble and advanced in years.

Also, anticipate complications when treating influenza, and watch very carefully for the development of a possible pneumonia, often present in severe cases. The rest of the treatment of the influenza is purely symptomatic, while the treatment of shock follows the regular schedule.

Pneumonia

Shock may occur with the sudden onset of pneumonia among the aged. Shock in pneumonia may also follow a few days of vague malaise and a mild febricula. The disease itself may start with a shaking chill and stabbing pain in the affected side of the chest. The pain is increased by movements or effort, and referred to the shoulder, the flank, or the abdomen; to avoid it the patient tries to lie on the affected side to restrain movements. There may also be noted abdominal distention, jaundice, symptoms similar to appendicitis or cholecystitis, painful tachypnea, tachycardia, delirium, convulsions, and cough. Sputa arc usually characteristic, but at times difficult to expel. If obtainable, useful information can result from culture and sensitivity tests. Physical examination reveals râles, impaired resonance, disturbed breath sounds, tubal respiration, pleural friction rub, tachycardia, cyanosis, and, finally, the characteristic X-ray picture. In short, the disease will be suspected in patients with fever, chest pain, cough, sputum, weakness or delirium, and auscultatory signs of consolidation.

Pneumococcal pneumonia shows a particular bloody sputum at the start, which soon becomes the characteristic rusty sputum, to end in a yellowish mucopurulent excretion during resolution. Sputum cultures and bacterial cultures make the diagnosis and indicate the treatment.

Hemophilus influenzae pneumonia is relatively rare among the elderly. The clinical signs are the common symptoms of pneumonia, but cyanosis is more marked, and the sputum is of an apple-green color and very tenacious. Laboratory reports will disclose the causative organism.

Viral pneumonia is a frequent disease, due to influenza and many other similar viruses. In most instances it results in a relatively mild infection, but it may be very serious (some influenza strains). Pneumonic symptoms are not characteristic, ranging from those of a common cold to severe respiratory insufficiency, in many instances resembling a bronchopneumonia, with auscultatory and X-ray signs noted only in a few restricted areas of the lung. The sputum is mucopurulent, at times with some blood. Serologic tests may help the diagnosis.

Streptococcal and staphylococcal pneumonias are usually due to complication of a previous disease, as influenza or pharyngitis, the streptococcal type representing a very severe disease among the elderly. Symptoms are always marked, the pharynx is inflamed and the tonsils are covered with exudate, and patients are severely ill. The sputum is abundant and of a salmon color. Diagnosis is made by laboratory means.

Other forms of pneumonia may be seen. In *Klebsiella pneumonia* the start may be more gradual; but, once established, the disease itself appears almost fulminant. The sputum is viscid and cherry red in color, and consolidation rapidly spreads from lobe to lobe. In *fungal pneumonia* the attack may appear in the classical form or as a chronic respiratory process. In *rickettsial pneumonia* there is no typical clinical picture, nor is there one in *mycoplasmal pneumonia.*

Most important, in *aspiration pneumonia* there is the history of accidental passage of a foreign body into the larynx and trachea, as in anesthesia, oily medications, acute alcoholism, epilepsy, profuse vomiting, mental impairment, or simply the inattention of old age.

Other pneumonic entities are diagnosed by laboratory means (*Pneumocystis carinii, tularemia,* etc.).

Treatment is essentially the same for all types of pneumonia and for shock, differing only in its etiological aspect. Patients will be confined to bed, with good hydration, comfortable feeding, oxygen administration, analgesics for pain (codeine preferred because it can also control coughing), and the basic treatment in each instance.

> Codeine, 30 mg, by mouth, every 4 to 6 hours; a little more if needed and tolerated.
>
> Acetylsalicylic acid, 300 to 600 mg, in tablets, every 4 hours, preferably with meals.
>
> *Aspiration pneumonia:* apply endotracheal tube or bronchoscope for aspiration of foreign material to wash the affected parts; give

cortisone, particularly if there is suspicion of aspiration of gastric juice (vomiting); give oxygen and watch for septic complication.

Pneumococcal pneumonia: penicillin, 300,000 units, by intramuscular injection, every 12 hours (intravenously, if so needed).

H. influenzae pneumonia: ampicillin, 1000 mg, by intravenous injection, every 4 to 6 hours (can be also given by mouth).

Viral pneumonia: symptomatic treatment.

Streptococcal and staphylococcal pneumonia: oxacillin, 2000 mg, by intramuscular injection, every 4 to 6 hours; either alone or with cephalothin, same schedule (for streptococcal, penicillin may accomplish the same results).

Klebsiella pneumonia: check sensitivity, but start with cephalothin, 8000 to 12,000 mg in 24 hours, and gentamycin, 1 mg for each kilo of body weight, every 8 hours (other antibiotics may work as well, i.e., tetracyclines, etc.).

Fungal pneumonia: amphotericin B for most forms—initial dose of 0.25 mg for each kilo of body weight in 24 hours, to be given by intravenous infusion lasting from 2 to 6 hours; dosage increased every few days by 0.25 mg for each kilo of body weight in 24 hours until it reaches 1 mg; always dissolved in 5% dextrose. *Actinomyces* infection responds to penicillin; and *Nocardia,* to sulfadiazine.

Rickettsial pneumonia (usually Q fever): treat with a tetracycline.

P. carinii pneumonia: give pentamidine isethionate, 4 mg per kilo in 24 hours, by intramuscular injection.

Mycoplasmal pneumonia: give a tetracycline or erythromycin.

Tularemic pneumonia: treat with streptomycin, and add a tetracycline if there is no improvement.

Legionnaires' Disease

Some patients with this disease (recently discovered in Philadelphia) will go into shock and even die after a few days with an acute flu- or pneumonia-like syndrome with elevated fever, chills, chest pain, and cough. Most cases do not show such a dramatic outcome. Diagnosis is assumed when the disease affects patients over 50 years of age (though younger patients may be affected), generally in small epidemics of only a few cases. X-ray examination may reveal lung or pleural involvement, with more or less marked consolidation or signs of pleuritis. In some instances, and in most recent times, the bacterium-like causative organism has been isolated from pleural fluid cultures; otherwise, no causative germ is found.

Treatment is palliative and symptomatic; but some good effects have been noted with the use of erythromycin.

> Erythromycin, 250 or 500 mg tablets; 250 mg every 6 hours, or 500 mg every 12 hours; but larger doses will be given in more severe cases.

Septicemia (Bacteremia)

A state of shock may occur when bacteria invade the circulating blood causing weakness or a confusional state; or fever of the hectic (septic) type, with chills, at least at the onset, and headache, or skin rashes, often purpuric or petechial. Bacteremia may spread from a known infected area, and is suspected when from such an infection there is no improvement in due time, or if, instead, there is an exacerbation of septic symptoms. The site of origin may be unknown (cryptogenic bacteremia), but most commonly bacteremia follows: erysipelas (a well-delineated red area with swollen borders, located mainly around the mouth or the eyes, but also on limbs or trunk), tonsillitis, otitis, urinary sepsis, or tooth abscess. In turn, bacteremia may produce new focal sites of infection, particularly in the heart. Check continuously for early detection of endocarditis and central nervous system manifestations, mainly meningitis. Also monitor the vascular system (thrombophlebitis), lungs (abscess, pneumonia, infarct), and skeletal system (osteomyelitis). Cultures will establish the diagnosis.

Treatment depends on the offending infective organism and its sensitivity to *antibiotics,* which will be administered accordingly. Control of the infection will result in the control of all secondary symptoms. Shock will be treated as usual.

Appendicitis

Regularly, elderly persons will start an appendicular attack with mild symptomatology, or with confusion and lethargy; but they may soon become unconscious, an occurrence that will necessitate the physician's help. Think of the common clinical pattern with an acute colicky pain, first noted in the epigastric area but aggravated by pressure over the right iliac fossa, where it is located thereafter. The skin of that area is hypersensitive; and the local muscles tend to be rigid. Fever rises slowly; there are tachycardia and leukocytosis. The appendicular points (McBurney, etc.) are very sensitive, and may provoke a rebound pain when pressure is exerted over a distant point (left iliac fossa) and suddenly released. A few gastrointestinal symptoms may be present, as nausea, vomiting, anorexia, or constipation. According to the anatomical location of the appendix, symptoms may vary:

if retrocecal or retroperitoneal, muscle rigidity will be less marked; if in the pelvis, tenderness will be elicited almost only by rectal or vaginal examination. The location of the pain, the increasing leukocytosis, and moderate fever are good diagnostic signs.

Ask for surgical advice, since a good approach is to remove the appendix at the earliest possible time. Keep the patient in bed, combat shock, maintain continuous suction (nasogastric tube), work for good hydration and electrolyte balance, and use antibiotics (specific, if known, and at a high dosage). Meperidine or codeine will help to control severe pain (not to postpone surgery!).

> Chloramphenicol, 100 mg per kilo of body weight in 24 hours, in divided doses, every 6 hours (dosage to be decreased and discontinued as soon as possible), either by mouth or intravenously.

> Ampicillin, 500 mg, every 4 to 6 hours; intravenously or intramuscularly; may use oral route afterward.

> Cephalothin, 500 mg to 1 g, every 6 hours; by intravenous injection (intramuscular route is painful, but may be used).

> Meperidine, 100 mg, by intramuscular injection, repeated as needed and tolerated.

> Codeine, 60 mg, by subcutaneous injection, every 4 to 6 hours.

Typhoid Fever

Shock will be present not only in cases complicated with hemorrhage or perforation, but in severe infections and those presenting neurological symptoms of a meningitic character. The disease usually starts gradually; symptoms worsen daily until a peak is reached the second week; then they recede gradually during the third week. The fever rises from 38°C (100°F) to about 39.5°C (103°F) or above; there are malaise, headache, and other pains, gastrointestinal discomfort, and the characteristic stupor. A large number of patients will show bradycardia (as related to temperature) with a dicrotic pulse. At the beginning there may be constipation or diarrhea; but as the disease progresses, there is always an intense diarrhea ("pea-soup"). The well-known rose spots appear at about the end of the first stage of the disease (seventh to tenth day), on abdomen and chest. Small macules of a pink color appear, which fade on pressure. Unfortunately, a large number of patients will fail to show this rash. Coincident with the rash splenomegaly develops. Pain is not always present in typhoid fever, but it may reach severe intensity. Some patients may suffer pain suggesting peritonitis, which is actually due to acidosis. And in cases of typhic perforation of the intestines, pain is really alarming. The laboratory will reveal leukopenia, but leukocytosis in complicated cases. Also diagnostic are *Salmonella typhosa* in the blood during the first week or in feces or urine at the end of the third week, and the agglutination reaction (Widal) starting during the second week. In all cases watch for the onset of intestinal hemorrhage, signaled by a fall of fever, rapid pulse, hypotension, and sweating; and for intestinal perforation, suggested by abrupt onset of abdominal pain and other symptoms, as with hemorrhage. In both instances shock may occur. Also watch for the atypical clinical picture with predominantly respiratory symtoms (pneumotyphus), urinary symptoms, resembling nephritis, or neurological symptoms, with psychotic or meningitis-like syndromes.

Shock is to be treated symptomatically whenever present. Patients have to be isolated and kept in bed, with the urine and feces well-disinfected; they are kept thoroughly clean, with dehydration avoided and nutrition and electrolyte balance well-maintained. Exercise the legs to avoid thrombosis. In cases of severe constipation use only mild laxatives; for diarrhea, use paregoric or other antidiarrheal drugs. Transfusions may be needed. Corticoids will be given to the severely ill patient, particularly one in stupor. The infection will be treated first with chloramphenicol, and ampicillin will be used as a second choice. Start antibiotics as soon as possible, to improve the prognosis.

Lactic Acidosis

This is only a form of metabolic acidosis with hyperlactacidemia, usually secondary to vascular collapse or hypoxia in cases of diabetes mellitus, heart insufficiency, acute infections, diseases of the lungs or the liver compromising their functions, or patients receiving certain medications (phenformin). There will be shocklike symptoms, such as hypotension, and a somewhat characteristic *hyperventilation*. The laboratory will give a positive diagnosis, with low pH and low bicarbonate concentration in blood; and the revealing hyperlactacidemia, over 7 mmol in each liter of blood. Ask the laboratory for advice about collection of blood samples.

The regular treatment for shock will emphasize the use of alkalinizing solutions to bring the pH to 7.2 or more in as short a time as possible. Give sodium bicarbonate solution, as needed and tolerated, even to doses of some 2000 mEq in 24 hours, that is, about 12 liters in total. Hemodialysis has also been advised, particularly when phenformin is involved.

Anaphylactic Shock

Anaphylactic shock consists of a very impressive and rapid reaction of the body occurring seconds or minutes after the administration of a foreign protein, any of the known allergenic drugs (curative or for diagnosis), or certain insect stings. Patients become apprehensive, agitated, cyanotic, with rapid pulse; complain of a choking sensation, throbbing in the ears, paresthesias, and itching; start sneezing, coughing, and wheezing; and are incontinent. Three main syndromes may appear: vascular collapse, laryngeal edema, or bronchospasm, leading to shock. Pupils are dilated, fever rises, loss of consciousness and convulsions occur, and the patient may die, all this happening in a lapse of 5 to 10 minutes. Cyanosis and tachycardia are the main guidepoints for an early diagnosis.

Sensitizing substances should not be given to patients presenting other allergies, but if they are necessary, try to desensitize the patient first, and be ready for an emergency treatment, including the use of emergency resuscitation equipment. With *no delay,* as soon as the first symptoms appear, give epinephrine. Patients will be recumbent and warm, with a patent airway. Use an endotracheal tube or perform a tracheostomy, if needed. Positive or regular oxygen administration will follow, as well as the administration of an antihistaminic, if advisable. To avoid or to shorten prolonged reactions use corticoids, though their value is not yet proved. Intravenous administration of saline or a colloid plasma expander, such as plasma protein fraction 5% solution or dextran 6%, will help to restore venous pressure, and indirectly arterial pressure. Vasopressor drugs, such as metaraminol or levarterenol, may be given by intravenous injection; aminophyllin may be of some value.

> Epinephrine, 1:1000 solution; give 1 ml, by intramuscular injection, immediately following appearance of symptoms.

> Epinephrine, 1:1000 solution; give 0.5 ml in 10 ml saline infusion, slowly by vein, starting rapidly if symptoms do not subside after the first 1-ml injection.

> Diphenylhydramine hydrochloride, 5 to 20 mg, in aqueous solution; give intravenously.

> Hydrocortisone, 200 mg, in aqueous solution, by intravenous injection, to be repeated in 4 hours, if needed; or:

> Dexamethasone, 8 mg, in aqueous solution, by intravenous injection, to be repeated in 4 hours, if so needed; or:

> Prednisolone, 50 or 100 mg, in water or saline, by intravenous injection, over a period of 30 seconds.

CARDIOGENIC SHOCK

General Considerations and Diagnosis

This is a variety of regular shock, as presented in the above section. In older books it was called collapse, as it is still being called in other languages, at least by some authors. As that word implies, it consists of a sudden, usually prolonged weakening of heart function, noted mainly by a decreased blood pressure, almost imperceptible pulse, shallow respiration, sweating, pallor, and partial unconsciousness, which may be, instead, some sort of confusion or delirium. Its main difference from regular shock is its lesser intensity of nervous involvement, together with the more severe implications when it is related to a previous important heart disease, such as myocardial infarction, tamponade, or late stages of heart failure.

Cardiogenic shock may be due to the following causes:

Disorders of the heart muscle, as in myocardial infarction, fibrillation, myocarditis, or heart failure.

Disorders extrinsic to the heart, as in terminal cases of congestive heart failure, cardiac tamponade, or pulmonary edema.

Also to be considered are post-myocardial infarct, severe stages of valvular disease, and heart failure in pneumonia, peritonitis, typhoid fever, intoxication (mainly cocaine and sulfas), rapid decompression, Addison's disease, and as a natural reaction to hemorrhages and pain.

General Treatment for Cardiogenic Shock

See the above section on "Shock," since the essentials of treatment are the same for both types.

Heart Failure

Actually, heart failure is the cornerstone of cardiogenic shock, an accident that may happen to a patient with a previously normal heart as well as to one with an established congestive heart failure. The outstanding symptomatology consists of marked arterial hypotension and extremely weak, almost imperceptible, rapid radial pulse; pale, moist and cool skin; and other evidence of low cardiac output. Patients with a previous congestive heart failure will also show exertional dyspnea, ankle edema, persistent asthenia, lung congestion and enlarged and tender liver, later ascites and cyanosis, and finally signs of cerebral impairment. Frequent causes of heart failure are listed below.

Myocardial infarction, with sharp retrosternal pain.

Fibrillation, with rapid irregular pulse.

Myocarditis, with fever, dyspnea, tachycardia, faint first heart sound, changing systolic murmurs, and EKG changes.

Acute pericarditis, with fast, shallow respirations, nonproductive cough, anxiety, asthenia, and the characteristic pericardial friction rub.

Valvular diseases, with the characteristic murmurs and accompanying symptomatology.

Cardiac tamponade, with a previous penetrating wound or established heart disease, followed by increased diastolic blood pressure, narrowed pulse pressure, increased venous blood pressure, and distant heart sounds.

Pulmonary edema, with more or less distressing cough, wheezing, tachypneic dyspnea, anxiety with or without chest oppression, and râles starting at the bases and ascending thereafter.

Tachycardia, with more than 100 heart beats a minute, which will very easily cause heart failure in older, debilitated patients.

Premature contractions or *escape beats,* which, when they become numerous and overwhelming, will cause heart failure in the old and feeble.

Complete heart block, with bradycardia and EKG changes.

Cardiac arrest, with sudden loss of consciousness, apnea, and lack of heart beats (no auscultatory sounds, no pulse).

Bacterial endocarditis, with evidence of a previous infective disease, secondary valvulopathy, skin hemorrhages (petechiae), and other symptoms of bacteremia.

Septic shock, with evidence of a previous infective disease plus symptoms of peripheral vasodilation (hypotension, weak pulse).

Hemolytic anemia, which in a crisis may lead to cardiogenic shock.

Dissecting aortic aneurism, with symptoms more or less similar to those of myocardial infarction and lower blood pressure in the legs than in the arms.

Pulmonary infarction, with sudden side pain, dyspnea, and cough.

The first steps in treatment will be those needed to take care of shock, with emphasis on the use of cardiotonics (digitalis) or vasodilators (sodium nitroprusside), as appears more advisable; use caution in overloading the patient with intravenous solutions.

Myocardial Infarction

It is not rare, after 60 years of age, to start a myocardial infarction either without symptoms or with an impressive cardiogenic shock which may strike during bed rest or after exertion. The majority of patients complain of a sudden retrosternal discomfort, or oppression. Usually, there is a very severe seizure, together with apprehension and fear. The pain may be referred to the neck, shoulder, or mandible instead of the classical retrosternal location. Other symptoms are: dyspnea, sweating, weakness, symptoms of congestive heart failure, edema or hepatomegalia, a fall in blood pressure (more noticeable with a previous hypertension), weak rapid pulse or, at times, a slow pulse at the beginning, and possibly arrhythmias. Shock may occur after the disease has been definitely established (post-myocardial infarction shock). The diagnosis is based on the characteristic pain, the electrocardiographic finding of initial elevation of the S-T segment and later inversion of the T wave, and the laboratory reports of leukocytosis and elevation of SGOT and LDH. Pain in angina is as in infarction, differentiated in that it lasts only a few minutes to less than 1 hour, with rapid relief obtainable on administration of nitroglycerin or amyl nitrate; there is little or no pain relief in infarction.

Patients are better referred to a cardiologist in a coronary unit. Complete rest is needed, and may be achieved by narcotic analgesics.

An important drop in blood pressure calls for the administration of pressor drugs by carefully monitored intravenous infusion:

> Isoproterenol hydrochloride, 1:200 solution (5 mg for each ml); add up to 10 mg (better lesser amounts) to 500 ml of 5% glucose, for intravenous infusion.

Anticoagulants can be used to begin treatment: heparin and warfarin, to continue with the latter, if anticoagulants are later chosen; and oxygen may also be used.

> Heparin (aqueous sodium), 7000 to 12,000 units, to start by intravenous or subcutaneous injection; to be followed by 5000 to 9000 units, every 4 hours, until warfarin starts to work (check the clotting time).

> Warfarin, 30 to 40 mg, by mouth, once the first day; 10 to 20 mg, once the second day; thereafter, 5 to 10 mg (more or less, as needed), every day (check the prothrombin time).

Bradycardia below 60 beats a minute requires atropine, larger doses if rate is slower; tachycardia requires lidocaine, and quinidine when the former is discontinued or reduced in amount. Quinidine is also given for auricular flutter, fibrillation, and premature beats. Digoxin may be used for flutter, fibrillation, and tachycardia. If needed, to quiet the patient, tranquilizers should also be given. To complement treatment, give only a liquid diet the first few days; a bland diet will follow; resume normal activity at a slow pace—and avoid invalidism!

> Morphine, 10 to 15 mg by subcutaneous injection, or 5 to 10 mg intravenously, if needed; repeat in 30 minutes. When necessary, watch for induced bradycardia or hypotension.

Meperidine, 50 mg by intravenous injection, or 100 mg subcutaneously; repeat in 30 minutes, if needed.

Atropine, 0.5 up to 1 mg, by intravenous injection.

Lidocaine, 100 mg in 5 ml, to inject intravenously 2.5 to 5 ml; followed by an intravenous infusion, at a rate of 1, 2, or 4 mg per minute.

Quinidine, 200 mg tablets; give 4 to 6 tablets a day, in three or four installments.

Digoxin, started by intravenous injection (0.75 to 1.25 mg in divided doses, during a 30-minute period), to be followed by quinidine by mouth.

Phenobarbital, up to 30 mg, every 6 hours, by mouth.

Diazepam, 5 to 10 mg, in tablets, one every 8 hours.

Acute Pericarditis

Shock will occur whenever tachypnea, with shallow respirations (particularly if the pleura is also involved), nonproductive cough, anxiety, and weakness are intense enough, or when pericardial effusion is sufficient to cause cardiac tamponade. Fever and chills are usual, but are not always present. Pain (the main symptom) is felt substernally or in the precordial area, radiating to the shoulders or neck; it is more or less intense, increased by some positions, as recumbent or prone, and relieved by others, as leaning forward or sitting; it is also increased by movements, as cough or respiration. At times, it is mistaken for myocardial infarction because of its duration. On auscultation, the characteristic friction rub is heard during the complete cardiac cycle (except, at times, only with the first or second sounds). Pain and friction rub will almost give the diagnosis, confirmed by electrocardiographic findings of elevated S-T and flattened or inverted T waves, and laboratory reports of leukocytosis and elevated erythrosedimentation rate.

With effusion (more than 250 ml), the X-ray findings will show an enlarged heart; also the auscultation sounds will change, diminishing or even disappearing. Large effusions may induce cardiac tamponade: the veins of the neck are notably distended, dyspnea appears or increases, pulse amplitude decreases during inspiration, pulse pressure narrows, and after some time there is enlargement of the liver, and ascites.

Treat the causative disease appropriately, if it is known (infectious disease, rheumatic fever, and the like). Analgesics are given for pain, barbiturates, for anxiety; corticoids may help (not only in rheumatic fever, but for effusions, pain, and fever). Pericardiocentesis may be life-saving when the pressure of the effusion becomes dangerous. The help of a cardiologist is necessary, since pericardiocentesis will be better performed by a specialist in a well-equipped hospital.

Codeine, 60 mg, by injection or by mouth, repeated every 4 to 6 hours, as needed.

Phenobarbital, 30 mg, by mouth, every 4 to 6 hours.

Prednisolone, to 60 mg a day, in divided doses, by mouth, for 3 to 5 days; thereafter, decrease and discontinue the drug gradually, as is feasible.

In an emergency, for pericardiocentesis, infiltrate with procaine 2% solution after thorough sterilization of the area; sit the patient upright on a chair; use a 16- or 18-gauge needle with a short bevel and fitting stylet (the needle connected to rubber tubing to prevent excessive movement and also to a well-grounded electrocardiograph); puncture 1 cm within cardiac dullness, pushing slowly inward and slightly upward; withdraw liquid slowly and avoid touching the myocardium, as warned by the EKG machine (sudden elevation of ST5).

Myocarditis

This disease can be almost symptomless (mild forms), usually associated with a previous, causative disease. More severe, acute cases will show dyspnea, together with fever, weakness leading to a syncopal state, chest pain, and final shock. Physical findings include: faint heart sounds, low systolic blood pressure, tachycardia, faint first heart sound, systolic murmurs which may change from time to time, arrhythmias, and electrocardiographic changes, such as conduction defects, abnormal T waves, low QRS, and so on.

When shock occurs, treat it vigorously. Also, take care of the previous disease; but the general therapy will only be supportive, for cardiac failure and anemia. Corticoids are beneficial during the first stages of the disease, particularly in the case of collagen diseases.

Valvular Diseases

These diseases are more frequent among younger people than among the elderly. Symptoms and treatment are similar in either instance, the diseases being mainly characterized by the corresponding murmur:

Mitral stenosis: presystolic murmur followed by a mid-diastolic rumble accompanied by thrill or tapping noted on palpating the apex. The face is usually flushed. Blood pressure is normal, but the pulse is feeble. Not rarely fibrillation will accompany mitral stenosis. Radiologic studies will show a straight left heart border; and the EKG, broad P waves.

Mitral insufficiency: murmur heard during the whole systole and spreading toward the left axilla. At the apex forceful beats will be noted on inspection, and a thrill will also be evident. Atrial fibrillation may be present. X-ray inspection will show an enlarged left ventricle; also broad or notched P waves will be seen in the electrocardiogram.

Tricuspid stenosis: presystolic murmur heard at the upper left border of the heart, better heard during inspiration. Some patients are jaundiced, and may show liver pulsations. X-ray shows enlarged right atrium; and there are tall peaked waves in the electrocardiogram.

Tricuspid insufficiency: a murmur heard at the upper left border of the heart; there is hepatomegaly, and enlarged right heart.

Aortic stenosis: systolic murmur heard at the upper right border of the heart, spreading toward both the clavicle and the neck on the right. A thrill may be palpated at the site of the murmur. There may be an elevated diastolic blood pressure. There is radiologic and electrocardiographic evidence of left ventricular hypertrophy.

Aortic insufficiency: diastolic murmur heard at the upper right border of the heart, but also at the apex and the right mid-border. Patients are pale, the pulse is strong (water-hammer pulse), and there are also capillary pulsations noted. Blood pressure shows low diastolic and moderately elevated systolic pressures. There is left ventricular hypertrophy noted in X-ray and EKG studies.

Pulmonic stenosis: systolic murmur heard at the upper left border of the heart.

Pulmonic insufficiency: diastolic murmur heard at the upper left border of the heart.

Not too many patients with valvular lesions reach advanced age; and these patients should be watched for the possibility of thrombotic episodes ending in a stroke. Many will develop atrial fibrillation, and then the possibility of pulmonary edema. Most patients with mitral lesions are female; and those with aortic lesions, male.

In case of stroke or shock, emergency treatment will be provided. For the treatment of the heart conditions, a radiologist and a surgeon will be consulted about the advisability of valvular correction.

Arrhythmias

Disruption of the normal cardiac rhythm is not a rarity in older people. Most healthy persons will tolerate most of these conditions with meager symptomatology, but only until the cerebral circulation is compromised, and shock is the consequence of severe lack of oxygen. A patient in shock may present a previously known cardiac arrhythmia, or this will be assumed when checking the pulse.

Bradycardia: heart beats below 60 a minute; a condition prone to cause loss of consciousness when it affects the elderly.

Tachycardia: heart beats over 100 a minute; prone to cause heart failure in weak hearts.

Atrial fibrillation: the pulse irregular in frequency and intensity; the diagnosis is made electrocardiographically; longstanding fibrillation may cause cerebral thrombosis.

Ventricular fibrillation: only diagnosed when monitoring the heart because in a very short time it will cause death.

Heart block: usually due to sclerosis or digitalis overdosage; shows bradycardia and dizziness or more conspicuous loss of consciousness.

The main therapeutic efforts will attempt reoxygenation of the central nervous system and other organs. Thereafter, each form of arrhythmia will be treated on an individual basis. (See other sections of this book for more details.)

Cardiac Tamponade

The diagnosis is based on the triad: increased venous blood pressure, increased diastolic pressure with narrowed pulse pressure, and distant heart sounds. There are distended neck veins (more evident during inspiratory movements), and, finally, edema, hepatomegaly, and ascites. Other symptoms of shock are also present. It follows a penetrating wound of the heart or is secondary to other heart disease.

As soon as the diagnosis is made, the patient will receive an injection of morphine or meperidine, and a pericardiocentesis will be carried out for the slow removal of blood. The site for puncturing the pericardium (avoid touching the ventricle!) is at the level of the 5th or 6th left interspace, 1 cm inside the area of cardiac dullness or 7 to 8 cm to the left of the corresponding sternal line, the needle going inward and slightly upward, with frequent checking for withdrawal of liquid. Also, access may be gained from between the xiphoid and the left sternal margin, inserting the needle directed upward at a 30° angle, pointing to the midline. From either side, the pericardium is reached at a distance of about 3 to 5 cm; or, more rarely, at a distance of about 7 to 8 cm, when the first point of entrance is used. If things are done properly (which is not always possible, particularly in rural areas), the needle should be connected to a well-grounded electrocardiograph (for warning against entering the myocardium); the patient will be well-grounded, too (to avoid inducing fibrillation). A rubber tube between the needle and the syringe will facilitate the procedure.

Morphine, 10 to 15 mg, subcutaneously.

Meperidine, 100 mg, by intramuscular injection.

Aortitis and Aortic Aneurism

Pain referred to the aorta is very similar to anginal pain; it may follow effort, emotion, or a heavy meal, but is less severe than the pure anginal attack. Some believe that aortalgia will occur when there is an obstacle to the blood flow through the coronary arteries (true anginal pain). In dissecting aortic aneurism, the clinical picture is similar to that of myocardial infarction, with pain and shock; a lowered blood pressure in the legs, to levels equal to or lower than that in the arms, occurs in this form of aneurism (also in coarctation of the aorta, aortic embolism, and so forth). X-ray examinations will support the diagnosis in many cases.

Treat shock as needed. If the coronary arteries are affected, treatment will be that of angina pectoris (q.v.). Patients with dissecting aortic aneurism will experience pain; then the final treatment is surgical, no matter that the results of the procedure are in doubt. If there is hypertension, propranolol must be given.

Propranolol, 20 mg, by mouth, every 6 hours; or 1 to 2 mg by the intramuscular route, every 6 hours.

Bacterial Endocarditis

Older people may have afebrile periods, but fever, chills, and other toxic symptoms are usually present. Some patients will tell about a previous heart disease (rheumatic endocarditis, atherosclerosis), but more frequently of an acute infection, surgery, or drug addiction. Patients usually suffer varied embolic phenomena; and previous heart murmurs change in nature, particularly with the acutely ill. If disease is due to an infection, shock will be present in many of these instances. Symptoms worsen, and a complicating meningitis is not rare. A good diagnostic hint is given by the valvular involvement and embolic phenomena (petecchiae) occurring during the course of any infective disease. Blood culture may disclose the causative organism and its sensitivity to antibiotics (do at least two or three cultures!). The clinical picture is that of *septicemia* (bacteremia) with *superimposed cardiac symptoms,* particularly murmurs, louder second sound of the pulmonic valve, and retrosternal pains.

Treat shock (see previous discussion on septic shock) and bacteremia. Penicillin is the antibiotic of choice, and will be given whenever possible, including to patients sensitive to it if desensitization can be successfully carried out.

Hemolytic Anemia (Crisis)

There is usually an abrupt onset with fever, chills, malaise, nausea, vomiting, and, at times, pain in the back or abdomen. Unusually severe cases may lead to prostration or shock with acute renal failure. Most patients are pale and jaundiced, showing tachycardia and weakness. Splenomegaly and dark (black or red) urine will be present. The abrupt febrile onset will give the clincial impression of the start of an infective disease, and if pains are severe, of a surgical condition. Marked paleness and jaundice will suggest anemia and will call for laboratory investigation of the blood. It will be found profoundly anemic with serum tinted pink, brown, or yellow, and red cells of normal size, shape, and coloring. The urine and feces show products of destruction of red blood cells, and the urine may be scanty.

Try to find the causative hemolyzing agent and eliminate it. Give sodium bicarbonate or lactate to alkalinize the urine; give blood transfusion to combat anemia (watch for increased hemolysis when autoantibodies are present), and treat for shock.

Arterial Hypotension

Patients with low blood pressure at times may show asthenia, dizziness, cyanosis and coolness of extremities, bradycardia, and occipital headache. Sudden efforts or change of position (orthostatic hypotension) may cause a syncopal accident or frank shock. Hypotension does not constitute a disease; it accompanies a number of medical conditions and is one of the principal factors of shock. A list of provoking diseases follows.

Hypoadrenalism: with the characteristic profound asthenia and hyperpigmentation.

Cachexia hypophysaria: with marked loss of weight, great asthenia, and other evidence of decreased endocrine function; Simmon's or Sheehan's disease (the latter following parturition).

Cancer: when reaching depauperating stages.

Chronic alcoholism: usually accompanied by polyneuritis.

Liver diseases: most of them will cause hypotension, particularly hepatic cirrhosis.

Debilitating diseases: any acute or, more frequently, chronic disease may reach a devastating stage in which hypotension is an important symptom. Include here most acute infections.

Anaphylactic shock: with a rapidly developing shock after the injection or ingestion of the offending substance.

Treat shock as usual, with particular emphasis on hypertensive drugs. For the chronic treatment of the condition, check each causative disease, and try fludrocortisone. For anaphylactic shock give epinephrine without delay!

Dopamine hydrochloride, 200 mg ampoules diluted in 500 mg of 5% dextrose in saline, thus having 400 μg in each ml, to start giving from 2 to 5 μg for each kilo of body weight every minute, and increasing gradually to a maximum of 30 or 40 μg for each kilo a minute, or as needed and tolerated.

Levarterenol (may be given together with dopamine), 4 to 6 mg added to 1000 ml of dextrose in water, to be infused in about 1 day.

Fludrocortisone acetate, 0.1 mg a day, by mouth.

Epinephrine, 1:1000 solution, 0.5 ml in 10 ml saline, by slow intravenous injection, or 1 ml by intramuscular injection.

Pulmonary Infarction

Symptoms of shock occur in the late stages of the disease; but elderly persons frequently go into shock immediately after the sudden onset of side pain, followed by dyspnea, cyanosis, and cough (with bloody sputum), symptoms resembling pneumonia, myocardial infarction, pleurisy, or pericarditis. On auscultation, râles, decreased pulmonary sounds, and increased second heart sound are noted. The diagnosis is suggested very strongly when venous thrombosis is present elsewhere in the body (more frequently in the legs). Small infarcted areas will show few symptoms. If an electrocardiogram is made (myocardial damage suspected), only signs of right ventricular strain will be found (cor pulmonale); but other signs are not uncommon (S-T depression, T inversion, and so on). It is to be noted that the location of pain may vary with the location of the pulmonary infarction; at the left lower lobe, the pain is precordial or retrosternal; pain may be referred to the shoulder, the abdomen, and so forth.

The first choice in the treatment of pulmonary infarction has to be given, in most cases, to morphine, or meperidine as an alternate.

Morphine, 5 mg, by intravenous injection; or 10 or 15 mg, by the subcutaneous route, to repeat as needed.

Give oxygen, digitalize if right-side heart failure occurs, and maintain adequate blood pressure with isoproterenol or metaraminol. Surgical embolectomy will be evaluated by a chest surgeon.

Metaraminol; add 100 mg to 1000 ml of 5% glucose, for slow infusion.

Isoproterenol, 2 (to 4) mg in 1000 ml of 5% glucose, for slow infusion capable of maintaining adequate blood pressure.

Anticoagulation is started immediately and continued for 3 to 6 weeks.

Pulmonary Edema

Cough is very frequently the first symptom, rapidly followed by dyspnea with wheezing, pallor with or without cyanosis, sweating, and finally a frothy pink sputum. Those with elevated blood pressure also show intense anxiety and a sensation of pressure in the chest. On auscultation râles are heard in the dependent areas of the lungs; and as the disease progresses, in upper segments. The diagnosis depends more on the clinical history than on X-ray studies: cough, tachypnea, râles, and frothy, bloody sputum developing in the course of a known previous disease (left ventricular failure, pulmonary embolism, cardiac arrhythmias, myocardial infarction, hypertension). It should not be mistaken for lung infarction, bronchopneumonia, or a severely acute asthmatic attack.

The basic treatment of pulmonary edema depends on the causative factor. Otherwise, the general rules for the treatment of shock will be followed. Place the patient in a semi-Fowler position, and give morphine (if there is no contraindication), oxygen (with antifoaming agents?), soft tourniquets to obstruct venous—not arterial!—return (to be rotated every 15 minutes and gradually removed when condition improves), diuretics, digitalis, and aminophylline. Venesection for the removal of about 500 ml of blood may be of good and prompt help, unless the patient is debilitated or anemic. In cases of marked hypertension, vasodilation with sodium nitroprusside may succeed in giving relief.

Morphine, 5 mg (rarely up to 10 mg), by intravenous injection.

Furosemide, 40 to 60 mg, intravenously.

Digitalis, as needed.

Aminophylline, 250 mg, by slow intravenous injection.

Bacteremia (Septicemia, Pyemia)

Bacteremia occurs following surgical manipulations (incisions, catheterization, and so on) or infective diseases, as primary abscesses in the skin, teeth, pharynx, adenoids, and sinuses; prostatitis, pyelitis, and phlebitis; subphrenic abscess, appendicitis, diverticulitis, and others; subacute bacterial endocarditis, puerperal fever, pneumonia, osteomyelitis, meningitis, and gonococcal infections. In each particular instance germs must be identified and their sensitivity to antibiotics established. (Blood cultures will be taken several times, preferably at the onset of a chill.) Among the elderly, the clinical picture may start with confusion, lethargy, or loss of consciousness, before the final complications due to relocation of the infection. There will be spiking fever (septic type) with chills, the character of the fever varying according to the initial source and the general condition of the patient (sustained, remittent, intermittent, irregular, or only febricular), and the chills being irregular in occurrence. There are: tachycardia, with a very weak pulse, thus prone to cause shock; distant heart sounds; nausea, frequently with vomiting; a mild splenomegaly; and any other symptoms, mostly belonging to the initial disease or the subsequent foci. In most instances, particularly in meningococcal septicemia, there are skin eruptions, mainly purpuric or petechial, but also papular, vesicular, or pustular, which are a very good help for diagnostic purposes. Finally, the secondary locations may result in endocarditis (check the heart daily, for murmurs or any other change), myocarditis, pericarditis, bronchopneumonia, pulmonary abscess, pleuritis, meningitis or meningoencephalitis, glomerulonephritis, or other localizations in the urinary system, the bones, or any other part of the body. Any secondary location will cause an increase of the general symptomatology.

Once the diagnosis of septicemia is established, general hospital care should be enforced, and the help of a specialist sought (surgeon, cardiologist, or otorhinolaryngologist). Whenever a purulent focus is found, it will be drained; and antibiotic therapy will be as specific and vigorous as possible. Avoid delay, in the interval while reports are awaited, by starting treatment with oxacillin or methicillin if a staphylococcal infection is suspected; or penicillin with gentamycin for possible gram-negative infections.

> Oxacillin, 1.5 g, by intravenous injection, four to six times a day, according to tolerance (nephrotic or anaphylactic reaction).

> Methicillin, 1.3 g, four times a day, by intravenous injection, freshly prepared in 5% dextrose to be given within 30 minutes (watch for marrow suppression or nephritis).

> Crystalline penicillin G, 1 million to 3 million units, every 3 hours, by intravenous injection (larger doses may be given if needed).

> Gentamycin, 5 mg per kilo of body weight in 24 hours, in four installments, by intramuscular injection (watch for 8th nerve injury—dizziness, etc.).

Influenza

Unconsciousness and delirium are not symptoms related to influenza, but present when fever or toxemia is severe, or the patient is old and debilitated. Prostration is marked, and all the usual symptoms are also intense, as noted by the physician or complained of by the patient during lucid intervals: sore throat, cough, headache, generalized pains and weakness. Weakness, when prolonged after subsidence of the general clinical picture, confirms the diagnosis, which may be proved by isolation of the virus from throat washings if that is done early in the disease. Positive serology tests are also obtained, later. Laboratory tests are the only possible way to differentiate influenza from para-influenza and other viral respiratory diseases.

Watch very carefully for complications, particularly pneumonia, almost always present in these severe cases. Keep patients in bed, maintain good nursing care, treat cough when it is bothersome, and use antipyretics and analgesics, if needed. For delirium give paraldehyde. For pneumonia use the appropriate antibiotic.

> Codeine, 30 or 60 mg, by mouth or by injection, repeated as needed and tolerated.

> Acetylsalicylic acid, 300 mg, plus codeine, 30 mg, to take by mouth every 4 or 6 hours, as needed and tolerated.

> Paraldehyde, 5 ml, by intramuscular injection, repeated after 30 minutes, when needed.

Pneumonia

Only in severe pneumonias will the patient reach the shock stage. This will happen only after the clinical picture has passed the initial symptoms of pharyngitis and bronchitis, and after the sudden elevation of temperature, the shaking chill, the stabbing pain in the side, and the painful cough accompanied by an almost characteristic sputum have occurred. Then the toxic phase may come. The sputum often is diagnostic:

> Rusty, in pneumococcal pneumonia.

> Tenacious and apple-green, in *H. influenzae* pneumonia.

> Mucopurulent, with some blood, in viral pneumonia.

> Abundant, salmon-colored in strepto- or staphylococcal pneumonia.

> Viscid, cherry-red, in *Klebsiella pneumoniae;* and bloody, in mycoplasmal pneumonia.

The physical examination shows: râles, suppressed breath sounds, tubal respiration, pleural friction rub, tachycardia, cyanosis, a characteristic X-ray picture with evidence of consolidation, and the finding of the causal bacteria in the sputum. Pneumonia will be suspected in persons with an acute chilly fever, chest pain, cough with sputum, and the auscultatory signs of consolidation. The later phase may include: delirium, convulsions, abdominal distress, jaundice, and finally shock.

Patients will be under good hospital care, particularly for the control of shock, with adequate hydration, electrolyte balance, oxygen, and the proper antibiotic:

Penicillin, for pneumococcal or streptococcal infection.

Ampicillin, for *H. influenzae* pneumonia.

Oxacillin, for staphylococcal or streptococcal infection.

Cephalothin and gentamycin for *Klebsiella* pneumonia.

Amphotericin B, for fungal infections.

Tetracycline, for rickettsial and mycoplasmal organisms.

Maintain a patent airway; give oxygen and intravenous fluids, phenobarbital for convulsions, and mannitol for elevated intracranial pressure.

Phenobarbital, 30 mg, every 6 hours.

Mannitol, 15% solution; give 1500 to 2000 ml, in 24 hours.

Peritonitis

Shock may follow a severe peritonitis or appear earlier in exceptionally toxic infections, in debilitated elderly persons or those suffering prolonged diseases. The clinical picture presents abdominal pain as the outstanding symptom. It is severe, diffuse, and unabating, increased by any sort of movement, thus forcing the patient to remain quiet and breathe shallowly, all this noted even in unconscious patients. The pain is acutely felt over the underlying epigastric, hepatic, appendicular, or other focus of the disease; and there are a marked rebound reaction and muscle guarding, nausea, vomiting, and at times diarrhea, high fever, chills, tachycardia, abdominal distention, hiccups, shoulder pain, and finally toxemia with dehydration and acidosis. Radiologic examination will show generalized dilation of the intestines, with gas and fluid. The laboratory will reveal leukocytosis and other evidence of infection, and possibly the identification of the infective microorganism.

Call a surgeon, to check and solve the source of infection. Put the patient on continuous gastric suction, with intravenous infusions for hydration and electrolyte balance, analgesics, and the specific antibiotic, if not known. Start immediately with a combination of penicillin and streptomycin, or with gentamycin or kanamycin, until antibiotic sensitivities are found.

Meperidine, 100 mg, by injection, repeated as needed and tolerated.

Gentamycin, 5 mg for each kilo of body weight in 24 hours, intramuscularly, in divided doses, every 6 hours.

Typhoid Fever

Typhoid patients may go into shock when severely ill, but when this happens, the diagnosis has usually been made. After a few days of what may look like an upper respiratory infection, as malaise, sore throat, nonproductive cough, or epistaxis, the symptomatology becomes gradually more and more severe: the fever rises steadily with bradycardia, headache, and abdominal distress until the appearance of the characteristic "pea-soup" diarrhea, splenomegaly, and increasing stupor, which may end in shock, and the well-known rose spots on the trunk, which clear under pressure. The final diagnosis depends on blood cultures (first week), stool cultures (third week), and the Widal reaction (second week).

When shock is present, efforts will be made to control it, following the usual pattern, and to give—if not yet given—the adequate antibiotic. The first choice is ampicillin or chloramphenicol. Put patients in bed, disinfect all excretions, give good nutrition and hydration, and control diarrhea. Give corticoids to the severely ill.

Ampicillin, 6000 mg, every 4 hours, by mouth.

Chloramphenicol, 1000 mg, every 6 hours, by mouth, until control of fever; then, half dosage, for 15 days.

Prednisone, 40 to 60 mg, in divided doses, to start; decrease dosage as soon as possible; and discontinue at a gradual rate.

Poisoning

In most instances of poisoning the diagnosis is obvious, and the treatment for shock will be carried out together with the specific treatment for a given poison. But accidental poisoning, or poisoning with the intent of suicide or murder, may present a very arduous problem because the physician cannot rely on apparent facts, which must be patiently and carefully collected, not only for diagnosis, but also for legal purposes. All available containers, remnants of foods or drinks, and excretions or secretions from the body are checked and saved for further examination. The following data will be of some help.

Underweight: suspect chronic poisoning (arsenic, lead, mercury, or some medications).

Dry mouth: atropine and derivatives.

Excessive salivation: mercury, lead, other heavy metals, insecticides.

Painful, loose teeth: mercury, phosphorus.

Bloody diarrhea: salicylates, anticoagulants, iron and corrosive substances.

Dyspnea: salicylates, physostigmine, atropine, strychnine, insecticides, botulism, cyanides.

Anuria: mercury, formaldehyde, phosphorus, sulfonamides, oxalic acid, carbon tetrachloride, trinitrotoluene.

Polyuria: lead.

Unconsciousness: alcohol, barbiturates, atropine, opium, cyanides, paraldehyde, insecticides, antihistaminics, salicylates, chlorpromazine, phenols, and final stages of any severe poisoning.

The treatment of shock will be carried out vigorously, giving special emphasis to checking fluid loss (electrolytes), hypotension (levarterenol), cerebral edema (mannitol), poison concentration in blood (dialysis), and evacuation of the stomach (gastric lavage), and to using the adequate antidote. A few poisons and antidotes are given here.

Acids: egg albumin, milk, milk of magnesia, magnesium oxide; avoid gastric lavage and carbonates.

Alcohol: lavage with sodium bicarbonate; give glucose and thiamine.

Alkalis: vinegar and water, equal parts; citrus fruit juice; olive oil or melted butter (also, margarine).

Antihistaminics: symptomatic treatment of shock.

Arsenic: milk (after gastric lavage), dimercaprol (BAL).

Barbiturates: treat shock vigorously.

Atropine: gastric lavage followed by activated charcoal.

Carbon monoxide: 100% oxygen, mannitol.

Cocaine: use tourniquet on injected extremity, or perform gastric lavage with potassium permanganate (1:10,000 solution).

Cyanides: amyl nitrite inhalation followed by sodium nitrite intravenously (300 mg in 10 ml of water), and immediately, also intravenously, sodium thiosulfate (25 ml or more, as needed, of a 50% solution).

Digitalis: gastric lavage or emesis followed by oral potassium chloride (3 or 4 g).

Formaldehyde: 0.2% ammonia water (200 to 240 ml).

Lead: calcium disodium edetate, either alone or with dimercaprol (BAL).

Mercury: milk or egg albumin.

Nitrites: emetics or gastric tube.

Opium and derivatives: gastric lavage with 1:10,000 solution of sodium permanganate; give 30 g of sodium sulfate in water before removing the tube, in the case of morphine intoxication.

Phenols: olive oil (better used as gastric lavage) or activated charcoal.

Salicylates: emetics or gastric lavage; give sodium bicarbonate or lactate intravenously.

Addison's Disease

Addisonians may go into shock during the stages of acute adrenal insufficiency, which shows some resemblance to the well-known acute abdomen: symptoms of dehydration together with a marked hypotension, abdominal pain with vomiting and diarrhea, fever; all this happening to a patient with hyperpigmentation (skin, pressure sites, creases, mucosae), sparse body hair (axillae), and small heart. Should the patient be a known Addisonian, there will be no diagnostic trouble; otherwise, differentiation from acute abdomen, diabetic accidents, and other possible causes of shock may be difficult. The laboratory will report elevated potassium and blood urea nitrogen, decreased natremia and glycemia, and very low levels of cortisol (in both blood and urine) and other adrenal hormones. Acute adrenal crises are to be suspected when this sort of clinical picture occurs after surgery, any stressful situation, adrenal injury, very severe infections, or withdrawal of corticotherapy.

Patients in this critical situation will immediately be hospitalized to treat shock according to the accepted measures. Emphasis will be put on the administration of intravenous plasma and fluids (with sodium), dopamine (with or without levarterenol), antibiotics, and hydrocortisone. Oxygen will be needed in most instances. Do not delay the administration of fluids or corticoids, and do not give sedatives or narcotics.

Isotonic saline, for infusion.

Plasma (or Dextran 40), for infusion.

Dopamine hydrochloride, 200 mg ampoules reconstituted to provide 400 μg in each ml of solution (put 200 mg in 500 ml of 5% dextrose): start with 2 to 5 μg for each kilo of body weight every minute; increase as needed and tolerated (about 30 to 40 μg for each kilo every minute).

Hydrocortisone, 100 mg intravenously at a relatively rapid rate, thereafter 50 to 100 mg by infusion (every 6 hours the first day, every 8 hours the second day; thereafter, gradual reduction). Be careful about the body volume of the patient!

Rapid Decompression

When persons, particularly divers, have been subject to elevated atmospheric pressure, a rapid decompression will provoke: headache, itching, arthralgias, with subsequent weakness or paralyses, visual disturbances, vertigo, dyspnea, and final unconsciousness. All these symptoms will appear in from 30 minutes to 6 hours after the subject has emerged at the surface. Diagnosis must be made as soon as possible, and the adequate treatment started immediately.

Start with plasma and oxygen, give acetylsalicylic acid for pains, and transport the patient promptly to the nearest decompression center.

Hemorrhages

See "Blood Loss" in the preceding section on "Shock."

SYNCOPE

General Considerations and Diagnosis

By definition, syncope is a sudden loss of strength and transient suspension of consciousness, usually due to cerebral anoxia, that is, a short cardiogenic shock. Consequently, the symptoms are: unconsciousness, marked hypotension, bradycardia (at least during the first stages; thereafter tachycardia may occur), intense pallor, usually followed by cyanosis, at times minor convulsions, and extreme muscular weakness while still conscious. There may be other syndromes with shock or coma; but syncope is always transient, while stroke is an enduring complex ending in complete paralysis of the affected muscles. The rapid recovery of consciousness confirms the diagnosis.

Syncope is usually due to: emotional crises, cardiovascular diseases (arteriosclerosis, valvular diseases, initial myocardial infarction, vasovagal syncope, carotid sinus syncope, hypotension, orthostatic hypotension), adrenal insufficiency, central nervous system disease, severe anemia, diabetes mellitus, hypoglycemia, hyperventilation, acute alcoholism, and some instances of very severe pain.

Because the patient ordinarily falls when stricken by syncope, once the head is placed in a recumbent position, reoxygenation will take place, and consciousness will be rapidly recovered—rarely will the physician arrive in time to treat these accidents. But unfortunately a large number of the elderly are injured by the fall, with either a severe cerebral lesion or fracture of a bone, circumstances that will be carefully evaluated in all instances. For this reason we shall add to the above list other, no less frequent causes of falls: vertebral basilar occlusion, cervical spondylosis, subclavian artery stenosis, Parkinson's disease, and epilepsy.

General Treatment for Syncope

Place the head on a level with or below the heart. This will usually suffice to help the patient recover from a syncopal attack. If the situation is unusually severe, the treatment will follow the schedule advised for shock. Otherwise, each causative condition will be treated according to accepted rules.

Pain

An earlier chapter of this book was entirely devoted to the diagnosis and treatment of pain. Any of the diseases studied there may cause syncopal states whenever the pain reaches intolerable proportions. A succinct listing of the principal causes of pain causing syncope follows; but the reader is referred to a more complete review of this interesting and very practical subject under the title "General Diagnosis of Pain," in the chapter on "Pain."

Anginal pain: retrosternal in location, and relieved by the use of nitroglycerin.

Myocardial infarction: more severe than the former, and not relieved by the use of nitroglycerin.

Pulmonary infarction: substernal pain, with abrupt fever, dyspnea, and anxiety.

Pneumothorax: dramatic onset with sharp side pain, dyspnea, and dry cough.

Appendicitis: colicky pains in the right iliac fossa, with fever and local muscle spasm.

Pancreatitis: located at the left side of the epigastrium and accompanied by local muscle rigidity.

Renal colic: excruciating pain from the costovertebral angle to the groin of the same side.

Peritonitis: agonizing, constant pain in the abdomen, exaggerated by motion; legs are flexed and the face reveals intense anguish.

Influenza: showing an upper respiratory or gastrointestinal involvement, with headache, generalized muscle pains, and profound asthenia.

Dengue: with symptomatology similar to influenza, but the pains reach disabling proportions.

Meningitis: with a very severe headache, rigid neck, and high fever.

Brain tumors and cysts: intense headache, projectile vomiting, papilledema, bradycardia, seizures, and behavioral changes.

Heart failure: with dyspnea, edema, and other cardiovascular symptoms.

Limb pain: may reach very intense proportions in some instances of bursitis, arthritis, neuritis, and gangrene.

Gout: with the typical pain in the great toe.

Anal pain: caused by hemorrhoids, strictures, etc.

Cancer: any form of cancer, particularly at the final stages, may cause very intense pain.

Under these circumstances, pain should be relieved with morphine or meperidine, and the treatment of each causative disease will be reinforced to avoid further critical pains.

Meperidine, 50 to 100 mg, by intramuscular or intravenous injection, to be repeated as needed and tolerated.

Anxiety Neuroses

Syncope is not a usual symptom of these conditions, but occasional patients may faint when the neurotic components reach an unbearable level. Anxiety is diagnosed because of tachycardia with palpitation, increased blood pressure (longstanding cases), sweating, hyperventilation, gastrointestinal disturbances, apprehension and indefinite fears, and tenseness.

A good psychiatric approach will try to solve the basic problems causing the reaction. For the medical prevention of repeated anxiety attacks, some sedatives might be given.

Diazepam, 2 mg tablets; take one every 8 hours; 5 mg may be given at the start.

Stress

Any situation stressing the pituitary–adrenal axis will cause some sort of shocklike symptomatology, with hypotension, tachycardia, possible dyspnea, and other symptoms that will bring on a reactive syncopal attack. Any debilitating disease, cachectic states, convalescence, and the like will be considered a cause for syncope, provided other more frequent or obvious causes are not present.

The treatment will be directed to the causative condition. To stimulate personal reactions, small amounts of corticoids may be given for short periods (slow decrease in dosage and early discontinuance is sought).

> Prednisone, 2 to 4 mg every 8 hours; decrease and discontinue as soon as possible.

Cardiovascular Diseases

Any cardiovascular disease capable of decreasing blood circulation to the brain may cause not only shock, but also a less alarming syncope. This may happen in the following situations.

Myocardial infarction: a syncopal attack may be among the initial symptoms.

Pulmonary infarction: with substernal pain, fever, dyspnea, and anxiety.

Heart failure: with dyspnea, edema, and other cardiovascular symptoms.

Paroxysmal tachycardia (more common among those on digitalis, not too frequent among the elderly): the heart rate rises abruptly to about 200 beats a minute, with occasional initial syncope (or the syncopal state arises after prolonged tachycardia) and very meager additional symptoms. The start and the end of the attack are abrupt, and each attack may last a few hours.

Stokes-Adams syndrome: characteristic of prolonged lapse between systoles in complete heart block is the occurrence of a syncopal state, with or without convulsions. The attack occurs if the asystole lasts longer than is tolerated by the brain. The heart rate is fixed at about 50 beats a minute, not changed by exercise (which may cause the syncopal attack).

Aortic stenosis: there is usually an elevated diastolic blood pressure, a systolic murmur is heard at the upper right border of the heart, and a thrill palpated at that site.

In most instances, symptomatic treatment will be given for residual complaints after the syncopal attack, which usually subsides before the physician can see the patient. As soon as the head has been put at the same level as the heart, the attack usually subsides. Prevention will be attempted whenever feasible. The treatment of the basic cause is a must for the total relief of symptoms. Myocardial infarction and pulmonary embolism will be treated as usual. Heart failure will be treated as for shock, with emphasis on cardiotonics. For paroxysmal tachycardia attacks use mechanical measures first (carotid sinus pressure, with continuous auscultation of the heart, to stop as soon as the attack ceases, but with extreme care in frail elderly persons), or give propranolol (edrophonium is a good alternate); quinidine or digitalis is used for specific treatment; cardioversion will be evaluated by a specialist. Heart block may respond to corticoids, if it is of recent appearance; otherwise it will require a pacemaker, particularly when isoproterenol, ephedrine, or epinephrine proves useless; intracardiac epinephrine may solve a prolonged cardiac standstill. Valve replacement is the only procedure advisable for aortic stenosis, whenever feasible; otherwise, routine treatment will be employed for heart failure.

> Propranolol hydrochloride; administer 1 to 3 mg (1 mg a minute) intravenously, in desperate cases, well-monitored and better evaluated by a specialist.

> Edrophonium chloride, 10-ml vials; inject intravenously 5 (up to 10) ml with due caution as to cholinergic reactions—particularly bradycardia or cardiac standstill.

> Quinidine, 200 mg tablets; give one every 8, 12, or 24 hours.

Encephalic Diseases

When there is impaired blood circulation within the brain, syncope may occur at the slightest increase of hypoxia. This is a relatively common happening among the elderly, particularly those affected with cerebral arteriosclerosis. Also, brain tumors and cysts will cause a similar symptomatology, because of decreased blood flow to the brain.

Cerebral arteriosclerosis will cause a gradual deterioration of affected elderly persons, usually starting with dizzy spells or frank syncopes that appear at varying intervals, mental changes (mainly poor memory for recent events, but also forgetfulness, confusion, and behavioral and personality alterations), blurred vision, and finally other evidence of localized lesions, until a complete stroke takes place, not rarely preceded by "little strokes" in which there is a transient weakness or numbness of a limb (contralateral), together with an also transient ipsilateral amaurosis (partial or complete).

Hypertension may accompany these symptoms. Arteriography is the best procedure in order to reach a complete diagnosis.

Intracranial tumor has a symptomatology that includes not only syncope but other more typical symptoms, such as headache, projectile vomiting, personality changes, papilledema, and progressive increase of the spinal fluid pressure and occurrence of neurological symptoms. Electrocardiographic and radiologic studies will give a complete diagnosis. According to the location of the space-occupying mass (tumor or cyst), other symptoms will be noted.

Temporal lobe: convulsive psychomotor seizures, a contralateral homonymous visual field defect plus aphasia if the left side is involved.

Frontal lobe: symptoms similar to the foregoing, plus anosmia if the base of the lobe is affected, and also more marked symptoms of altered personality.

Parietal lobe: again, a similar symptomatology, but seizures are usually focal, with a contralateral hemiparesis, hyperreflexia, and other neurological signs.

Occipital lobe: predominance of visual alterations.

Cerebellar: disturbances of coordination and equilibrium.

Residuals of cranial injury may present syncope following rapid and forceful movements of the head, which tendency is added to the history of the previous accident (whenever known).

Migraine will present the common symptomatology of the disease, but occasionally there will be a more or less marked and more or less permanent lightheadedness which may be followed by syncope.

Arteriosclerosis will be treated prophylactically with a low-fat diet (no more than 20% of the total caloric intake) consisting mostly of polyunsaturated fats, and an antilipemic drug (clofibrate, thyroid extracts, or estrogens, the latter only for women).

Clofibrate, 500 mg capsules; take one four times a day.

Thyroid extract (thyroglobulin) tablets; take 15 to 30 mg, according to effects and tolerance.

Conjugated estrogens, 0.625 or (better) 0.3 mg tablets; take one a day for 21 days, with no use for 7 to 10 days.

For brain tumors and cysts, discuss surgical procedures with a neurosurgeon. Otherwise, treat symptomatically. The same advice will be sought for residuals of cranial injuries.

Migraine attacks may be aborted with a sedative or with ergotamine (the latter, if there are no cardiovascular contraindications). Methysergide may be tried for the chronic state.

Phenobarbital, 15 (or 30) mg, every 6 to 8 hours.

Ergotamine tartrate, 0.25 mg in 0.5-ml ampoules, by subcutaneous injection.

Methysergide, 2 mg tablets, to take one every 8 or 12 hours (watch for side effects).

Valvular Diseases

These diseases were reviewed in the previous section on "Cardiogenic Shock," q.v. for more information. A short summary follows.

Mitral stenosis shows a presystolic murmur and thrill at the apex of the heart, together with flushed face and feeble pulse.

Mitral insufficiency presents a systolic murmur at the apex which spreads toward the axilla, forceful heart beats, and thrill.

Aortic stenosis murmur is systolic and is heard at the upper right border of the heart area; there is a thrill at the same site, and elevated diastolic blood pressure.

Aortic insufficiency shows a diastolic murmur heard at the same upper right side of the heart area, paleness, forceful pulse, and blood pressure with ample pulse pressure.

Tricuspidic and *pulmonic* lesions are less frequently noted.

A large number of patients with valvular defects do not reach advanced age; but those who do come to senescence carrying these lesions will be carefully watched for thrombotic episodes, which may end in a stroke syndrome. Pulmonary edema is also a threat to those who develop atrial fibrillation. Most patients with mitral lesions are female; and those with aortic ones, male.

Symptomatic treatment will be given to these patients, whose only hope for amelioration lies in the performance of some sort of valvular surgery, under the guidance of a cardiologist and a chest surgeon, who will evaluate the advisability of the procedures. In case of shock or stroke, emergency treatment will be provided, following the accepted rules.

Bradycardia

A slow pulse is not the best way to obtain adequate blood flow to the brain. A rate of less than 60 beats a minute constitutes bradycardia. This situation is usually well tolerated without any outstanding symptomatology; but when it becomes more marked, syncope with or without convulsions may occur. Elderly persons are more likely to react with syncope and convulsions than younger people. The increase in vagal tone may be due to a previous meningitic reaction, any disease increasing intracranial pressure, reflex irritation of the vagal system by gastrointestinal diseases, a hypersensitive carotid sinus, or the use of beta-adrenergic blocking drugs (propranolol). A more recently described syndrome of bradycardia–tachycardia should be noted. Patients present alternate episodes of bradycardia and tachycardia (or fibrillation). Different arrhythmias may also be present.

No treatment is generally required; but if there are syncopal episodes, try to control them with atropine or atropine derivatives. In general, these patients should learn to avoid the influences that may provoke syncope, particularly dietary excesses. As usual, lying down will help in most instances. For the tachycardia–bradycardia syndrome the only acceptable treatment is the implantation of a pacemaker, which should be thoroughly discussed with a cardiologist and a chest surgeon.

> Atropine, 0.3, 0.4, or 0.5 mg tablets; give 0.15 to 0.25 mg, two or three times a day, before meals, as needed and tolerated.

Hypotension

This condition was reviewed in the section on "Cardiogenic Shock," q.v. for more information. Syncope, of course, is more easily found than true cardiogenic shock. During the critical stage there will be asthenia, dizziness, cyanosis and coolness of the extremities, bradycardia, and occipital headache. Hypotension may accompany the following diseases: chronic adrenal insufficiency (asthenia, hyperpigmentation), cachexia hypophysaria (weight loss, asthenia and other decreased endocrine functions), cancer at its depauperating stage, chronic alcoholism (with polyneuritis), liver diseases (of the cirrhotic type), debilitating diseases of any kind, and anaphylactic shock (sudden onset following the injection or ingestion of the offending substance).

Since syncope does not require the aggressive treatment that is given in case of shock, only symptomatic measures will be carried out in these cases. But the basic disease must be aggressively treated, to avoid further more serious complications. Fludrocortisone should be given in some instances. Anaphylactic shock, no matter how simple it may appear at the start, should be treated immediately with epinephrine.

> Fludrocortisone acetate, 0.1 mg a day, by mouth.

> Epinephrine, 1:1000 solution; inject 0.5 ml in 10 ml of saline by slow intravenous route; or 1 ml by intramuscular injection, which will suffice in most of these instances.

Orthostatic Hypotension

This condition is also called postural hypotension because it occurs by a change of position. When the patient changes from a resting position to an active upright one, syncope may supervene. Falls are not rare, and among the elderly may cause additional injuries. Causative, or at least contributory, factors may be any debilitating condition, anxiety, a previous sympathectomy, peripheral venous stasis, or the use of excessive antihypertensive medication. There is a complex and variable association of postural hypotension with rigidity, tremor, dysarthria, diplegia, vertigo, incontinence, lack of inflection in the voice, and other neurological symptoms, thus constituting the Shy-Drager syndrome.

When there is a known causative factor it will be treated accordingly. Otherwise, recommend that the patient not change too rapidly from the supine to the upright position. If antihypertensive drugs are being used, reduce dosage; and advise the use of elastic stockings if there is peripheral venous stasis. Ephedrine and fludrocortisone will be tried.

Ephedrine sulfate, capsules containing 25 mg; tablets containing 25 mg; give one three times a day, or as tolerated and needed.

Fludrocortisone acetate, 0.1 mg once a day.

Adrenal Insufficiency

Addison's disease may be the cause of shock when the patient goes into an acute crisis, but because of the low blood pressure natural with the process syncope may also occur. A second cause for syncope is the hypoglycemic condition usually common to these patients. The outstanding, almost diagnostic, symptom of chronic adrenal insufficiency is marked asthenia and hyperpigmentation of the skin. Patients complain of tiredness even when they get up from bed in the morning, after a good rest. There is a diffuse hyperpigmentation of the skin and mucosae, more marked on exposed areas, pressure sites, and nipples and of a very early occurrence on the knuckles of the fingers. Other symptoms include: anorexia, diarrhea, nausea and vomiting, scanty body hair better noted at the axillae, and irritability. Syncope may follow unusual stress or prolonged periods without eating. Blood pressure is low, the heart size is small, the lymphoid tissue is enlarged, and actue crises may occur with some clinical resemblance to an acute abdomen, particularly if the patient is subject to some sort of surgery, any stressing situation, adrenal injury, or severe infection. The laboratory will report very low levels of cortisol (and other adrenal hormones) in the blood and urine; also elevated potassium and blood urea nitrogen, plus decreased natremia and glycemia.

The basic treatment is that for chronic adrenal insufficiency. Cortisone is enough for the milder cases. Otherwise, it will be given together with desoxycorticosterone or fludrocortisone. The diet has to be rich in proteins and carbohydrates, given at small, frequent meals. Protect the patient from stressful situations and all infections. Check electrolytes frequently.

Hydrocortisone, 10 mg a day, one dose on arising and the second at noon (better not given near bedtime).

Fludrocortisone, 0.05 to 0.1 mg, given in the morning, once a day or every other day (check blood pressure and ankle edema).

Vasovagal Syncope

This is simple fainting, related to a sudden drop of blood pressure caused by a sudden emotion or pain. Elderly persons are prone to react this way: first, there is a feeling of anxiety and weakness with paleness and cool extremities, sweating, a need to yawn or sigh, and restlessness; this is followed in a few minutes by blurring of vision, lightheadedness, decreased muscle tone, and final collapse. Syncope is accompanied by a fall because in most instances it occurs when the patient is in an upright position. Differently from orthostatic hypotension, there is not necessarily a sudden change from lying down to the erect position. The systolic blood pressure, if checked at this time, is usually below 70 mm Hg.

Place the patient in a recumbent position, with the head at the level of or below the heart line. Inhalation of strong odors (aromatic spirits of ammonia) may help some persons.

Carotid Sinus Syncope

The elderly are perhaps more reactive to carotid sinus syncope than to vasovagal syncope. Between the attacks they usually complain of spells of weakness or dizziness. The attack generally follows a rapid movement of the head (turning or rising) or may happen when the patient is using a tight collar, and can be elicited by pressing for a few seconds over the carotid sinus (stimulate only one!), but this maneuver is not advisable for elderly persons who may react with a cerebrovascular accident. Among the elderly, the vagal response is usually accompanied by bradycardia; younger people may show a reactive hypotension; other cases do not show any of these changes.

Syncope accompanied by bradycardia will respond to atropine; ephedrine with phenobarbital is good for those responding with hypotension (as well as for those responding with bradycardia). Patients who do not react with either bradycardia or hypotension will not respond to drug treatment; these persons will take care to avoid all situations that may precipitate the crisis.

Atropine sulfate, 0.3, 0.4, or 0.5 mg tablets; give 0.25 to 0.4 mg about three times a day, always as tolerated and needed.

Ephedrine sulfate, 25 mg capsules; give about three times a day, as tolerated and needed.

Phenobarbital, 15 mg tablets; give one tablet together with ephedrine medication.

Hot or Crowded Places

It is well known that standing in hot or crowded places for a relatively long time can cause syncope, which happens more easily to elderly people than to younger adults. Under the circumstances, the diagnosis will try to establish whether or not this is a transient episode of little importance, or a more important situation that needs treatment.

Anemia

Persons who react with syncope to effort or other circumstances, are pale and asthenic, and complain of dizziness, headache, tinnitus, and spots before the eyes, will be suspected of having anemia. A blood examination will be required. Any of the following types of anemia may be present.

Post-hemorrhagic anemia: there is a history of acute bleeding, and the diagnosis corresponds to that of blood loss (q.v.).

Sideropenic anemia: usually due to an occult blood loss; iron in the blood is low (hypochromia, microcytosis).

Hemolytic anemia: with increased bilirubin in blood and urobilinogen in feces and urine; it is normocytic anemia (with evidence of increased hematopoiesis); the patient is usually jaundiced and has splenomegaly.

Pernicious anemia: patients are pale and mildly jaundiced, complain of limb paresthesias, anorexia, and dyspepsia (achlorhydria), show a smooth painful tongue, and have large oval red cells.

Hypoplastic anemia: also aplastic, mostly due to exposure to toxic agents (when present in the elderly); it is normochromic and normocytic, with leukopenia and thrombocytopenia.

Thalassemia: patients come from countries bordering the Mediterranean Sea or Southeast Asia; blood count is normal, but hemoglobin is very low; patients have splenomegaly.

Secondary anemia: usually present with chronic, longstanding diseases, particularly of endocrine organs, liver, or kidney.

Lead poisoning anemia: history of exposure; characteristic basophilic stippling of erythrocytes.

Symptomatic treatment will be given whenever needed; but only the basic treatment for the specific type of anemia will be established. For posthemorrhagic anemia give blood transfusions, if needed; and take care of the causative disease. Iron deficiency anemia poses the need for finding a hidden bleeding spot, which will receive the necessary care; but iron is the specific drug for it. Pernicious anemia requires permanent treatment with cyanocobalamin; if not treated, it will cause death. Hypoplastic and aplastic anemia require a search for the toxic cause, which must be eliminated; recently packed red cells are given every 6 weeks (5 or 6 units in a couple of days), with platelets occasionally required; androgenic steroids are effective stimulants of the bone marrow. Thalassemia (major type) must be treated with blood transfusions at regular intervals. Secondary anemias call for treatment of the basic conditions. Finally, lead poisoning anemia needs no treatment if mild; but in other, more severe instances it will be treated with penicillamine or calcium disodium edetate.

Blood well-matched for transfusion, to be given as needed.

Ferrous sulfate, 200 mg tablets, to take three a day, with meals.

Cyanocobalamin; give 100 μg by intramuscular injection, starting three or more times a week; to stabilize a treatment with 100 μg once a month.

Packed red cells, well-matched for transfusion.

Testosterone enanthate; give about 300 mg for each kilo of body weight in 24 hours, twice a week by intramuscular injection.

Penicillamine, 250 mg, by oral route, three or four times a day.

Calcium disodium edetate, 500 to 1000 mg, by intravenous injection, once a day.

Cough Syncope

A syncopal state may follow prolonged irrepressible coughing, or just a simple and somewhat violent coughing, particularly among frail elderly persons. The increased intrathoracic pressure causes a fall in blood pressure sufficient to cause cerebral parlyzing hypoxia. This accident occurs relatively easily when the patient suffers from arteriosclerosis and the brain vessels are already damaged. Most patients with cough syncope are males, middle-aged or older, not rarely plethoric, and with emphysema. After the patient coughs violently for a while, or only after a few moderate coughs, he falls unconscious for a few seconds, or only presents a more or less marked vertiginous reaction. Needless to say, the great majority of these patients present a chronic pulmonary condition, usually due to smoking.

No treatment is needed for cough syncope, nor would it arrive in time if needed; but repetition of these attacks should be avoided. Naturally, that requires treatment of the condition causing coughing, and patient should quit smoking, since this is the trigger element. Also, these patients are to be retrained in coughing gently. Bechics may be of transitory help, but are not a basic feature of treatment.

Syncope During Micturition or Defecation

Reflex sensations during micturition or straining at stool may provoke a syncopal reaction. The elderly are relatively prone to syncopal attacks during micturition, with the risk of injuries on falling. These patients usually suffer from a prostatic disease, hypertrophy, or malignancy. Those who faint after straining at stool actually cause their syncope, perhaps in the same way as those who faint after coughing.

If there is a prostatic disorder, care will be taken of the disease. Meanwhile, these patients should be advised to pass urine while sitting on the toilet. Patients who fall into syncope when straining at stool should be given laxatives and taught not to strain for defecation.

> Cascara, tablets containing about 300 mg; take one or two every night, or as needed and tolerated.

> Milk of magnesia, 1 tablespoonful every night, the dosage to be adjusted for each individual.

Syncope Due to Drugs

Syncopal states (even shock) may be due to the use of certain drugs, which will be carefully sought when dealing with these patients. Just a reminder of a few of these drugs will be given here. First think of antihypertensives and vasodilators, namely, veratrum alkaloids (cryptenamine, veratrum viride), Rauwolfia alkaloids (Rauwolfia, reserpine, deserpidine, and so on), monoamine oxidase inhibitors (pargyline), thiazide derivatives, sympatholytic drugs (these two last groups representing a large number of known medications), nitrites and nitrates, pentaerythritol, isosorbide, erythritil, papaverine, propranolol, cyclandelate, and others. Second, all allergenic substances will also be considered (pollens, insect venoms, serum, food, antibiotics, and so forth). For more details, see "Anaphylactic Shock."

Hypoglycemia

There is no need for the hypoglycemic reaction to reach the state of shock; many patients will only faint with a syncopal attack. Typically, there will be headache, moist skin, pale or flushed face, paresthesias (numbness), tremors, tachycardia (rarely, bradycardia), palpitations, emotional instability, initial dizziness, and final syncope. The diagnosis of hypoglycemia is difficult because of its varying causes and courses. There are paroxystic hypertension caused by pheochromocytomas, anxiety states, and others. The attack may occur early in the morning or some time after the last meal, which is a fasting hypoglycemia; or it may be reactive to a relatively recent meal, that is, a postprandial hypoglycemia. In the first case there may be a reaction to insulin produced by a pancreatic tumor or given by a previous injection, or it may be reactive to oral hypoglycemic drugs or other sulfonylureas; also, other tumors may cause hypoglycemic attacks (adrenocortical carcinomas, hepatomas, or some sarcomas). Postprandial hypoglycemia may be due to a previous gastrectomy, intense vagotony, or initial diabetes, and it might occur from 2 to 5 hours after the previous meal. The diagnosis is made by the finding of about 40 mg of glucose, or less, in each 100 ml of blood. For more elaborate diagnostic procedures, request insulinemia levels and perhaps adrenal hormones as well. Any patient with syncope (or in shock), moist skin, and low glycemia, who improves following the administration of glucose (by mouth or intravenously) must be considered to have hypoglycemia. Other tests can be performed for the diagnosis of pancreatic beta cell tumors.

The critical stage is immediately relieved by the administration of sugar or glucose; patients should carry sugar for these emergencies. If it is given by mouth, it is better to complete the meal with additional food, to prevent recurrence of the attack. A total of 10 to 20 g of glucose is to be given either by mouth or intravenously, if needed. Other causes of hypoglycemia are to be treated individually.

Glucose, 25% solution, for intravenous administration.

Diabetes Mellitus

There are patients who, before a clear onset of the diabetic disease, present a period of "latent," "hidden," or "chemical" diabetes with a meager symptomatology, but are prone to develop evident hypoglycemic attacks. These attacks can also be therapeutically caused by excessive dosage of insulin (or the lack of sufficient food after the injection). In each case, the diagnosis to be made is that of hypoglycemia, which is not too difficult after the use of insulin, but may pose a threat to the sagacity of the diagnostician during the pre-diabetic stage. Nevertheless, the symptomatology of these hypoglycemic attacks does not differ from that of the above-mentioned hypoglycemia, q.v.

Give glucose (10 to 20 g) by mouth or intravenously, readjust carefully the amount and the timing of insulin and food, and, in the case of pre-diabetes, control diet and exercise. Most persons with non-overt diabetes are obese individuals who should be restored to their ideal weight by a reduction in carbohydrate intake (particularly simple sugars) and a moderate increase in exercise. Once at the ideal weight level, they will maintain it thereafter. No insulin or oral hypoglycemic drugs are used at this stage. These patients must be carefully followed because the great majority will develop a regular clinical picture of diabetes and will need special individual care.

Falls

When the above inductive factors for falls are ruled out among the elderly, a search will be carried out for parkinsonism, epilepsy, or any of the following organic conditions: vertebrobasilar syndrome, cervical spondylosis, or subclavian artery stenosis.

Vertebral-basilar occlusion: usually partial in nature, provokes intermittent transient episodes of cerebral symptoms, including syncopal attacks, confusion, unilateral weakness and numbness of muscles, and at times slurred speech or blindness. When the occlusion is complete, there are dysarthria, dysphagia, and other corticospinal symptoms, as well.

Cervical spondylosis: more frequently diagnosed among the elderly because of a local pain or pain radiating to chest and upper limbs, paresthesias, and even paresias or paralysis; occasionally, patients may present large osteocartilaginous proliferations capable of causing syncope.

Subclavian stenosis: also known as "subclavian steal syndrome," will cause a syncopal attack whenever blood supply to the brain is sufficiently reduced. There will be symptoms of claudication of an extremity together with other symptoms due to impairment of the central nervous system, namely, pain, paresthesias, paresia, or extreme weakness of muscles.

Parkinson's disease: see appropriate entries in this book, for more complete information; but note that these patients may present episodes of blurred consciousness, which may cause a fall.

Epilepsy: see also appropriate entries for better information, but keep in mind that the majority of persons with a seizure will fall to the ground.

Good radiologic studies will solve diagnostic doubts in many instances by showing the bone structures and the condition of arteries as seen in arteriograms. Other procedures may also be of help, as plethysmography, venography, and the like. But in all instances the help of a specialist must be requested, since these diagnostic procedures may require practiced skill.

Anticoagulant therapy is advised at times, but there is always a risk involved, particularly of intracranial hemorrhage among hypertensive patients. Surgery may also be beneficial, but it also carries a risk. More conservative measures may give some relief, as exercise, bracing, bolstering the position in bed, and avoidance of efforts that may induce symptoms. Early consultation is desirable.

COMA

General Considerations and Diagnosis

Coma is a state of unconsciousness from which the patient cannot be aroused even by the most powerful and painful external stimuli. It is well to say that coma is a final outcome of shock or stroke, when the patient becomes unable to respond. In stroke there is paralysis of one side of the body, while in shock there is a marked drop in blood pressure. The comatose patient seems to be in a very deep sleep, without any conscious reaction, and with a total lack of sensitivity and motility. The worst situation occurs when a patient is found comatose in the street, and there is no help from anyone to give a history. A careful physical examination is crucial at this time, and reports from the laboratory and the radiology department, as described at the beginning of this chapter (q.v.), will help. The most frequent findings are listed here:

Cranial injuries: lesions of scalp or bone structures; initial symptoms of shock possibly followed by others of stroke (paralyses). The final diagnosis may be made by angiography. There is a slow increase in symptoms in extradural hemorrhage; stiff neck and bloody spinal fluid in subarachnoid hemorrhage.

Bodily injuries: require a watchful attitude when affecting frail elderly persons, as there is always the possibility of brain reaction or massive hemorrhage.

Diabetic coma: is suggested because of a previous diagnosis of diabetes. It is otherwise characterized by dry skin and other symptoms of dehydration, irregular deep and superficial respirations, hypotonic muscles, normal or mydriatic pupils, strong pulse, feeble or abolished patellar reflexes, acetone odor to the breath, hyperglycemia, and marked ketonuria.

Hypoglycemic coma: is suspected when it is known that the patient is being treated for diabetes, particularly using insulin. It will be thought of if the skin is moist or perspiring freely, with the eyeballs soft, pale or flushed face, tachycardia, and low values (less than 40 mg%) for blood glucose, corrected by the injection of glucose.

Uremic coma: most older persons reaching uremic coma are actually cachectic, and many are known to suffer kidney disease (glomerulonephritis or the like). Symptoms are: paleness, hypothermia (or hyperthermia), miosis, Cheyne-Stokes respiration, hypertension, retinopathy, and a urinous odor to the breath and sweat, plus laboratory findings of elevated urea, and evidence of acidosis and anemia.

Infections: may go into coma when the toxemia is intense, or the defenses are weak. This applies particularly to the elderly with influenza and pneumonia, but with other infections as well.

Encephalitis: severe neurological symptoms will occur as in Eastern encephalitis; with stiff neck, vomiting, convulsions, myoclonus, tremors, ocular paralysis or other palsies, as hemiplegia, as well as loss of consciousness. The spinal tap may show an elevated pressure, albumin, and possibly the causal virus.

Meningitis: may cause coma in addition to its other symptoms.

Epilepsy: may incur a deep residual sleep, a true coma when reaching the status epilepticus stage; or coma may be the consequences of injuries received during the attack. The typical convulsive crisis will orient the diagnosis.

Hemorrhage: when severe, can cause shock and coma (see the corresponding entry in the foregoing section).

Hepatic coma: occurs in patients with previous disease of the liver, as viral hepatitis or cirrhosis; the patient becomes irritable and confused, goes into a stuporous state, and finally reaches the comatose stage.

Addison's disease: may provoke final coma following an acute crisis.

Hyperthyroidism: may present a final coma, frequently preceded by dysphagia. It may follow a thyroid storm.

Hypothyroidism: with severe myxedema; coma may occur.

Cranial hypotension: may follow a spinal tap, dehydration, or intracranial hemorrhage, or may be idiopathic; the diagnosis is difficult, and spinal tap is not advisable for this purpose. Respirations are of the Cheyne-Stokes type, and the pulse is hypotonic and irregular.

Toxic substances: several different toxic substances may be incriminated as causes of coma, and a careful search will be made for alcoholism, barbiturates, cocaine, opium, and others.

Physical agents: those that may produce coma are high altitude, coldness, sunstroke, heatstroke, and others.

Bradycardia: syncope, shock, or coma may be present in cases of permanent slow pulse, including the Stokes-Adams syndrome.

The handling of the comatose patient will follow the same pattern as that indicated at the beginning of this section for general unconsciousness, which should be consulted for more information.

Treatment is also similar. It will be both for the emergency and for the basic state, as the cornerstone of care. Emergency treatment preferably is given in the hospital; provide for a patent airway, even performing artificial respiration, if so needed, and monitor vital signs. It is well to change the patient's body position frequently, placing him on his side to avoid passage of secretions or excretions into the respiratory tract. Pass urinary catheters; give blood expanders (blood, plasma, dextran, electrolyte solutions) as needed to restore blood and pulse pressures to normal; give epinephrine or isoproterenol to increase blood pressure if needed. Make every effort to start the basic treatment as soon as possible.

Diabetic Coma

When a diabetic patient goes into coma, ascertain at once whether it is due to the diabetes or to an intracranial hemorrhage, or of another type of injury as indicated in the paragraphs opening this section (q.v.). The hypoglycemic type is entirely different from diabetic coma. Finally, the lactic acidotic coma also must be kept in mind. In diabetic coma there is a previous stage of increasing symptomatology: weakness, vomiting, excessive thirst and urination, and final unconsciousness; with evidence of dehydration, as very dry skin, irregular deep respirations, hypotonic muscles, normal or mydriatic pupils, strong pulse, acetone odor to the breath, marked hyperglycemia, and glycosuria, together with increased ketonemia and ketonuria. The hypoglycemic coma differs because of the moist or freely perspiring skin, pale or flushed face, soft eyeball, tachycardia and low glycemia, and the rapid relief after glucose administration. Lactic acidosis follows a stage of hyperventilation and mental confusion, with no cyanosis, and no changes of blood pressure or of the peripheral circulation. In the nonketotic hyperglycemic coma there are hyperglycemia and glycosuria, but no acetone is present in blood or urine.

The treatment of diabetic coma creates an emergency situation. It must be carried out in the hospital, the patient well-monitored for vital signs, and an intravenous catheter immediately inserted. As soon as the diagnosis is made, give regular insulin at a rate of 5 to 10 units an hour intravenously (alternate schedules are 15 units to start, followed by 15 units every hour; or 25 to 50 units by vein and by intramuscular injection, every 1 or 2 hours). Insulin-resistant patients require larger amounts, usually a double dose, but these patients are better treated by a specialist. It is better to start fluid replacement with normal saline solution, 1 liter during the first hour, and 300 to 500 ml an hour thereafter. Nevertheless, if the blood pH is below 7.1, or the blood bicarbonate is below 9 mEq for each 1000 ml, give instead the same amounts of hypotonic saline with 44 or 88 mEq of sodium bicarbonate (45 mEq in each 50-ml ampoule). Also, in cases with glycemia over 500 mg%, use a 0.45% saline solution; and when glycemia reaches a lower concentration of 250 mg% or less, use 5% glucose solutions and reduce insulin to half the amount. Some 3 or 4 hours after starting treatment, also give potassium (about 40 mEq every hour). Any other concomitant disease (e.g., infection) will be vigorously treated.

For nonketotic coma start with hypotonic saline, and be sure you are giving the necessary amount of liquid (4 or more liters in the first 10 hours) to obtain the right amount of urine output (no less than 50 ml an hour). Start insulin therapy with 15 units of regular insulin intravenously plus 20 units subcutaneously, to continue with about 20 units subcutaneously every 4 hours. No more than 20 mEq of potassium an hour will be given, but its administration can be started at the very beginning of treatment.

Lactic acidosis is treated with sodium bicarbonate infusions, to bring the blood pH above 7.2.

Regular insulin, 100-unit vials (100 units in each ml).

Normal saline solution, for intravenous infusion.

Saline solution, 0.45%, for intravenous infusion.

Sodium bicarbonate, 7.5%, for intravenous infusion, 45 mEq in each 50-ml vial.

Potassium phosphate, 40 mEq in each 20-ml ampoule.

Hypoglycemic Coma

When patients reach this stage, blood glucose is well below 40 mg%, and some previous symptoms of hypoglycemia have already occurred: flushed or pale face, moist or frankly freely perspiring skin, tremors, tachycardia, or more rarely bradycardia, and there may be the history of a previous administration of insulin or any other hypoglycemic drug. Today, most diabetics carry with them an identifying card with enough data to suggest a diagnosis. Care will be taken to determine whether the hypoglycemic coma is due to the use of sulfonylureas or to any other disease capable of causing a lowering of blood sugar, namely, adrenocortical carcinomas, hepatomas, a previous gastrectomy, or a very intense vagotony. Patients may also be fasting, or a large interval may have elapsed since the last meal. The diagnosis is given by glycemic figures, below 40 mg%. Other more elaborate diagnostic criteria shoud be reserved for a specialist. A good orientation is given by the rapid improvement following the injection of glucose, particularly if the person in coma was perspiring abundantly.

There are patients who react readily with unconsciousness to the slightest transgression of their regimen; these persons should always carry sugar with them, which will be taken at the first indication of an approaching reaction. In these cases, it will be better to complete the meal with some additional food, to avoid a recurrent attack. The amount required is about 10 to 20 g of glucose, by mouth or intravenously, according to individual need. Treat other causes of hypoglycemia individually.

Glucose, 25% solution, for intravenous administration.

Uremic Coma

Elderly persons with uremia are usually in a cachectic state due to a previous kidney disease, which has provoked a precomatose stage with rapid loss of weight, sensations of extreme weakness and coldness, itching, dry mouth with intense fetor hepaticus, vomiting, diarrhea, paresthesias, and mood changes. Patients in uremic coma are pale, with low or elevated temperature, Cheyne-Stokes respirations (apnea—increasing depth of inspiratory movements—decreasing depth of respiratory movements—apnea), increased ammonia odor to the breath (fetor hepaticus), miosis, not rarely hypertension and oliguria or anuria (prostatic hypertrophy), gallop rhythm of the heart, and other evidence of dehydration and infection. The most important signs for diagnosis are the very low concentration of the urine (with more or less notable amounts of protein and red blood cells) and the elevated levels of urea and other wastes in blood. Uremic coma is usually a late stage of any of the following diseases.

Glomerulonephritis: the chronic stage is noted by proteinuria, hematuria, and urine casts.

Nephrosclerosis: evidence of renal insufficiency plus hypertension.

Chronic pyelonephritis: persistent bacteriuria.

Obstructive uropathies: due to prostatitis or renal stones.

Others: infections, metabolic diseases, nephrosis, polycystic kidney, and so on.

Each causative disease will be treated individually. Proteins in diet will not surpass 500 mg for each kilo of body weight in 24 hours, with addition of essential amino acids (new approach: to give alpha-keto or alpha-hydroxy acid analogs). Otherwise, diet will be complete in calories and vitamins; and fluids will be given according to established diuresis. Also give the needed amounts of sodium, potassium, calcium, and phosphate. The use of dialysis or kidney transplants will be discussed with specialists in these fields.

Infectious Coma

Because of a very aggressive infectious disease or poor organic defenses, any person but particularly the frail elderly, will go into coma in a matter of hours. Among these patients, pneumonia following influenza is a relatively frequent occurrence, and should be watched for carefully. Gram-negative organisms, such as *E. coli, Pseudomonas, meningococci, Proteus,* and others; bacteroides; and infections of the central nervous system can easily induce a comatose state. In all instances the etiological factor has to be uncovered and the sensitivity of the offending organism determined in order to give the adequate treatment.

A symptomatic approach will be carried out for immediate relief, but the basic treatment will be an aggressive one against the causative factor. Usually, antibiotics will be given in huge amounts, according to effects and tolerance.

Encephalitis

Eastern encephalitis and encephalitis lethargica may induce shock and a final comatose state. Patients may show fever and the common neurological traits of either disease. Symptoms include: stiff neck, vomiting, convulsions, tremors, myoclonus, ocular paralysis, hemiplegia, and unconsciousness. There may be exaggerated deep tendon reflexes or superficial reflexia. The spinal tap will show elevated pressure and hyperproteinemia. In sleeping sickness, particularly the Gambian type, the disease has a longstanding previous course, and there is a pronounced adenopathy. The incidence among the elderly is low.

For the treatment of encephalitis there are almost no remedies, except those antibiotics effective against known microorganisms. In other instances, reduce cranial hypertension with mannitol, control convulsions, give oxygen, and maintain a good nutrition. For sleeping sickness, consult the Center for Disease Control, in Atlanta, Georgia.

Epilepsy

Only in rare instances will the disease start at an advanced age; the diagnosis depends mainly on the typicality of the seizures because the electroencephalographic records are not always convincing. When it occurs, most cases will reveal a causative factor, which will be sought. Cause may include the following:

Expanding lesions of the brain: tumors are suspected first, but also hemorrhages, cysts, and abscesses.

Intracranial pressure: because of cerebral edema, or hypertensive encephalopathy.

Hyperpyrexia: due to heatstroke, sunstroke, or very acute infections.

Injuries: usually with an obvious history.

Others: the list is relatively long—infective or parasitic diseases of the central nervous system, hypocalcemia, hypoglycemia, permanent bradycardia, anaphylactic reactions, or toxic agents.

Anticonvulsant drugs should be given to patients with seizures, according to the type lf epilepsy, if it is of the idiopathic type, or according to the causative factor, if secondary. Check for more details in other sections of this book.

Blood Loss

If severe enough, shock provoked by blood loss may progress into coma. After a lapse with dizziness, weakness, profuse sweating, tachycardia with feeble pulse, and hypotension (there may be a previous phase of hypertension), the patient faints; and little by little a deep sleep characterizes the outcome of coma. Then, the patient will not respond to any exterior stimulation, even a painful one. The laboratory will report the extreme anemic condition, not rarely after a previous phase of apparent blood concentration.

External hemorrhages are easily detected because the blood is seen flowing from a wound or a natural opening: injuries, epistaxis, hematemesis, or hemoptysis. *Internal hemorrhages* usually are linked to symptoms of shock (see above lines) plus a possible previous history of gastrointestinal or cardiovascular disease.

Injuries: are most commonly noted by inspection, helped by a history of an accident.

Epistaxis: blood flowing from the nose, rarely enough blood to cause shock (less often, coma); but at times flowing backward into the pharynx.

Hematemesis: usually blood coming from esophageal varices or gastric ulcerations; the former regurgitated, rather than vomited like the latter.

Hemoptysis: the blood "coughed" out, usually frothy.

Gastrointestinal hemorrhage: may show a syncopal attack followed by hematemesis or melena; with other symptoms of peptic ulcer, gastritis, or gastric cancer.

Ruptured aneurisms: provoke a rather rapid course of events, with pain, shock, coma, and, not rarely, death, when they are located in the aorta.

Since coma represents an extremely severe stage of the hemorrhagic condition, drastic measures are to be taken, particularly in regard to blood replacement and surgical attempts to stop bleeding. Consider that large amounts of blood will be needed in the great majority of cases; and that if a satisfactory control of symptoms does not take place in a short time, surgical repair will be an immediate need.

Blood for transfusion, well-matched for each individual patient, to be given at reasonable speed to control the situation.

Calcium gluconate, 10% solution; give 10 ml for every liter of blood, always injected intravenously at a slow rate.

For more details see other sections of this book.

Hepatic Coma

The diagnosis is relatively easy because of a history of previous liver disease. Liver cirrhosis, cancer, abscess, and hepatitis are the common causes of hepatic coma. It may also be due to yellow fever, drugs, anesthetics, poisoning by fungi, and other toxic substances. In most instances there is a full clinical picture of the causative disease, to which there are added slight behavioral changes, irritability, confusion, tremors (particularly *asterixis* of the outstreched hands), increased fetor hepaticus, and usually hyperventilation. In coma, the patient seems to be in a very deep sleep, with no conscious reactions even to potent external stimulation, with a total lack of sensitivity and motility. The laboratory will report elevated transaminases, phosphatases, and bilirubin, and decreased cholesterol and serum albumin. Be on the alert for patients treated with chloramphenicol, streptomycin, isoniazid, phenylbutazone, sulfamethoxipyridazine, and also other drugs. For more diagnostic details see the beginning of this section.

Emergency care will consist of providing a patent airway (artificial respiration, if so needed); frequent change of position, the patient lying on one side to avoid pressure ulcers and swallowing of secretions; placement of urinary and blood catheters; and monitoring vital signs carefully; all this is best done in the hospital. Start as soon as possible with blood expanders (plasma, dextran, electrolyte solutions), to restore to normality the blood pressure and pulse; and epinephrine or isoproterenol, to help to increase blood pressure. Give potassium if there is hypokalemia. The diet will consist of only parenteral solutions while the patient is in coma, and avoidance of proteins for a short period thereafter. Give phenobarbital to the agitated patient, and vitamin K to those prone to bleed. Corticoids have been reported to be helpful in most of these cases. Needless to say, the causative disease will be treated as aggressively as possible, particularly infections.

Human plasma protein fraction, 500 ml flask, to be given according to need.

Dextran 40, 10% solution in saline.

Isotonic saline (0.9% solution), to be given as needed.

Epinephrine, 1:1000 solution; give 0.05 to 0.1 ml intravenously; repeated as tolerated and needed.

Isoproterenol, 0.2 mg in each ml, to add from 10 to 15 ml in each 1000 ml of electrolyte solution (preferably 5% glucose in water), and to administer according to blood pressure response.

Potassium phosphate, 20-ml ampoule with 40 mEq.

Lactulose, syrup, 2 or 3 tablespoonfuls, three or four times a day, adjusting the dose according to intestinal action.

Vitamin K, 1 mg in each ml, adjusting the dose according to prothrombin time.

Prednisolone, 25 or 50 mg in each ml, to start with 20 or 30 mg a day, to be reduced and slowly discontinued thereafter.

Adrenal Insufficiency

During an acute adrenal crisis coma may occur. It will present the common traits of deprivation of motility and sensitivity, as in a deep sleep from which not even powerful external stimulation can rouse one. This situation is usually preceded by extreme asthenia, headache, abdominal pain (almost always present, and capable of giving the wrong impression of an acute abdomen; but in this situation there are more localized symptoms and signs), pain and tenderness at one or both costovertebral angles, vomiting, and perhaps diarrhea. There is dryness of the skin and mucosae, possibly with cyanosis with or without petechiae, fever, and low blood pressure. Also, there may be a history of a previous adrenal injury (surgery, hemorrhage, septicemia); surgery to the brain, lung, or prostate; or discontinuance of corticoid therapy. The diagnosis results if the patient is a known Addisonian, with hyperpigmentation, asthenia, scanty body hair, hypotension, and a small heart. The laboratory will report low amounts of cortisone in blood and urine, low amounts of other adrenal hormones, hyponatremia, hyperkalemia, hypoglycemia, and the positivity of special tests when performed.

In the presence of an impending or more likely an overt crisis suggesting acute adrenal failure, there is no need to wait for the laboratory reports to confirm the situation, but there is need for immediate intravenous administration of hydrocortisone followed by infusion of adequate amounts of the same hormone. Cortisone is a good alternate if there is no hydrocortisone available. If there is a psychotic reaction, instead of corticoids give an aqueous adrenocortical extract, no matter that its efficiency is of dubious value. Watch for hypokalemia during the second couple of days, and give potassium if needed.

> Hydrocortisone, 25 or 30 mg in each ml, to start with 100 mg intravenously—immediately—followed by infusion of 50 to 100 mg every 6 hours the first day, every 8 hours the second day, then to continue every 8 hours, but reducing the dose gradually.

For more details, see entries in preceding sections.

Hyperthyroid Coma

This type of coma is extremely rare, but may occur following a very severe thyrotoxicosis—particularly of the "storm" type—with cachexia, extreme asthenia, *dysphagia,* and final comatose state.

Treat as for thyroid storm: absolute bed rest, oxygen therapy, cold packs to reduce hyperpyrexia, sedation with phenobarbital, intravenous propranolol, propylthiouracil, and corticoids. Sodium iodide and cholestiramine may be added.

> Phenobarbital, 30 mg, by intramuscular injection.

> Propranolol, 1 mg in each ml, to give intravenously 1 mg in 1 minute; maximum dosage for each administration should be 3 mg or less, with time given for it to reach an effective action; second dose may be given after 2 or 3 minutes; always carefully monitoring the heart function and the central venous pressure to avoid drastic lowering of the blood pressure (may reach cardiac standstill).

> Propylthiouracil, 50 mg tablets; to give by nasogastric tube in amounts of 100 to 200 mg, every 6 hours.

> Hydrocortisone, 25 or 50 mg in each ml, to start immediately with 100 mg given intravenously, and to continue according to response, about 50 mg, every 8 hours; decreasing the dosage as soon as possible, to discontinue gradually.

Sodium iodide, ampoules containing 100 mg in each ml; give 10 ml intravenously, every 12 or 24 hours.

Cholestyramine resin; give less than a teaspoonful (some 4 g) with meals, when the patient is able to swallow.

Hypothyroid Coma

This is also a rare occurrence, which may happen with severely myxedematous patients. It may be an adrenal crisis due to thyroid therapy in cases of pituitary myxedema. Hypothyroid coma may occur in insufficiently treated myxedamatous patients. It usally starts with intense hyperpnea, which may result in deep sleep leading to real coma. The knowledge of a previous hypothyroid condition, obvious as in the case of myxedema, makes the diagnosis of hypothyroid coma easy. The prognosis is usually grave.

Emergency treatment requires the intravenous use of levothyroxine sodium, together with hydrocortisone and adequate pulmonary ventilation. When the patient recovers from coma, liotrix may be given by mouth.

Levothyroxine sodium, 500 μg in each 10-ml vial; give 4 to 6 ml (200 to 300 μg) intravenously, repeating half the dose in 12 hours.

Hydrocortisone, 25 or 50 mg in each ml; give about 100 mg every 8 hours during the first day, then reduce and slowly discontinue this medication.

Liotrix preparations; give 15 but no more than 30 mg to elderly persons on thyroid medication; but the dosage must be carefully adjusted to response and tolerance.

Acidosis

In *respiratory acidosis* there is drowsiness going into stupor and finally coma, which may occur in patients with pulmonary emphysema and those with depressed respiratory center (nervous system disease, drugs, anesthesia), myasthenia gravis, congestive heart failure, pneumonia, lung disease, and laryngeal obstruction (edema, foreign body), and as an accident in assisted respiration, leading to an excess of carbon dioxide.

In *metabolic acidosis,* as in diabetic acidosis, there is some evidence of dehydration, and the coma is preceded by abdominal pain, asthenia, headache, and hyperpnea. This condition may be due to diabetes, diarrhea, salicylate poisoning, renal failure, or any form of dehydration. Severe forms lead to coma.

Laboratory reports will indicate a decreased pH in the blood for both forms of acidosis, but the CO_2 is decreased in metabolic acidosis and increased in respiratory acidosis.

In respiratory acidosis try to improve respiratory movements by using aids or bronchodilators. Care must be used when giving oxygen because it may lead, paradoxically, to CO_2 narcosis! In other cases, restore acid–base equilibrium of the blood by means of sodium bicarbonate solution given intravenously, better in 5% glucose solution. The condition causing acidosis will be treated aggressively.

> Sodium bicarbonate, 7.5% solution, for intravenous infusion, 45 mEq in each 50-ml vial; add one or two vials (rarely three or four) to 1 liter of 5% glucose in water. The correct amount to be given can be calculated by multiplying the blood bicarbonate deficit expressed in mEq by 25% of the body weight.

Intracranial Hypertension

Patients with intracranial hypertension will present a very intense headache, projectile vomiting without accompanying nausea, and papilledema followed by coma. These symptoms are practically diagnostic, either when presented together or in any possible combination. A few patients will show bradycardia, sleepiness, ocular palsies, seizures of the epileptic or the Jacksonian type, dizziness, diplopia, and perhaps other manifestations of focal neurologic disorders. The great majority of cases will correspond to an expanding lesion within the skull.

> *Brain tumor:* symptoms of cranial hypertension, plus evident symptomatology of location of the tumor, which diagnosis will be better referred to the neurologist.

> *Brain cyst:* usually as above.

> *Cerebral abscess:* with symptoms of cranial hypertension, plus symptoms of the causative infection, usually with fever (not rare in cases with brain tumor), and history of a previous infective disease.

There are also cases due to pure arterial hypertension (with vomiting, headache, and papilledema).

For the relief of symptoms due to intracranial hypertension the best procedures to follow are: administration of mannitol; urea; glucose, or, better, invert sugar.

> Mannitol, 10% solution, by intravenous drip.

> Urea, 30% solution; give 1 g of urea for each kilo of body weight, also by intravenous infusion.

> Glucose, 50% solution, for intravenous drip.

> Invert sugar, 10% solution; give by intravenous infusion.

Intracranial Hypotension

This is a rare occurrence, not easy to diagnose, which may appear without any known cause or may follow spinal tap, dehydration, hemorrhage in the meninges, meningitis, or other diseases. Initial symptoms are: headache, dizziness, stiffness of the neck, pain along the spine, and mood changes; symptoms of established intracranial hypotension are: cardiac arrhythmias, feeble pulse, Cheyne-Stokes respiration, and evidence of impending coma. If a spinal tap is inadvertently performed, all symptoms worsen. The final diagnosis and treatment are usually reserved for the neurologist.

Traumatic Coma

All severe injuries will cause shock, and if severe enough, a following coma. The diagnosis will be obvious in the majority of cases. Such a reaction may even occur immediately following an injury when the patient appears in good condition. For this reason, it will be very desirable to hospitalize all these patients and to check them with the aid of a neurologist.

The immediate treatment will be as for stroke or shock, which will be found in previous sections of this chapter.

For more complete information see the corresponding entry "Injuries," in the section devoted to "Shock."

Meningitis

As stated before (see corresponding entry in the section on "Stroke"), older persons suffering from meningeal infections may go rapidly into coma, with loss of motility and sensitivity, not responding to strong external stimuli, with evidence of paralyses of the limbs and face, contracted pupils, stiff neck, and positivity of such reflexes as Babinski (extension of toes on plantar irritation), Brudzinski (legs flex when the neck is forced to flexion), and Kernig (the legs flexed as above resist attempts to restore them to extension). In other words, a patient with evidence of meningeal reaction will go into coma, and the best help for diagnosis will be the examination of the spinal fluid. The fluid will show hypertension in bacterial meningitis, along with an increased number of cells and protein, and decreased glucose. In viral meningitis the amount of glucose is normal and there are fewer cells. In both instances the causative factor can be identified.

Try to normalize blood volume and pressure with electrolyte solutions and perhaps with levarterenol; the basic procedure is to treat the causative infection very aggressively and to give cortisone.

Isotonic electrolyte solution, to be given at a rate sufficient to maintain an adequate blood volume.

Levarterenol, 4 to 6 mg, added to the above solution or to 5% glucose in water (1000 ml).

Ampicillin, 200 mg for each kilo of body weight in 24 hours, in divided doses every 3 or 4 hours, intravenously.

Kanamycin, 15 mg for each kilo of body weight in 24 hours, intramuscularly, in two or three installments (not to surpass 1500 mg a day).

Hydrocortisone, 50 mg to start, followed by the same amount in the intravenous drip every 6 or 8 hours; to reduce and discontinue its administration as soon as possible.

Alcoholic Coma

When the patient reaches the coma state, it is not too deep, ordinarily, because most cases respond to painful stimuli. There are alcoholic breath, red face and eyes, equally moderately dilated pupils with conjugate deviation of the eyes, deep and noisy respirations, decreased body temperature if there is hypoglycemia (other patients may present fever or normal temperature), and evidence of nervous depression and gastric irritation, with positive Babinski reflex, trismus, and vomiting. The laboratory will report concentrations of alcohol in blood over 200 mg%.

Try to recover as much alcohol as possible from the stomach by means of lavage with warm tap water containing activated charcoal. Do not give ipecac to the unconscious patient. Maintain a patent airway, and keep the patient warm. Assist respiration, if necessary. Give hypotonic sodium chloride solution together with 5% glucose solution by intravenous infusion, to maintain a good urine output (which should be measured). Other blood expanders should be given if necessary. Give diazepam to the excited patient.

Sodium chloride, 0.45% solution, at sufficient speed to maintain an adequate urine outflow.

Glucose, 5% solution, to be given with the above.

Dextran 40, 10% solution in any of the above.

Diazepam, 10 mg, added to the intravenous drip.

Barbiturate Poisoning

This poisoning is due to suicidal intent in the great majority of instances. Coma may occur with only moderate drugging and will almost always be present with severe poisoning. These patients will present shallow and slow respirations, cyanotic cold clammy skin, dilated and nonreactive pupils, decreased or abolished reflexes (including corneal) with muscle twitching, and other symptoms of circulatory collapse. There are low blood pressure, feeble irregular pulse, and the final coma, usually deep. The laboratory will report barbiturates in the urine.

Stomach lavage (tap water with charcoal) will be helpful if performed within 4 hours after the ingestion. Maintain a patent airway, and assist respirations whenever needed. Try to reexpand blood volume with an electrolyte solution, plasma, or other expanders; and to increase blood pressure with vasopressors. Dialysis is required in severe cases.

Sodium chloride, 0.45% solution, for intravenous infusion.

Plasma, for intravenous infusion.

Dextran 40, 10% solution in the above sodium chloride solution.

Levarterenol, 0.2% solution containing 1 mg in each ml; give 4 (up to 8) mg in any of the above solutions.

Cocaine Poisoning

Cocaine is usually injected. Following symptoms of stimulation, there are symptoms of depression and final stupor and coma. The patient sweats, but the mouth is dry; there is mydriasis, and elevated temperature; bradycardia is followed by tachycardia, and hypertension by hypotension, respirations appear difficult, and there may be convulsions.

Put a tourniquet proximal to the site of the injection. If the drug was swallowed, perform gastric lavage with permanganate; give oxygen or assist respiration, as needed. Give phenobarbital for excitement.

Phenobarbital, 30 mg, by intravenous injection, as sedative.

Potassium permanganate, 1:10,000 solution, for gastric lavage.

Poisoning with Opium or Derivatives

Here we shall consider opium, morphine, meperidine, methadone, codeine, and heroin—which drugs are given either by mouth or by injection. Initial symptoms are those of stimulation of the nervous system, followed by those of depression and final stupor and coma. There are sweating and dry mouth, pale skin (possibly with rashes), tachycardia preceding bradycardia, characteristic miosis (but the pupils may dilate at a later stage), relaxed muscles and absent reflexes, slow respirations (shallow, irregular, stertorous, and of the Cheyne-Stokes type), low temperature and low blood pressure, and after the symptoms of shock a deep coma.

Naloxone seems to be the drug of choice for poisoning with this kind of narcotic; levallorphan or nalorphine is an acceptable alternate (but not to be used in poisoning with pentazocine). If the drug is injected, apply a proximal tourniquet; if swallowed, give a stomach lavage with potassium permanganate, 1:10,000 solution; inject sodium sulfate before removing the tube. A high enema may also be given. Keep the patient warm, change his position frequently, maintain a free airway, assist respiration when necessary, expand blood volume with electrolyte solutions, and monitor vital signs.

Naloxone hydrochloride, ampoules containing 0.02 or 0.4 mg in each ml (ampoules of 2 and 1 ml, respectively); give intravenously 0.005 mg for each kilo of body weight; repeating *only* when needed to maintain a response to external stimuli.

Levallorphan, solution containing 1 mg in each ml, in 1- or 10-ml containers; give 0.02 mg for each kilo of body weight by the intravenous route, repeating twice (at 10- or 15-minute intervals) if so needed.

Potassium permanganate, 1:10,000 solution, for stomach lavage.

Sodium sulfate, 30 g in water solution.

Carbon Dioxide (CO_2)

Respiration in poorly ventilated spaces will cause symptoms starting at a 2% concentration of CO_2 and becoming lethal when a 10 to 15% concentration is reached; there are elevated blood pressure, extreme weakness of muscles, red throat, dyspnea, and palpitations; but with the progression of the poisoning there will be hypotension and coma. Before going into coma these patients complain of headache, general discomfort, and ringing in the ears.

The administration of oxygen is the only acceptable treatment, which will be assisted in many instances. Cardiorespiratory resuscitation is frequently required to save these patients.

Carbon Monoxide (CO)

This poisoning is another way to commit suicide (starting the car engine and staying in the garage with the doors shut). Symptoms include elevated blood pressure and full bounding pulse, vomiting, and changed skin color (dusky, flushed, or cyanotic) in only about half of the patients. There are paralysis, muscular twitching followed by rigidity (jaw), accelerated and stertorous dyspnea, and final coma.

Remove patient immediately from the toxic air, with as little effort on his part as possible; loosen his clothes, and keep his body warm. Complete rest for many hours is mandatory, and 100% oxygen the basic therapy. In very severe cases some advocate a phlebotomy followed by blood transfusion. Glucose, 50% solution, and prednisolone, both intravenously, are used to control cerebral edema.

Blood, well-matched, for transfusion.

Glucose, 50% solution, to give 50 ml intravenously.

Prednisolone, 25 or 50 mg in each ml; start by giving 20 or 30 mg a day; reduce the dosage and slowly discontinue it thereafter.

Lead Poisoning

More frequently encountered with children, it may occur at any age. The adult comatose patient may be a known sufferer from industrial chronic lead poisoning, who may have developed toxic encephalopathy or may have had a cerebral accident of hemorrhage or thrombosis. The "lead-line" may be present in the gums of some patients. The laboratory usually gives good clues for diagnosis, namely, increased amounts of lead in the blood and in the urine (over 0.01 m%), microcytic anemia, and an almost typical basophilic stippling of the erythrocytes.

Basic treatment of this stage is carried out with dimercaprol (BAL), either alone or combined with calcium disodium edetate. Cerebral edema is treated with glucose or mannitol and corticoids.

Dimercaprol, 3-ml ampoules containing 100 mg in each ml, to give 3 mg for each kilo of body weight every 4 hours by deep intramuscular injection; the third day, give it every 6 hours; and thereafter, every 12 hours, for about 10 days.

Calcium disodium edetate (also, calcium disodium versanate), 20% solution in 5-ml ampoules; give 15 to 20 mg for each kilo of body weight every 12 hours by slow intravenous infusion, for only 5 days; if necessary, may repeat after a 2-day interval.

Glucose, 50% solution; inject 50 ml intravenously.

Mannitol, 10% solution, for intravenous administration.

Sunstroke and Heatstroke

Persons with a large portion of the body exposed to the damage caused by heat (either from the sun or any other source) will rapidly go into shock, usually following the regular symptoms of this kind of injury, and then into coma. Dermic symptoms appear, with the bullae of second degree burns in sunburn or of second or third degree burns in other instances. In all instances the diagnosis is easily made because of the history of exposure.

Treat shock, and try to decrease body temperature with a tub bath or iced sheets (not below 38.5° rectally—checked every 10 minutes). If overtreated, the patient has to be rewarmed with blankets or hot drinks. Treat local lesions (avoiding oily preparation), and control fever, and pain if present.

Sodium bicarbonate, 2 or 5% solution; apply locally, ad libitum.

Calamine lotion; apply locally after using the above solution, three or four times a day.

Acetylsalicylic acid, 600 mg, tablets; take every 4 to 6 hours.

Electrolyte solutions, to expand blood volume, as needed.

Plasma or dextran 40, to expand blood volume, as needed.

Levarterenol, 4 to 6 mg, added to 1000 ml of 5% glucose, or to same amount of electrolyte solution.

Hydrocortisone; start with 50 or 100 mg given intravenously; follow with same amount every 6 hours the first day, and every 8 hours thereafter, trying to decrease the amount as soon as possible, and to discontinue this therapy slowly.

Accidental Hyperthermia After Exposure to Cold

We have all heard the unfortunate stories of elderly persons who, having been deprived of the means to keep their homes warm, have frozen to death. The elderly have little resistance to lower temperatures, and in situations that could be tolerated by others they rapidly develop symptoms of intolerance, which include confusional states, vascular collapse with slowing of blood circulation, decreased oxygenation of tissues, and edema. The most damage, probably, comes from multiple thrombosis, provoking myocardial infarction, pancreatitis, and gastric ulcerations; and also from secondary pneumonia, due to the damage to the lungs, which may also cause impaired ventilation and resultant metabolic acidosis. Peripheral vasoconstriction leads to gangrene of the distal areas. As a consequence of all those alterations, the patient shows changes of mood and behavior, dysarthria, and ataxia; develops intense asthenia; and goes into coma. The skin becomes pale and very cold, its dryness evident together with some edema. Also noted are sluggish reflexes and stiff neck. There is low blood pressure, with bradycardia, arrhythmias (beware of ventricular fibrillation), and slow respirations. A characteristic *J wave* (may be present also with low pH, or elevated pCO_2 or calcemia) in the electrocardiogram confirms the diagnosis (appears at the junction between S and T in left chest leads).

Muscles become rigid, gangrene of distal parts may appear (nose, ears, toes, fingers), epigastric tenderness may result from pancreatitis, and, finally, the temperature drops considerably, to less than 35°C (95°F). Below 32.2°C (90°F), the prognosis is extremely poor, with death occurring in most instances. Other factors contributing to development of hypothermia are: the use of certain drugs (salicylates, phenothiazines, barbiturates, diazepam, reserpine, imipramine, alcohol), injuries, steatorrhea, and hypothyroidism. The diagnosis will not be too difficult because of the history and the findings; the J wave may confirm it. Many patients suffer repeated reactions of this type!

Certain special steps should be taken for the total treatment of these cases. In the first place, rewarm patients, but *not too actively* (0.5° to 0.7°C an hour); it is enough to cover them with a single blanket in a room heated to about 26° to 32°C (78.8° to 89.6°F). Recool if there is a fall of blood pressure; start rewarming after stabilization. Try to expand blood volume with 5% glucose in water warmed to 37°C (98.6°F), or use dextran 40. Do not give thyroid preparations to the elderly, as has been suggested for the treatment of frozen people. Hydrocortisone is a very good additional help. If the patient stops breathing, perform a cardiorespiratory resuscitation, and give oxygen therapy. Others claim any medication unnecessary and advocate a simple rewarming of the patient as explained in the above lines. Since pulmonary infection is almost sure to occur in the elder patient, protect these patients with a broad-spectrum antibiotic of the type of tetracycline.

Glucose, 5% solution in water, warmed to body temperature (37°C); give by intravenous infusion.

Dextran 40, 10% solution, in 5% glucose or isotonic saline (500 ml).

Hydrocortisone, 100 mg by intravenous drip, every 8 hours during the first day, thereafter reducing the dosage gradually and discontinuing medication at a slow rate.

Tetracycline, 250 mg by intravenous drip every 6 hours; or 500 mg every 12 hours.

High Altitude Sickness

Persons rapidly transported to places located at high altitudes may present headache, asthenia, drowsiness, chilliness, vomiting, dyspnea, and cyanosis, followed by irritability, vertigo, visual and auditory disturbances, flushed face, Cheyne-Stokes respirations, and perhaps other evidence of cerebral edema. Symptoms may clear in one day, but they may progress to a comatose condition. Before this happens, the patient should be returned to a lower altitude.

As soon as symptoms start to be of some intensity, give oxygen therapy, which will relieve them very rapidly. Those who do not become adjusted to the new altitude should be returned to sea level as soon as possible.

IV. MENTAL DETERIORATION

HANDLING THE MENTALLY DETERIORATED PATIENT

Evidence of mental deterioration is far from a rarity among older people. It may indicate a purely psychiatric disease, or it may be a reaction to a disease alien to psychiatry. Included in this last group is what is considered as senility, the main factors being failing memory, emotional irritability, confusion of the mind, or anxiety, depression, delusions, or hallucinations, and the final grouping of symptoms characterizing dementia. Evidence of both types of mental deterioration is described as follows:

Failing memory, mainly for recent events, is one of the earliest symptoms of mental deterioration, present even with persons who still are perfectly alert and oriented in all other senses.

Emotional states presenting fear, apprehension, sadness, loneliness, and the like, in a previously normally oriented person, may follow drastic changes in life, namely, retirement, new environment, or loss of close relatives, or be apparent without a known cause.

Irritability as a reaction to futile causes, particularly in previously friendly personalities, will suggest some internal change.

Confusional states characterized by disorientation as to person, place and time constitute an individual psychopathic condition.

Anxiety evidenced by apprehension, tension, fatigue, palpitations, tachycardia, sweating, hyperventilation, or aerophagia, also suggests a mental change.

Depression, differing from anxiety because of irritabiltiy, boredom, poor concentration, and the idea of helplessness and lack of any future interest, is another symptom of change.

Delusions may represent more serious diagnostic problems, since they occur in patients of otherwise normal mental functions, with good intellectual capability, but who present erroneous beliefs not due to true mistakes, not always evident to the interpreter, but evident by themselves when discovered, because of the reluctance of the patients to accept them as a mistake.

Hallucinations are easily determined when the patient refers to unreal perceptions of the eyes or the ears.

Dementia constitutes a summation of several of the above symptoms, thus integrating an irreversible deterioration of most, if not all, intellectual functions, namely, memory, attention, emotions, judgment, and so on.

Any of these reactions may indicate the presence of a psychiatric condition or the initial stage of a different disease, as stated above. Efforts will be made with older persons first to rule out organic diseases, such as an infection, a prostatic problem, a thrombosis or hemorrhage affecting the brain, and many others. In this section of the book emphasis will be on the medical aspect of mental deterioration. The psychiatric aspect will be better appreciated and treated by a specialist. Thus, we shall consider the situations described in the following list.

Initial phases of syncope, shock, and coma may be accompanied by behavioral changes, irritability, or confusion and followed by the common symptoms of the causative condition plus the lowering of blood pressure and unconsciousness.

Chronic brain syndrome is the established sequence of an acute organic brain syndrome with impairment of memory, emotional responses, orientation (confusional states), and other intellectual functions: usually leading to or being the product of presenile or senile dementia, chronic alcoholism and other toxics, arteriosclerosis of brain vessels, brain tumors, local or systemic infections, and other chronic diseases as well.

Anemia is at times evidenced only by paleness, weakness, and change of mood, irritability, or depression; diagnosis is backed by the hemogram findings.

Lung diseases may also start by showing some sort of mental deterioration, for instance, pneumonia starting with a confusional state. All older persons presenting mental impairment have to be very carefully checked for a lung condition.

Hypoventilation will be evidenced by weakness and change of mood (irritability, depression) and possibly other symptoms of hypoxia.

Carbon dioxide poisoning is but a form of hypoventilation.

Myocardial infarction is to be feared when dealing with elderly persons presenting only symptoms of mental deterioration, particularly if symptoms are of sudden appearance; under these circumstances, all elderly persons will be checked for this condition, regardless of the symptomatology shown by them.

Heart failure is usually already known to exist, to its symptoms being added others of mental deterioration.

Arrhythmias will cause mental symptoms because of hypoxia; so check for them (bradycardia, permanent slow pulse, fibrillation).

Aortic stenosis presenting elevated diastolic blood pressure and a systolic murmur at the upper right border of the heart may also present mental impairment.

Hypertension of the encephalopathic type presents recurrent attacks of mental changes (confusion, irritability, behavior, mood), together with elevated or rapidly rising blood pressure, headache, vomiting, and convulsions.

Polycythemia may exist when mental symptoms appear, but the disease is diagnosed because of its complications (cerebral hemorrhage or thrombosis, myocardial infarction, bleeding peptic ulcer). In any event, among the earlier symptoms of polycythemia are lassitude and dizziness.

Disseminated intravascular coagulation may be revealed by slight initial mental impairment, but sooner or later the common symptoms of each particular impaired location will alert the physician to the possibility of this generalized occurrence.

Endocarditis may start clinically among the elderly like any other form of disseminated intravascular coagulation.

Systemic lupus erythematosus starts with mental impairment (psychoses of different types) not too rarely, particularly among patients over 60 years of age, thus making the diagnosis complex and delayed until the butterfly erythema appears on the face, and the lupus erythematosus cell, in the blood.

Hypoglycemia starts with its usual symptomatology, but early symptoms could be irritability, incoordination, dysarthria, and particularly disorientation, behavioral changes, and perhaps convulsions. If the patient is on antidiabetic therapy, the diagnosis is practically sure to be hypoglycemia; otherwise, it will be suspected as soon as hypoglycemia below 40 mg% is reported.

Hyperglycemia occurs mainly in known diabetic patients who become weaker, dizzy, and confused or irritable before going into coma.

Hypocalcemia causing latent or overt tetany is also accompanied with some frequency by evidence of irritability and psychotic changes; one of us has described a syndrome of "hypoparathyroidism with mental changes and ectodermal disorders" usually starting at younger ages, but which may be prolonged into or become evident in later years (the accompanying ectodermal disorders are early cavities and erosion of the free borders of the teeth).

Hypercalcemia shows disorientation, asthenia, lethargy and collapse during acute crises.

Hyperthyroidism starts in older people either with tremor, irritability, excitability, nervousness, exhilaration, or delirium changing into depression; or with apathy, indifference, sluggishness, and cachexia.

Hypothyroidism may reach the state of "myxedema madness" with paranoid delusions or other forms of psychoses; the diagnosis depends on obvious evidence of myxedema—not obesity!

Hypopituitarism of the cachectic type (Simmonds' disease or Sheehan's syndrome) may start with confusion and thereafter weakness, extreme fatigability, and the corresponding laboratory and X-ray evidence of the glandular involvement.

Hyperpituitarism may show insomnia and psychoses whenever it causes adrenal hyperfunction (Cushing's syndrome).

Dehydration presents confusion as one of the frequent symptoms, together with skin and tongue dryness, hypotension, oliguria, and final shock.

Hyponatremia due to "water intoxication" causes lethargy, stupor, and confusion before reaching the comatose state.

Hypernatremia also causes confusion, stupor, and final coma.

Alkalosis, both the metabolic and the respiratory type, may cause excitation and agitation because of generalized irritability.

Infections, either systemic or localized ones affecting the elderly, may show a confusional state or marked irritability of sudden onset as the first symptom in a person previously in better mental condition. Consequently, the search for symptoms of infection has to be carefully made. Fever is not too reliable a symptom in these patients. Check systemically for generalized infections (influenza is number one), then for localized infections (lungs, abdomen, circulatory system, central nervous system, in this order—and for men include the prostate).

Meningitis and *encephalitis* can induce any reaction from the central nervous system, including psychologic ones. Most probably other evidence of nervous involvement will appear to aid the final diagnosis.

Intracranial hemorrhages will be noted by clinical evidence of a stroke. If the stroke develops insidiously, symptoms of confusion are most likely to occur.

Poisoning will cause, beside the specific symptomatology, some sort of mental derangement; for which reason it will be safest to check geriatric patients for poisoning whenever the onset of mental impairment points out the occurrence of an abnormal situation.

Other diseases of any kind, namely, of the liver, the kidney, and so on, may present mental troubles together with their specific symptomatology; but at times the mental troubles will be most prominent symptoms.

This long list of possibilities makes obvious the need for a complete plan for examination of the patient. In all instances it should be a complete physical together with all needed secondary help from the laboratory, radiology department, or any other resource. In other words, all organs and systems are to be examined, and special emphasis is to be put on those phases of the examination that should appear suspicious. This is the only way really to serve our patients.

Naturally, treatments will vary widely in accordance with any possible cause of disease, for even sedation will be somewhat different from patient to patient. The reader is referred to each particular instance in the following pages.

Personality Changes

These changes are not easily detected because they start gradually, in many cases being only a slow increase in emphasis of previous personal traits. The main symptoms are: exaggerated introspection, apathy, lack of interest and initiative, obsessions, and obscenity. Two main problems may arise: the first is the obsessional neurosis, with unwanted, anxious, insistent, and repetitive thoughts of any kind (of having a disease, being parasitized, killing someone, committing obscene acts, and so on); the second, occurring in those in institutions, the institutional neurosis, with a total personal inhibition regarding the surroundings, lack of interest and initiative, apathy, and not rarely a bizarre posture or gait.

Determining how to cope with these problems is the crucial point in the care of the elderly. In general, the social approach is the better help that can be given to these persons. Loneliness is the most important situation to combat; it is better if it can be done at home, but at least it is also to be done with those in institutions, where the attendants cannot always give the needed personal attention. Therapeutically, some benefit may be obtained from the regular administration of thioridazine.

Thioridazine, tablets containing 10 or 25 mg each; start with 10 mg three times a day, increasing at relatively slow steps to 25 mg, also three times a day.

Confusional States

A number of diseases among elderly people will present only confusion, usually accompanied by some sort of malaise; any confused elderly patient previously alert and active may be developing a disease. It is to be noted that confusion is not always acute, except when it is due to injuries, hyper- or hypoglycemic crises, cerebral infarction or hemorrhage, cardiac failure, infectious diseases, dehydration, urine retention, or intoxication with drugs, alcohol, or other toxins. The clinical picture consists of wrong appreciation of the surroundings, as well as of time and persons. Patients will not be aware of where they are, or their own home or closer relatives, and will have no idea of the time in which they are living. Confusional states may follow a well-known and already diagnosed disease; but they may also appear with unknown connection to a causative factor, which may exist no matter how difficult it is to find. The list of causes given under "Handling the Mentally Deteriorated Patient" is a help in achieving this goal. Nevertheless, a brief list of the more frequent causes of confusion is given here.

Senility: this condition develops more or less slowly, with decreased memory, first for recent events; also, ever-lessening attention, diminished brightness and resistance, greater intolerance, and marked evidence of involutional changes (skin, arteries, lens, muscles, and others); there is no evidence of a disease causing confusion.

Diabetes mellitus: this disease is to be suspected first if the patient comes from a family with several cases of diabetes, is obese and/or hypertensive, and presents itching or any of the frequent reactions of peripheral nerves, cardiovascular system, kidneys, or skin.

Organic brain syndrome: there may be a history of intoxication (alcohol, drugs, environmental) or drug withdrawal, a chronic or acute infection, trauma to the head, frank symptomatology of metabolic changes, tumors, cardiovascular disease, or any other disease. Besides confusion there are also other cognitive failures (defective reasoning, poor perception), affective changes (mood, emotion), and usually some evidence of depression.

Fever: this symptom together with confusion may indicate the existence of an infective disease, particularly encephalitis, brain abscess, meningitis, or even heat- or sunstroke after exposure to elevated temperature.

Injuries: following a trauma to the head check for fracture, contusion, concussion, brain laceration, or some of the hemorrhages within the skull; patients will soon become unconscious.

Metabolic diseases: these diseases may or may not be accompanied by specific symptoms, namely, uremia detected by elevated BUN or a worsened prostatitis; electrolyte imbalance also revealed by laboratory reports; hyper- or hypothyroidism diagnosed by the corresponding thyroid tests; Addisonian crisis with great asthenia plus low levels of adrenal hormones.

Vascular diseases: not rarely these diseases present confusion as the main symptom. Myocardial infarction is the most important one to keep in mind, which may or may not show EKG changes. Any form of cardiac insufficiency will cause confusion if there is some cerebral hypoxia. In hypertensive encephalopathy there are usually additional headache, blurred vision, and nausea, the diagnosis is based on an elevated diastolic blood pressure and retinal vascular spasm.

Hypoxia: any condition capable of causing hypoxia will provoke confusion. This is the case of many of the above-mentioned diseases, and also of some tumors (particularly intracranial), anemia, hypothermia, and intoxications (alcohol, carbon dioxide fumes, drugs).

Intracranial tumors: such tumors are usually accompanied by headache, but the blood pressure is not excessively high.

Hypothermia: this condition is noted by coolness of the skin and confirmed by checking body temperature.

Intoxications: the greatest difficulty in diagnosing these conditions among the elderly consists of the outstanding effects caused by minute amounts of the offending substance acting on sensitive patients; nevertheless, anamnesis plays a very important role, whenever available.

Anemia: this condition may be revealed by unusual pallor and asthenia; but at times the diagnosis is difficult, particularly in the case of B_{12} deficit, which should be looked for in all dubious cases of mental confusion.

Diseases causing confusion are to be treated basically, in all instances. Confusion itself will be treated with sedation, with paraldehyde or a major tranquilizer such as thioridazine, since other sedatives may make things worse. Chlorpromazine may also be employed. In other words, to the basic treatment of the causative disease, add any of the following:

Paraldehyde, ampoules containing 2, 5 or 10 ml; inject from 5 to 10 ml, intramuscularly, the dose in accordance with age and corporal volume, and also according to response (some patients may refuse to take fluids and stay drowsy the following day); give it only if absolutely necessary.

Thioridazine, 10 or 25 mg tablets; give 25 mg three or four times a day, according to response and tolerance.

Chlorpromazine, containers of 1, 2, or 10 ml, with 25 mg in each ml; start with small doses—12.5 to 25 ml—when injecting intramuscularly to the frail patient, giving up to 50 or 100 mg in total, according to tolerance and response.

Depression

Depression may be related to a previous causative disease (which might be any of those discussed in the above lines) or may be an independent affective disorder. The main symptoms are hypochondriacal in character, usually in this order: complaints of constipation, insomnia, anorexia, or fear of having a cancer. Together with these complaints the patient will present apathy, withdrawal, evident anxiety, lack of initiative, and other similar symptoms. The combination of depression with anxiety makes it at times difficult to recognize he existence of true depression; which may also be difficult to do in the presence of delusions. There are also patients who are agitated and show paranoid defensiveness, oversensitiveness, suspiciousness, or maniacal symptoms. Because of the intricacies of these symptoms, it will be better to seek the advice of a psychiatrist.

The family physician will take care of the patient until the psychiatrist takes over; or if the case is only a mild one, treatment of causative disease will be carried out immediately and with intensity by the attending physician. In all instances, check carefully for a basic disease, if it is not already evident or known. Try to improve the nutritional state of those who appear to be undernourished (extra food, vitamins, and minerals). Electrotherapy will be advantageously given to many of these patients. Drug therapy may be also beneficial in many instances, with imipramine or amitriptyline (the latter has the advantage of its secondary tranquilizing effect). Depressed patients are better kept in the hospital because the evident risks of undernourishment and suicide exist.

Amitriptyline hydrochloride, in 10-ml vials containing 10 mg in each ml; give 10 to 20 mg (some patients may require up to 30 mg) by intramuscular injection, three or four times a day, according to response and tolerance; resort to oral administration (tablets containing 10, 25, 50, 75, 100, or 150 mg each) as soon as possible.

Imipramine, 2-ml ampoules containing 25 mg each; give about one (or two) ampoules a day, readjusting dosage according to response and tolerance.

The Paranoic Aggressive Elder

Paranoics are oversensitive, suspicious, defensive individuals who cannot adjust well to their peers, who are extremely introverted, and finally tend to blame those around them for personal failures. This condition makes them resentful and aggressive. When dealing with the elderly, mainly unmarried women over 60 or 65 years of age, paranoia will be suspected as soon as a suspicious, resentful person becomes aggressive; nevertheless, the diagnosis has to be left to the psychiatrist, since it is not easy to differentiate paranoia from mania or even schizophrenia. Check for visual impairment, which at times increases reactive paranoia. Also, check for bothersome symptoms, which are at times capable of causing this sort of reaction in those previously predisposed.

If there is a basic cause, namely, deafness, an intercurrent infectious disease, or the like, it will be intensively treated. Nevertheless, the paranoic symptoms do not always recede when the causative disease improves. A very tactful relationship will be established with these patients, because of their suspiciousness and resentfulness; the general care is better directed by a psychiatrist. For amelioration of paranoic symptoms trifluoperazine or thioridazine has been recommended. A final try will be given to electrotherapy, always under the direction of the psychiatrist.

> Trifluoperazine hydrochloride, 10-ml vials containing 2 mg in each ml, or tablets containing 1, 2, 5, or 10 mg each; give 1 mg (0.5 ml) at no less than 4-hour intervals, to reach no more than 6 mg in 24 hours, according to response and tolerance; resort to the oral route as soon as possible, and give 5 mg every 12 hours, the dosage readjusted, usually increased, according to response and tolerance; thereafter, decrease and stop medication.

> Thioridazine, 10 or 25 mg tablets; give 25 or 50 mg three times a day, according to response and tolerance.

Initial Phases of Syncope, Shock, or Coma

It is not rare among the elderly that before syncopal or comatose conditions are fully developed some sort of mental impairment will announce the impending clinical picture. Patients may present irritability, confusion, emotional changes, anxiety, or depression. The diagnosis will not be easy, since these symptoms of mental deterioration may also indicate any other pathologic condition in course. On the other hand, syncope, shock, and coma may be due to several different causes. Consequently, the physician facing this situation actually must solve a very complicated puzzle: first, to know that the mental symptomatology announces syncope, shock, or coma; second, to know the cause of the impending syncope, shock, or coma. The first clue to the development of any of these states may be given by falling blood pressure; at times paleness and sweating with or without arrhythmias (tachycardia or bradycardia, mainly) may occur; also dizziness and light-headedness may complete the picture. Finally, unconsciousness will point out the final diagnosis for syncope, shock, or coma. The way to solve the second part of the puzzle will be found in the corresponding sections on syncope, shock, and coma, which need not to be repeated here.

First steps to be followed are to put the patient in a horizontal position, with a slight elevation of the legs; to be sure that there is a patent airway and to help with the administration of oxygen; and to catheterize the vein to draw blood for adequate tests and for giving blood, plasma, or any other form of blood volume expander. Vasoactive drugs will be considered later, particularly dopamine and isoproterenol. Thereafter, the basic treatment will be carried out.

> Blood, well-matched for transfusion.

> Dextran 40, 10% solution in saline or 5% glucose.

> Dopamine hydrochloride, prepare a 400 μg/ml solution. To administer, start with 2.5 μg a minute intravenously for each kilo of body weight, increasing to 20 μg a minute for each kilo of body weight, according to response.

> Isoproterenol, to give up to 2 mg in 500 ml of 5% dextrose, intravenously, according to response and tolerance.

Chronic Brain Syndrome

Organic brain syndrome, either acute or chronic, may occur at any age, but it is perhaps more frequent at older ages. Patients present a confusional state, with marked disorientation in time and space, diminished attention, increased impairment of memory for recent events, as well as impaired judgment and reasoning, evidence of depression, and the addition of hallucinations and delusions. Disorientation is an important diagnostic clue, as are the visual hallucinations and the deterioration of other intellectual functions. The list of causative factors given under "Handling the Mentally Deteriorated Patient" (q.v.) applies here; nevertheless, let us present a brief reminder.

> *Initial phases of syncope, shock, and coma* with hypotension and other symptoms of the causative condition will cause mental symptoms.

Myocardial infarction presenting a sudden onset of symptoms, plus those corresponding to the disease itself (not always well noted), must be considered.

Disseminated intravascular coagulation, another possible cause, is also of sudden onset, usually accompanied by other symptoms of stroke.

Intracranial hemorrhage developing slowly is more likely to cause mental symptoms.

Infections of any kind, either acute or chronic, general or localized, may cause symptoms of organic brain syndrome.

Intoxications of all sorts (consider in this order: alcoholism, sedatives and tranquilizers of any kind, anticholinergics, antidepressants, or any other chemical of wide use) will cause, together with the specific symptomatology, other symptoms of mental impairment.

Endocrine and metabolic diseases may provoke, sooner or later, besides the usual symptoms, other symptoms of mental impairment (consider in this order: diabetes, hypoglycemia, hypoventilation, carbon dioxide poisoning, hypocalcemia, hypercalcemia, hyperthyroidism, hypothyroidism, hypopituitarism, hyperpituitarism, dehydration, hyponatremia, hypernatremia, alkalosis).

Drug withdrawal, particularly for sedatives and tranquilizers, will cause evidence of mental deterioration.

Alcohol withdrawal will cause reactions as above.

Other causes of organic brain syndrome should also be considered, namely, injuries, tumors, epilepsy, parkinsonism, multiple sclerosis, systemic lupus erythematosus, and perhaps others.

Together with the evidence given by the usual work-up for the causative disease, there may be some abnormalities noted in the electroencephalogram.

Naturally, the basic treatment is that for the causative disease. Disorientation may be ameliorated by the use of tranquilizers (only the major tranquilizers because the minor ones may worsen the situation). The rest of the care is purely symptomatic. A decision has to be made about whether to keep these patients at home or to send them to an appropriate center.

Thioridazine, tablets containing 10 or 25 mg; start with 10 or 25 mg at bedtime, and increase dosage according to tolerance and response of the psychotic symptoms.

Presenile and Senile Dementia

The so-called presenile dementias usually occur before age 60 and mostly constitute Alzheimer's or Pick's diseases. Older patients, with senile dementia, are self-centered and usually present a marked confusional state, particularly noted because of difficulties in adapting to new experiences and surroundings, emotional instability, particularly with irritability, depression, and some paranoic symptoms (defensiveness, oversensitiveness, suspiciousness). In other words, this situation actually becomes a part of the organic brain syndrome. The worst part of it consists of outbursts of anxiety and fear of death.

This is an extremely sad subject, let us state, because of its very close relationship to the vicious, *ominous,* and sinister discrimination against age carried out by employers of all kinds. Most elderly persons confined at home because of age must feel deeply that the waste of their abilities and experiences is like a waste of precious material; indeed, that they are wasting the fuel that maintains their life. On the other hand, the care of the needy elderly should not be a matter of wording, advertising, and political propaganda worth almost nothing to their welfare. A restructuring of laws, rules, and customs is needed to allow them the opportunity to perform their duties—as long as they can do so adequately—in the same way that the disabled are now beginning to be treated more justly. This social injustice is, in fact, the beginning of deterioration for many persons; to it will be added—besides inherited characteristics—all other social circumstances leading to loneliness, such as their children moving away from home, the loss of close relatives and friends who die, and all other changes in surroundings and economy that usually accompany aging.

Let us not talk about the psychological or the social aspects of treatment, which are strongly suggested in the foregoing statements. Medically, if there is a basic pathologic condition contributing to the development of senile dementia, it will be aggressively treated. Irritability may respond to thioridazine or haloperidol; delusions and paranoic symptoms, to fluphenazine or trifluoperazine. Do not give these patients antidepressants or minor tranquilizers, which may worsen the condition. By the way, it will be rewarding, in a large number of cases, to check for self-medication, usually carried out by many of these patients looking for the relief of unpleasant symptoms, particularly insomnia and constipation. Some of these self-administered drugs are really deleterious to them; be sure their use stops.

Thioridazine, tablets containing 10 or 25 mg each; start with 25 or 50 mg at bedtime, adjusting dosage and timing as needed and tolerated.

Haloperidol, tablets containing 0.5, 1, 2, or 5 mg each; give 1 or 2 mg at bedtime, and same dosage—if needed—in the morning; but adjust medication to response and tolerance.

Fluphenazine, long-acting tablets containing 1 mg each; give one or two every day.

Trifluoperazine, tablets containing 1, 2, 5, or 10 mg each; give 1 or 2 mg every day, adjusting dosage to response and tolerance.

Arteriosclerosis

Early diagnosis is usually very difficult, depending mostly on the onset of true arteriosclerotic complications, such as thrombosis, embolism, stenosis, aneurism, or minor evidence of organic brain syndrome. In some instances a good suspicion of sclerotic changes may arise from finding enlarged, tortuous, and somewhat hard peripheral arteries (forehead, arms, legs), which may be seen or palpated; or finding calcified vessels in X-ray films. Also, plethysmographic or oscillometric abnormalities will indicate arterial involvement of the limb vessels. Perhaps, among the earlier symptomatology of affected elderly persons, we can count on precocious evidence of forgetfulness and personality changes and, later, symptoms of impaired memory and confusion. Consequently, when the elderly start with any evidence of mental deterioration, check as carefully as possible the condition of the arteries flowing into the brain to detect more or less advanced symptoms and signs of sclerosis before a major catastrophe occurs. Look first for a lesion in the carotid bifurcation, where a murmur could be heard on auscultation, and positive arteriography will be the final proof—making the search almost compulsory whenever episodes of cerebral ischemia have previously occurred in the form of so-called little strokes. In most instances, particularly if there have been, together with the confusional state, headache and dizziness, and, more important, any minor evidence of focal symptoms (numbness, tingling, diplopia, scintillating scotomas—these in those patients who did not present the condition in earlier years), a more complete cerebral angiographic study will be carried out, including serial brain scans whenever they are considered necessary. If a stroke occurs, the diagnosis will be easier (q.v., in the corresponding section on ''Stroke'').

For good treatment, consideration of the well-known causative factors of arteriosclerosis is a must, namely, diabetes mellitus, hypertension, obesity (including fat-rich diets), heavy smoking, sedentarism, and others. Otherwise, the general treatment for arteriosclerosis becomes mostly preventive. In the first place, regulate the diet carefully, and be sure that the patient follows instructions. A drastic reduction in saturated fats of animal origin will be the first step, that is, bacon and other fat meats, butter, cheese, regular milk, and, most important, cream, egg yolk, chocolate, and all sorts of fried foods. Because of this reduction in fats, a surplus of fat-soluble vitamins will be given, especially vitamin A. Diets will consist of fruits, cereals, bread, skim milk, potatoes, vegetables of all kinds, lean meat, fish, chicken, egg white, cottage cheese, or any other food poor in saturated fats. This diet will be the only treatment, or will be better reinforced (or those medications used when the diet alone fails to decrease blood cholesterol and blood lipids) with clofibrate, thyroid and estrogen preparations, nicotinic acid, and perhaps the pharmacologic administration of unsaturated fatty acids. Cholestyramine has also been recommended. Life can be drastically prolonged whenever some sort of surgery is available for the replacement of the affected vessels; so, the advice of a specialist will be requested.

Clofibrate, capsules containing 500 mg each; give one capsule four times a day, readjusting the dosage to the personal response.

Thyroid extract, tablets containing about 15, 30, or 60 mg (exactly ¼, ½, or 1 grain) each; give some 30 mg to start, readjusting the dosage to response and tolerance, not forgetting that thyroid is not recommended when a serious heart problem is involved.

Conjugated estrogens, tablets containing 0.625 mg each, to give one a day for 20 days, with pauses of 7 to 10 days. Men treated with estrogens may react with gynecomastia.

Nicotinic acid, tablets containing 50 or 100 mg each, to start with one a day, readjusting dosage to response and tolerance (watch for acral vasospasm).

Cholestyramine, packet containing 9 g or cans containing 378 g, to use before each of the three main meals of the day, one packet mixed with water or any other liquid food (before stirring, allow the powder to become moist).

Cerebrovascular Accidents

Before the full accident of a stroke takes place, at times there are premonitory symptoms of the confusional type together with dizziness and headache. These symptoms have been described in more detail in the preceding paragraph on arteriosclerosis, q.v. After the stroke accident, again symptoms of confusion, lack of memory, disorientation, and other forms of mental deterioration occur. The stroke may be due to brain infarction by thrombosis or embolism, or by hemorrhage. Clinically, there is a more or less rapid obnubilation and the patient falls more or less unconscious, with stertorous respirations (may be of the Cheyne-Stokes type), flushed face, bradycardia with a full pulse, not rarely initial hypertension followed by hypotension, and the characteristic flaccidity of one side of the body. With large thrombi the onset is usually acutely violent; with hemorrhage, symptoms are more generalized, and stiff neck is frequently noted. The complete clinical picture also includes dysarthria, fever, vomiting, convulsions, and the focal evidence corresponding to each particular vessel, as follows:

Aortic arch: different blood pressure in both arms.

Subclavian steal syndrome: dizziness and collateral vertebral artery circulation.

Basilar artery: a very extensive symptomatology, with dizziness, paralysis or paresia, staggering gait, dysarthria, confusion, decreased memory, and perhaps blindness or deafness.

Posterior cerebral arteries: ocular signs and symptoms.

Internal carotid: contralateral symptoms.

Middle cerebral artery: also contralateral symptoms.

Anterior cerebral artery: again contralateral symptoms.

In cases of subdural hemorrhage there is usually a previous injury to the head, and radiologic studies are informative. Transient episodes of "little strokes" are not rare with hypertensive encephalopathy, where elevated blood pressure is an important part of the clinical picture. Brain tumors run a slower course; symptoms include evident papilledema and focal signs, and the spinal fluid presents elevated pressure and proteins. Once the acute stage is over, evidence of mental deterioration (confusion, disorientation, decreased memory, and so on) reappears.

The treatment of the acute episode was reviewed at the beginning of the chapter on "Unconsciousness," q.v. Mental deterioration may improve during rehabilitation. There is no need for a very active medication. In the first place, remember that it is agreed that drugs which depress the central nervous system usually worsen the mental condition of these patients. Only small amounts of mildly stimulating drugs are advised for treatment of mental confusion and allied states. Dextroamphetamine has been recommended for this purpose, and will be used according to response and tolerance.

Dextroamphetamine, long-acting tablets containing 10 or 15 mg each, to give one in the morning, not to interfere with sleep, readjusting dosage in accordance with response and tolerance.

Brain Tumors

Evidence of some form of mental deterioration, particularly among the elderly, is the first warning of intracranial tumor. Soon, headache and vomiting will be added, and progressive neurologic symptoms will indicate the location of such a tumor. On clinical examination there will be noted papilledema and increased pressure of the spinal fluid. Focal symptoms usually are the following:

Parietal lobe: there are contralateral symptoms of the hemiplegic type, with motor or sensory seizures, and aphasia if the left side is involved.

Temporal lobe: psychomotor seizures are frequent, usually with aphasia or visual defects.

Frontal lobe: mental deterioration is paramount, at times with convulsive seizures, aphasia, or anosmia.

Occipital lobe: there are mainly visual symptoms (hemianopsia, hallucinations, papilledema).

Cerebellar: there are disturbances of coordination and equilibrium.

Radiologic studies, spinal tap, electroencephalography, and other tests will strongly help in diagnosing cranial tumors. Since many of these tumors are metastatic in origin, the site of the primary lesion has to be found, if not already known.

Surgery, and, in its absence, chemotherapy, are the only advisable therapeutic resources for the treatment of intracranial tumors. However, for symptoms due to intracranial edema and in the interval before surgery, mannitol will be given.

Mannitol, 10% solution, to be given intravenously.

Anemia

Being more or less anemic is a rather frequent situation among the elderly. In most instances there will be a meager symptomatology, and the condition will pass unnoticed unless medical examination is made for some other cause. Only when the anemic state becomes more intense will symptoms become apparent, such as paleness of the skin and mucosae, dizziness, asthenia, tinnitus in the ears and spots seen before the eyes, sometimes headache, and, what is more important for us at this time, other symptoms of mental deterioration, particularly irritability and psychotic changes. A helpful orientation will be to search for blood status whenever an elderly person begins to present a bizarre attitude and is pale. Types of anemia include:

Acute blood loss: the problem is created by an external or an internal hemorrhage, a topic reviewed to some extent in the preceding chapters, q.v. The external hemorrhage is obvious. The internal hemorrhage may start with forgetfulness and confusion, before other symptoms become manifest.

Iron deficiency: usually the symptomatology starts very slowly, but irritability is one of the earlier symptoms among the elderly, together with asthenia, anorexia, gastrointestinal discomfort, dysphagia, and some neurologic symptoms as well (pain, numbness).

Pernicious anemia: B_{12} deficit will also start slowly with asthenia, paresthesias, soreness and smoothness of the tongue, anorexia, other gastrointestinal complaints, and evident mental deterioration, showing symptoms of depression, confusion, and also paranoia.

Folic acid deficiency: rarely, a case will show demential symptoms together with other neurological disorders in a way similar to those noted in pernicious anemia, but these patients are not improved by the administration of vitamin B_{12}.

Other anemias: any form of anemia of sufficient intensity will cause similar mental deterioration.

For the relief of mental symptoms due to anemia, the best treatment is to attack the anemic state itself. An initial transfusion of whole blood or at least packed cells should be given immediately. This is a must in acute blood loss, and will be followed by the closing of the leak site, and other measures against shock, if it is present. Plasma is a good substitute for blood, if the latter is not available. For iron deficiency anemia there is need for some help to relieve mental reactions: inject paraldehyde intramuscularly in acute cases, or give thioridazine by mouth; but start administration of iron immediately, which is specific for this condition. In cases of pernicious anemia, cyanocobalamin (vitamin B_{12}) furnishes the basic and radical therapy, though symptomatic help has to be given at times with paraldehyde, thioridazine, or chlorpromazine; but always remember that this sedative therapy is not always well tolerated by the elderly. Folic acid deficiency will respond to the parenteral or oral administration of this vitamin, though some patients also need the help of corticoids. Finally, all other anemias will be treated according to etiology and the need for symptomatic help.

Blood, well-matched, for transfusions.

Paraldehyde, ampoules containing 2, 5, or 10 ml; inject about 5 or 10 ml intramuscularly, the dosage according to age, corporal volume, tolerance, and response; give it only if absolutely necessary.

Thioridazine, 10 or 25 mg tablets; give 25 mg three or four times a day, according to response and tolerance.

Ferrous sulfate, tablets containing 200 or 300 mg each, or elixir containing 220 mg in each teaspoonful (5 ml); give 300 mg three times a day, according to response.

Cyanocobalamin (vitamin B_{12}), 10-ml ampoules containing 1000 μg in each ml (also repository preparations), to inject intramuscularly 100 μg every other day at the start, to continue once a month as soon as results are obtained; oral maintenance may also be provided, with 2 mg once a week.

Folic acid, 1 mg tablets, to give one a day.

Respiratory Diseases

Sooner or later, a number of respiratory diseases will cause symptoms of mental deterioration. The problem starts when these symptoms herald the respiratory manifestations. Ronchi or râles heard on auscultation will alert the physician to pulmonary diseases, unless the patient presents chronic coughing and expectoration, in which case pulmonary signs will be heard at all times. Nevertheless, cough is a very important early symptom of respiratory diseases, together with sputum production, which perhaps comes next. Pain, dyspnea, and wheezing appear later on. If any of these symptoms and signs appear together with or following mental deterioration, it will be wise to think of a respiratory ailment. In most instances the mental reaction will be due to hypoxia or infection. Respiratory conditions may include:

Chronic bronchitis: late in the disease, or during its acute exacerbations, the patient may present confusion, irritability, or other evidence of mental deterioration; but the diagnosis has usually already been established, years earlier, because of cough and sputum.

Acute bronchitis: some confusion or other mental troubles will be present in very acute attacks; but the symptomatology is evident from the beginning: cough starting dry and turning productive, expectoration, and wheezing and sibilants heard first, turning into ronchi and râles later.

Pneumonia: the disease may start with confusion, irritability, or other emotional changes, before fever and pulmonary symptoms become evident. Convulsions and delirium are not rare. The fever, side pain, sputa, special characteristics, auscultation, and X-ray findings will give the final diagnosis.

Emphysema: this disease may be primary, but it usually accompanies chronic bronchitis.

Lung infarction: the acute onset of this disease with chest pain, dyspnea, and cough with or without hemotysis, usually occurs with a very intense anxiety reaction and a not too rare confusional state.

Atelectasis: together with its acute symptoms (dyspnea, cyanosis, fever, pain, hypotension, tachycardia, wheezing, and cough) there are almost always, with the elderly, irritability, confusion, and finally syncope or shock.

Lung abscess: the mental derangement usually follows a well-established syndrome with septic fever, sweats, cough, and expectoration of pus.

For the final diagnosis of most of these conditions there is a need for good laboratory and X-ray studies, which in most instances will give sufficient supportive evidence. Bronchoscopic studies are advisable quite often.

Only when the mental symptoms are intense or troublesome will some help for them be given with adequate medication. Otherwise, the treatment of the causative disease will solve all the problems. Always remember that the use of sedative medication is not advisable for these elderly pulmonary patients because the secondary depression of the respiratory centers will increase the retention of pulmonary secretions, particularly because of the decreased cough reflex. Oxygen therapy will improve a large part of the symptomatology.

Hypoventilation

This is another form of decreased oxygen supply to the brain capable of provoking symptoms of mental deterioration such as confusion, restlessness, depression, or irritability, or other emotional or psychological changes. Together with the mental depression there will be a lowering of blood pressure, tachycardia, and headache; and if there is acidosis added (respiratory acidosis), there will also be miosis, papilledema, and intermittent contracture of a group of muscles. The usual causes of this respiratory failure are obstructions to the normal air flow, or restrictions to the normal movements of respiration. Let us review the most important situations:

Chronic bronchitis: symptoms present late in the disease or during its acute exacerbations to a patient with chronic cough and sputum.

Emphysema: this disease usually runs its course together with chronic bronchitis.

Asthma: symptoms are mostly a late occurrence in a known asthmatic patient.

Injuries to the chest or cranial trauma may be followed by restricted respiratory movements, and thereafter the mental changes.

Atelectasis and pneumothorax: elderly persons may show mental symptoms together with the acute manifestations of dyspnea, cyanosis, possible fever, pain, hypotension, tachycardia, and pulmonary symptoms.

Pleural effusion: symptoms may occur when it is large enough to cause respiratory restriction.

Heart insufficiency: this condition may cause hypoventilation by itself or because of massive pulmonary congestion restricting gaseous exchange.

Other cases of hypoventilation are due to depressive drugs or diseases acting upon the central nervous system.

Under these circumstances, a good study of arterial blood gases is needed to confirm the diagnosis. Oxygen and carbon dioxide will be the target of these studies. There is oxygen deficit if its partial pressure (Pa_{O_2}) in arterial blood is below 50 mm Hg, either with or without hypercapnia. Also, CO_2 partial pressure (Pa_{CO_2}) above 50 mm Hg is diagnostic.

In all instances the treatment of the causative disease is essential, and will be carried out aggressively. Either acute attacks or chronic states of respiratory failure will be basically treated with oxygen therapy and the relief of the obstruction. In acute crisis oxygen will be delivered at a rate sufficient to keep Pa_{O_2} at about 55 mm Hg (watch for respiratory acidosis); in acute states the Pa_{O_2} may reach 60 mm Hg and is checked at adequate intervals. Obstruction may be relieved by giving aerosol bronchodilators or aminophylline by injection. If intubation and other measures are needed, it is best to have the patient in a specialized center. Do not spare antibiotics or other needed measures.

Isoproterenol, 1:200 solution, to be put in the respirator by placing 0.5 ml of the solution in 3 ml of saline, to be delivered in a 15-minute period, and repeating at needed intervals (from 15 minutes to 2 hours).

Aminophylline, ampoules containing 25 or 250 mg in each ml; inject intravenously (at 10-minute intervals), 250 (up to 500) mg, carefully checking for cardiac reaction (arrhythmia); for maintenance use the same amount in 50 ml fluid (in 30-minute intervals) every 6 hours.

Carbon Dioxide Poisoning

This represents a sort of hypoventilation, and will also provoke asthenia and change of mood, namely, irritability, depression, restlessness, confusion, or other changes. There is also heaviness of the head, dyspnea, hypertension followed by hypotension, and if it is prolonged, a final coma. The diagnosis is obvious when it is found that the patient has been exposed to a poorly oxygenated atmosphere.

Oxygen therapy is the rational care for these cases, following artificial respiration if necessary.

Myocardial Infarction

Any sudden evidence of mental deterioration, particularly of the confusional or the irritability type will alert the physician to search for the development of some basic disease, myocardial infarction being one of the more important ones to consider. Many older persons will start the disease this way, even without any chest pain. So, the physician will not wait until the classic symptoms take place, no matter that perhaps some of them may appear— that is, arrhythmia, hypotension (rarely absent), and later on fever, leukocytosis, and elevated erythrosedimentation and transaminases. Most patients will go into shock sooner or later. Have an EKG done as soon as possible. For more detailed information, see other entries in this book.

These patients should be taken immediately to an intensive care unit. They will be put at rest as the first precautionary care, given oxygen if so needed, and started with anticoagulant therapy if the case is severe enough for it. If there is pain, give meperidine.

> Heparin, to start therapy by injection, giving the aqueous sodium preparation, 100 units for every kilo of body weight, to be followed every 4 hours by 75 units, adjusting dose to have a clotting time of 20 to 30 minutes. Start warfarin at the same time, by mouth.

> Warfarin, give 10 to 20 mg, adjusting dosage for continuation of therapy to about 5 or 10 mg a day, according to prothrombin time.

Heart Failure

In most instances the disease is already diagnosed when mental deterioration starts. That is, the patient also presents dyspnea (exertional, paroxysmal during the night, orthopnea), asthenia, enlargement of the heart and evidence of a congestional situation in the lungs and the liver (hepatomegaly), râles, and ronchi, with the legs showing dependent edema; and these symptoms, together with the positive diagnosis of some sort of organic heart disease, some variations of the arterial pulse, and elevated venous pressure, alert the physician to diagnose heart failure, differentiating it from other conditions such as neurocirculatory asthenia, kidney or pulmonary diseases, or tumors of the lungs or mediastinum. Laboratory and other tests are not very informative in most instances.

Treat the cause, if known, and improve the heart condition. Rest is mandatory to start with. This usually includes the use of hypnotics to help sleep. Only when there is evident improvement will the patient be allowed gradually to resume physical activity. While he is resting, give only small, low-calorie, low-sodium (1 to 2 g), and low-residue meals; these will be bland and repeated four to six times a day. Again, gradually resort to more normal feedings. Give vitamins and mineral supplements whenever needed. Naturally, the basic treatment for heart failure consists of the use of digitalis and diuretics. The use of vasodilators, paracentesis, or peritoneal dialysis has to be reserved for very severe cases.

> Digoxin, tablets containing 0.125, 0.25, or 0.5 mg each; or injectable containing 0.25 mg in each ml; to start with 2 to 3 mg a day (intravenously, 0.75 mg), to continue a maintenance dose of 0.25 to 0.75 mg a day, according to response and tolerance.

> Chlorothiazide, tablets containing 250 or 500 mg each; give 250 to 1000 mg a day, readjusting the dosage according to response and tolerance.

Heart Block and Arrhythmias

Syncope or at least momentary faintness will be present when the interval between heart beats is prolonged more than the cerebral hypoxia will stand. In the case of sino-atrial block, at auscultation no sound is heard between the audible beats. In auriculo-ventricular block, symptoms depend on the type of blocking: with advance blocking there will be palpitations, or dizziness with the possibility that syncope may supervene at times, accompanied by convulsion in the case of Stokes-Adams crises. Other forms of bradycardia or arrhythmia will cause similar symptoms. The electrocardiogram will give an exact diagnosis of the condition encountered: complete lack of waves in a sino-atrial block; prolonged to dissociated P-QRS sequence in auriculo-ventricular block.

Atropine or ephedrine will be given for sino-atrial block; ephedrine or isoproterenol, for incomplete auriculo-ventricular blocks; and the use of a pacemaker for complete auriculo-ventricular block.

> Atropine sulfate, tablets containing 0.4 mg, to take one or one and a half, four times a day, readjusting dosage according to response and tolerance.

> Ephedrine sulfate, 25 mg tablets, four times a day; a double dose may be given, if needed and tolerated, in cases of Stokes-Adams crises.

> Isoproterenol hydrochloride, from 5 to 15 mg, three or four times a day, by the sublingual route.

Aortic Stenosis

Elderly persons, mainly males, with an aortic stenosis previously well-tolerated, will start to present some symptomatology, not rarely including syncopal attacks and other forms of mental impairment. Other common symptoms are asthenia, dyspnea (exertional), anginal pain, the typical murmur (systolic, at the upper right border of the heart) accompanied by thrill, and narrowed differential blood pressure. X-ray studies will show an enlarged left ventricle. EKG studies will reveal left hypertrophy. Extreme care will be taken with these patients, since they are prone to die within the 3 years after developing a frank symptomatology.

Surgical correction of the defect, whenever feasible, is the best solution for this serious problem. It will be decided by the specialist. Meanwhile, the management of these patients will be the same as for those with angina pectoria or heart failure, q.v.

Endocarditis

In the acute stage there will be elevated temperature, chest pains, and a toxic state in which mental impairment is prone to occur (confusion, irritability, or depression). Some of these patients have had a previous operation, an infection, or accidents due to drug addiction. The skin may present petechiae; previous heart murmurs change in character, or new sounds may appear. In subacute endocarditis there may also be mental impairment, fever, generalized pains, anemia, weight loss, splenomegaly, or heart murmurs. In both instances embolic phenomena will complete the clinical picture and worsen the mental condition.

Start immediately an aggressive antibiotic therapy with the specific antibiotic—if known—or with penicillin, cephalothin, methicillin, erythromycin, or any of the tetracyclines.

Arterial Hypertension

Normal blood pressure, as accepted by most authorities, is in the range of 120–80 mm Hg, for, respectively, systolic and diastolic phases. For persons over 60 years of age, a 90 mm Hg diastolic pressure is permissible; but persons with the limits, also accepted by some groups, of 160–95 perhaps should be rechecked every 6 to 12 months. There is no doubt that all those with a diastolic blood pressure of 105 or over do require immediate treatment; below this figure, treatment will be given whenever convenient according to each particular case and considering individual risks.

High blood pressure may exist without causing any symptoms, detectable only by readings of the sphygmomanometer. Usual complaints of these patients are: headache (mainly in the morning, but occurring at any time), palpitations, asthenia, tinnitus, or lightheadedness. Specific complaints of asthenia, cramps, and polyuria may account for hyperaldosteronism; while palpitations, headache, and sweating account for pheochromocytoma. Check for a history of diabetes, heavy smoking, abuse of salt in food, or any other of the known causes of hypertension. In longstanding cases there will also be cardiac involvement (left ventricle hypertrophy due to overwork, paroxysms of nocturnal dyspnea, anginal pains, and possible terminal myocardial infarction), renal involvement (nocturia, hematuria), cerebral symptoms of the stroke type (hemorrhage, thrombosis), and peripheral lesions (pain, cramps, intermittent claudication, impotence in men). In *malignant hypertension* of the *hypertensive encephalopathy* type symptoms are more severe: intense cephalalgia, blurred vision, nausea, vomiting, confusion, convulsions, some of the neurologic symptoms, and even coma. The examination of the patient will reveal narrowing of the retinal arteries, which in more advanced cases will consist of flame-shaped hemorrhages and final papilledema. This is always present in malignant hypertension. Cardiac findings will be evident in advanced cases, with loud second aortic sound, congested lung bases, and some forms of arrhythmia, as well as other findings in the peripheral vessels, as pulse or bruits. It will be convenient to check also, in all instances, height and weight, the thyroid gland, abdomen (particularly for kidneys and aorta), and the extremities. From the laboratory request: urea nitrogen, creatinine, glucose, cholesterol and uric acid in blood, a complete blood count, urinalysis, serum potassium, radiologic studies of the chest or the urinary tract if so advisable, and the adrenal hormones when this gland becomes suspect.

The main goal of treatment is to lower diastolic pressure to a sustained range below 90 mm Hg, or as close to it as possible in other resistant cases. Patients with diastolic pressures below 105 will be treated if the systolic readings are high, if they are heavy smokers, diabetics, or males, or show heart hypertrophy, hypercholesterolemia, hypertriglyceridemia, or a family history of complications of hypertension. These patients will be treated with a thiazide diuretic (hydrochlorothiazide, chlorthalidone) or a potassium-sparing diuretic if symptoms of hypokalemia are easily developed (spironolactone, triamterene)—either alone or in combination with a thiazide. Always be careful when digitalis is used together with a diuretic (increased toxicity), in which instance a potassium-sparing diuretic should be used, or additional potassium given. Patients with diastolic blood pressure between 105 and 130 mm Hg should be initially treated with a diuretic; but if there is no response, a second drug will be added, namely, propranolol, methyldopa, or reserpine. Consider individual side effects of each drug, starting with small dosages which will be increased as needed. Those with diastolic blood pressure over 130 mm Hg, and all those resistant to the above-scheduled regimens will receive an additional hydralazine, to be used with caution in anginal patients. Should the above plans fail, first of all check for the reason for the failure: usually disobedience on the part of the patient, very frequently also excessive sodium intake, and at times the use of other drugs; inquire about the use of "cold remedies," particularly vasoconstrictors, or the occurrence of a secondary cause of hypertension. The last step in the treatment of hypertension is the addition to the plan already followed of guanethidine (instead of or together with hydralazine). In all instances, try to reduce dosage and medication whenever good results are being achieved.

Hydrochlorothiazide; give 50 to 100 mg a day.

Chlorthalidone; give 25 to 100 mg a day.

Spironolactone; give 50 to 100 mg a day.

Triamterene; give 50 to 150 mg a day.

Propranolol hydrochloride; give 40 mg a day to start, increasing gradually to 320 mg a day (rarely 480 mg a day).

Methyldopa; start with 500 mg a day, increasing gradually to 2000 mg a day (rarely 3000 mg a day).

Reserpine; give a daily dosage of 0.1 mg, increasing to a maximum of 0.25 mg a day.

Hydralazine hydrochloride; start with 50 mg a day, to a maximum of 250 mg by slow increases.

Guanethidine sulfate; start with 12.5 mg a day, increasing gradually to 100 mg a day (rarely a maximum of 300 mg will be given).

Polycythemia

In polycythemic conditions the occurrence of mental impairment (confusion or other changes) is mainly secondary to minute thromboses. As in polycythemia vera, most patients will complain of headache, dizziness, marked asthenia, postprandial somnolence, and occasional pains in the muscles of the legs; and will present a dusky-red complexion (perhaps the outstanding symptom), hemorrhages due to hemorrhoids or epistaxis, and hypertension as a rule. The red cells of the blood are increased to above 6 to 7 million.

Polyglobulia due to diseases of the circulatory system (mitral stenosis, cor pulmonale) or to dehydration will be treated according to the basic cause. Leg pain, mostly of the gouty type, will be treated with colchicine, probenecid, sulfinpyrazone, or allopurinol. Polycythemia vera is treated with periodical venesections (remove enough blood—500 to 1500 ml—to keep the hematocrit at 45%) or radiophosphorus therapy given by a specialist. As an alternative to this therapy, chemotherapy with chlorambucil, melphalan, or a similar drug will be considered.

Colchicine, tablets containing 0.5 or 0.6 mg each; give 0.5 mg every hour until control of pain or provoking nausea or diarrhea; alternate schedule, 1 mg every 2 hours; not to exceed a total of 4 to 6 mg in 24 hours.

Systemic Lupus Erythematosus

Among the symptoms selected by the American Rheumatism Association for the diagnosis of SLE, those related to the central nervous system are listed, which may include psychoses (depression, confusion) or convulsions. Four of these 14 symptoms must be noted to make the diagnosis of SLE: butterfly rash, discoid lupus, alopecia, photosensitivity, ulcers in the mouth, Raynaud's phenomenon, arthritis, lupus erythematosus cells, false positive syphilis tests, CNS symptoms, proteinuria, cell casts, serositis, hematologic changes.

Patients with a mild form of the disease need no treatment; others need corticoids, which, however, may worsen mental impairment.

Diabetes Mellitus

Mental confusion is not too rarely the initial symptom of diabetes among patients over 70 or 80 years of age. They may be obese (66%) and/or hypertensive (50%). Other symptoms may be pruritus, asthenia, retinopathy, neuropathy, nephropathy, or a less characteristic arteriosclerotic complex.

Because of the poor symptomatology available to arouse suspicion of diabetes at this advanced age, it is better to check for it whenever an elderly person appears confused: fasting glycemias will be over 120 mg%; and the 2-hour postprandial test, over 245 mg%. Many other diseases also present confusion as the main symptom in many instances. Among them, the diagnostician has to be careful first of all with cases of pure senility (other psychological and physiological changes due to actual aging). An organic brain syndrome will be due to intoxication, drug withdrawal, infection, trauma, or cardiovascular diseases; and the patient will show other cognitive, affective, or depressive symptoms. Confusion with fever mostly corresponds to infective diseases or exposure to elevated temperature. After head injury look for fracture, contusion, concussion, brain laceration, hemorrhage, and possible subsequent unconsciousness. Uremia also presents elevated BUN or a worsened prostatitis. Laboratory reports will help in differentiating electrolyte imbalance, hyper- or hypothyroidism, and Addison's disease. Myocardial infarction is revealed by EKG changes (not always present). Hypertensive encephalopathy shows high systolic blood pressure and other additional symptoms. Intracranial tumors present headache, but no hypertension. Anemia shows unusual skin pallor. Hypothermia causes coldness of the skin and low bodily temperature. Finally, anamnesis will help the diagnosis of intoxication, even when small amounts of the offending substance are given to a sensitive patient.

Diet will be helped with insulin, in most instances. Give no less than 150 g of carbohydrates and 80 g of protein; and as much insulin as needed, starting with about 20 units of Lente or NPH insulin; or 15 units of this slow insulin plus 5 units of regular insulin. Adjustment will be made at short intervals, usually increasing insulin as needed. Only after reaching satisfactory control will one consider an easier treatment with oral hypoglycemics.

Diabetic Acidosis

Usually, the onset is gradual, but soon symptoms become obvious and the patient seems to be very ill. By this time mental symptoms may have occurred in the form of confusional states, depression, or the like. Not rarely, there is abdominal pain simulating an "acute abdomen," with vomiting, meteorism, fever, and leukocytosis. Naturally, a diabetic may have a real "acute abdomen." There are also other revealing symptoms, such as dry and flushed skin, dry mouth, intense thirst, hyperventilation (air hunger) with acetone odor of the breath, tachycardia with weak pulse, and the characteristic hyperglycemia, glycosuria, and decreased CO_2 combining power of the blood serum. Coma may follow. In the great majority of instances this accident will occur to a known diabetic; but beware of the possibility of the disease starting with the patient going into a diabetic coma.

When mental symptoms start the clinical picture, there is no need of giving sedatives or the like; the physician will start insulin therapy immediately and the infusion of hypotonic saline with sodium bicarbonate. The rest of the treatment belongs to a specialist.

> Regular insulin, 200 to 700 units or even more during the first 24 hours; starting with 50 units by subcutaneous injection together with 50 units by vein; and repeating 50 to 100 units every hour until a beneficial effect is achieved, noted in symptomatology or in laboratory findings; then, decrease the frequency.

> Hypotonic saline, with one or two ampoules of sodium bicarbonate (7.5%) added in 1 liter; to infuse at a relatively rapid rate to reach about 2 liters in some 4 hours, checking the effects carefully according to laboratory reports.

Hypoglycemia

It is well known that patients going into hypoglycemia resemble those with an acute alcoholic intoxication. In other words, mental impairment may be the first warning of the impending situation. Most patients will be those on insulin or other hypoglycemic agent for treatment of a known diabetes; or those who neglect to have food at the due time, particularly following the administration of the hypoglycemic drug. Others, who are not diabetics on insulin therapy, may also present hypoglycemic bouts, such as those with pancreatic tumors, following gastrectomy, and others. The symptoms will be, besides those of mental impairment, moist and pale skin, frequently hunger, shallow respirations, full and bounding pulse, frequent tremors, and possibly convulsions before coma occurs. Hypoglycemia below 60 mg% is pathognomonic (below 40% reveals impending coma).

The objective of the treatment is to restore immediately the lost balance of blood sugar concentration. A patient still alert, or semialert, will be able to take some sugar by mouth or any beverage with sugar (fruit juice, with added sugar), honey, candies, and so on. For this reason, all patients potentially subject to hypoglycemia should carry with them lumps of sugar at all times. Those who are not able to swallow will be immediately given an infusion with dextrose. Thereafter, these patients should be under the guidance of a specialist in diabetes.

> Dextrose, 25% solution; inject intravenously 40 to 80 ml (equivalent to 10 or 20 gr of glucose).

Hyperthyroidism

Regular cases presenting overactivity, irritability, sweating, tremors, diarrhea, tachycardia, exophthalmos, and goiter are very easy to diagnose at any age; but the elderly who become apathetic and lethargic, perhaps with a more or less marked confusion, may be starting a hyperthyroid disease. In these cases the diagnosis depends mostly on laboratory findings, particularly an increased uptake of radioiodine or of serum protein-bound iodine. Tachycardia is present in all patients; and a goiter (either apparent or retrosternal) is likely to be found. The skin will be hot and moist even in the apathetic quiet patient. If checked, tremor will be noted in most instances, particularly if a paper is placed over the extended hand. Weight loss will not be too rare, nor will dyspnea and hypersensitivity to heat (the reverse is also true, tolerance to cool surroundings). Diarrhea or frequent defecations are relatively frequent in patients living in hot countries. Hyperthyroidism is more frequent among women; after the menopause care will be taken to differentiate it from anxiety neurosis, which will not show the metabolic changes.

Radioiodine therapy is the treatment of choice for older persons with hyperthyroidism; but the advisability of surgical removal for large or obstructive tumors will be discussed with an endocrinologist and a surgeon. Bed rest is advisable for severe cases; diet will provide large amounts of calories, proteins, carbohydrates, and vitamins (particularly of the B group);

sedatives or sympathetic blocking agents will be given only to the very nervous and irritable.

Hypothyroidism

Mental depression, marked apathy, or hallucinations may be the outstanding symptoms of hypothyroidism for older patients—mostly women, as always happens with diseases of the thyroid gland. Other symptoms may be entirely absent, or only gradually appear, namely, asthenia, nervousness, pallor, intolerance to cool surroundings. Later in the course of the disease evidence of myxedema will be apparent, that is, the peripheral edematous tissues, puffiness of face and eyelids, thickening of the tongue, yellowish hue of the skin, slow speech with hoarse voice, and a host of other symptoms. Thyroid hormones are always on the low side when checked. Blood cholesterol is elevated, and a macrocytic anemia may contribute to paleness. Note that the patients are puffy, but not obese. Low body temperature may denote hypothermia.

When treating hypothyroid, aged patients, the administration of thyroid hormones must be very carefully evaluated, starting with low or very low doses and increasing the amount gradually before the active dosage is reached. A too rapid treatment may cause anginal reactions or even heart failure. For the average case use thyroxine or thyroid extracts; for the hypothyroid patient with hypothermia use triiodothyronine, which has a more rapid activity.

> Thyroxine, tablets containing 0.1, 0.2, or 0.4 mg each; give 0.025 mg to start, slowly increasing by 0.05 mg every 10 or 15 days to reach the maintenance dose of about 0.2 to 0.3 mg.

> Thyroid extract, tablets containing 15, 30, 60, 120, 180, 240, 300, or more mg each; to start by giving 15 or 30 mg, increasing dosage by 15 mg every 1 or 2 weeks until the active maintenance dosage is reached; the pulse should not increase more than three to five pulsations a minute at every change of dose, until it reaches the normal speed of 70–75 a minute.

> Triiodothyronine, give 20 μg intravenously every 4 hours, until recovery from hypothermia—better administered together with a corticoid.

Hypopituitarism

This is not frequent at older ages, but may occur, and at times the mental derangements will be the first symptom, either due to the cachectic state or to hypoglycemia. Usually, the diagnosis is very difficult. Corticosteroids, which are the only available medication for hypopituitarism, may cause psychotic reactions.

Hyperpituitarism

As in the case of hypopituitarism, hyperpituitaric syndromes are rare in advanced ages. The possible diseases are acromegaly and Cushing disease. In either case mental derangements may occur; but, again, this is a rare instance among the elderly. The diagnosis is easier than with hypopituitarism, but it should be left to a specialist.

Surgery may help in many cases; but the final decision will be left to a neurosurgeon and an endocrinologist. Some efforts are being made to develop a medical treatment, but results are not yet encouraging.

Dehydration and Electrolyte Imbalance

These subjects have been reviewed in some detail in previous pages, q.v. for more information. A very succinct account is given here.

Dehydration: decreased skin turgor, shrunken eyes, dry tongue, oliguria, hypotension, asthenia, confusion, and other mental derangements.

Hyponatremia: with evidence of a causative disease, such as heart failure, cirrhosis, nephrosis, adrenal insufficiency, and so on.

Hypernatremia: accompanied by confusion, stupor, and shortly by coma.

Alkalosis: with irritability in the case of metabolic alkalosis, and with hyperventilation and tetany in cases of respiratory alkalosis.

In these instances the diagnosis has to depend on the laboratory reports, which will be essential to scheduling the best treatment with adequate infusions.

For dehydration give isotonic saline by intravenous infusions. Hyponatremia is corrected by restoring exactly the depleted amount of sodium, which is calculated by multiplying the deficit of sodium expressed in mEq by 55% (males) or 50% (females) of the body weight. Hypernatremia requires the administration of water by mouth or intravenous administration of 5% glucose in water. Only in extreme cases of metabolic alkalosis will ammonium chloride be given; otherwise, no specific treatment is required. In respiratory alkalosis rebreathing from a paper bag usually suffices.

Hypocalcemia

This condition is mainly due to hypoparathyroidism, but also to malabsorption, rickets, and renal insufficiency. Personality changes are prone to occur, which will be accompanied by neuromuscular excitability, cramps, tetany, convulsions, dyspnea with stridor, and cataracts. There is a little-known syndrome of hypocalcemia, ectodermal disorders, decalcified teeth, early cavities, and mental troubles, possibly true psychoses, which may start in adult life and be prolonged into older ages. The diagnosis is given by the low values of calcium in the blood, which may be checked repeatedly together with hyperphosphoremia.

Basic treatment is carried out with calcium salts (intravenously in acute tetany), with dihydrotachysterol or calciferol, or any of its metabolites if calciferol does not elicit a clear response.

Calcium gluconate, 10% solution; give 10 or 20 ml in electrolyte solution by slow drip; to be followed as soon as possible by oral administration of 4 to 6 g a day.

Dihydrotachysterol, 1.25 mg in 1 ml of the oily solution; give 4 ml a day during the first 2 or 4 days, decreasing to a maintenance dose of about 1 ml (check blood calcium).

Calciferol, usually to be preferred, in doses of 2 or 3 mg a day.

Hypercalcemia

Depression and psychoses may occur in cases of hypercalcemia, but in most instances these occur late in the disease, when other symptoms are already present to disclose a positive diagnosis. Hypercalcemia is due, in the first instance, to hyperparathyroidism, but also to some malignant tumors, longlasting immobilization of patients in bed (acute bone atrophy), hyperthyroidism, or hypoadrenalism.

The treatment will be addressed to the causative condition.

Septic Shock

During the course of any infective disease, particularly when it presents a severe clinical picture, there will be added to the characteristic symptoms of such a disease those corresponding to shock. But before this occurs there will be hypotension, very weak pulse, cadaveric pale face, sweats, superficial respiration, anoxia, apathy, immobility, hypasthenia, and at times, irritability, restlessness, or delirium and a worsening of the primary symptoms. In most instances the diagnosis of the causative infection has been previously established. Not rarely, among the elderly, the infection may start with or rapidly run into shock; then, the diagnosis and treatment of shock come first, but do not preclude the diagnosis of the causative disease, starting with the finding of fever, chills, malaise, or prostration and other particular symptoms.

Treatment must start immediately: absolute bed rest with the head below the body level and turned to one side, and the legs elevated. Correct water and electrolyte balance, raise the blood pressure (epinephrine, levarterenol), increase or reinforce anti-infective therapy, and give meperidine for the nervous overtone.

Meningitis

Patients with meningitis may present delirium; or in other cases, confusion. The diagnosis will depend on the suggestive grouping of symptoms as follows: fever with chills, stiffness of the neck and back, headache and other pains in the body, nausea and vomiting, convulsions, a petechial or ecchymotic rash, and abnormal reflexes (Kernig, Brudzinski, Marañón). The spinal fluid examination will give the final diagnosis.

Encephalitis

Symptoms and signs of encephalitis are similar to those of meningitis, namely, confusion or delirium, fever, stiff neck, nausea and vomiting, convulsions, and abnormal reflexes. In fact, encephalitis may include meningitis, when mainly a viral infection spreads over all parts of the encephalon. The clinical picture also shows sore throat, malaise, lethargy, stupor, tremors, cranial nerve palsies or spastic paralyses of the limbs, exaggerated deep tendon reflexes, absent superficial reflexes, or pathologic reflexes. The spinal fluid shows increased pressure and protein, normal glucose, and possibly the corresponding causative pathogen.

There is no specific treatment for viral encephalitis, but the following measures will help: mannitol for increased intracranial pressure, phenobarbital for convulsions, maintenance of patent airway, oxygen therapy, intravenous nutrition. For known pathogens, give the specific treatment.

> Mannitol, 15% solution, for intravenous infusion; give 1500 to 2000 ml, in 24 hours.

> Phenobarbital, 30 (to 50) mg, every 6 hours, as needed and tolerated.

Sunstroke or Heatstroke

Persons debilitated by age, intoxications, or diseases may react with heatstrokes when exposed for a time to elevated temperature from the sun or other form of heating. The first stage includes: headache, dizziness, nausea, visual disturbances, and mental impairment, possibly with convulsions. This stage is followed by: sudden loss of consciousness, very high body temperature, arrhythmic tachycardia, dryness of the skin for lack of sweating, the skin appearing flushed and hot, and hypotension and delirium, at times.

Once a person has had an attack of heatstroke, there is a tendency to repeat the situation when reexposed, even to a less excessive temperature.

Lower patient's temperature by placing him in a cool, shady place, without clothing, sprinkled with water, and moderately fanned. After a while, put the person in an ice bath—until his temperature falls to 39°C (102°F). Maintain circulation by massaging the extremities. Give symptomatic help whenever needed.

Typhoid Fever

Stupor, as a more or less confusional or delirious state, is an outstanding feature of typhoid fever, reached gradually. The disease starts with an indefinite malaise, sore throat, nonproductive cough, epistaxis, and other symptoms suggesting an upper respiratory infection. Symptomatology gradually becomes more and more severe: the fever rises steadily with relative bradycardia, headache, abdominal distress with distention, constipation, and finally the "pea-soup" diarrhea, splenomegaly, and rose spots, which appear on the trunk and fade on pressure. The diagnosis depends on positive blood cultures (first week), stool cultures (third week), or positive Widal test (second week).

Give the specific antibiotic, but start immediately with ampicillin or chloramphenicol. Patients will be isolated in bed, and will be well fed and hydrated; the diarrhea must be controlled, all excretions disinfected, and the severely ill treated with corticoids.

Ampicillin 6000 mg, every 4 hours, by mouth.

Chloramphenicol, 1000 mg, every 6 hours, by mouth, until fever is controlled; then, half the dosage for 15 days.

Prednisone, 40 to 60 mg, in divided doses, to start; decrease dosage as soon as possible; discontinue it gradually.

Typhus and Other Rickettsial Diseases

Delirium or confusion will be present only in late stages of severe forms of these diseases, but the elderly may start it earlier. Other symptoms are: a high temperature, chills, prostration, pains in the head and other parts of the body, and the skin rash, as follows.

Epidemic (classic) typhus: rash starts on trunk and axillae; spreads to limbs, sparing face, palms, and soles; and may become confluent or purpuric.

Endemic (murine) typhus: rash is slightly petechial.

Rocky Mountain spotted fever: rash starts on wrists and ankles.

Rickettsialpox: rash is all over the body.

Trench fever: rash is on the chest and abdomen.

The diagnosis depends on the Weil-Felix reaction and the finding of specific antibodies.

Give symptomatic help, together with tetracyclines.

Tetracycline, 500 mg, every 3 to 6 hours, by mouth, for 7 to 10 days; in severe cases, the first dose of 1000 mg is given by intravenous injection.

Pneumonia

Among the elderly and alcoholics, unconsciousness with delirium or confusion is not unusual in pneumonia. The disease starts with symptoms of an upper respiratory infection with pharyngitis or bronchitis. The temperature rises suddenly or in steps, with a shaking chill and sharp pain on the affected side of the chest, rapid and dyspneic respiration, profuse sweating, and coughing (may appear with some evidence of provoked pain), accompanied by a sputum (not always expectorated under the circumstances), peculiar to each variety of pneumonia:

Pneumococcal: sputum initially bloody, rapidly turning into the well-known rusty sputum.

H. influenzae: tenacious, apple-green sputum.

Viral: mucopurulent sputum, may be tinged with blood.

Staphylococcal or streptococcal: abundant sputum of salmon color.

K. pneumoniae: viscid, cherry-red sputum.

Mycoplasmal: a bloody sputum.

Malaria

Cerebral malaria occurs with confusion, delirium, headache, and convulsions, usually ending in coma. Elderly persons may not suffer so seriously, but will appear delirious during the acute paroxysm. The clinical picture presents periodic attacks, lasting for a given lapse of time, in which fever rises abruptly, and there are shaking chills and profuse sweating, splenomegaly, anemia, leukopenia, and the causative *Plasmodium* identified in the blood. Paroxysms occur every 48 hours in *P. vivax* and *P. falciparum* malaria; and every 72 hours in *P. malariae* disease. *P. falciparum* causes most cases with serious complications, including cerebral malaria.

Acute attacks for all three types of plasmodia are treated with quinacrine, chloroquine, chlorguanide, or pyrimethamine.

Quinacrine, 200 mg, every 5 hours, to a total of five doses; thereafter, 100 mg, every 8 hours, for 6 days.

Chloroquine, 1000 mg, to start; 500 mg, 6 hours later; thereafter, 500 mg, once a day, for 2 days.

Chlorguanide, 300 mg, every 12 hours, for 10 days.

Pyrimethamine, 50 mg, the first dose; thereafter, a daily dose of 25 mg, for 2 days.

Influenza

Frail elderly persons may become confused or delirious when fever, toxemia, or either one, is severe. Prostration is marked, and all the usual symptoms are also intense, namely, sore throat and other pharyngeal symptoms, cough, headache, generalized aches, and weakness. Weakness when prolonged after subsidence of the general clinical picture, confirms the diagnosis, proven by isolation of the virus from throat washings if done early in the disease. Mental impairment worsens or appears when pneumonia complicates the clinical picture. Positive serology tests are obtained later. Laboratory tests are the only possible way to differentiate influenza from para-influenza and other viral respiratory diseases.

Watch for complications (pneumonia), keep patients in bed, maintain good nursing care, treat cough when it is bothersome, and use antipyretics and analgesics, if needed. For delirium give paraldehyde.

Codeine, 30 or 60 mg, by mouth or by injection, repeated as needed and tolerated.

Acetylsalicylic acid, 300 mg, plus codeine, 30 mg, to take by mouth every 4 to 6 hours, as needed and tolerated.

Paraldehyde, 5 ml, by intramuscular injection, to repeat after 30 minutes, when needed.

Rheumatic Fever

This disease will very rarely be found among the elderly, who may present marked confusion or delirium as a nervous complication. These patients have previously shown a streptococcal infection, most frequently a streptococcal pharyngitis with fever, followed by any of the important complexes of rheumatic fever. These complexes are: articular pains; cardiac involvement, with murmurs, enlargement, and insufficiency; nervous reactions, usually chorea; and dermic symptoms, such as nodules or erythema marginatum. The diagnosis depends on finding one or more of the complexes.

Observe bed rest and watch for complications. Salicylates are the basic drugs to be given, but penicillin may be of good use. Paraldehyde may control delirium.

> Sodium salicylate, 1000 to 2000 mg, every 2 to 4 hours at the start of treatment; continuing with a daily dosage of 6000 mg a day, in three or four installments (30 mg of thyroid extract a day may increase tolerance).

> Penicillin, 200,000 to 250,000 units, twice a day, by mouth; or benzathine penicillin, 1.2 million units, intramuscularly, once a month.

> Paraldehyde, 5 ml, by intramuscular injection, repeated in 30 minutes, if needed.

Alcoholism

No matter how important they are, the social and familial implications of alcoholism are of no significance for our purposes here. Usually, the diagnosis is obvious because the family brings the patient to be treated, or the patient comes on his own or has been involved with a police matter. In other instances the diagnosis has to be made by the consulting physician, in spite of the fact that a number of alcoholics will strongly deny their addiction. During an acute intoxication there is marked evidence of mental deterioration: slurred, hesitating speech; lack of appropriate coordination in movements, ataxia, drowsiness, errors of commission, nystagmus, flushed face, tremors, and a marked alcohol odor to the breath. If the situation reaches the point of poisoning, there will also be other symptoms of central nervous system depression, such as conjugate deviation of the eyes, trismus, repetitive and automatic movements, trend to violence, gastric irritation with nausea and vomiting, and other symptoms of hypoglycemia. Alcohol concentration in blood will give the diagnosis. The legal upper limit is 50 mg%, and intoxication is agreed to start at 150 mg%; from 300 mg% up, there is unconsciousness, and this level is lethal in many instances.

Treatment of alcoholics is really a major problem because of the poor cooperation they usually give. Personal and social implications will be solved through adequate centers and institutions. The physician has to be aware of the many complications caused by chronic alcoholism and to treat them; namely, nutritional impairment, gastrointestinal irritation, cirrhosis, pancreatitis, anemia, heart lesions, neuromuscular disorders, and the like. Moderate intoxication will be treated by keeping the patient warm and maintaining a patent airway after removing all residual alcohol by gastric lavage, leaving in the stomach a water solution containing 4 g of sodium bicarbonate. The comatose state requires catheterization to infuse hypotonic saline or 5% glucose solutions to maintain blood pressure at the necessary level. Dialysis will be performed in extremely severe instances. An attempt to use vitamin B_1 (thiamine) will not always be totally fruitless.

Depressant Drugs

Mental deterioration is not rarely due to the use of some sort of depressant drugs, whether prescribed by the physician or bought by the patient OTC. In many instances the diagnosis has to be made by elimination of other causes. Occasional use may become very difficult to detect; drug dependence or addiction will be easier, since patients do not try to cover their habit. Only when dealing with the use of morphine and hallucinogens will one encounter a denial on the part of the patient, in most cases. Epileptic patients on *anticonvulsant drugs* may develop intolerance to the medication, showing mental derangements such as drowsiness, dizziness, ataxia, nervousness, and nystagmus, which may increase to mental dullness and psychoses. In addition to these more or less general symptoms, each drug may cause other reactions, such as gum hypertrophy (hydrophenylhydantoin), exfoliative dermatitus (mephentoin), bone marrow depression (carbamazepine and trimethadione), and so on. Neuroleptic antipsychotic *major tranquilizers* will cause mental derangements either directly or indirectly; for instance, it is not rare that the elderly react with urinary retention capable of provoking mental reaction. Other symptoms of this type are extreme anxiety or terror crises, restlessness, parkinsonian signs, diskinesias, or other forms of depression. *Minor tranquilizers* or sedative drugs cause more marked behavioral reactions, as well as ataxia, lack of coordination, error of commission, and other forms of excessive sedation leading to depression. *Opiates* and similar drugs present drowsiness, mental confusion, hypotension, bradycardia, miosis, hypothermia; and in those using these drugs by injection, scars on the arms and legs; or those using them by nasal insufflation, erosion of the mucous membranes.

As with alcoholism, drug dependence poses two different sorts of problems, namely, social and medical. Withdrawal represents a socio-medical approach because of the complexities of its handling. In cases of acute intoxication a gastric lavage will be performed for extraction of residual toxics; in case of injection, a tourniquet should be applied (following the accepted technique). Because of respiratory depression, keep a patent airway and assist respiration, if so needed. And, maintain an adequate blood volume by using infused electrolytc solutions. When symptoms of excitement or delirium occur, use a short-acting barbiturate or chlorpromazine by intravenous injection. Nalorphine or levallorphan may correct respiratory depression. Hallucinatory psychotic states, such as those provoked by marijuana, may respond to chlorpromazine, a short-acting barbiturate, or haloperidol. Opiate intoxication should be treated with antagonists, such as naloxane.

Electrolyte or plasma solutions, given intravenously to expand blood.

Sodium pentobarbital, ampoules containing 50 or 100 mg; inject intravenously 100, 200, or more mg, to relieve excitement.

Chlorpromazine, containers of 1, 2, or 10 ml, with 25 mg in each ml, starting with small doses—12.5 to 25 mg—and increasing up to 50 or 100 mg in total, according to tolerance and response; injections to be given intravenously, but only intramuscularly to the frail older person.

Levallorphan, 1 mg in each ml, in ampoules with 1 or 10 ml; give 1 mg intravenously; followed by 0.5-mg doses, if so needed and tolerated, according to respiratory response.

Haloperidol, with 5 mg in each ml, in 1- or 10-ml ampoules; give intramuscularly from 2 to 5 mg, according to response regarding psychotic reactions, repeating the doses as needed and tolerated.

Naloxane, 0.4 mg in 1-ml ampoules, or 0.02 mg in 2-ml ampoules, to start with 0.4 mg intravenously, and follow according to response and tolerance.

A summary of drugs that may cause these syndromes is given here:

Anticonvulsant drugs: acetazolamide, carbamazepine, chlordiazepoxide, clonazepam, dextroamphetamine, diazepam, ethosuximide, ethotoin, mephenytoin, mephobarbital, meprobamate, methamphetamine, metharbital, methsuximide, paramethadione, phenacemide, phenytoin, phenobarbital, primidone, and the bromides.

Major tranquilizers: butaperazine, chlorpromazine, fluphenazine, haloperidol, loxapine, mesodirazine, molindone, perphenazine, piperacetazine, thioridazine, thiothixene, and trifluoperazine.

Minor tranquilizers: amobarbital, chloral hydrate, chlordiazepoxide, clorazepate, diazepam, ethchlorvynol, flurazepam, glutethimide, hydroxyzine pamoate, meprobamate, methaqualone, methyprylon, oxazepam, paraldehyde, pentobarbital, phenobarbital, and secobarbital.

Opiates: opium and also alphaprodine, codeine, heroin, meperidine, methadone, morphine, and propoxyphene.

Atropine and Other Belladonna Derivatives

Mental symptoms may reach stupor, delirium, and delusions, associated with extreme dryness of the mouth, difficulties in swallowing, blurred vision, flushed skin, dilated pupils, tachycardia, and fever.

For treatment use stomach lavage or a tourniquet; and inject short-acting barbiturates to counteract excitement. Cool the patient; maintain a patent airway.

Digitalis

This substance also provokes delirium, together with vomiting and bradycardia, which are the outstanding symptoms. Finally, there is a fall of blood pressure and ventricular fibrillation. The EKG indicates a long P-R interval, depressed ST segment, and evidence of blocking and ventricular irregularities.

Give milk, and perform a gastric lavage immediately, preferably with powdered charcoal. The best medication will be potassium chloride, 0.3% solution in 5% glucose, by intravenous infusion, with careful monitoring of blood levels of potassium and effects upon the EKG. Defibrillation may be required.

Iron

Mental symptoms consist of lethargy followed by coma, all coming after nausea, vomiting, diarrhea, tachycardia, hypotension, and evidence of acidosis and dehydration. A second stage is characterized by cyanosis, pulmonary edema, anuria, coma, and death.

Perform gastric lavage (better with half-strength Fleet's enema solution). Infuse isotonic saline or 5% glucose solution. The drug of choice for treatment is deferoxamine mesylate, which will be given immediately.

> Deferoxamine mesylate, ampoules containing 500 mg each, to be dissolved in 2 ml of water and then to be added to an infusion with saline, 5% glucose, or the like, at a speed of 15 mg for each kilo of body weight every hour. The amount of medication to be given is 80 mg for each kilo of body weight. After 12 hours a second similar dose may be given if needed. It is advisable to check blood pressure in order to reduce the speed of administration if the blood pressure falls.

Salicylates

Delirium, restlessness, excitement, and convulsions will precede coma whenever it is present, or will occur without coma. The face is flushed; there are hyperpnea, hyperthermia, abdominal pain, profuse perspiration, headache, tachycardia with hypotension, vomiting, and other evidence of dehydration or of acidosis or alkalosis. Rarely the patient will deny having taken aspirin or other salicylate. The urine will give the salicylate reaction with ferric chloride (port-wine color).

Perform stomach lavage, and take the patient to the hospital for monitoring the blood pH, sodium, chloride, and potassium while infusing the adequate solution for these cases (containing sodium bicarbonate or lactate and potassium).

Other Analgesics

In the case of intoxication due to the administration of antipyrine, aminopyrine, phenylbutazone, or the like, symptoms will be dizziness, cyanosis, and final coma; and the treatment practically the same as for salicylate poisoning.

Amphetamines

Maniac symptoms may occur with other evidence of irritability, tremors, hyperreflexia, fever, sweating, tachycardia with hypertension, arrhythmias, mydriasis, and finally convulsions and coma.

First, sedate the patient with chlorpromazine intravenously or at least intramuscularly; and then perform a gastric lavage.

> Chlorpromazine; give 1 mg for each kilo of body weight, repeated according to response and tolerance (from containers with 1, 2, or 10 ml, at a concentration of 25 mg for each ml).

Nitrites

Mental deterioration is not too marked, but there are almost always dizziness, faintness, muscular relaxation, tremors, dyspnea, hypotension and other symptoms of circulatory collapse, at times cyanosis, and the history of treatment for angina or post-infarction.

Perform gastric lavage; administer epinephrine or levarterenol for blood pressure; and give oxygen therapy plus methylene blue for metahemoglobinemia (noted by cyanosis).

> Epinephrine, 1:1000 solution, to inject 1 ml subcutaneously.

> Methylene blue, 1% solution, to inject intravenously from 5 to 25 ml, very slowly.

Warfarin and Anticoagulants

Symptoms depend on the site of the hemorrhage caused by these drugs; the reader is referred to the entries dealing with this topic.

Perform gastric lavage, preferably with activated charcoal; and administer vitamin K intravenously to counteract the effects of the anticoagulant.

> Vitamin K, 10-ml vials containing 10 mg in each ml; give 1 mg for each kilo of body weight, by intravenous injection.

Other Diseases

Again it is necessary to mention that any disease occurring in an older person may present, together with its proper symptoms, some evidence of mental deterioration, particularly of the confusional type. Thus before a diagnosis of a purely psychiatric character is made, it is imperative to eliminate all possible basic causes of disease in any of the organic systems of the body. We have devoted a great deal of space to respiratory and cardiovascular diseases, these diseases perhaps being among the most frequently encountered in this age group. Others are to be considered, as well.

> *Injuries:* usually with a previous history of an accidental trauma and turning into a cerebrovascular accident.

> *Prostatic diseases:* of great importance among older males because they may end in renal disease or urinary retention, which will provoke unequivocal symptoms of mental derangement plus the particular symptoms of prostatic hypertrophy, cancer of the prostate, glomerulonephritis, and final uremia.

> *Urinary retention:* not rarely the cause of a confusional syndrome affecting a male with prostatic problems, or any other person with bladder or urethral problems.

> *Glomerulonephritis:* in which mental symptoms become apparent only after longstanding disease, and are mainly due to uremia; urinary changes will give the main clues for diagnosis.

> *Pyelonephritis:* accompanied by symptoms of infection.

> *Uremia:* the final stage of renal failure, characterized by mental changes (not rarely the first evidence of the condition), the diagnosis made by the elevated blood levels of nitrogenous products (BUN, urea, creatinine).

> *Hepatitis:* confusion and shock or coma coming after other symptoms of the disease have been evident; so, the diagnosis is already made before this late stage.

Cirrhosis: either due to alcoholism or diseases of the liver; the symptoms of the disease are evident before the mental reaction occurs.

Actually, it is unnecessary to go further with this review, since it might embrace almost all that we know about medical problems. It need only be emphasized once more that in the presence of an older patient with any form of mental impairment, before we state it to be a psychiatric problem, it is mandatory to make a complete search for a possible basic cause of the problem, which may be a different disease.

It is mandatory that the diagnosis of the basic ailment be made because the treatment depends entirely on the elimination of this cause. Each different disease will be treated instead of giving symptomatic care, which might improve a symptom but not cure the patient.

V. NEUROLOGICAL SYMPTOMS

PAIN

This symptom is so important that we devoted an entire chapter to it, entitled "Pain" (q.v.).

UNCONSCIOUSNESS

Again, this is a very important topic by itself, which we discussed in a separate chapter entitled "Unconsciousness" (q.v.).

TREMOR

Tremors are involuntary and rhythmical alternate movements of opposing muscles, which may be rapid or slow, fine or coarse, intentional or rest tremors. Athetosis, myoclonus, or convulsions are different involuntary movements of a more ample range. In athetosis the movements are ceaseless, slow, sinuous, and more marked in the hands; myoclonic contractions are shocklike; and convulsions involve almost the entire body.

In each instance, the treatment is that of the causative factor.

Parkinsonism

This condition is characterized by coarse tremors, alternate relatively slow movements of the fingers, the "pill-rolling" gesture of the hands and upper limbs; but also including the head, eyelids, and tongue. The tremor is present at rest and diminishes or totally disappears with purposeful movements or during sleep. Rigidity may impair associate movements, force the patient to move slowly, and give his face a blank expression; it also causes a special slow but festinating gait. When a limb is moved passively, it proceeds as by small steps (cogwheel phenomenon). Speech is slow and monotonous. It has to be differentiated from senility, hyperthyroidism, and other tremors. Parkinsonian tremors are noted in Parkinson's disease, and also in some cases of encephalitis, meningitis, or tetanus. In encephalitis there are fever, stiff neck, nausea and vomiting, sore throat, malaise, lethargy or stupor, paralysis of some of the cranial nerves, spastic paralyses of the limbs, exaggerated tendon reflexes, and convulsions. In meningitis twitching or convulsions are more frequent, with fever, chills, stiff neck, confusion or delirium, usually a skin rash, dyspnea (Cheyne-Stokes' or Biot's respiration) and abnormal reflexes. In tetanus the clinical picture usually follows a known wound, and the symptoms start with stiffness of the jaw, spasms of other muscles of the neck and back, slight fever, dysphagia, irritability, hyperreflexia, and convulsions.

Encephalitis, meningitis, and tetanus will be treated accordingly, each one with the proper medication. In pure parkinsonism, tremors may respond to atropine-like drugs, trihexphenidyl, cycrimine, amantadine, and levadopa.

> Tincture of belladonna, to start with 15 drops every 6 to 8 hours, increasing gradually according to response and tolerance.

> Levadopa, 500 mg every 8 hours, by mouth, to start; increasing gradually by increments of about 500 mg a day, according to response and tolerance.

Senility

Deterioration caused by age, without other pathologic implications, may show an intentional tremor, at times very similar to that noted in parkinsonian syndromes, but no other focal abnormalities will be found. In senile dementia tremors are inconspicuous among a number of severe symptoms, such as marked confusion, emotional instability, irritability, depression, and other paranoiac tendencies.

Rarely will any treatment be needed or afford relief. A try may be given to belladonna, in small amounts.

> Tincture of belladonna, to start with 10 drops, three times a day, increasing dosage according to response and tolerance.

Chorea

Huntington's chorea may start in adult life and last for about 15 years; few cases are to be seen among the elderly. The disease usually starts with mental symptoms (personality changes), and then the jerky movements appear in the face, neck, and arms, disappearing during sleep. In other forms of chorea there are less marked serious mental symptoms, or no symptoms at all, and no history of similar cases in the family. Finally, there is a possibility that when this syndrome appears in old age it does not belong to the same type as Huntington's chorea.

Sydenham's chorea will very rarely be seen in old age because it is a disease usually present in younger groups, mostly females. It is associated with rheumatic fever, and appears even after subsidence of the disease, with involuntary, purposeless, nonrepetitive movements of the face, trunk, and extremities, that is, any muscle in the body, except the eyes. The diagnosis is made by the typical movements.

There is no treatment for Huntington's disease, only a minor improvement noted at times with chlorpromazine or reserpine; nor is there any for Sydenham's chorea. For the latter, and only if there is a concomitant heart involvement, salicylates and corticoids should be given.

Multiple Sclerosis

The disease is characterized by bouts and remissions of symptoms, namely, visual and sensory disturbances (impaired vision, transient weakness, varied paresthesias, dizziness), lack of bladder control, some form of ataxia, and at a later stage, nystagmus, intention tremor, and scanning speech (Charcot's triad). Many patients will present mental impairment, convulsions, hemiplegia, and other disturbances; for the findings in multiple sclerosis are extremely variable and manifold, thus giving the clinical picture great variability.

There is no treatment for multiple sclerosis, but trials should be given to the use of corticoids, vasodilators, cyanocobalamin, procaine, isoniazid, tolbutamide, blood transfusions, and low-fat diets. There is nothing to lose, and some authors have claimed to have improved their patients with some of these remedies.

Cerebrovascular Accidents

Early diagnosis is that of arteriosclerosis, which is not an easy diagnosis to make. Good hints are the finding of enlarged, tortuous, and somewhat hard peripheral arteries, or calcified vessels in X-ray films; plethysmographic or oscillometric abnormalities; and, perhaps above all, the precocious evidence of forgetfulness, personality changes, and late symptoms of impaired memory and confusion. Tremors are usually present, but are not of paramount importance. Finally, there come the undesirable complications of thrombosis, embolism, stenosis, aneurism, or other evidence of organic brain disturbances. Stroke accidents are characterized by a more or less rapid obnubilation, the patient falling more or less unconscious, with stertorous respirations (may be of the Cheyne-Stokes type), flushed face, bradycardia with full pulse and not rarely initial hypertension followed by hypotension, and the characteristic flaccidity of one side of the body. With large thrombi the attack starts acutely and violently; with hemorrhages, symptoms are more generalized, and a stiff neck is frequently noted; all is completed with dysarthria, fever, vomiting, convulsions, and the focal evidence corresponding to each particular vessel. For more details see other entries on cerebrovascular accidents.

Usually, this sort of tremor needs no special treatment; but for the other associated cerebral disease the reader is referred to the chapter on unconsciousness.

Cerebellar Diseases

Intentional tremor together with ataxia is a good indication of cerebellar diseases, particularly tumors of the cerebello-pontine angle and those of the fourth ventricle. Vertigo is also of diagnostic interest, namely, with persistent imbalance but rare paroxysms, almost always accompanied by deafness and tinnitus. Cerebellar tremor is rapid and fine, dependent on the ataxic condition. Ataxia is the basic symptom: with exaggerated, ample movements, always excessive for their purpose, lacking coordination and strength. This cerebellar syndrome appears in the following instances.

Cerebellar tumors: with added symptoms of cranial hypertension; when of an angiomatous nature, may improve with age.

Cerebellar abscess: usually secondary to an ear infection, with local symptoms, fever, mental derangement, and nystagmus.

Cerebellar hemorrhage: with an initial apoplectic attack; thereafter, the cerebellar syndrome is noted.

Cerebellar injuries: rarely will cause the cerebellar syndrome, but usually are of a very poor prognosis.

Other cerebellar reactions: in which a true cerebellar syndrome may be present, together with symptoms of an infection, intoxication, or specific diseases of the nervous system with cerebellar implication (Friedrich, Marie).

The treatment, surgical in most instances, will be addressed to each particular disease. Tremors will not need any special measure.

Drugs

Phenothiazines are capable of inducing tremor together with drowsiness and hypotension. These patients will also show tachycardia, ataxia, nasal congestion, fever, blurring of vision, dryness of the mouth, and stiffness of the neck, and may go into coma. The phenothiazines may be detected in the urine. The diagnosis is easy in most instances, when the patient is a known phenothiazine user.

Provide gastric lavage. Treat shock if hypotension is marked, but do not use pressor drugs. If there are convulsions, give pentobarbital, but not other depressant drugs. Treat any infection present. For intolerable ataxic symptoms give diphenhydramine.

Blood, well-matched for transfusion.

Dextran 40, 10% solution in saline or 5% glucose; or other electrolyte solutions to expand blood volume.

Isoproterenol; give 2 mg in 500 ml of 5% dextrose, intravenously, according to response and tolerance. It is better to avoid pressor drugs.

Pentobarbital, injectables containing 50 mg in each ml; give intravenously 100 mg or more, according to response and tolerance.

Diphenhydramine, injectables containing 10 or 50 mg in each ml; give from 1 to 4 mg for each kilo of body weight, intravenously; do not oversedate.

General Paresis

Not as frequently found as in the past, general paresis may still be noted in some cases of late syphilis, presenting memory loss, headaches, poor concentration, severe personality changes, dysarthria, and tremors of the tongue, lips, and fingers. In short, suspicion will arise when a patient becomes irresponsible, confused, and slovenly, has speech difficulties, and shows tremor.

Treatment for general paresis consists of the use of short-acting penicillin in large doses and for a relatively prolonged time. Spinal fluid should be checked every 3 or 4 months, changes of which, together with reversal of clinical symptoms, will serve to evaluate the effects of therapy.

Aqueous crystalline penicillin G; give from 1 to 20 million units a day, intramuscularly or intravenously, for no less than 10 days, up to 20, according to response and tolerance.

Hyperthyroidism

Tremor is one of the most constant and specific symptoms of hyperthyroidism. It is a fine, rapid tremor noted all over the body (when the patient is touched) but particularly in the fingers. To make it more noticeable, put a piece of paper over the extended hand. Other symptoms of hyperthyroidism are: nervousness, asthenia, weight loss (in spite of a good feeding schedule), hot sweating skin, overactivity and irritability, palpitation, and tachycardia; all this together with a possible goiter and exophthalmos. The classical and typical picture of irritability and overactivity may be reversed in the older person who presents, instead, apathy and lethargy, perhaps with heart failure or cachexia. Under the circumstances, request from the laboratory the corresponding figures for protein-bound iodine in the serum (will be above 8 μg%), triiodothyronine uptake (will be over 35%), and perhaps other substances (T_4, butanol-extractable iodine, free thyroxine, cholesterol, basal metabolic rate, and others). Do not mistake hyperthyroidism for any of the following diseases.

Anxiety neurosis: frequent in post-menopausal women, with evident psychological symptoms but lacking the basic organic symptoms of hyperthyroidism, and basically the laboratory findings.

Thyroiditis: with the main difference tenderness of the gland, which is not found in hyperthyroidism; in thyroiditis the radioiodine uptake is low, around 5% or less in 24 hours.

Administration of thyroid hormones: evident by history, and because of a low radioiodine uptake (about 5% or less in 24 hours).

T_3 thyrotoxicosis: with elevated triiodotyronine and normal or low values for other thyroid tests.

Tachycardia: when due to heart diseases; will not present other symptoms of the thyroid series.

Consequently, the final diagnosis depends on the evaluation of pure thyroidal symptoms (tremor, irritability, tachycardia, hot sweating skin, and goiter and exophthalmos—if present) and the results of laboratory tests.

As stated before, radioactive therapy is the treatment of choice for the older person with hyperthyroidism. Surgical removal will be discussed with an endocrinologist and a surgeon when there are large, obstructive goiters. Relatively severe cases will be treated with bed rest, at least at the beginning; a diet high in calories, carbohydrates, proteins, and vitamins; and sedatives or sympathetic blocking agents if nervousness and irritability are too prominent.

Radioiodine, to be administered by authorized specialists.

Phenobarbital, 15 to 30 mg, three or more times a day, according to response and tolerance.

Propranolol, tablets containing 10, 40, or 80 mg each; give 10 mg, three or more times a day, according to response and tolerance, but being careful with increasing the dosage when treating early heart failure.

Vertigo

Dizziness is the lay word for vertigo, the condition characterized by the subjective sensation of rotatory movement in space, either of the person or of surrounding objects, usually accompanied by the tendency to lose one's balance. The main cause of vertigo is a disease of the labyrinth, including the vestibular portion of the 8th cranial nerve. Patients with vertigo may also present deafness and tinnitus (often unilateral), nystagmus, positive Romberg's sign, inability to walk in a straight line, and perhaps a nauseous sensation.

Symptomatic treatment of vertigo may be accomplished by bed rest and the administration of perphenazine or dimenhydrinate. Provide the basic treatment for the causative disease.

> Dimenhydrinate, tablets containing 50 mg each, or injectables with 50 mg in each ml (1 or 5 ml); give 50 mg every 4 to 6 hours, by mouth or by injection, according to response and tolerance.

Otitis

Many patients will complain of vertigo, but the main symptoms refer to the ear itself, with local pain, deafness, and fever with chills; on otoscopy the eardrum bulges, loses its landmarks, and finally may rupture and allow pus to drain, at which stage the secretion will provide the diagnosis of the infective organism and its sensitivity to antibiotics.

The basic treatment includes bed rest, analgesics, and the specific antibiotic (or an ample-spectrum one in other cases). Myringotomy may be performed by the internist, but is better left to the otologist.

> Penicillin, give 600,000 or more units every day, for at least 7 to 10 days, according to response and tolerance.

Labyrinthitis

All forms of labyrinthitis are accompanied by an intense vertigo, as the main symptom. If it is due to a disease of an adjacent part of the auditory system, other local symptoms will also be present. There may also be deafness, tinnitus, nausea, and at times visual disturbances. Most patients tend to fall in a certain direction. In acute labyrinthitis there is also fever, at times with sudden deafness and paralysis of the facial nerve.

When an infection is the cause, the use of antibiotics, usually with adequate drainage performed by a specialist, is the proper management. Noninfective cases respond better to bed rest in a dark room, and the administration of sedatives (phenobarbital), antihistaminics (chlorpheniramine), and perhaps chlorpromazine in the early phases of the disease.

Phenobarbital, 15 to 30 mg, three or more times a day, according to response and tolerance.

Chlorpheniramine, long-acting capsules containing 8 or 12 mg each, to give one every 12 hours, dosage adjusted according to response and tolerance.

Chlorpromazine; inject 50 mg, intramuscularly, at the beginning of symptoms.

Ménière's Disease

This disease is characterized by intermittent attacks of vertigo together with deafness, tinnitus, nausea and vomiting, profuse sweating, headache, and nystagmus, all lasting from a few minutes to several hours and recurring after variable periods—even for the same patient. During dizziness, the patient tends to fall toward the affected side. The final, positive diagnosis has to be made by a specialist, following a few specific tests.

Surgery is frequently the last resort for the treatment of this disease. Medically, a try will be given to dimenhydrinate, atropine, or diuretics with a salt-free diet and ammonium chloride. A psychological approach must be used in some overly apprehensive patients.

Dimenhydrinate, tablets containing 50 mg each, or injectables with 50 mg in each ml (1 or 5 ml); give 50 mg every 4 to 6 hours, by mouth or by injection, according to response and tolerance.

Atropine sulfate, 0.6 mg, given by subcutaneous injection.

Ammonium chloride, tablets containing 500 mg each; give 1000 or 2000 mg four times a day.

Drug-Induced Vertigo

Some drugs are well known causes of vertigo, in the first place streptomycin, and also alcohol, salicylates, opiates, and others. Usually the diagnosis becomes obvious because of the history of the patient's medication.

Streptomycin: be careful of the onset of tinnitus, deafness, loss of equilibrium, and vertigo, when administering this antibiotic, which will be discontinued at the first sign.

Neomycin: is another aminoglycoside, like streptomycin, also capable of injuring the 8th cranial nerve.

Kanamycin: same as the above.

Gentamycin: same as the above.

Alcohol: acute intoxication causes vertigo, central nervous depression, incoordination, ataxia, gastric irritation (nausea and vomiting), hypothermia, tachycardia, dyspnea, flushed face, and alcoholic odor to the breath.

Salicylates: vertigo is accompanied by profuse sweating, epigastric pain and vomiting, restlessness, excitement, dyspnea, tachycardic feeble pulse, hypotension, visual and auditory disturbances, delirium, and possibly convulsions.

Narcotics (opium and derivatives): vertigo occurs together with headache and weariness after an initial phase of exhilaration and physical relaxation. The pinpoint pupils are characteristic. A rich symptomatology accompanies this intoxication.

Barbiturates and similar sedatives: a vertiginous state is accompanied by headache and mental confusion, ataxia, somnolence, or other similar symptoms, all ending in coma at times.

Basic care will be directed to the causative factor. Symptomatically, vertigo may be treated with bed rest and dimenhydrinate.

Dimenhydrinate, tablets containing 50 mg each, or injectables with 50 mg in each ml (1 or 5 ml); give 50 mg every 4 to 6 hours, by mouth or by injection, according to response and tolerance.

Acoustic Neuroma

Acoustic neuromas as well as other tumors of the cerebellopontine angle usually provoke vertigo, but the main impairments are tinnitus and local hearing difficulties. Because they may cause pressure on adjacent structures, other symptoms may appear: facial paralysis and anesthesia, paresis of the soft palate, corneal arreflexia, and possibly hemiplegia or hemianesthesia of the contralateral side. Diagnosis is helped by finding an elevated protein level in the spinal fluid, enlarged porus acusticus in X-ray films, and no vestibular response to caloric stimulation.

The treatment will be discussed with a specialist.

Cerebellar Lesions

The cerebellar syndrome consists of: ataxia (without Romberg's sign) and a frequently staggering gait with ample movements (dysmetria) that will cause one to touch the eye instead of the nose, or the leg or thigh instead of the knee, when asked to use a finger, or heel, to perform these maneuvers; adiadochokinesia, evident when one is asked to rapidly perform alternate movements, for instance, of the hand up and down; absence of synergistic movements (asynergia), for instance, flexing the legs to avoid falling when pushed backward; nystagmus; and a fine rapid tremor, either at rest or intentional, closely related to ataxia. Vertigo is an important part of the syndrome, characterized by persistent imbalance and rare occurrence of paroxysms, almost always accompanied by deafness and tinnitus. This syndrome may appear in the following cases.

Cerebellar tumor: plus symptoms of cranial hypertension; may improve with age when due to angioma.

Cerebellar abscess: with fever, mental symptoms, and other local symptoms of ear infection.

Cerebellar hemorrhage: initial stroke followed by cerebellar syndrome.

Cerebellar injuries: previous history of trauma.

Other conditions: general infection, intoxication, or specific diseases, such as Friedrich's or Marie's syndromes.

Specific treatment for each basic cause will be carried out (infection, toxic), but it will be kept in mind that surgery is required for the great majority of patients, which will be discussed with a neurologist and a neurosurgeon. An annoying vertigo may respond to dimenhydrinate, but will not always do so.

Dimenhydrinate, 50 mg tablets; take one every 4 to 6 hours, adjusting the dosage to response and tolerance.

Eye Diseases

Because of visual impairment, vertigo is frequently provoked by initial glaucoma, cataracts, or retinitis, which diseases will be sought for diagnosis in patients of advanced age.

Initial glaucoma may cause vertigo, but the main warning is the progressive loss of vision because of narrowing visual fields; this coming with headaches, halos around lights, frequent changes of glasses, impaired dark adaptation, and the evidence given by tonometry findings or elevated intraocular pressure. The acute attack is rather easily diagnosed because of the glaucoma already known to exist: the pain is often extreme, and the vision blurred.

Cataracts develop insidiously and may cause mild vertigo associated with the progressive blurring of vision; the opacified lens is seen through the ophthalmoscope.

Retinitis provokes vertigo because of the distortion in size and shape of objects, decreased visual acuity, and other forms of ocular discomfort; the diseased retina is seen through the ophthalmoscope. It is to be noted that retinal reactions occur following choroiditis, alcoholism, diabetes, tobaccoism, arterial hypertension, sarcoidosis, and many infectious diseases. For more detailed information see other entries in this book.

Treatment has to be addressed to the causative factor. Since these causes vary greatly, no details will be given here, but the reader is referred to the corresponding entries in other parts of this book. Nevertheless, if vertigo becomes too annoying, a try will be given to dimenhydrinate, by mouth or by injection; but this will not at all preclude the use of adequate treatment.

> Dimenhydrinate, tablets containing 50 mg each, or injectables containing 50 mg in each ml (container with 1 or 5 ml); give 50 mg, every 4 to 6 hours, by mouth or by injection, according to response and tolerance.

Hypertension

Many patients with hypertension complain of lightheadedness, which may become severe enough to be called vertigo. Other symptoms will be headache (mainly in the morning), palpitation, asthenia, and tinnitus; and in longstanding cases there will also be cardiac involvement (left ventricle hypertrophy, nocturnal dyspnea, anginal pains), nocturia, hematuria, intermittent claudication, or other symptoms as well. Blood pressure readings will be above 160/95 mm Hg.

> *Hyperaldosteronism* will give specific complaints of asthenia, cramps, and polyuria; the laboratory findings will help diagnosis.

> *Pheochromocytoma* will give specific complaints of palpitation, headache, sweating, and abnormal laboratory reports.

> *Abnormal history* to be disclosed: check for a history of diabetes, heavy smoking, abuse of salt in the food, or any other of the known causes for hypertension.

Try to bring blood pressure reading to a diastolic pressure of 90 mm Hg or less. Those with readings below 105 diastolic will be treated with a diuretic if they present any of the known factors causative of high blood pressure. Above 105 diastolic requires the use of a diuretic; and if no response is obtained, propranolol, reserpine, or methyldopa will be added. More severe cases, the diastolic blood pressure over 130 mm Hg, will follow the above schedule, but if there is no adequate response, hydralazine will be added (with extreme caution in anginal patients). The last resource will be the use of guanethidine together with or instead of hydralazine. In all instances, adjust dosage to response and tolerance.

Hydrochlorothiazide; give 50 to 100 mg a day.

Propranolol hydrochloride, to start with 40 mg a day, increasing gradually to 320 mg a day.

Hydralazine hydrochloride, to start with 50 mg a day, gradually increasing to 250 mg a day.

Guanethidine sulfate, to start with 12.5 mg a day, gradually increasing to 100 mg a day.

Hypertensive Encephalopathy

This is just a form of malignant hypertension, with intense cephalagia, blurred vision, nausea, vomiting, confusion, convulsions, at times intense vertigo or other neurological symptoms, and final coma. The eyes will show narrowed retinal arteries with flame-shaped hemorrhages and papilledema in advanced cases. Note that papilledema is always present in malignant hypertension. Other symptoms will also be present, namely, elevated systolic and diastolic pressures, the latter largely over 105 mm Hg, palpitations, asthenia, tinnitus, evidence of left ventricle hypertrophy, nocturnal dyspnea and orthopnea, nocturia, hematuria, peripheral involvement (pain, cramps, intermittent claudication, impotence in men), and congested lung bases; and helpful laboratory reports with values for BUN, urea, creatinine, cholesterol, potassium, glucose, and uric acid in blood, a complete blood count, urinalysis, adrenal hormones, and X-ray studies. For more complete information see the entry on ''Arterial Hypertension'' in the chapter on ''Mental Deterioration.''

Since this represents a real medical emergency, the treatment will be immediately and aggressively given. It will start with diazoxide together with furosemide; alternate drugs are hydralazine, reserpine, methyldopa, or nitroprusside for diazoxide, and ethacrinic acid for furosemide. The effects on blood pressure have to be carefully monitored, to maintain the systolic phase between 150 and 170; and the diastolic, between 100 and 90. Some authors advise the use of mannitol or a spinal tap to alleviate intracranial pressure.

Diazoxide, 300 mg in a 20-ml container, to be given rapidly in the vein (avoid extravasation!), repeating every 4 to 6 hours, according to response and tolerance; to resort to oral antihypertensives as soon as possible.

Furosemide, injectables containing 10 mg in each ml (2 or 10 ml), to give 40 to 80 mg by vein, repeating as needed and tolerated.

Hypotension

Asymptomatic in a good number of cases, hypotension may also be characterized by vertigo accompanied by asthenia, easy fatigability, and a tendency to syncopal episodes. Acral parts of the body are usually cool, at times cyanotic; there are a slow pulse and occipital headache, and postural hypotension may occur when the patient changes from a supine to an erect position. A systolic blood pressure below 80 mm Hg represents an emergency situation. Hypotension is usually a part of any of the following conditions:

Syncope: presents irritability, confusion, emotional changes, anxiety or depression; the main characteristic of syncope is its transiency.

Shock: occurs with altered sensorium, pale and clammy skin, tachycardia, dyspnea, thirst while the patient is conscious, oliguria, and final unconsciousness (not transient as in syncope).

Coma: the patient is totally unconscious, as in a deep sleep from which there is no arousal even after painful stimulation.

Adrenal insufficiency: is characterized by extreme asthenia, hyperpigmentation, and hormonal evidence.

Liver cirrhosis: ascites is the main clue for diagnosis.

General infections such as influenza, salmonellosis, and many others will present hypotension together with their characteristic symptoms.

Toxics: there are a number of intoxications that may cause hypotension, but chronic alcoholism is the most important among the elderly.

Other: any debilitating disease will cause hypotension.

Needless to say, in each particular instance the treatment will be that of the causative disease. Vasoconstrictor drugs may be tried in emergency situations.

Hyperventilation

Rapid and deep respirations—usually due to anxiety states, hypoxic or anoxic conditions, anesthesia, or respiratory devices—cause a fall in blood carbon dioxide with increased alkalosis and elevated blood pH. Symptoms will consist of more or less marked tetanic contractions of muscles, intermittent postural changes due to sustained contraction of groups of muscles (asterixis), or other forms of neuromuscular irritability. Not rarely, vertigo accompanies these states.

Rebreathing from a paper bag (not plastic) will improve the situation in most instances. The causative condition will be treated accordingly.

Bradycardia

A rate of less than 60 heart beats a minute is considered bradycardia. In most instances there will be a very sparse symptomatology, or no symptoms at all. Other patients may present some evidence of hypoxia or anoxia, in which instances vertigo results, together with a syncopal reaction in many cases, even reaching convulsions, as often occurs in Stokes-Adams crises. The electrocardiogram may point out the cause of bradycardia. Some occurrences of bradycardia are summarized here.

Sinusal bradycardia: with less symptomatology than in heart block, this abnormality usually stays between 40 and 60 pulsations a minute; the rate may become more rapid with exercise or by pressing on the eyes or the carotid sinus, and there is a complete cardiac complex in the EKG.

Heart block: symptoms are usually more marked; heart beats are usually below 40 a minute, and do not change by exercise or by pressing on the eyes or the carotid sinus; the EKG reveals the block site.

Digitalis intoxication: there is a history of use of the drug because of a previous heart condition; there will be nausea, abdominal pain, marked asthenia, salivation, low temperature, and perhaps varied forms of arrhythmia.

Uremia: this condition follows a known kidney disease, and is easily diagnosed because of anorexia, dry tongue, nausea, bad breath, loss of weight, headache, asthenia, mental changes, and many other symptoms, backed by laboratory findings of elevated BUN, urea, and creatinine in the blood.

Infections: notable ones include influenza, typhoid fever, streptococcal infections, and others.

Hypertensive encephalopathy: other symptoms are intense headache, blurred vision, nausea, confusion, convulsions, and final coma. Diastolic blood pressure is well over 105 mm Hg.

Others: check also for drug abuse (salicylates, etc.), cerebrovascular accidents, intracranial tumors and cysts, meningitis, lesions of the mediastinum, carotid sinus irritation, hypothyroidism, and some heart diseases.

The use of atropine, epinephrine, or ephedrine may improve the bradycardic stage when not due to heart block; but the real treatment of this condition has to be addressed to the basic causative disease in each particular case. Of course, in most instances symptomatic treatment will be useless, as in the case of typhoid fever. Nevertheless, atropine or ephedrine will be tried in cases of sino-auricular block; and ephedrine or isoproterenol, for incomplete auriculo-ventricular block. In other cases a pacemaker is needed.

Atropine sulfate, tablets containing 0.4 mg; take one or one and a half, four times a day, readjusting dosage according to response and tolerance.

Ephedrine sulfate, 25 mg tablets, four times a day, readjusting dosage according to response and tolerance.

Isoproterenol hydrochloride, sublingual tablets containing 10 or 15 mg; give from 5 to 15 mg three times a day, readjusting dosage according to response and tolerance.

Anemia

Patients who complain of vertigo together with paleness of the skin and mucosae, asthenia, tinnitus, spots before the eyes, headache, irritability and psychotic changes among other symptoms of mental deterioration, are to be suspected of being anemic, and a complete blood count will be requested for confirmation. A brief orientation for the diagnosis of anemia is given, again, in the following lines.

Acute blood loss: is the consequence of an external or an internal hemorrhage.

Iron deficiency: there is a slow onset of symptoms, mainly irritability, asthenia, anorexia, gastrointestinal discomfort, dysphagia, pain, numbness, and other minor symptoms.

Pernicious anemia: there is also a slow start, with asthenia, paresthesias, a sore, smooth tongue, gastrointestinal symptoms, depression, confusion, and possibly paranoiac symptoms.

Folic acid deficiency: the symptomatology is similar to that of pernicious anemia, but not improved by the administration of cyanocobalamin.

Other anemia: vertigo and mental deterioration will be symptoms of any form of anemia, if it is sufficiently severe.

An initial transfusion of whole blood or at least packed cells will afford relief. In acute blood loss it will be followed by surgical closure of the bleeding site. In all instances with evidence of shock, this condition should be treated aggressively. Other anemias will be treated according to established rules: iron therapy (ferrous sulfate), cyanocobalamin, folic acid. For more details, if needed, see other entries.

Infections

Any infection of significant intensity may cause vertigo. Usually, the particular symptoms of each disease will be evident, making the diagnosis relatively easy. The fever syndrome, concurrent with most infections, includes an elevation of temperature, with or without chills, general malaise, asthenia, tachycardia (bradycardia or relative bradycardia in some instances), polypnea, pallor or flushing, variable sweating, anorexia, nausea, and possibly other reactions. Also of good diagnostic help are skin rashes, so characteristic in many instances, localized pains, and other symptoms from the blood, the kidneys, and other systems. A brief review of only the most frequent infections diagnosed in old age is given here.

Influenza: occurring during epidemics, with rapid onset, marked asthenia, and generalized pains and fever.

Pneumonia: not rarely a complication of influenza; rapid onset with side pain, cough, and sputum suggestive of the variety involved; in Legionnaires' disease a pneumonic clinical picture occurs in small epidemics with fever.

Chronic and acute bronchitis: with marked cough, fever, and expectoration.

Hepatitis: viral hepatitis may cause not only vertigo but also coma (hepatic coma), the diagnosis made almost only after development of jaundice, dark urine, gray stool, and some itching and fever.

Bacteremia: with septic fever, chills, frequent skin rashes, the germs spreading from a previous septic area.

Shigellosis: diarrhea (with pus, blood, and mucus), cramps and prostration, with fever.

Salmonellosis: usually presented as an acute gastroenteritis (fever, nausea, vomiting, colicky pains and diarrhea); in *typhoid fever* the onset gradually increases to a serious clinical picture, with "pea-soup" diarrhea the second week.

Malaria: precise cycles with sudden fever, shaking chills, and sweating.

Brucellosis: with gastrointestinal upsets, joint pains, and characteristic lymphadenopathy and splenomegaly. Fever is undulant.

Rickettsial diseases: a common subsyndrome of high fever, malaise, headache, pains along the spine and legs, and conjunctivitis; and a characteristic rash in the principal varieties of *typhus,* as well as in cases of *Rocky Mountain spotted fever.*

Meningitis: suggested if there is a stiff neck.

Encephalitis: headache, convulsions, myoclonus, hemiplegia, and backache in various combinations.

Tuberculosis: reactivation of an old disease; cough, evening fever, night sweats, X-ray evidence.

Rheumatic fever: with carditis (pericardial rub, murmurs, enlargement and heart failure, in varied combinations), polyarthralgia, a previous beta-hemolytic streptococcus infection or history of rheumatic fever; chorea is extremely rare among adults.

Tetanus: with characteristic trismus.

Infections of the abdominal organs: usually with signs of acute abdomen, particularly localized pains of extremely severe character.

For more details see corresponding entries in other sections of this book.

Psychogenic Vertigo

The diagnosis of psychogenic vertigo requires a careful evaluation of the patient to eliminate all possible causes of organic origin. In the elderly it may intermix with the so-called benign positional vertigo, when there is not any organic explanation for a mild form of orthostatic vertigo: the patient feels vertigo following a sudden positional change, particularly with the head looking upward, turned aside, or lowered. Other psychoneurotic symptoms are usually present when the patient suffers this kind of complaint.

Psychologic treatment is always appropriate. Symptomatically, the vertiginous state may be alleviated with dimenhydrinate.

Dimenhydrinate, tablets containing 50 mg each; take one, every 4 to 6 hours, adjusting the dosage to response and tolerance.

Secondary Vertigo

Other possible vertiginous reactions, from a variety of other diseases, may also occur, the diagnosis depending on the regular symptomatology for each of these diseases. For example, a good number of abdominal diseases are prone to cause vertigo, particularly diseases of the stomach, the liver, or the appendix.

Gastric diseases: symptoms are mostly related to the digestive process, either when the stomach is empty or following ingestion of food.

Liver: symptoms are extremely variable; jaundice is frequent, but pain at the right upper quadrant is revealing.

Appendix: principal symptom is pain at the right lower quadrant.

PARESIA AND PARALYSIS

Stroke

Unconsciousness and paralysis of one side of the body are the main characteristics of stroke. An entire section of this book has been devoted to this subject, which the reader should consult, in the chapter on unconsciousness.

Facial Paralysis

During the first month of the paralytic disease there is a flaccid paralysis of the affected side; but following this lapse, the paralyzed muscles become contracted, and there is a spasmodic deviation of facial structures toward the affected side, contrary to the way it happened during the paralytic stage, with deviation toward the sound side. Paralyzed muscles lose the natural sulcus running from the nose to the side of the mouth; all facial structures become attenuated and do not agree in movement. The expressions of emotion are lacking—laughter, grief, and the like. If the patient is requested to blow, the paralyzed cheek inflates excessively; if asked to close his eyes, the affected eye will close imperfectly, which happens even when sleeping; tears will constantly be seen running from the affected eye.

Supranuclear paralysis: is seen in hemiplegia due to stroke, with little impairment to eye movements; also seen in some cases of pernicious anemia.

Nuclear paralysis: the eye is involved as usual, and is also accompanied by hemiplegia, but on the opposite side; this form is frequent in lesions of the brain stem.

Peripheral facial paralysis: is like the above, but usually accompanied by hypoesthesia, paresthesia, local pain, and other symptoms.

Peripheral facial paralysis is the most frequent form. If due to exposure to chilling or trauma, and no other cause is found, it will be considered to be a case of Bell's palsy. If it follows, by hours or days, an acute otitis media, or is related in any way to problems within the ear, it will be considered due to edema within the bony facial canal. Other causes of peripheral paralysis are: systemic infections, toxic polyneuritis, diabetes, injuries, and so on. The diagnosis is easy because of the typical expression of the face.

Those lesions within the skull causing facial paralysis will receive the required treatment for each particular instance. Other causes of facial paralysis will also receive the due care: diabetes, intoxications, infections, trauma. The very frequent cause of otic lesions will be treated with antibiotics, myringotomy, and any other adequate measure. Bell's palsy may respond to corticoids. In most instances supportive help with massage, electric stimulation, or taping the deviated structures may give encouraging results. It is best to consult with a specialist.

> Penicillin, to start, until the selected specific antibiotic is known; as an alternate, use broad-spectrum antibiotics.

> Prednisone; give 10 mg, four times a day, for the first 4 days, decreasing dosage thereafter to reach 8 mg a day; and finally discontinuing the drug very slowly.

Paralysis of Limbs

In hemiplegia all one side of the body is paralyzed. In paraplegia, not too rarely diagnosed, both legs are paralyzed, perhaps together with the interior parts of the body. Very rarely diplegia (paralysis of the arms) will be diagnosed. In monoplegia only one limb is paralyzed; and this may occur with paralysis of muscles innervated by only one injured nerve.

> Hemiplegia: following or accompanying stroke due to any of the different forms of cerebrovascular accidents, q.v.

> Paraplegia: due to lack of movement of the muscles, not to interference with movement, as in arthritis, and the like; it may be central in origin, with troubles of sphincters, local anesthesia, no atrophy of muscles, and positive reflexes; in peripheral paraplegia there are no tendon reflexes, muscles are atrophic, sphincters are intact, and there is no or very little local anesthesia. If the muscles are spasmodic (hard to touch), paraplegia may be central. The most frequent form is due to injuries to the spine, but it may also be due to tumors, cysts, vertebral tuberculosis, or other myelitic infections, particularly *rickettsioses,* the Guillain-Barré syndrome, other lesions of the spinal cord, and even encephalic lesions. Because of

the complexity of the etiological factors, these problems are better left to a neurologist.

Diplegia: very rare, usually due to specific diseases (Aran-Duchenne, and the like) but also to cervical ribs or peripheral lesions.

Monoplegia: mostly due to traumatic lesions, particularly to the upper limbs; with paralysis of the radial, the cubital, the median, or other nerves, also including the legs.

Most of these problems belong to the domains of neurologists and surgeons, and the final evaluation of the problem will be left to them. In most instances the only task left to the internist is to alleviate pain, whenever present.

Meperidine, 50 to 100 mg, by injection, repeating according to response and tolerance.

Guillain-Barré Syndrome

Recently, this disease received wide publicity because of its occurrence after vaccination against influenza. It is also known to occur following gastroenteritis or even a mild respiratory infection, and might be described as a motor polyneuritis. Symptoms are: paraplegia (or marked paresis), particularly of the proximal muscles, which are hypotonic and show very slow electric reactions; uni/or bilateral facial paralysis, rarely with diplegia or the need of a respirator, frequently with dysphagia, dysarthria, and paresia of the lateral rectus, local paresthesias or true pains of the eye, abolished tendon relfexes, and little or no involvement of sphincters; possibility of edema of the legs; and in some instances mental symptoms. The spinal fluid shows little change in cells, but a very marked elevation of protein, a very typical alteration.

No treatment is known, but there are reports of some benefit obtained with the administration of corticoids. Give symptomatic support.

Prednisone; give 10 mg, four to six times a day; reduce the dose in 4 or 5 days, to reach gradually 8 or 10 mg a day; thereafter, discontinue the drug very slowly.

Polyneuritis

This is a widespread sensory and motor impairment of peripheral nerves affecting the distal portions of limbs, with weakness, pain or lesser paresthesias and tenderness, hypoesthesia or even anesthesia (particularly of the vibratory sense) involving hands and feet, depressed or absent tendon reflexes, and a glossy red skin with disturbed sweating, all beginning gradually. A search for the causative factor is a must: alcohol, sulfonamides, other toxics, diabetes mellitus, gout, porphyria, meningitis, pneumonia, tuberculosis, rheumatism, systemic lupus erythematosus, polyarteritis nodosa, Guillain-Barré syndrome, beri-beri, cancer and other cachetic states.

It is necessary to control the causative factor. For the polyneuritic condition itself keep the patient in bed, with rest for the affected extremity (avoid pressure over the feet); advise a high caloric diet and a surplus of vitamins of the B group, particularly thiamine; control pain with regular analgesics, and as soon as possible advise massage and active exercise.

> Thiamine hydrochloride, give 10 to 20 mg, three or four times a day, starting by the parenteral route, soon to be followed by oral administration.

> Meperidine, 50 to 100 mg, by injection, adjusting dosage to response and tolerance.

Cerebral and Spinal Tumors

Symptoms of cerebral tumors develop slowly with evidence of intracranial hypertension and localized disturbances. Intracranial hypertension is characterized by intense headache, vomiting with nausea (projectile vomiting), papilledema, frequent bradycardia, vertigo, and perhaps mental derangements. Local disturbances depend on the location of the tumor.

> *Parietal lobe tumors:* contractures of the hands, convulsive seizures, monoplegia, sensory focal seizures, localized paresthesias, and also speech disturbances, agraphia, and other disturbances.

> *Frontal lobe tumors:* may cause aphasia or anosmia (left side or base as site of tumor), psychic disturbances (irritability, poor memory, mood changes), amimia, mild facial paralysis, and nystagmus.

> *Temporal lobe:* convulsive seizures, unpleasant sensations (taste, smell), and possibly aphasia or homonymous visual field defect of the opposite side.

> *Occipital lobe:* homonymous hemianopsia of the opposite side, with visual hallucinations or other disturbances, disturbances of taste sensations, seizures, and other symptoms.

In spinal tumors symptoms depend on the site of the lesion, namely, extramedullary or intramedullary. In all instances the spinal cord or its roots become compressed.

> *Extramedullary tumors:* start with pain and paresthesia corresponding to a particular root, followed by hypoesthesia and anesthesia and paresia; symptoms are at times unilateral, at times bilateral.

Intramedullary tumors: cause less pain and earlier sphincter symptoms.

For a complete diagnosis of these tumors, special radiologic procedures are required, which will be better evaluated by specialists, for both diagnosis and treatment.

Injuries

Paresic or paralytic conditions evolving after more or less serious injuries are manifold, affecting the central nervous system or the peripheral nerves. The most frequently encountered of these injuries are the following:

Head injury: usually causes unconsciousness, which lasts for a short time when it is classed as a cerebral *concussion;* symptoms are similar to those of intracranial hypertension, q.v., and may be due to hematoma or hemorrhage. Emergency surgical treatment is usually required.

Spinal cord injury: injuries to the cervical area, such as of the whiplash type, may not involve the spinal cord because of the amplitude of the canal; but at lower levels of the cord it is not rare to find paralyses below the injured site, which becomes severely painful, usually with stiffness of the neighboring muscles. Note that a reactive paralytic ileus or a retroperitoneal hematoma may mask the evidence of vertebral involvement. Low back pain may be due to injury.

Limb injury: injuries to the limbs or their roots do not cause a true paralysis, but the corresponding movements will be sharply limited, even reaching complete immobility.

Nerve injury: local injuries to nerves will paralyze the muscles innervated by them.

A complete physical examination is required in all instances, using all helpful measures, to decide the extent and importance of each particular injury. In all these cases the help of a surgical specialist is of great importance, since practically all require surgical intervention.

Posterolateral Sclerosis

Older patients are not rarely affected by this "combined systemic disease" (another name used for it), a progressive degeneration of the posterior and the lateral columns of the spinal cord. It starts with paresthesias of toes, feet, and finally fingers (numbness, feeling of pins and needles, and so on), and unsteady gait because of weakness and sensation of heaviness of the legs;

some patients reach the stage of flaccid paralysis with hyporeflexia or occasionally hyperreflexia, and mental deterioration with memory impairment, psychotic stares, and loss of equilibrium and vibratory sense. Many of these patients also present pernicious anemia, which diagnosis in the presence of all these symptoms makes the final diagnosis of posterolateral sclerosis almost certain.

Treatment is the same as for pernicious anemia, with cyanocobalamin.

> Cyanocobalamin, 100 μg by injection, three times a week to start, and thereafter, 100 μg once a month.

Diseases of the Spine

Diseases of the spine may affect bones or nervous structures, but even when mainly bones are diseased, neurologic manifestations are usually important. They may be characterized by paresthesias, pain, paresias, or paralyses. Of course, local symptoms will be decisive in many instances.

> *Injuries:* following a trauma, there will be local pain and tenderness, muscle spasm, and also the possibility of local deformation and neurologic symptoms due to injuries to the spinal roots or to the spinal cord itself (as happens in the well-known Brown-Séquard syndrome with paralysis on one side and anesthesia on the other side, as occurs in cases of lesions affecting one side of the spinal cord).

> *Herniated disk:* true paralysis will rarely occur, but some sort of paresia is not rare, at least a marked weakness of the extremities; symptoms are noted in the arms in the case of a herniated cervical disk, but are more marked in the legs in the case of a lumbosacral disk.

> *Vertebral tuberculosis:* see below, following "Diseases of the Spine."

> *Spinal osteoarthritis:* this frequent condition of the elderly very rarely—if at all—will present neurologic implications, which will be of the type of weakness or paresis. Cervical lesions are more numerous than other types, perhaps, with pain and paresthesias as the main symptoms (upper limbs), but even reaching paraparesis or paraplegia.

> *Spinal tumors:* in extramedullary tumors unilateral or bilateral symptoms may end in anesthesia and paresis, preceded by pain and paresthesias corresponding to the injured root; in intramedullary tumors earlier sphincter symptoms accompany a clinical picture similar to any found in the above diagnoses.

Peroneal muscular atrophy: this usually starts before 30 years of age, but the clinical picture may evolve very insidiously, to be diagnosed at a later age, with weakness and eventual paresis of peroneal and tibial muscles (''stork leg'' because of atrophy below knees). In *hypertrophic interstitial neuropathy* the clinical picture is almost the same, but with pupilar and gastrointestinal symptoms.

Hereditary muscular atrophy: symptoms are similar to those of muscular dystrophy (weakness of pelvic muscles terminating in paralysis of the lower limbs), but starting later in life, even in old age.

Radiologic studies, including plain films, myelographic tests, and other procedures will give the final diagnosis in most instances. Each case has to be evaluated individually, and the final handling discussed with specialized teams, since surgical or neurological approaches are always needed.

Although surgical or neurological procedures are needed for most patients, symptomatic care may be given to decrease discomfort, particularly pain. Other physical measures (massage, electrotherapy, and so on) may also be used. But it will not be forgotten that for the great majority of inherited diseases there is no effective treatment available at this time.

Vertebral Tuberculosis (Pott's Disease)

At times, paraplegia may start the symptomatic picture of Pott's disease. In this instance, the diagnosis may become difficult, the paralytic condition usually due to compression caused by an infected vertebra suddenly dislocated or compressed by neighboring vertebrae. In all cases the final and characteristic gibbous will give the diagnosis, which may be anticipated by radiologic studies. Other general symptoms of tuberculosis are present (evening febricula, night sweating), as well as local symptoms (pain elicited by pressure or motion, some rigidity, perhaps swelling). It is very important to make a positive diagnosis before the spine becomes deformed. X-ray and laboratory procedures detecting vertebral disease and tuberculosis infection are of great help.

Careful evaluation of each case will be carried out to decide a good medico-surgical approach. Of course, general measures for good diet, rest, and so forth, will be observed. Symptomatic help will be given in each case. A combination of ethambutol with isoniazid or with rifampin will be tried first.

Ethambutol, 15 mg for each kilo of body weight, in one oral dose, always watching the state of visual acuity.

Isoniazid, 5 to 10 mg for each kilo of body weight, in one or two daily doses (watch particularly the patient with liver dysfunction).

It will always be very helpful to add pyridoxin, 50 mg a day, orally, for better tolerance.

Encephalitis

Most forms of encephalitis are viral in origin and affect young patients, but at times elderly persons will present cranial nerve or peripheral nerve palsies together with fever, stupor going into coma, convulsions, stiff neck, other symptoms of infection (sore throat, vomiting, lethargy), and tremors; and on physical examination exaggerated deep tendon reflexes, other abnormal reflexes, and spinal fluid showing elevated pressure, higher amounts of protein, lymphocytic pleocytosis, and possibly the causal organism. Watch for complicating pneumonia or urinary retention. This clinical picture may be confused with stroke, brain abscess or tumors, or meningitis.

There is no known specific treatment for these viral infections, but patients may be helped with an adequate symptomatic treatment and general hospital care. Provide the best possible parenteral or nasogastric nutrition in the event of coma; give mannitol for cerebral hypertension; give phenobarbital for convulsions; be sure there is a patent airway (use oxygen if needed); and avoid decubitus ulcers, urinary retention, pneumonia, or other infections.

Mannitol, 10% solution; inject intravenously.

Phenobarbital, 15, 30, or more mg, intravenously, as tolerated and needed.

Syringomyelia

Loss of pain and thermal senses is the most characteristic feature of syringomyelia. Other senses are usually normal. The hypoesthesic reactions are mainly noted in the hands and around the shoulders. Also, the fingers, hands, and arms may show hypotrophy or frank atrophy of muscles, particularly the small muscles of the hands or those around the shoulders. Other usual symptoms are: nystagmus, Horner's syndrome, Charcot joints, vasomotor and trophic changes, spasticity with ataxia, neurogenic bladder, and absence of deep reflexes (particularly upper limbs); and when the proximal parts of the central nervous system are particularly involved, there are: atrophy and fibrillation of the tongue, dysphonia, nystagmus, and loss of sensation (pain, temperature) in the face; but with involvement of the distal portions, there will be more marked symptoms in the lower extremities. Myelography is a very good diagnostic help, showing partial or complete block at the site of the lesions. Do not mistake syringomyelia for tabes dorsalis (Argyll Robertson pupils) or multiple sclerosis (intermittent symptomatology). Rule out the presence of spinal cord tumor, which is not rare in these cases.

Treatment is not too encouraging, but patients may be helped in avoiding invalidism or delaying it until as late as possible. X-ray therapy has been recommended, but results are useless or very poor. Laminectomy and decompression may afford some relief, at least in selected cases, for which reasons specialists will always be consulted. Watch for aspiration pneumonia in long-lasting cases: and always treat aggressively any intercurrent infection.

Hodgkin's Disease

Adenopathy (firm, painless, and large nodes) together with itching, sweating, asthenia, fever, and weight loss—with remissions of the clinical picture—characterizes Hodgkin's disease. But not too rarely other symptoms may become prominent, among them paresias or paralysis (of the paraplegic type, mostly), which occur when the spinal cord in squeezed by extradural compression. Other manifestations may be: laryngeal paralysis, Horner's syndrome, neuritic pains, symptoms of brain involvement (depending on the affected site), splenomegaly, hepatomegaly, and abdominal, mediastinal, and any other manifestations due to the evolved masses. The final diagnosis is made by lymph node biopsy, since hemograms may appear relatively normal during the early stages of the disease. Radiographic studies (plain films, angiographic tests, and others) are also of help in determining the extent of the disease, which is a crucial factor in scheduling treatment. The finding of Reed-Sternberg cells is valued by many authors.

Depending on the stage of the disease, the therapeutic approach varies. Radiation will usually suffice in stages I and II, and not rarely in stage III. Nonresponding patients in stage III and those in stage IV will be subject to chemotherapy with mechlorethamine, vincristine, prednisone, and procarbazine as a first approach, given in 14-day cycles with 14-day pauses, for a total of three to six cycles.

Mechlorethamine, 6 mg for each square meter of body surface, by intravenous injection, on days 1 and 8 (may be 0.3 mg/kg).

Vincristine, 1.4 mg for each square meter of body surface, by intravenous injection, on days 1 and 8.

Procarbazine, 100 mg for each square meter of body surface, by mouth, spread over 14 days.

Prednisone, 40 mg for each square meter of body surface, by mouth, spread over 14 days, but only in cycles 1 and 4.

Cerebral Arteriosclerosis

Problems related to arteriosclerosis have been reviewed in more detail elsewhere in this book, to which sections we refer the reader. Paresias or paralyses will occur mainly when the carotid vessels are involved, thus provoking symptoms of supratentorial origin: paresia or paralysis of the face or extremities, even reaching the stage of hemiplegia, mental changes (confusion, poor memory, behavioral changes), aphasia, and areas of anesthesia; all this occurring as a final stroke or, more frequently, in transient attacks of "little strokes." Subtentorial symptoms of vertigo, ataxia, and altered vision will occur mainly when the vertebral and basilar arteries are involved. Subclavian artery stenosis has been discussed in this section of the book dealing with syncope, q.v. X-ray studies of the arteries will give the final clue to diagnosis; but these arteriograms are to be done by specialists.

Advice for prophylactic measures must be given to all persons suspected of having cerebral arteriosclerosis, particularly if they have been subject to "little strokes." This will include: moderate exercise; diet with low amounts of animal fats; avoidance of active nervous system depressant drugs, particularly major sedatives and the like, as well as avoidance of smoking, alcohol and other toxics, and stressful living conditions; treatment of any coincident disease (obesity, diabetes, hypertension, syphilis, chronic infections, hypothyroidism); and the use of anticoagulants or vasodilators whenever found advisable. The use of antihyperlipidemic drugs will be considered when diet alone fails to control cholesterolemia. Surgical procedures may save many a life. For more detailed information see other entries in this book.

Myasthenia Gravis

Ptosis of the eyelids is the most frequent initial symptom of myasthenia gravis; but there is also increasing fatigability and weakness of muscles innervated by bulbar nuclei, thus causing other symptoms noted from the extraocular muscles (such as strabismus or diplopia), from muscles used to talk and swallow (such as impaired tongue movements and high-pitched nasal voice), from facial muscles (such as the so-called myasthenic smile, nasal and snarling), and other muscles as well (muscles of the extremities, the very serious paralysis of respiratory muscles). Reflexes and sensory perception are normal; but symptoms may worsen slightly during the day and improve after rest. Episodic crises of severe paralytic reaction occur from time to time. The paresic reaction responds almost specifically to the administration of cholinergic drugs: edrophonium chloride for cranial muscle symptoms, or neostigmine for muscles of the extremities. Most patients are females and may also present hyperthyroidism. Interesting experiments have been done with plasma exchange or "plasmapheresis."

Pyridostigmine bromide is presently the drug most frequently used for continuous treatment, though neostigmine may also be prescribed. Additional help may be given with the use of ephedrine, potassium, or corticoids. Side effects may improve with atropine-like medication. Attacks of respiratory paralysis are to be treated immediately with the intramuscular injection of neostigmine, a drug that all patients at risk should always carry with them; in this instance assisted respiration and hospital care are a must.

Pyridostigmine bromide, 5 mg in each ml for injection (2-ml ampoules), and tablets containing 60 mg each, or 180 mg in slow-release tablets; dosage to be individualized for maximal response and minimal side effects. Usually a daily intake of about 1000 mg is average, but adjust to smaller or larger dosage at adequate intervals; the 180 mg slow-release tablet is advisable for night administration.

Neostigmine methylsulfate, 1-ml ampoules containing 0.25 or 0.5 mg each; or vials containing 10 ml with 0.5 or 1 mg in each ml; give 1 mg intramuscularly as soon as respiratory insufficiency is noted; additional 1-mg doses may be given two or three times during the first hour if there is not a good response. Assisted respiration may be needed in spite of the neostigmine administration.

Ephedrine sulfate, tablets containing 22.5 mg each; give half a tablet with each dose of neostigmine.

Potassium supplement, as needed.

Tincture of belladonna, as needed and tolerated.

Edrophonium chloride, 10 mg in each ml, in 1-ml ampoules or 10-ml vials; give 0.2 ml intravenously, at a 15- to 30-second rate, only adding the remaining 0.8 ml if no response is obtained in 45 seconds.

Myotonia Atrophica

This is not a true paralytic disease, but the muscle hypertonus prevents adequate muscle movement, particularly of the hand (fist-making muscles) and tongue, face, jaw, leg, and so on. When the patient grasps an object, it is not possible to release it immediately. Other symptoms also may be present, such as baldness, testicular atrophy, cataracts, or other endocrinopathy.

A try will be given to quinine sulfate, procainamide, or diphenylhydantoin.

Quinine sulfate, 300 or more mg, two or three times a day.

Periodic Paralysis

This familiar disease may also be seen occasionally among the elderly. Patients suffer periodic crises of flaccid paralysis, from a mild form with only a few muscles involved to almost a complete paralysis of the whole body. Such attacks last for a few minutes or may be prolonged for a few hours; they appear most frequently upon waking from sleep, but may also be precipitated not only by rest but also by coldness or overeating, and may be preceded by thirst, sweating, paresthesias, or cramps. Care will always be taken for a possible paralysis of respiration. Fortunately, attacks are less frequent and severe among aged people. Blood potassium may be increased, decreased, or normal during the attacks, the treatment depending on these findings.

Hypokalemic periodic paralysis will respond fairly well to a diet low in sodium and with potassium supplementation. Hyperkalemic attacks (also hypokalemic) respond to acetazolamide.

> Potassium chloride, 2 to 3 g, three or four times a day; in acute attacks increase the oral dose to 5, 10, or more g; the dosage is adjusted to response and tolerance.

> Acetazolamine, tablets containing 250 or 500 mg each; give a daily amount of 250 to 1000 mg, according to response and tolerance.

PARESTHESIA AND NEURALGIA

Any abnormal sensation felt without the corresponding stimulus or responding differently to such stimulation is a paresthesia. Strictly speaking, neuralgia is a paroxysmal pain along the path of one or more nerves, while neuritis is true inflammation of a nerve attended by pain, local tenderness, paresthesia or anesthesia, paralysis, and altered reflexes; nevertheless, it is customary to refer to neuralgia as a pain in a nerve, as in the case of sciatica neuralgia, alveolar or tooth neuralgia, and the like. Consequently, here we shall refer to abnormal sensations or nerve pain as the initial symptom.

In *arteriosclerosis* abnormal sensations of the hands may occur, acroparesthesia not rarely heralding hemiplegia when localized more intensely in one hand; other symptoms will call attention on this diagnosis, such as the hardening and tortuosity of peripheral arteries, and their increased density on X-ray films. If there is also *arterial hypertension,* acroparesthesias will occur more frequently, such as numbness of fingers, intermittent claudication, meralgia paresthetica, little strokes or other evidence of hypertensive encephalopathy, and so on. *Raynaud's disease* usually starts with crises of acroparesthesia and change of color of the distal part of the affected limb, followed by the characteristic more or less extensive gangrene. *Postmenopausal* reactions may also cause acroparesthesia, particularly when there is also intense flushing, often with added pain. Several *neuropathies* will occur with paresthetic symptoms: multiple sclerosis, tabes, brain tumors (particularly cortical tumors, with localized paresthesia usually with paresia and mild myoclonus), and all forms of *neuritis,* including meralgia paresthetica, trigeminal neuralgia, scalenus anticus syndrome, and others. In *pernicious anemia* paresthesias of the tongue and of the limbs may be early symptoms of the disease, preceding other neurological manifestations such as ataxia, loss of vibratory sense, and others. Chronic *alcoholism* may show paresthesias before a clear syndrome of polyneuritis becomes evident, which paresthesias may occur with tremor, flushed face, or a more complex organic brain syndrome. Consider poisoning with *methyl bromide* or *methyl chloride* if a person close to the place of fumigation complains of an intense feeling of burning, chills, or formication in addition to dizziness, hypotension, convulsions, evidence of pulmonary edema, and final coma. The neurological complications of *diabetes mellitus* are well known; but the disease is usually already diagnosed when evidence of peripheral neuritis arises. In *hypoglycemia* the critical stage is not rarely preceded by formication in the skin of the fingers or the scalp. *Chronic glomerulonephritis* may run for years with almost no symptomatology, but even at this time persistent paresthesias may occur, which will call for investigation of the renal function whenever other logical cause is not found. In latent *tetany* paresthesias are not exceptional, but the diagnosis will rely on evidence of neuromuscular hyperirritability and other possible trophic changes (a syndrome characterized by latent tetany and ectodermal disorders—decalcified distal portion of teeth, brittle nails, and early cavities—together with a psychopathic disturbance, as mania or schizophrenia, is not a rare finding). *Pellagrins* usually complain at early stages of the disease of severe paresthesias in the mouth and the skin, and not too infrequently of burning feet.

Arteriosclerosis

Acroparesthesias may be among the earlier symptoms of arteriosclerosis; when localized in one hand, they may herald an oncoming hemiplegia, since relatively frequently some sort of paresia is added to the paresthesia, which may end in a true paralysis. A good suspicion of sclerotic changes may arise from the finding of peripheral sclerotic vessels (enlarged, tortuous, hard to touch), calcified vessels in X-ray films, or poorly working arteries as detected by plethysmography or oscillometry. Among the elderly, early evidence also arises from little strokes, forgetfulness, personality changes, and later impaired memory and confusion. A lesion in the carotid bifurcation may be heard on auscultation. Angiographic studies are needed for a complete final diagnosis. A stroke (q.v.) may be the final outcome of arteriosclerosis.

Prophylaxis for arteriosclerosis includes the treatment of any coincidental (which could be causative) disease—such as obesity, diabetes mellitus, arterial hypertension, syphilis, any chronic infection, and hypothyroidism, diseases that are among the most frequently found. The diet will be carefully regulated, with little or no animal fat (this requires a surplus of fat-soluble vitamins, such as vitamins A and D) and assurance that the patient faithfully follows it. Advise moderate exercise, avoidance of major depressant drugs, an end to smoking or use of alcohol or any other substance toxic to the addict, and avoidance of stressful life conditions. Anticoagulants and vasodilators will be used if needed, as well as antihyperlipidemic drugs when diet alone cannot control hypercholesterolemia. Life can be drastically improved if some sort of surgery is advisable for the particular patient.

Clofibrate, 500 mg, four times a day, adjusting the dosage.

Thyroid extract, 30 mg to start, readjusting dosage as advisable.

Cholestyramine, one package before each of the three daily meals.

Raynaud's Disease

Crises of paresthesia and change of color of the fingers or the toes are usually the starting symptoms of Raynaud's disease. In this instance the symptoms are symmetrical; in the case of Raynaud's phenomenon, they are unilateral. At the beginning of the disease only one or two fingers may show symptoms; but this stage is relatively soon followed by involvement of all other fingers, except the thumbs. Color changes occur, from pallor or cyanosis to rubor of the skin, followed by throbbing and some swelling, numbness, stiffness, and pain. Atrophic changes occur in long-lasting cases, with fat atrophy of the tips of the fingers, and ultimate gangrene. Strictly speaking, this is not a true gangrene, but gangrenous ulcers that may heal when the patient experiences warmer weather, since it is well known that cold precipitates the attacks, which are perhaps also activated by emotional upsets. The disease is usually mild and its course slow. Females are more frequently affected than males.

In mild cases patients only need some protection from cold, namely, to avoid extreme temperatures, to wear good warm gloves and have good body coverage, and to stop smoking if they smoke. Hands must be strictly protected from injuries and infections, because both heal badly and slowly. If the skin is dry, advise the use of softening and lubricating lotions. Severe cases may respond to surgery, if done early (sympathectomy). Vasodilators will be used only when the above measures fail to control symptoms, but they are not always as efficient as desired. Discuss further action in all troublesome cases with a neurosurgeon, and do so before it is too late.

Papaverine hydrochloride, 150 mg sustained-release capsules, to take one every 12 hours.

Pentaerythrytol tetranitrate, 80 mg sustained-release tablets, to
take one every 12 hours.

Postmenopausal Syndrome

During the late climacteric there are usually very few symptoms still present;
flushes rarely stay for long periods, menses may return once or twice without any other implication, and the nervousness, asthenia, irritability, arthralgias, and other minor annoying symptoms gradually diminish. At times
an itching, formication, numbness of extremities, or other paresthesias may
last longer than usual or appear late in the course of the physiologic process.
Also, paresthesias due to atrophic changes occurring in the urethra and
external genitalia occur late and may be extremely severe; but fortunately
these problems respond well to cyclic administration of estrogens. Naturally, good care has to be taken to rule out malignancies that can appear at
this time of life.

For 20 days every month (that is, medication is given for 20 days, with
pauses of about 10 days) estrogens can be administered, for long periods of
time. Warnings against the use—or abuse—of estrogens during the late years
of life, because of undesirable side effects such as thrombosis or malignancies, are perhaps well founded, but most probably they apply more to the
synthetic products or prolonged uninterrupted administration. Large numbers of physicians have been using estrogens in this cyclic way with no
regrets.

Conjugated estrogens, tablets containing 0.625 mg; take one a day,
for 20 days a month; with pauses of about 10 days. Larger doses, up
to 1.25 mg could be given for restricted periods of time.

Meralgia Paresthetica

This is a disturbance of sensation from the external cutaneous femoral nerve
noted in the outer surface of the thigh as formication, burning, tingling,
stabbing or any other form of pain, or numbness, varying from slight feelings
to almost complete anesthesia. There may also be a sensation of tightness or
moistness; and not rarely the hair may fall out. Symptoms may worsen with
exercise, to a point that a confusion with intermittent claudication may
occur; but in the latter condition symptoms disappear after a short rest.
Check for a possible causative condition, such as diabetes, infection, spinal
lesions (at the level of 2nd and 3rd lumbar roots), trauma to the nerve (tight
girdles, truss, and the like), and other possibilities (obesity, flat feet, and
even hypertension).

If a causative factor is found, it should be treated intensively; and all forms of direct trauma to the nerve avoided or corrected. Otherwise, the treatment is as for any other form of neuritis, including a diet rich in vitamins of the B complex, direct administration of thiamine, and analgesics when pain is troublesome.

Thiamine hydrochloride, tablets containing 15 mg; take three or four every day; also, thiamine can be given by injection.

Acetylsalicylic acid, 300 to 600 mg in tablets, as needed and tolerated, better after meals.

Meperidine, 50 to 100 mg, by injection, in the case of unbearable pain.

Trigeminal Neuralgia

Women more frequently than men complain of sudden attacks of short-lasting but excruciating pain felt at one side of the face, in any of these areas: infraorbital, the jaw, ophthalmic, or the tongue. Attacks are initiated by irritation of a specific trigger zone usually located in the painful area, which the patient avoids stimulating in any form because the pain usually reaches enormous proportions. It feels as if the skin is rent, pierced, or burned; if it affects the tongue, mastication is impossible; it occurs intermittently, with exacerbations when prolonged beyond a few minutes, and is repeated several times a day, a week, or a month, or yearly, the intervals being shorter and shorter with advancing age. During the intervals, many patients complain of unpleasant paresthesias (formication, burning sensation), which in some instances constitute the whole disease, and the area remains hypersensitive; pressure in some points causes pain (foramina supra and infraorbital, inframental, etc.). In long-lasting or very severe cases trophic changes may also occur, such as atrophy or edema of the skin, hair falling out, and the like. Also, it is not too rare that the painful attack is accompanied by contracture of the muscles of the face ("tic douloureux"). In all instances check for a causative factor such as diabetes, intoxications, infections, lesions of bones of the skull or the face, or any other chronic disease of the surrounding structures.

Treat any possible causative disease aggressively. In all instances first try a medical approach; if that fails, consider percutaneous electrocoagulation of the preganglionic roots. Use, in order, thiamine, alcohol injection into the nerve, carbamazepine, or diphenylhydantoin.

Thiamine hydrochloride, intramuscularly, 1000 mg a day, for 10 days.

Carbamazepine, 200 mg tablets; start with two a day, adjusting dosage to tolerance and response.

Sciatica

Pain occurs along the sciatic nerve, usually due to a true neuritis, and attended by paresthesia of both thigh and leg, wasting of the muscles of the calf and tenderness on pressure over the nerve, which responds with pain when the leg is forced straight while the thigh is flexed over the abdomen. Pain presents different characteristics, and may be dull or lancinating, severe or bearable, worse while standing; it extends from the buttocks to the ankle all along the back of the extremity. Usually, the pain is steady, but it may also be paroxysmal. Points tender to pressure are present along the nerve at the buttocks, the popliteal area, and at the ankle. Most patients try to move the leg to avoid pain: the leg is flexed and rotated externally, and there is some claudication while walking. Trophic changes may occur. Avoid confusion with arthritis (coxofemoral), diseases of the foot or knee, and others. Efforts will be made to diagnose the causative disease, almost always present. Check for diseases of the spine, particularly herniated discs and cancer (not rarely a metastasis from the prostate); but also find a history of an injury, alcoholism, diabetes, chronic infections, and other usual causes of neuritis.

Always treat the causative factor; and the treatment of sciatica itself will be tried as well. Advise bed rest, immobilization of the leg, application of heat, and analgesics for pain. Thiamine and carbamazepine deserve a trial.

Acetylsalicylic acid, 300 to 600 mg in tablets, some four times a day, according to response and tolerance.

Thiamine hydrochloride, intramuscular injection of 1000 mg once a day, for about 10 days.

Carbamazepine, 200 mg tablets, start with two a day, thereafter adjusting dosage to response and tolerance.

Scalenus Anticus Syndrome

Because of pressure caused by cervical ribs, fibrous bands, or a tight scalenus muscle on the brachial plexus and the subclavian artery, arm acroparesthesias, possibly with neuralgia and edema, will occur. The nervous manifestations mainly occur on the ulnar side, and they may increase to show also impaired sensitivity to pain and touch, muscular weakness, cold and blue hands, at times a Horner's syndrome, and not rarely diminished pulsations noted at the wrist. A positive sign consists of disappearance of or increased pulsations on one side when the patient sitting with the hands resting on the thighs inhales deeply, holds the breath, hyperextends the neck, and turns the head forcibly to one side and then to the other.

Conservative treatment will be tried before resorting to surgery, involving the removal of the abnormal rib, or section of the fibrous bands or of the scalenus anticus. The conservative approach consists of the use of a sling, traction of the neck while resting on the bed, or the less complicated use of pillows arranged to support the shoulder the correct way. Analgesics may be used occasionally for pain.

Intercostal Neuralgia

Of easy diagnosis, intercostal neuralgia usually affects one of the lower intercostal nerves, with pain and paresthesias, either permanent or paroxysmal, and due to herpes zoster or pleurodynia in the majority of cases. Other causes may be vertebral diseases or injuries, aortic aneurism, or tumors of the mediastinum.

The treatment depends on the cause; but symptomatic help with analgesics, thiamine, or physical measures will always be welcomed.

Cervical Neuralgia

Cervical neuralgia may start as a common torticollis lasting for a few days and extending thereafter to the arms; or may start with pain in the arm. There are paresthesias and pain along the arm to the fingers, with or without weakness of the corresponding muscle segments, and stiffness of the fingers, with or without edema. On examination, the movements of the neck are impaired; there is local tenderness on palpation, with diminished reflexes, different blood pressure readings in the arms, and possibly dilation of one of the pupils. The main cause of cervical neuralgia is a herniated cervical disk; but also consider other vertebral diseases, a supernumerary rib, other forms of injury, and diseases of the thorax. The diagnosis is given by a good history and X-ray findings in most instances, including myelography whenever needed.

If the disease is due to a known cause, this cause should be treated as indicated; but regarding the treatment of cervical neuralgia itself, conservative measures will usually be adequate. These consist of avoidance of stressful conditions that might aggravate cervical neuralgia, including massage or other forms of manipulation on the site, which might be more damaging than helpful. Nevertheless, some benefit may be expected from moist heat applications, ultrasound, motorized intermittent hand-controlled traction (starting with 6 to 7 kg and gradually increasing to 16 or 20 kg), isometric exercises, and, above all, wearing a collar during the day and using a cervical contour pillow during the night. Protracted pain may require the local injection of an anesthetic, but usually regular analgesics and muscle relaxants will suffice. Arterial spasms will respond to vasodilators. Inflammation may subside under the influence of phenylbutazone or anti-inflammatory enzymes.

Lidocaine, 1% solution, to inject 5 to 10 ml.

Codeine, 30 to 60 mg, by mouth, every 4 or 6 hours.

Phenylbutazone, 100 mg tablets; give one every 4 to 6 hours, according to response and tolerance.

Other Neuralgias

Practically speaking, any nerve may cause pain, usually responding to local irritation. The above entries referred to the most important forms of neuralgia; here a brief account of other forms of neuralgia is given.

Polyneuritis: mostly present as acro-esthesia, the pain is slowly progressive with tenderness, paresthesia, and muscle weakness; sensory perception of pain or vibrations is diminished; and there are final trophic local changes. Note that most polyneuritis originates from a known cause: alcoholism, intoxication (arsenic, lead, and even drugs), hypovitaminoses (beri-beri, pernicious anemia, pellagra), diabetes, and infectious diseases (diphtheria, leprosy, encephalitis, poliomyelitis, syphilis, and many others). There is an important *senile polyneuritis,* which is a regular polyneuritis possibly due to, or to a combination of, arteriosclerosis, hypovitaminosis, and infection.

Lumbago, or low back pain, starts at the lumbar area, with either dull or marked intensity, impairing the erect position and at times radiating, perhaps along the sciatic nerve; usually is due to injury or any other local mechanical insult, including disk or vertebral diseases; but also may be due to any infectious disease (influenza, meningitis, and so forth), any possible form of rheumatism, and—particularly interesting for our purpose—the well-known forms of *climacteric* and *senile osteoporosis,* of an easy radiologic diagnosis.

Suboccipital neuralgia: pain in the back of the neck, at times more marked on one side and perhaps with muscle spasm; there is a sensitive point on pressure at the midpoint of a line from the mastoid to the first cervical apophysis when the posterior branch of the second nerve root is injured.

Coccygodynia, also called coccyodynia, refers to pain in the coccyx and neighboring areas, not rarely accompanied by annoying spasms of the levator ani muscle; at times it is a residual of parturition, but it usually is a reaction to previous injury (a fall, or repeated small injuries).

Foot neuralgia: relatively frequent, referring to the heel, the sole, or the metatarsal area, gout being the most important form of all.

Neuralgia of the phrenic nerve: usually manifested as retrosternal pain, very similar to anginal pain; it may immobilize the corresponding hemithorax, cause hiccup, increase with respiration and swallowing, and present several tender points (supraclavicular, several vertebral points, sternum, and costodiaphragmatic); it is mainly due to peritonitis, subphrenic abscess, gall bladder diseases, pleurisy, pericarditis, and other diseases of the mediastinum.

Glossopharyngeal neuralgia: recurrent attacks of very severe pain affecting the pharynx (posterior area), the tonsils, the back of the tongue and the middle ear, strongly suggestive of an attack of trigeminal neuralgia; the pain is increased by swallowing or talking, which is a good clue for diagnosis.

Pernicious Anemia

Different forms of neuritic pain are constant findings, sooner or later, in patients suffering from pernicious anemia. Paresthesias of the hands and feet, numbness and tingling, are among the initial symptoms of the disease. Ataxia, possibly ending in a true paraplegia, may occur, resembling tabes dorsalis in the first instance, or multiple sclerosis, in the second. Ataxic patients will not show pupillary signs, but may present particular difficulties in walking during the night, astereognosis, pallanesthesia, diminished reflexes, and other evidence of implication of the posterior columns of the medulla; paraplegics may also show amyotrophy and sphincter disturbances. Some patients will present early asthenia, a positive Romberg sign, hypertonicity or hypotonia, a confusional state (usually with a paradoxical euphoria), and also evidence of impairment of the gastrointestinal tract (glossitis, dyspepsia, and diarrhea), an anemic systolic murmur, ankle edema, moderate hepatomegaly and splenomegaly, and perhaps other complaints corresponding to a complex clinical picture. The positive diagnosis is made when the abnormal large oval erythrocytes, hyperchromia, and achlorhydria are reported; but at times these abnormalities occur late in the disease, and a medullogram is almost mandatory. Other tests are also available, and may be of use for a final decision. Response to cyanocobalamin confirms the diagnosis.

If the diagnosis is made when the patient is in a precarious condition, blood transfusion and bed rest are needed. Otherwise, vitamin B_{12} will be ordered as permanent medication during the rest of the life of the patient. Folic acid is formally contraindicated when the neurological manifestations are of paramount importance.

Cyanocobalamin, intramuscular injection; give 100 μg every other day, until hemogram returns to normal and neurologic symptoms frankly improve or disappear; for maintenance therapy use 100 μg intramuscularly once a week, or give 250 to 500 μg daily by mouth.

Chronic Alcoholism

A relatively characteristic sign of chronic alcoholism is the corresponding toxic polyneuritis, with acro-esthesia and paresthesia, the pain slowly progressive with tenderness on pressure, hypesthesia and pallanesthesia, and final trophic changes with muscle weakness and skin hypotrophy. Other symptoms are: an almost characteristic tremor of hands and tongue; evidence of chronic gastritis, with emesis and weight loss, and unmistakable signs of cirrhosis; a chronic pharyngotracheobronchitis with matinal expectoration; and also mental deterioration with loss of memory, changes of mood and behavior, and at times a typical psychotic condition (Korsakoff's pyschosis, with confusion, disorientation, fabrication, and mild delirium). An ordinarily late event, conditioned by infections (pneumonia or a less serious one), injuries, and the like, is an attack of delirium tremens, with exaggerated tremors of the hands, lips, and tongue, and hallucinations causing great irritability, possibly ending in convulsions and coma. Other diseases also associated with chronic alcoholism are cerebellar degeneration and coagulation disorders. The withdrawal syndrome will occur from 1 to 10 days after the last drink, and is characterized by exacerbations of the mental symptoms. Diagnostic clues are the flushed alcoholic face, ethylic breath, the tremors and neuritic pains, and confessed or implied alcohol dependence.

Treatment of alcoholism is a major problem, usually because of the poor cooperation given by the patient. Solve personal and social implications through adequate centers and institutions; and use the adequate measures in each particular instance for the complications, namely, nutritional, digestive, cirrhotic, anemic, and the like. Disulfiram therapy will be discussed with the patient, and given only with full cooperation.

Disulfiram, 250 or 500 mg tablets; give the first 250-mg morning dose only 12 hours after the last drink; not to exceed 500 mg a day, for 2 weeks; maintenance dose, 250 mg a day, until full recovery.

Diabetes Mellitus

Paresthesias, particularly of the acroparesthetic type, are not too rare symptoms of diabetes mellitus, and are almost indicative of an oncoming acidotic crisis: there will be numbness, formication, burning sensations, coldness, or any other abnormal sensation, perhaps felt more frequently at the tips of the fingers. These symptoms may be associated with neuritic pains, caused by the usually present peripheral neuropathy, of which the symptoms are: acro-esthesia, hypesthesia of hands and feet at times reaching true anesthetic proportions, pallanesthesia (mostly noted in the lower extremities), hyporeflexia, ulterior muscular wasting of the interosseous (muscles of the hands), and outstandingly painful sensations characteristic of the affected nerve or nerves. Any elderly person presenting these vague complaints will be suspected of being diabetic and checked accordingly. First, seek other symptoms of diabetes, such as polydypsia and polyuria, obesity or weight loss (no matter that there is usually increased appetite), asthenia, blurred vision, itching of the skin, particularly in the vulva, frequent and variable refractive changes, cataracts, characteristic diabetic retinopathy (micraneurisms, hemorrhages, hard exudates), possible evidence of occlusive vascular disease affecting mainly the feet, hypertension, dermic diseases (infective disease, xanthomatosis, necrobiosis lipoidica, vitiligo), and confirmation or extension of the neurologic complaints. Second, resort to laboratory confirmation of the disease, with a simple measure of fasting glycemia, or more elaborate procedures capable of detecting milder forms. Fasting glycemia will be over 120 mg%; and the 2-hour postprandial findings, over 215 mg%, or 245 mg% after age 70. Once the diagnosis of diabetes mellitus is established, watch for the usual complications, namely, keto-acidotic accidents, arteriosclerosis (mainly noted in feet, retina, or coronaries, or renal or cerebral), infections, or any other possible complication.

Always try a simple dietetic approach first. The diet will include no less than 150 g of carbohydrates and 80 g of protein. A satisfactory control will show fasting glycemia of 130 mg% or below, or 2-hour postprandial glycemia of 150 mg% or below. If after a reasonable trial of a few days these acceptable levels are not reached, insulin should be added. If the case is not too severe, and those starting at older ages are not usually severe, oral antidiabetics may be used for convenience. In this last instance, care will be taken regarding cooperation, tolerance, and mixed medications.

> Lente or NPH insulin; give 10 units before breakfast if glycosuria (with no renal impairment) is + or ++; or increase up to 20 units if the findings are +++ or ++++; further adjustments will be carried out (generally for increased amounts of insulin) to obtain a satisfactory control of the disease, which may include the use of more rapidly acting insulins.

> Tolbutamide, 500 mg tablets; take up to 1500 mg a day, preferable in divided doses after meals.

> Acetohexamide, 250 mg tablets; take up to 1000 mg a day, preferably in only one dose before breakfast, in two installments.

> Tolazamide, 100 or 250 mg tablets; give from 100 to 1000 mg in one or two installments.

Chlorpropamide, 100 mg tablets; give 100 to 400 mg a day, with breakfast.

Hypoglycemia

Unless the symptomatology is known because of previous attacks of the same nature, isolated acroparesthesias will not be sufficient clinical evidence for the diagnosis of hypoglycemia. But whenever a diabetic patient who uses insulin or active oral hypoglycemic drugs feels numbness, tingling, formication, burning, or any similar sensation, notably at the tip of the fingers, be on the alert for the oncoming hypoglycemic attack. Before syncope or shock occurs, there will be headache, moist skin, tremors, pale or flushed face, tachycardia (on some occasions, bradycardia), palpitation, emotional instability, and dizziness closely preceding the syncopal stage. Of course, diabetics treated with hypoglycemic drugs are not the only subjects of hypoglycemia; check also for pancreatic insulinogen tumors, adrenocortical carcinomas, hepatomas, post-gastrectomy syndrome, or a very severe vagotony. The diagnosis is given when glycemic levels are below 40 mg%; but other more elaborate laboratory procedures are also available, such as determining blood levels of insulin or adrenal hormones. Improvement after the ingestion of glucose is almost diagnostic.

While the patient is still alert, give sugar by mouth, in the form of sugar tablets or glucose solution. It is a good precaution for persons who may suffer hypoglycemic attacks always to carry with them a few lumps of sugar. After this initial treatment, it will be better to complete the meal with additional food, to avoid recurrences of the attack. The unconscious patient will receive 20 g of glucose by intravenous infusion. The cause of hypoglycemia will always be considered.

Glucose, 25% solution, for intravenous administration.

Chronic Renal Insufficiency

Aged patients who previously suffered from some renal disease may present at this time of their lives a clinical picture of renal insufficiency. Check for it whenever a patient reveals a history of any of the following:

Acute glomerulonephritis	Infection of the urinary tract
Pyelonephritis	Renal vascular disease
Chronic obstructive uropathy	Diabetic nephropathy
SLE uropathy	Gout
Tubular diseases	Periarteritis nephropathy
Amyloid disease	Hypercalcemia
Toxic substances (drugs)	Radiation nephropathy

or any other similar condition capable of damaging the kidneys. Frequent complaints are those of peripheral neuropathy with acro-esthesia, hypesthesia of hands and feet (at times reaching proportions of true anesthesia), pallanesthesia mostly marked in the lower extremities, headache, pruritus, myoclonus, hyporeflexia, and pain of the affected nerve or nerves. Other complementary symptoms are: weakness and lethargy of a progressive nature, which together with asthenia and dyspnea sharply limit previous levels of activity, anorexia (weight loss) and thirst, diarrhea, hiccup, purpura, and bleeding. Most patients have arterial hypertension and are prone to its frequent complications, namely, cerebral hemorrhage, pulmonary edema, and heart failure. There is uremic breath, and many patients complain of an annoying metallic taste in the mouth. Signs of dehydration are usually present, the skin is dry with frosty (urea) crystals and excoriated, the retina may be damaged, and finally the classical picture of uremia appears in full. The findings of anemia, azotemia, and acidosis give the laboratory diagnosis of the condition. The anemia is normochromic and normocytic. Nitrogen retention is noted because of the elevated figures for blood urea, BUN, and creatinine. Acidosis is usually moderate, with CO_2 between 10 and 15 mEq/liter. At this time in the disease the urine shows a fixed specific gravity of about 1.01 and a fixed elimination of 1 to 3 or slightly more liters per day, and presents a mild proteinuria, hyaline casts, and few hematic cells, white and red. In addition, the laboratory usually finds low calcemia and proteinemia, and elevated kalemia and phosphatemia.

There is always the possibility of an acceptable improvement of the insufficiency if something can be done to cure or improve the causative obstruction, infection, noxious drug administration, hypercalcemia, and so forth. Renal transplants and extracorporeal dialysis are being used successfully in the treatment of renal insufficiency. These possibilities will be discussed with specialists. In all instances, put these patients on a diet with a protein load of 500 mg for each kilo of body weight every 24 hours, with the other dietary elements present in adequate amounts. Liquid intake must be enough to maintain an adequate diuresis without water retention; diuretics are to be given only if edema is prominent. Sodium will be restricted and electrolytes monitored. Hypertension also calls for sodium restriction, but in other instances sodium should not be curtailed; moreover, at times an extra amount will be given (including sodium chloride and sodium bicarbonate) when there are weight loss and decreased urine volume. Potassium intake will be restricted, with avoidance of foods rich in this salt: orange, grapefruit, banana, pineapple, hamburger, beef (chuck, round, and ribs), turkey, apricots, strawberries, melons of all kinds, tomato, artichoke, brussel sprouts, raisins, dates, prunes, avocado—average portions of which supply from 200 to 1400 mg of the salt. Potassium supplementation is only occasionally needed. Giovanetti's diet is advisable for most patients (protein no more than 40 g, but below 35 g for most elderly persons, with inclusion of all essential amino acids). Phosphates and calcium will be handled as needed, according to their blood levels. Regarding other medications, do not forget that most of them are to be drastically reduced because of their slow elimination, though many are needed for the treatment of the causative disease or the accompanying symptomatology.

Tetany

Before the tetanic muscle spasms appear, or between the crises after the full disease is established, paresthesias and other evidences of the extreme irritability of the nervous system will occur. The tonic contractions will be seen mainly in the muscles of the extremities; but in the case of tetanus, in those of the face and back. Patients will complain of paresthesias, around the mouth or in the limbs, and these may be the first clinical evidence of the condition. A suspicion of tetany will arise whenever these paresthesias occur in patients also presenting trophic symptoms of the type or decalcified teeth (in adults, the free distal edge usually presents minute erosions), brittle nails, early cavities, and finally cataracts or bone hypercalcification. There is a syndrome which may start in adult life consisting of these minute "fractures" of the free edge of teeth, brittle nails, early cavities, hypocalcemia (absolute or relative to phosphorus content), and mental disturbances (manic or schizophrenic reactions), a syndrome that is not too rare and responds well to therapy directed to increasing calcemia. Other mental troubles may be irritability of mood, or psychoneurotic manifestations. The irritability of the nervous system is detected by a few well-known tests, such as Trousseau's, Chvostek's, or Erb's. The causes of tetany are the following:

> *Tetanus:* a rare infection today; the spasms are noted in the face (risus sardonicus) or the trunk (opisthotonus), and there is an infectious syndrome with fever and the history of a previous wound. There are no trophic changes.

> *Hypoparathyroidism:* patients show low calcemia and elevated phosphoremia, no calcium in the urine, and normal alkaline phosphatase; parathormone level in blood is low.

> *Alkalosis:* patients show normal serum calcium, blood CO_2 elevated (metabolic alkalosis) or diminished (respiratory alkalosis), high blood pH, lack of the usual trophic signs, and a positive history for the causal ailment (in metabolic alkalosis: diuretic therapy, violent gastric emptying, hyperfunction of the adrenal cortex; in respiratory alkalosis: usually follows anxiety hyperventilation, but also salicylate poisoning, hypoxia, and fever).

> *Pseudohypoparathyroidism:* there are bone anomalies (short stat-

ure, round face, microdactylia), possible parathyroid hyperplasia, elevated levels of parathormone in the blood, and lack of response to hormone therapy.

Hyperaldosteronism: rare in old age, it will present hypertension, hypokalemia, and at times hypomagnesemia (in this instance, there is no response to calcium therapy).

Laboratory reports will be a help in the diagnostic procedure, in accordance with the above indications.

As shown elsewhere in this book (q.v.), the treatment of hypoparathyroidism consists of the adequate use of calcium salts, parathyroid hormone, dihydrotachysterol, and calciferol, according to responses and reactions. If tetany is due to *C. tetani* infection, the treatment will include the adequate symptomatic care plus antitoxin (human tetanus immune globulin to be preferred), antispasmodics, anticonvulsants, and penicillin. For electrolyte imbalance, the corresponding correction will be needed. For primary hyperaldosteronism, surgical correction of the condition is the best procedure; in other instances, a trial will be given to spironolactone therapy.

Pellagra

Nicotinic acid deficiency is the main feature in the determination of pellagra, which may cause paresthesias in many patients. These paresthesias may occur early in the disease, and may be severe, noted mainly in the mouth and in the pellagrin skin, and also including a burning sensation of the feet in many patients. Following or coincidental with these paresthesias the characteristic erythema will be an almost definitive clue to the diagnosis, namely, a pink erythema that may become darker after a time, noted on the surfaces exposed to sunlight, particularly on the dorsum of the hands, but also on the face and neck. Always consider the possibility of the coincidence of pellagra with other diseases, particularly those impairing absorption of food and causing malnutrition.

Nicotinamide is the drug of choice for the treatment of these patients. Nicotinic acid can also be given, but its use is curtailed by its unpleasant vasodilating effects of the distal blood vessels (nose, ears, fingers). For most of these patients the diet has to be improved, by giving 2500 calories or more, with ample proportions of proteins and a good supplementation of vitamins, particularly those of the B complex.

Niacinamide, tablets containing 50, 100, or 500 mg each, to give 300 to 500 mg, or even more, according to response and tolerance; initial therapy with nicotinamide injectable (containing 100 or 200 mg in each ml) should be administered intramuscularly or even intravenously, in a dosage of about 50 to 500 mg, according to response and tolerance.

MYOCLONUS AND CONVULSIONS

Myoclonus is the involuntary shocklike jerk of a muscle, in its entirety, in part, or in a group. It differs from convulsions in that in the latter, larger portions of the body are involved, usually the entire body. Choreic and tetanic contractions are entirely different, though in tetany there may be myoclonus.

There may be myoclonus in *encephalitis,* perhaps among the earlier symptoms; also in *epilepsy,* in the stage immediately preceding the convulsive seizure. In *Parkinson's disease* there is bradycinesia, difficult to differentiate from true myoclonus, which may also occur. Myoclonus is relatively frequent in cases of *tabes dorsalis* and *general paresis,* causes which will be carefully searched for whenever it begins in relatively late adult life. Some patients with *acidosis* may present myoclonus, particularly if the acidotic condition is caused by diabetes, uremia, or adrenal insufficiency. Myoclonus will be present in *barbiturate intoxication* as well as during or after the clinical course of a few *infections* (influenza, typhoid fever, toxoplasmosis). Finally, there are other diseases in which myoclonus may appear, but there is no reason to include them here now.

Convulsions are the typical evidence of *epilepsy* in most of its forms, not only in cases of generalized seizures, but also in partial seizures and in cases of symptomatic epilepsy due to cranial injuries, brain tumors or abscesses, cerebral arteriosclerosis and cerebral hemorrhages, infections of the brain, cerebral edema, and so on, in a long list of possible incidences, which will be dealt with more detail in the next entry (q.v.).

Epilepsy

Epileptic seizures may be of a convulsive general character or only focal, myoclonic, or even noted by absences, without any muscle jerking. Usually they follow a heralding aura (with any particular sensation for each particular individual, usually similarly repeated each time); the patient falls unconscious, and convulsions appear as sudden, violent, involuntary contractions of large groups of muscles, first tonic (about 30 seconds) and thereafter clonic (about 2 minutes). Once the convulsive stage is over, there is a period of inert relaxation (about 10 minutes) with stertorous respiration, and finally a deep, almost comatose sleep. When the patient awakes from this sleep, he is very tired, and for a while somewhat confused ("crepuscular" state, as designated by many European physicians). But the epileptic seizure may be less impressive, with only focal convulsion, as in the case of jacksonian epilepsy, merely myoclonic jerks, or only transient loss of consciousness without convulsions or falls. The convulsive seizures may be, as indicated: (1) generalized, without any initial focal site, consisting of the classic grand mal seizures, or other seizures that may be called clonic, tonic, atonic, akinetic, or only myoclonus or absences; (2) unilateral or predominantly unilateral seizures; (3) partial seizures with or without loss of consciousness; and (4) other seizures which do not belong to any of the above groups. We must consider here "status epilepticus," characterized by recurrent seizures without a pause between them. When the attack is close to the classic picture, the diagnosis is relatively easy to make; but not so in other instances, when the help of the electroencephalogram is essential, provided that positive findings are noted. Other radiologic or laboratory procedures will help in finding a cause for the epileptic attack.

Primary idiopathic epilepsy presents grand mal seizures, with a complete clinical picture, or only petit mal seizures consisting of myoclonus, absences, and akinesia (both types may coexist); other forms of psychomotor seizures may also be present; the epileptic attacks may start in old age, but epilepsy is usually diagnosed earlier in life.

Cranial injury: jacksonian epilepsy is mainly the type present, with the attacks starting at a specific site, continuing only in focal convulsions, and not rarely unaccompanied by loss of consciousness.

Brain tumor or abscess: attacks may be generalized or of the jacksonian type, and these seizures may be the first symptom of the disease, which once established will present other symptoms of cranial hypertension, and fever in the case of an infection.

Cerebral arteriosclerosis: this will be the prime cause suspected when an aged patient with a previous good general condition or with minor symptoms of generalized sclerosis begins to have seizures.

Cerebral hemorrhage: convulsions may start the clinical picture, which will be rapidly followed by the classical symptomatology of a stroke.

Infections in the brain: both encephalitis and meningitis may start the clinical picture with seizures, but soon other diagnostic symptoms will appear as well. Consider also malaria, tetanus, toxoplasmosis, and so on.

Cerebral edema: there are convulsions of the grand mal type, but without an aura and of prolonged duration, usually accompanied by some sort of paralysis and not rarely ending in coma.

Hyperpyrexia: convulsions are due to a severe infection (rare among the elderly) or to heat or sunstroke.

Toxic substances: alcohol, strychnine, and other convulsant agents may be the cause of convulsions. Include here anaphylactic reactions.

Metabolic origin: convulsions may be a part of the clinical picture of hypoglycemia, tetany, cerebral hypoxia, and a few of the withdrawal syndromes.

The big problem with these convulsive seizures is that because of the falls that follow the attack, injuries are almost inevitable, at times severe ones. The tongue is almost always bitten in epileptic attacks (put a padded tongue depressor between the teeth at the beginning of the attack); bones may be fractured, and the head injured; so check carefully for any of these occurrences after the attack is over.

There is an absolute need to establish the etiologic diagnosis in all cases with convulsions, since the treatment varies accordingly. In each particular instance, treat the basic causes of secondary seizures. Only in the case of epilepsy, or when symptomatic anticonvulsive therapy is advisable, will anticonvulsant drugs be given. For grand mal seizures give diphenylhydantoin, phenobarbital, mephenytoin, mephobarbital, primidone, bromides, or ethotoin. For petit mal seizures advise the use of ethosuximide, paramethadione, methsuximide, phensuximide, mephobarbital, or acetazolamide. For psychomotor seizures the treatment is as for grand mal seizures, but higher doses are usually needed. For status epilepticus first try phenobarbital or paraldehyde intravenously, or use diazepam, diphenylhydantoin, or even general anesthesia.

Diphenylhydantoin, 100 mg tablets; start with 100 mg after supper, adjusting the dosage (usually higher) to response and tolerance. Injectables containing 100 or 250 mg each are given by slow intravenous drip, less than 500 mg, also according to response and tolerance. Care will be taken for gum hypertrophy.

Phenobarbital sodium, to be added to diphenylhydantoin if no results are obtained; tablets containing about 15, 30, or 60 mg; give 30, 60, or more mg at bedtime, adjusting dosage to response and tolerance; for intravenous use prescribe 120 mg in each ml, to give a total amount by slow drip of about 400 to 600 mg, according to response and tolerance.

Mephobarbital, tablets containing about 30 or 100 mg each; take up to 200 mg one to three times a day, according to response and tolerance.

Ethosuximide, 250 mg capsules; take a total amount of 500 to 1500 mg a day, in one or two installments, adjusting dosage to response and tolerance.

Paraldehyde; give from 6 to 10 ml intramuscularly; or, better, if possible, give intravenously 1 or 2 ml diluted in 3 or 6 ml of saline.

Diazepam; give about 10 mg intravenously, prepared as instructed, and repeated according to tolerance and response.

Anticonvulsant therapy will be prolonged for as long as convenient and tolerated; but efforts will be made to discontinue it as soon as possible, even in the case of idiopathic epilepsy. Nevertheless, treatment will be continued whenever needed, but with care taken to avoid or alleviate undesirable side effects.

Stroke

For more details consult the corresponding entry in the chapter on unconsciousness. Only the basic facts will be reviewed here.

A stroke consists of a sudden and enduring loss of neurological functions with unconsciousness accompanied by paralysis. Usually, the attack is heralded by headache, dizziness, nausea or vomiting, and paresthesias with weakness on one side of the body. Not rarely, this side will also present myoclonus or frank convulsions. Consequently, whenever such myoclonus or convulsions are followed by frank hemiplegia, a strong suspicion of stroke will arise.

Subdural hematoma follows an injury to the head and presents headache, spastic hemiplegia, spinal fluid tinged with blood, radiologic and electroencephalographic findings.

Subdural hemorrhage follows an unusual exertion, with headache, stiff neck, hypertension of blood vessels and of the spinal fluid, and among the elderly a history of recurrent attacks.

Intracerebral hemorrhage: the clinical picture is that of subdural hemorrhage occurring in a patient with a previous tendency to bleed (hemopathy, liver cirrhosis); other symptoms vary according to the involved artery: vertebral and basilar arteries, middle cerebral artery, posterior cerebral artery, anterior cerebral artery, or the internal carotid.

Cerebral thrombosis: there is a progressive onset usually following previous neurological complexes and marked evidence of arteriosclerosis.

Cerebral embolism: usually there is a fulminant onset, with symptomatology corresponding to the involved artery.

Arterial hypertension: among other symptoms, myoclonus,

cramps, or twitching of the muscles may occur, the clinical picture worsening until the stroke appears.

Other causes of stroke: these may be brain tumors or abscesses, cerebral arteriosclerosis, temporal arteritis, epilepsy, migraine, mitral stenosis, leukemia, and other diseases which will be considered in the following lines.

The final diagnosis will be completed in each particular case by the adequate accepted means, such as spinal fluid studies, X-ray films, electroencephalography, and so on.

Patients with a stroke, independently of the cause, will be confined to bed, with good care to avoid decubitus ulcers, and will receive parenterally both medications and nutrition. If they are agitated, some sedation will be given. Lumbar punctures will be carefully evaluated, since they may be helpful whenever there is increased intracranial pressure; but they may also be dangerous. The bladder must be catheterized in almost all instances. Anticoagulant therapy will be discussed with specialists, as well as the need for carrying out some sort of surgery, extremely helpful in many instances.

Cerebral Tumors and Cysts

Myoclonus and convulsions may be caused by irritation of the brain, the main symptoms belonging to the complexes of cranial hypertension and the localization of the new mass. An intense cephalalgia, which interferes with sleep, will increase with effort and may be more severe at the site of the lesion, and resistant to ordinary analgesics. This pain together with projectile vomiting and papilledema is characteristic of cranial hypertension. Also there may be bradycardia, ophthalmoplegia, and behavioral disorders. If the tumor localizes in the pituitary gland, the headache is mostly frontal, and the patient may complain of extreme weakness. The headache may resemble migraine.

Hydatid cyst of the brain, frequent in Europe, is relatively rare in the United States, where children are more frequently affected than adults. Headache may be the first manifestation of an expanding mass within the skull, even when it occurs in a patient in general good health. Diagnosis is made by X-ray examination and laboratory tests (eosiniphilia, Carson's test, complement fixation).

Surgery is the only approach to this problem. Persons over 80 years of age will not be treated surgically but may be given 50% glucose solution.

Glucose, 50% solution; inject intravenously 25 ml—most cases will respond well to this amount—up to 50 ml.

Analgesics are of little value. Narcotics are not advised and are not indicated for these patients, and lumbar puncture is not recommended.

Cerebral Abscess

When the irritation caused by a cerebral abscess reaches sufficient intensity, there will be unmistakable signs of progressive neurological symptoms, including myoclonus or convulsions and other evidence of increased pressure within the skull (headache, projectile vomiting, papilledema), as well as visual defects, paresia or paralysis of cranial or other nerves, sleepiness, fever, and also some meningeal irritation with stiffness of the neck and a positive Kernig's sign. A careful search for the initial infection will be made: sinusitis, otitis media, pulmonary infection, or any other sepsis. For a final diagnosis the use of several of the different radiologic procedures will be needed, such as cerebral angiography, pneumoencephalography, brain scan, and so on.

Any infection may cause a brain abscess, but staphylococci and pneumococci are found most frequently; consequently, oxacillin or a regular penicillin will be the antibiotic of choice to start therapy, before the most active one is known. Antibiotherapy will start as soon as there is any suspicion of a brain abscess because it may abort the infection or may make possible a better and safer operation. A neurosurgeon will always be consulted.

> Oxacillin, ampoules containing 250, 500, 1000, 2000, or 4000 mg each, to be reconstituted in the corresponding amount of normal saline or 5% glucose, to be given intravenously by slow infusion in amounts of 1000 to 4000 mg every 4 to 6 hours, for a total of about 10 days, always watching carefully for the development of resistant strains.

Encephalitis

In encephalitis backache, fever, headache, and neurological symptoms, in varied combinations, are common. Malaise, insomnia, convulsions, myoclonus, ocular paralysis, and hemiplegia might also mark its progress. Clinical pictures vary from very mild, as frequently found in St. Louis encephalitis, to very severe, with hyperpyrexia, convulsions, and coma, such as is common in Eastern encephalitis. Spinal fluid examination will differentiate encephalitis from meningitis—lacking meningeal characteristics—and will give the etiologic diagnosis.

Isolate patients in bed, giving the regular hospital care. Viral encephalitis has no specific etiologic treatment. Give the specific antibiotic when the infecting germ is known. Corticoids, early in the disease, will help headache and convulsions. Excessive intracranial pressure usually responds to mannitol or urea-invert infusions. Analgesics may be tried.

> Prednisone, 5 to 20 mg, every 6 hours, according to need and tolerance; to be reduced and discontinued at a slow pace.

Acetylsalicylic acid, 300 to 600 mg, in tablets, every 4 to 6 hours, preferably with meals.

Codeine, 30 mg, by mouth, every 4 hours; may be given together with acetylsalicylic acid. Increase to 60 mg if needed and tolerated.

Meperidine, 50 mg, orally or by intramuscular injection, every 4 hours. Increase to 100 mg if needed and tolerated.

Mannitol, 10% solution, by intravenous infusion.

Phenobarbital, 30 mg, by mouth or by injection, to control convulsions. Increase the dosage if needed and tolerated.

Meningitis

It is usual that convulsions form a part of the symptomatology of meningitis. Myoclonic twitching or convulsions usually follow the febrile chills, and the clinical picture is completed with headache, vomiting, confusion or delirium, pains all over the body (back, limbs, abdomen), stiffness of the neck, a rash that is petechial in nature, positivity of Kernig's, Brudzinski's, and other similar signs, dyspnea (Cheyne-Stokes or Biot type), and a possible final shock or frank coma. The spinal fluid will show hypertension, pus, and the well-known association of high protein and low glucose. The causative germ will be found in the spinal fluid, but at times only in the blood, or obtained from the pharynx. It will also be good to check for factors V and VIII, because intravascular clotting is not a rare complication of meningitis.

Meningococcal meningitis: epidemic or endemic; no evidence of a previous organic infection; classical clinical picture.

Pneumococcal meningitis: usually following a pulmonary infection.

Streptococcal or staphylococcal meningitis: following a previous otitis media, sinusitis, or similar infection.

H. influenzae meningitis: mostly only in very young children.

Tuberculous meningitis: with a known initial lesion, the clinical picture developing at a relatively slow pace.

Needless to say, a patient with meningitis should be hospitalized immediately and receive adequate care. Mannitol or 25% glucose will be given to combat elevated intracranial pressure; evidence of shock or impending shock will be treated with blood-expanding solutions (with dopamine or isoproterenol added if there is a poor response); assisted respiration is given whenever needed; and anticoagulants may control intravascular coagulation. Antibiotics are urgently needed, with the specific one given in each particular case; but in the meantime patients are treated as follows: for meningococcal meningitis, penicillin (chloramphenicol for allergic patients); for pneumococcal meningitis, also penicillin; for streptococcal meningitis, penicillin; for staphylococcal meningitis, oxacillin or methicillin; for tuberculous meningitis, a complex therapy with isoniazid, ethambutol, and rifampin, plus streptomycin and corticosteroids.

Mannitol 10% solution, to be given by intravenous infusion.

Normal saline, or 5% glucose, for intravenous infusion (with added dopamine or isoproterenol if needed).

Anticoagulation: start with heparin and continue with warfarin.

Aqueous penicillin G; give about 20 million units every 24 hours, preferably in divided doses, to be continued until 5 days after all symptoms of infection subside.

Chloramphenicol; give 100 mg for each kilo of body weight every 24 hours (if the patient is sensitive to penicillin).

Oxacillin, ampoules containing 250, 500, 1000, 2000 or 4000 mg each, to be reconstituted with saline or 5% glucose; give 2000 to 4000 mg every 4 to 6 hours.

For tuberculous meningitis treatment, see any entry referring to tuberculosis.

Bradycardia

A heart rate of less than 60 pulsations a minute constitutes bradycardia, which may be due to a heart sinus condition or to an auriculoventricular block. In either instance the consequence is the same, namely, cerebral hypoxia, which may induce a syncopal reaction, usually with convulsions. The elderly are not as resistant as younger people to the effects of cerebral hypoxia; they react relatively soon to oxygen deprivation, with asthenia, confusion, and then a convulsive syncopal state. This clinical picture does not occur frequently with sinus bradycardia as with auriculoventricular block, when the Stokes-Adams syndrome may develop, with dizziness and the full clinical picture. When the patient is checked, the very slow heart rate will provide the diagnosis; but the diagnosis cannot be complete without an electrocardiogram. In the "sick sinus syndrome" bradycardia alternates with tachycardia. For more details, see under the heading "Tremor," earlier in this chapter.

In general, the treatment for syncopal convulsions of this sort is the same as the treatment described for shock (q.v.), including rest, the head at a lower level than the heart, and blood expanders and cardiotonics if needed. For treatment of the general condition a try will be given to atropine or other belladonna products; but the final decision to use or not to use a pacemaker will be left to the specialist.

> Atropine, 0.5 or 1 mg ampoules, and 0.3 or 0.4 mg tablets; give 0.3 to 0.6 mg a day, according to tolerance and response.

> Tincture of belladonna, give 10 to 30 drops every 6 or 8 hours, according to response and tolerance.

Hypoglycemia

Many patients with hypoglycemic attacks regularly present myoclonus or convulsions as a part of the clinical picture, which also consists of hunger, sweating, asthenia, anxiety, paleness of the lips, dyspnea, tremors, confusion, irritability, and final syncope or coma. In other words, a convulsive attack accompanied by sweating, preceded by hunger, and occuring in a patient using hypoglycemic agents or presenting a disease capable of reducing blood sugar, will strongly suggest the diagnosis of hypoglycemia. Consider pancreatic or extrapancreatic tumors provoking hyperinsulinism, a post-gastrectomy condition, extremely increased vagal tone, and others.

An early diagnosis is essential—and not too difficult to obtain in the great majority of cases (because of the history—since the condition responds rapidly and efficiently to the administration of sugar or glucose, either by mouth (before unconsciousness occurs) or by intravenous administration. The rest of the treatment depends on the correction of the causative factor, namely, more careful administration of hypoglycemic agents, better timing of meals, or the complete treatment of the cause. After the administration of sugar or glucose, it is wise to give an adequate meal to prevent recurrence of the attack, and to observe a regular food intake.

> Glucose, 25% solution; give 40 to 100 ml, according to response, by the intravenous route.

Tetany

In tetany, tonic contraction is almost the rule, but nonetheless convulsions may be an important part of the regular clinical picture, which consists of extreme irritability of the nervous system, paresthesias around the mouth or in the limbs, trophic signs (eroded teeth, brittle nails, early cavities, cataracts, bone hypocalcification), psychoneurotic manifestations, and the positivity of signs (Trousseau, Chvostek, Erb). The causes of tetany may be: *tetanus* (an infective condition with spasms in the face and the body; no trophic signs), *hypoparathyroidism* (low calcemia, elevated phosphoremia, trophic changes), *alkalosis* (elevated pH and the history of a causative factor), *pseudohypoparathyroidism* (with bone anomalies), and *hyperaldos-*

teronism (with hypertension and hypokalemia, but rare among the elderly). Laboratory reports are a must for a complete diagnosis. For more details see under the heading "Paresthesia and Neuralgia," earlier in this chapter.

Each clinical type of tetany requires its own treatment. For tetanus give symptomatic care, human tetanus immune globulin, and penicillin. For hypoparathyroidism give calcium salts, parathyroid hormone, dihydrotachysterol, or calciferol, according to response and tolerance. For electrolyte imbalance, its correction is the root of the whole treatment. For hyperaldosteronism, a trial will be given to spironolactone, but surgery is usually the final resource.

Acidosis

In a few instances of acidosis, myoclonus or convulsions will be an important part of the clinical picture, together with asthenia, headache, paresthesias, dizziness, confusion, even meningeal symptomatology, and final coma. *Respiratory acidosis* follows pulmonary emphysema, depression of the respiratory center (diseases of the nervous system, use of drugs or depressants), myasthenia gravis, congestive heart failure, pneumonia, lung disease, laryngeal obstruction (edema or foreign body), or assisted respiration (excess of CO_2). *Metabolic acidosis* shows also some evidence of dehydration, abdominal pain, and hyperpnea, all following diabetes, diarrhea, salicylate poisoning, renal failure, or any other form of dehydration. In all instances there is a lowered pH, but the CO_2 in the blood will be high in respiratory acidosis and low in the other type.

For respiratory acidosis use bronchodilators or mechanical aids, but treat the causative factor basically. If oxygen is given, care will be taken not to provoke CO_2 narcosis. For metabolic acidosis restore acid–base balance by giving sodium bicarbonate solution in 5% glucose. Also, treat the causative condition well.

> Sodium bicarbonate, 7.5% solution containing 45 mEq in each 50-ml vial, one or two vials to be added to 1000 ml of 5% glucose in water. The amount to be given is estimated from this formula: blood bicarbonate deficit in mEq multiplied by 25% of the body weight.

Anaphylaxis

Convulsions will either precede or accompany shock when an anaphylactic reaction occurs. The very impressive accident consists of a rapid succession of symptoms, in a matter of seconds or minutes, following the administration of a foreign substance, particularly of proteic nature or a drug, or an insect sting. Patients become agitated and apprehensive; the pulse increases rapidly in frequency; there are cyanosis, sneezing, coughing, wheezing, possible incontinence, and complaints of choking, throbbing in the ears, itching, and other paresthesias; pupils are dilated, fever rises, and three main syndromes may appear, namely, vascular collapse, laryngeal edema, or bronchospasm; rapidly followed (after a total of 5 to 10 minutes) by loss of consciousness and convulsions. Early diagnosis will be guided by the appearance of cyanosis and tachycardia following the intake of the offending substance.

When administering any of the substances capable of causing anaphylactic reactions, the physician will always have readily available an ampoule of epinephrine to be given with *no delay* at the start of the first alarming symptom. Place the patient in a recumbent position, keep the body warm, maintain a patent airway (resort to endotracheal tube or tracheostomy if necessary), assist respiration if there is some trouble in this area, use antihistaminics or corticoids to shorten reactions, and restore venous pressure with blood expanders and vasopressors.

> Epinephrine, 1 : 1000 solution; give 1 ml by intramuscular injection, or 0.5 ml in 10 ml saline intravenously, if the first intramuscular dose has little effect.

> Diphenylhydramine hydrochloride, 5 to 20 mg in water solution, to be given intravenously.

> Hydrocortisone, 200 mg in water, by intravenous injection, to be repeated after 4 hours if so needed.

Alcoholism

In chronic alcoholism as well as in the acute poisoning, convulsions are usually present, but in neither case are they diagnostic. In the *acute attack* symptoms correspond to nervous depression and gastric irritation, namely, incoordination, asthenia, vertigo with ataxia, dyspnea, cyanosis, tachycardia, confusion or delirium, vomiting, abdominal pain, and final coma with convulsions and elevated fever. In *chronic alcoholism* a good guidepoint is the toxic polyneuritis with acro-esthesia and paresthesia, these troubles slowly progressive and accompanied by tremors (tongue and fingers), chronic gastritis, evidence of liver cirrhosis and mental deterioration, and occasional attacks of delirium tremens, ending in convulsions and coma. For more details see above in this chapter, under the heading "Paresthesia and Neuralgia."

When treating these patients take advantage of adequate centers and institutions. Try disulfiram therapy after a productive discussion with the patient; and regulate as carefully as possible the patient's nutrition, health, general condition, and behavioral mood.

Disulfiram, tablets containing 250 or 500 mg each, to start therapy only 12 hours after the last drink (very important!), by giving 250 mg in the morning; try to give 500 mg a day for 2 weeks, according to response and tolerance; and until full recovery (?) use 250 mg every morning.

Infections

It is impossible to complete this entry adequately. Convulsions may occur in any infection severe enough to cause nervous irritation, or in any patient sensitive enough (some are more sensitive than others) to this sort of irritation. Consequently, in a longer or shorter period of time a patient with a fever syndrome may reach a convulsive state. This will happen more frequently with very young patients; but the elderly may react similarly, particularly in cases of meningitis, encephalitis, syphilis, tetanus, malaria, rabies, toxoplasmosis, and perhaps some metabolic disease as well. But it must be stressed at this time that many older persons do not show high fever, even in cases of severe infections. The components of the fever syndrome, in addition to a temperature over 37°C (98.6°F), are generally malaise, weakness, anorexia, tachycardia (there may be a relative bradycardia in some instances), polypnea, concentrated urine with elevated nitrogen excretion, vasomotor changes (pallor or flushing), sweating, possible delirium or chills, and other symptoms characteristic of other organs or systems of the body, which may help in the diagnosis. Laboratory reports will show leukocytosis and the causative germ in many instances.

Meningitis and encephalitis: see corresponding entries earlier in this section.

Syphilis: there is usually evidence of a previous infection, such as chancre, secondary stage, and the like; but among the elderly late lesions are more frequently found, such as skin or bone lesions, visceral syphilis, cardiovascular syndromes (aortitis), and central nervous system involvement.

Tetanus: see "Tetany" earlier in this section.

Malaria: the disease is characterized by the sequence of chills (the tremors may reach the category of true convulsions), fever, and sweating; but during the course of the disease true convulsions will appear (particularly in the case of cerebral malaria), together with delirium, jaundice, gastrointestinal disorders, and final coma.

Rabies: when the irritability of the nervous system develops, there will be fear of drinking water (hydrophobia), due to spasms of the pharynx, paresthesias, accesses of extreme irritability (rabies), paralysis, and also convulsions, all following a history of an animal bite.

Toxoplasmosis: the disease may show only adenopathy, splenomegaly, and a maculo-papular rash; but in severe cases myocarditis and convulsions may occur.

Metabolic disorders: see other entries in this section relating to hypoglycemia and acidosis.

The help from laboratory, radiologic, and other possible tests is so abundant that it is impossible to give a useful summary of it here. Each instance will require individual investigation to determine the correct diagnosis.

The same thing can be said of treatment: each disease will be treated according to the accepted rules. The symptom, convulsion, will respond better to the basic therapy; but at times anticonvulsant drugs may help, such as phenobarbital, paraldehyde, diazepam, or even diphenylhydantoin.

Phenobarbital sodium, containers with 120 mg in each ml; give intravenously by slow drip a total amount of 400 to 600 mg, according to response and tolerance.

Senile Chorea

Paralysis agitans is also called senile chorea, but this condition is different from parkinsonism. Senile chorea is most probably an independent entity, starting in old age with the unceasing occurrence of rapid and ample jerky movements, involuntary in nature, apparently well-coordinated, but without any purpose, entirely different from myoclonus, convulsions, tremor, or athetosis. In this instance, it is a chronic condition not traceable to any form of heredity, which is possibly due to sclerosis principally involving the optostriate nuclei in the thalamus opticus and the corpus striatum.

Treat any disease that may help arteriosclerosis to develop, such as obesity, diabetes, hypertension, syphilis, hypothyroidism, or any chronic infection; advise moderate exercise, a diet with little animal fat and a surplus of fat-soluble vitamins, avoidance of major depressant drugs and sedatives, as well as avoidance of toxic substances (smoking, alcohol) and stressful life conditions. Anticoagulants, vasodilators, and antihyperlipidemic drugs will be given whenever needed. Discuss the advisability of surgery by a skilled neurosurgeon.

Parkinson's Disease

Tremor and rigidity are the essentials of parkinsonism, but at times apparent myoclonus may occur. Nevertheless, the alert physician will immediately recognize the tremor and rigidity, so that the identification of the disease will be relatively easy. For more details, see the beginning of this chapter on "Neurological Symptoms."

Pure parkinsonism will be treated with atropine-like medication, trihexyphenidyl, cycrimine, amantadine, or levadopa.

Tincture of belladonna; give according to results and tolerance.

Levadopa; start with 500 mg every 8 hours, increasing dosage according to response and tolerance.

Tabes Dorsalis

Among older adults, myoclonus may occur in some cases of tabes dorsalis, but the classic symptoms of fulgurant (shooting or lightning) pains, hypotonia, inability to walk in the dark, crises beginning suddenly and lasting for hours or days (gastric, laryngeal, urethral, anal, or rectal), and painless trophic ulcers will help one to reach the final diagnosis. Laboratory tests will decide it.

It is better to prevent than to treat the disease; but in the last analysis use large doses of penicillin, even to over 20 million units a day, intravenously.

General Paresis

Dementia paralytica or general paresis is another form of late neurosyphylis. Here also older adults may present myoclonus, but the common symptomatology will give the clue to diagnosis. There is a slow onset with decreased memory, poor concentration, speech disorders, irritability and tremors (better noted in the fingers), and characteristic behavioral changes (confusion, irresponsibility, psychotic manifestations). Again, the laboratory tests will decide the diagnosis.

Treatment will be as for tabes dorsalis, which is stated in the above entry (q.v.).

Toxic Substances (Saturnism and Others)

Convulsions may occur in alcoholism (q.v. above), saturnism, or intoxication by strychnine, digitalis, camphorated drugs, and other substances. Mild myoclonus may occur in intoxication by barbiturates. In most instances the history of administration or abuse of the noxious substance is evident. In *saturnism* the "lead-line" in the gums may be noted, and the basophilic stippling of erythrocytes is almost characteristic. In *strychnine poisoning* (including picrotoxin and nux vomica) jerks occur wherever the skin is touched, and all the remaining symptomatology is that of a severe case of tetany (q.v.). In *digitalis intoxication* convulsions occur when the disease is well established, with outstanding abnormalities of the pulse and no loss of consciousness until very late. In *camphorism* there are a typical camphor odor of the breath (and urine), tachycardia, delirium, and at times a burning pain in the stomach (due to the administration of large doses). In *amphetamine intoxication* convulsions may occur, with or without coma, but always with marked excitability of the nervous system (irritability, mania, tremor, and so forth). In *antihistamine intoxication* convulsions are preceded by depression followed by excitation. In *arsenic intoxication* (arseniasis) convulsions with or without coma come late; classic symptoms are the "rice-water" stools, intense thirst, abdominal pains, and the garlic odor of the breath. In *cocainism* choreic movements and convulsions are usually present, with excitement, hallucinations, dilated pupils, fever, changes of blood pressure (first high, thereafter low), cyanosis, and final coma. In *salicylism* neither convulsions nor other symptoms are too characteristic, except perhaps for the profuse sweating and tinnitus; the diagnosis depends mostly on the history. In *parathion intoxication* (an organic phosphate insecticide), convulsions will come relatively late, with coma in most instances, the diagnosis depending on the history. In *chlorinated organic insecticides intoxication* (DDT, chlordane, aldrin, and others) convulsions are usually followed by depression; there are also tremors, giddiness, respiratory failure, and other symptoms of little help for diagnosis. In *narcotic intoxication* convulsions are of little diagnostic interest because of their very late occurrence. *Barbiturate intoxication* may cause mild myoclonus. In *atropinism* caused by atropine salts or belladonna there may be convulsions, but other symptoms are of greater interest, namely, dryness of the mouth with husky voice, dilated pupils, excitement with confusion, flushed face, and others. In *carbon monoxide intoxication,* tetanic convulsions, together with a dusky reddened skin that also shows bluish red patches, are practically diagnostic when the person is found in a closed automobile with the engine running. In *cyanide intoxication* convulsions are usually violent, and there are a characteristic odor to the breath (bitter almonds or peach kernels), mental confusion, dyspnea, and final coma.

In all instances there is the need for emergency treatment. Treat the patient symptomatically; but try to use the appropriate antidote whenever possible.

Saturnism: use calcium gluconate or calcium chloride, and try to delead the patient with calcium disodium edetate (with or without dimercaprol).

Strychnine: use paraldehyde or diazepam.

Digitalis: use potassium salts; but if they are contraindicated (renal insufficiency), give atropine, quinidine, or procainamide.

Camphor: use a short-acting barbiturate or chloral hydrate.

Amphetamines: use chlorpromazine.

Antihistamines: use sedatives.

Arsenic: use dimercaprol.

Cocaine: relieve nervous excitement with a short-acting barbiturate or with chlorpromazine.

Salicylates: use sodium bicarbonate or lactate intravenously to correct acid–base balance.

Organic phosphate insecticide: use atropine, by injection.

Chlorinated organic insecticide: use a short-acting barbiturate.

Atropinism: use a short-acting barbiturate.

Carbon monoxide: give oxygen, and transfusion if necessary.

Cyanide: use amyl nitrate, and follow with sodium nitrite.

Narcotics: use levallarphan, nalorphine, and oxygen.

Barbiturates: use assisted respiration, intravenous fluids, and vasopressors.

SPASTICITY

Spasticity consists of the hypertonic stiffness of muscles, which are therefore resistant to stretching and awkward when moved. Spasms are long-lasting and usually not painful; cramps last a shorter time and usually hurt. Nevertheless, some cramps will be included here.

Torticollis (Wryneck)

This sort of contraction of the muscles of the neck (sternocleidomastoid and trapezius muscles) may be due to a disease of the basal ganglia or to an entirely unknown cause; or it may be due to fibromyositis. In the first instance check for postencephalitic parkinsonism or paralysis agitanus; and in the second for a previous injury, infection, unusual stress, or a physical influence. The clinical picture is the same in both instances; the muscles are contracted at the posterior quadrant of one of the sides of the neck, the head becomes rotated to the opposite side and flexed to the same side, movements are usually very painful, and there is also an exquisite tenderness to touch. The main difference between spasmodic and fibromyositic torticollis is the duration, with a longer duration in the first instance, with the possibility of a reactional hypertrophy of the muscle.

> *Spasmodic torticollis:* there is not only a sustained tonic spasm, but it may also be intermittent, and after a few months there may be muscle hypertrophy; there is a previous history of extrapyramidal

disease, such as parkinsonism or encephalitis, which will be carefully searched for, including diseases of the cervical spine.

Traumatic torticollis: the previous injury may even be a mild one; it may follow a vertebral luxation; and it may become permanent.

Torticollis due to an infection: any inflammation to the cervical spine (tuberculosis), to the muscles themselves, to the pharynx, or to the middle ear may also be the cause of wryneck; the diagnosis usually becomes obvious.

Stress torticollis follows unusual exertion of the corresponding muscles; the diagnosis is also obvious.

Physical torticollis: this condition is due to exposure to unusual coldness.

Other forms of torticollis are of relatively little interest here because they refer to earlier stages of life: abnormalities of the vertebrae, injury during birth, and so on.

The diagnosis will be relatively easy in most instances because the clinical picture is characteristic and almost unmistakable; the laboratory and radiologic procedures will give decisive help in reaching the exact diagnosis.

Causative factors are to be eliminated whenever possible, both in spasmodic or fibromyositic torticollis. In the first case, drugs of the type of belladonna may be helpful; and also meprobamate, chlorpromazine, or barbiturates. Surgery may be discussed in some instances. In the case of fibromyositic torticollis, massage, rest, and heat applications are of help; in some refractory instances, the local injection of procaine into the trigger nodules may become necessary.

Tincture of belladonna, 15 or more drops each time, adjusting dosage and timing to response and tolerance.

Meprobamate, 400 mg tablets; adjust dosage to response and tolerance.

Procaine, 1% solution; inject 0.5 ml or more into each nodule, according to response and tolerance.

Blepharospasm and Hemifacial Spasm

In hemifacial spasm, of which blepharospasm may be a part, there is a unilateral sudden contraction of facial muscles occurring without a cause or following some sort of trigger excitation (laughter, chewing, talking). There is no pain in most cases, but at times it may occur (do not take it for tic douloureux). In blepharospasm, the contraction is limited to the orbicularis; nevertheless, it may be bilateral, but usually responds to the same etiological factors as hemifacial spasm. In many instances hemifacial spasm corresponds to lesions of the facial nerve, but mostly it is due to cerebellopontine angle tumors, in which the more important symptoms are not the spasms but tinnitus, vertigo, facial palsy and anesthesia, and other evidence of cerebellar involvement. For an accurate diagnosis ophthalmologic, otologic, radiologic, electroencephalographic, and other similar studies are needed.

There is an emergency need for an early diagnosis, since surgery (or radiotherapy) is the only adequate means for an acceptable treatment. Specialists must be consulted in all instances.

Occupational Spasms

Also called cramps, at times, these spasmodic contractions of a group of muscles designed for a specific activity may appear during the exertion of the particular activity and strongly interfere with its execution. There may be a pure spasm, a painful spasm, a trembling spasm, or a paralytic spasm.

> *Writer spasm:* once established, it appears sooner or later whenever an attempt to write with a pencil or pen is made; the hand twitches on the pen or pencil, and the contracture may extend to the fist and even the whole forearm, so that it is impossible to write a word; after a rest the spasm may disappear, but it will be reactivated as soon as a new attempt to write is made.

> *Other hand spasms:* spasms similar to writer spasm may also occur when other activities are performed with the hands, by stenographers, musicians, drivers, and so on; the clinical picture shows the same results, that is, spasms preventing the completion of the regular activity.

> *Tennis elbow:* it is the proximal portion of the forearm, not the elbow, that hurts, this proximal area becoming painful close to the medial or lateral aspect of the elbow, the pain even radiating to the distal part of the arm; there is tenderness on pressure over the forearm muscles or about 2 cm below the epicondyle, and free movements of the arm may be impossible.

At times, treatment is unsatisfactory, and is mainly directed to the relief of pain. The first advice is rest for a time, perhaps with the aid of adequate bandaging, or application of a brace or splint. Local infiltration with anesthetic solution or with corticoids may give some help. Surgery may be needed in some selected cases, particularly when dealing with tennis elbow. A beneficial suggestion is to change the object grasped to a larger size, be it a pen or a paddle, since a different position of the muscles during the effort will tend to relieve the painful position.

Procaine, 1% solution, to infiltrate 0.5 ml or more into the affected areas.

Scalenus Anticus Syndrome (Cervical Rib)

Although this syndrome is usually due to a congenital anomaly (the cervical rib), symptoms may appear later in life, particularly among women. Only a few persons will present spasmodic contraction when intending to perform a regular kind of work ("intention tremors"). This spasm is similar to other occupational spasms. There are also local neuralgic pains along the arm, paresthesia, and not rarely an edematous reaction. The situation is worse at night in bed, and improves after the arm is moved. Some weakness of the muscles of the hand may occur. Horner's syndrome is not an exception. Disappearance of pulsations in one wrist when the patient is sitting with the hands on the thighs and hyperextending the head to one side while holding the breath is considered a positive sign.

Spontaneous remissions may occur; bed rest, with traction on the neck and the use of adequate pillows, may also help; some relief will be obtained by means of physical therapy; stress should be avoided; and local infiltration with anesthetic solution may solve problems for a relatively long time. Analgesics and muscle relaxants may be tried. Surgery may be a good solution for some cases, which will be discussed with specialists.

Procaine, 1% solution; inject 0.5 ml or more into the painful areas.

Codeine, 30 mg (up to 60 mg) by mouth, every 6 hours, adjusting dosage to response and tolerance.

Meprobamate, 400 mg tablets; take 400 mg or less every 8 hours, according to response and tolerance.

Myotonic Syndromes

Myotonia refers to tonic spasms of muscles, which organs present increased irritability and contractility while the power to relax is notably diminished. Following a voluntary movement of the affected muscles—for instance, the act of grasping an object—these muscles remain strongly flexed for a more or less prolonged period of time, resembling the situation of a tetanic attack; but once this hypertonic stage is overcome, the regular movements can be performed as usual. The repetition of these spasms may cause muscle hypertrophy, but no increase in strength, which is actually diminished. Some of the syndromes are congenital, while others appear later in life; they may also be present in older people. Electric examination will give the myotonic reaction in most instances, though not in all of them.

Myotonia congenita: is usually present from birth, affecting mainly males, in the legs, the hands, and the masseters; otherwise, the rest of the body functions and activity are not impaired.

Myotonia atrophica: combines the aforementioned myotonic situation and muscular dystrophy (atrophy and weakness) of other muscles; this condition appears late in life and is also accompanied by early baldness, loss of teeth, testicular atrophy, cataracts, and acrocyanosis.

Myotonia acquisita: is also similar to myotonia congenita, but with a later appearance in life, usually following an injury or a causative disease.

Paramyotonia congenita: also appears early in life, the myotonic reaction mainly provoked by cold.

There is no known specific treatment, but many patients respond to the administration of quinine salts; also, procainamide or diphenylhydantoin may be helpful.

Quinine sulfate, 120, 200, or 300 mg tablets; adjust to the lowest possible dosage, according to response and tolerance.

Tetany

Spasticity caused by the tonic contractions of all tetanic syndromes is almost characteristic and diagnostic. The regular clinical picture consists of a very advanced nervous irritability, which may add convulsions or clonic spasms to the tonic contractions. The tonic attack may affect a few muscles at a time to the whole body: the arms may acquire peculiar positions (obstetrician's hand, carpopedal spasm); or there may be opisthotonos, lateroflexion spasm, or even massive spasms. Many bizarre gestures may also be provoked, such as risus sardonicus; but we should pay particular attention to visceral crises, which include laryngeal spasm with dysphagia, gastric spasm with vomiting, intestinal spasms with diarrhea, and rectal, vesicular, appendicular, and similar spasms. The clinical picture is completed with paresthesias, usually around the mouth or in the limbs, different psychoneurotic manifestations, and the classic trophic changes of eroded teeth, brittle nails, early cavities, cataracts, bone hypercalcification, and others. Nervous irritability can be checked by means of the well-known tests: Chvostek's (contraction of muscles of the face on tapping the facial nerve), Trousseau's (obstetrician's hand provoked by pressure on the arm with the sphygmomanometer cuff), Erb's (excitability of muscles elicited by a galvanic current), and perhaps others as well. Causes of tetany are the following:

Tetanus: symptoms usually follow a previously known wound, starting with trismus due to contracted masseters, and then risus sardonicus, opisthotonos, or massive spasm, with extremely painful contractural attacks provoked by minimal stimulation provided by gentle touching of the skin, noise, or light; and also fever and other evidence of infection; there are no trophic changes, and the diagnosis is made by finding the causative germ.

Hypoparathyroidism: all symptomatology, active and latent, is usually present, with particular evidence of nervous irritability and trophic changes; the laboratory will report a low calcemia, elevated phosphoremia, low parathormone levels in the blood, normal alkaline phosphatase, and absence of calcium in the urine.

Pseudohypoparathyroidism: the disease starts early in life, with bone abnormalities (short stature, microdactylia, round face), possible parathyroid hyperplasia, elevated levels of parathormone in the blood, and a peculiar lack of response to parathormone.

Hyperaldosteronism: this disease is rare in old age; the patient will show hypertension, hypokalemia, and in some instances (these are not responsive to calcium therapy) hypomagnesemia.

Metabolic alkalosis: the tetanic syndrome will be present unless there is a marked hypokalemia with muscle hypotonia; the diagnosis is made by elevated CO_2 and pH; the cause will be searched for: excessive diuresis, vomiting, gastric drainage, excessive use of corticoids, or the presence of a frank hyperadrenocorticism.

Respiratory alkalosis: a tetanic syndrome may occur, but most frequently there will be nervous irritability leading to syncope; hyperventilation is almost always present; the blood pH will also be elevated, but the CO_2 content will be low; check for neurotic hyperventilation, hepatic coma, other lesions of the central nervous system, elevated fever, or excessive use of salicylates.

The laboratory will be requested to report blood levels of calcium, phosphorus, CO_2, parathormone, potassium, magnesium, or of any other interesting component; urinalysis; and also X-ray studies and electrocardiagraphic records.

The treatment of tetany varies according to its cause. Symptomatic treatment, with sedatives and anticonvulsant drugs, is of good help provided hypocalcemia is not the essential cause. Tetanus infection is treated with human tetanus immune globulin with added penicillin, chlorpromazine, or diazepam and phenobarbital. Hypoparathyroidism requires adequate amounts of calcium plus parathyroid hormone (not for more than 7 days), dihydrotachysterol, or calciferol, and for some refractory cases also phenytoin and phenobarbital. Pseudohypoparathyroidism is relieved with calcium salts and vitamin D. Hyperaldosteronism usually requires surgical removal of tumors, but a try may be given, in secondary hyperaldosteronism, to dexamethasone suppression or to spironolactone; surgical procedures will be carefully evaluated. Finally, in cases of alkalotic tetany correction of the metabolic imbalance will solve the situation.

Human tetanus immune globulin, 250 units in each container, to give a total treatment amounting to 3000 to 6000 units, better in fractional administration (500 units each time), adjusting dosage to individual needs.

Tetanus antitoxin may be an alternate when the above is not available, in intravenous doses of 100,000 units repeated as tolerated (check first for sensitivity!).

Aqueous penicillin G; give 20 million units a day, according to tolerance and response.

Chlorpromazine; inject 50 mg intramuscularly, to start, followed by oral administration of 50 to 100 mg every 6 hours.

Phenobarbital, 30 or more mg, by injection, adjusting dosage and timing to response and tolerance.

Calcium chloride, 10% solution, for slow intravenous administration until tetanic attacks are controlled (better not to surpass 10 ml); thereafter add 50 to 1000 ml of either saline or 5% glucose for slow infusion, adjusting dosage to urine or blood calcium determinations.

Parathyroid hormone; give 50 to 100 units by intramuscular or subcutaneous injection, repeating up to 5 times a day and discontinuing administration as soon as convulsions are under control, but not to be used more than 7 days.

Calciferol, tablets containing 1.25 mg (50,000 units); give one to four tablets a day, also checking for response. Also could be used initially by injection, intramuscularly.

Spironolactone, tablets containing 25 mg each, to adjust dosage to the lowest effective level, according to individual response.

Sodium chloride, to be administered orally (intravenously only if absolutely needed), with potassium chloride in most instances; will be enough for correction of metabolic alkalosis.

Breathing into a *paper* bag is usually enough for correction of respiratory alkalosis; in other instances assist respiration with oxygen and carbon dioxide.

ATAXIA

The lack of order characteristic of ataxia is noted by failure of muscular coordination, since voluntary movements become irregular, lacking harmony and measure. This holds true for all kinds of movements, but it appears clinically when the patient attempts to walk; there is enough strength, but a complete lack of adequate sequence, amplitude, and automatism for each step, as if the purpose, instead of walking, were playing football or violently hitting the floor with the heel. Other movements are also impaired, such as touching the nose with a finger, grasping a pen or piece of paper from a table, and so on. Romberg's sign will be positive in most instances; that is, the patient will fall, if not assisted, when asked to close the eyes while having both feet placed together. For this reason, patients are totally unable to walk in the dark. A summary of diseases provoking ataxia is given here, some of them reviewed afterward in somewhat more detail.

Alcoholism: the ataxic gait in acute alcoholism is characteristic of the condition, accompanying the other well-known symptoms.

Diabetes: ataxia will be present when the not rare polyneuritic reaction is well advanced, together with its corresponding symptomatology (care will be taken not to make the wrong diagnosis of tabes dorsalis) and the symptomatology of diabetes itself.

Multiple sclerosis: the disease usually presents the characteristic exacerbations and remissions, ataxia being, only at times, one of the symptoms, together with other sudden disturbances of motility and sensitivity, including visual problems, the attacks being provoked at times by intercurrent diseases or accidents.

Locomotor ataxia or tabes dorsalis: this form of neurosyphilis presents a typical ataxic gait with wide steps and most of the symptoms recorded in the opening paragraph, as well as the well-known "lightning" pains, the Argyll Robertson pupils (which react to accommodation but not to light), and others.

Acute ataxia: this is just a clinical picture of ataxia with a sudden onset, usually due to intoxications (as in the case of acute alcoholism, gas poisoning, aluminum poisoning, and so forth), infections (particularly encephalitis); or an unknown cause, as in the case of *Leyden-Westphal idiopathic acute ataxia.*

Pernicious anemia: together with the usual symptoms of pernicious anemia there will be evidence of ataxic features very similar to those of tabes dorsalis; but it is to be noted that the neurologic changes may open the clinical picture, before evidence of anemia.

Pellagra: although very rare, ataxia may occur in cases of pellagra, and it may also be the opening symptomatology.

Beri-beri: ataxia will be among the late manifestations of the disease, following formication, or other paresthesias, cramps, muscle tenderness (mainly the calf), and so on.

Cerebral ataxia: the different forms of cerebral ataxia present the typical features of incoordination but unilaterally and accompanied by symptoms indicating the location of the brain lesion: *temporal ataxia,* with difficulties in finding names, hemianopsia, mild hemiplegia progressing from legs to face, and so on; *motor area* of the brain, with irritability, contractures, local convulsions, hemiplegia, and aphasia if located in the left side; *cortical ataxia* due to lesions of the frontal lobe, causing an extreme instability, making it almost impossible to stand erect, with changes of mood and behavior with a trend toward joking and fatuity; *thalamic ataxia* or hemiataxia, which is strictly unilateral and follows a previous hemiparesis or frank hemiplegia.

Cerebellar ataxia: incoordination is extremely marked, but Romberg's sign is negative, that is, the patient will not fall when he closes the eyes; movements are excessively ample in all senses; it is almost impossible to perform alternate movements with some speed (adiadochokinesia); there may be tremor, nystagmus, muscle hypotonia, and other symptoms.

Hereditary cerebellar ataxia: the *Friedrich's* hereditary spinal ataxia starts at or before puberty, and very few cases will be seen in old age (of course, already diagnosed); cerebellar heredoataxia of *Pierre Marie* is similar to Friedrich's, but starts after 20 or more years of age, there are no bone abnormalities, muscles are mostly hypertonic, and there may be optic or labyrinthine manifestations. Other cerebellar ataxias are *Refsum's disease* with retinitis pigmentosa, sensory changes, ichthyosis, and electroencephalographic changes; and a similar *Bassen-Kornzweig's syndrome* with added scoliosis.

Ataxia telangiectasia: patients with this congenital syndrome will very rarely be seen at advanced ages; there is a cerebellar ataxia together with telangiectasia of cutaneous and ocular tissues.

Labyrinthine ataxia: there will be marked ataxia together with vertigo and a trend to fall in a specific direction; other otic symptoms may be present, such as, tinnitus, deafness, nausea, and at times visual disturbances; labyrinthitis and other similar local diseases may cause the same symptoms.

Radiculitis: pure radiculitis will rarely cause ataxia, but ataxia due to peripheral neuritis is relatively frequent, occurring in many of the above-mentioned examples.

In each particular instance there is almost always need for complementary studies to be done by pathologists, radiologists, or any other specialists, including, of course, electroencephalography and other similar procedures. It is not practical to try to review all these procedures at this time.

Again, in each particular instance the treatment will depend entirely on the causative factor, be it cerebral, cerebellar, or in any other location. For symptomatic relief, very little is to be done, except for the use of sedatives and muscle relaxants for stiffness or contractures, or the use of dimenhydrinate for vertiginous conditions.

Alcoholic Ataxia

The outstanding symptom of acute alcoholism is ataxia, that is, walking like a drunkard. From here, the physician will try to detect alcoholic breath, initial exhilaration rapidly followed by central nervous depression, incoordination, gastric irritation with nausea and vomiting, hypothermia, tachycardia, dyspnea, flushed face, paresthesias and polyneuritis caused by chronic intoxication (of which other symptoms will also be present), tremor, a more complex organic brain syndrome, and confessed or implied alcoholic addiction.

During the acute alcoholic intoxication try stomach lavage whenever possible, avoid emetics, use cathartics if advisable, give thiamine and 25% glucose solution intravenously, assist respiration, and change the patient's posture frequently; if symptoms are alarming, dialysis can be performed. Efforts will be made to treat chronic alcoholism.

Thiamine hydrochloride, 100 mg in each ampoule; give one or more ampoules, as needed and tolerated.

Glucose, 25% solution; give 20 g (8 ml) by intravenous injection, only if there are hypoglycemic symptoms.

Diabetic Ataxia

Only following acro-esthesia, hypesthesia of feet (may become complete anesthesia), pallanesthesia, hyporeflexia, ulterior muscle wasting, and annoying pains, which are the important symptoms of neuritic reaction of the lower limbs, will ataxia furnish one more symptom in the clinical picture of diabetes. In other words, it is no more than a secondary; but it is useful when other symptoms are not well marked. The logical approach, under the circumstances, will be to search for other diabetic symptoms and request laboratory reports.

For more details on diagnosis and treatment, see other entries with more information.

Multiple Sclerosis

A patient with ataxia who presents widespread neurological symptoms that come and go could be strongly suspected of having multiple sclerosis. Check carefully for intention tremor, nystagmus or other visual impairments, difficult speech, spastic paralyses, and increased tendon reflexes; and for exarcebations of these symptoms following injuries, infections, vaccinations, or other similar forms of stress. If checked, most patients will present increased gamma globulin in the spinal fluid. Watch for infections of the urinary system.

There is no form of efficient therapy for this condition, but some patients may respond to some of the following drugs: corticoids, cyanocobalamin, procaine, isoniazid, tolbutamide, and so on. The best policy is to keep the patient as well-protected as possible against stress, particularly hot weather.

Tabes Dorsalis

Ataxia, particularly noted when the patient tries to walk in the dark, is one of the most important symptoms of tabes dorsalis, a disease also called syphilitic posterior spinal sclerosis. Symptoms are: shooting or lightning paroxysmal pains of great intensity, other disturbances of sensation and of reflexes, myoclonus occurring in some patients, hypotonia, painless trophic ulcers, and sudden crises (which may last for only hours, but also for days) of disturbances of the stomach, the larynx, the urethra, the rectum, and the anal canal and retention of urine, lack of sex reactions, and so on. More males than females will be diagnosed as having tabes dorsalis. Laboratory tests will help to establish the final diagnosis.

As said before, it is better to prevent than to treat the disease because once established it very rarely will be cured completely. When necessary, use very large amounts of penicillin, even over 20 million units a day by the intravenous route.

Pernicious Anemia

Many patients with pernicious anemia will present ataxia, similar to tabes dorsalis, with notable difficulties in walking in the night, astereognosis, pallanesthesia, diminished reflexes, and perhaps other implications of the posterior columns; but there will be no pupilar signs. This form of ataxia may end in a true paraplegia, thus resembling a case of multiple sclerosis, also with amyotrophy and trouble with the sphincters. Needless to say, these situations occur because of the neuritic involvement almost always present in pernicious anemia: there will be pain, paresthesias of the hands and feet, numbness, and tingling, these symptoms occurring among the initial symptoms of the disease, possibly together with marked asthenia. Check for other symptoms, such as glossitis with a smooth tongue, dyspepsia, diarrhea, ankle edema, mild hepatomegaly and splenomegaly, hyper- or hypotonia, positive Romberg's sign, confusion with a paradoxical euphoria, and the classic anemic systolic murmur. Laboratory reports will confirm the diagnosis with the finding of abnormal and large oval erythrocytes, hyperchromia, and achlorhydria; but if these tests fail, a medullogram is mandatory. An efficient response to cyanocobalamin is also a positive sign of the disease.

Give transfusions only if the patient is in bad shape; otherwise, prescribe cyanocobalamin to be used as a lifetime treatment. Do not ever give folic acid:

> Cyanocobalamin, intramuscular injection; give 100 μg every other day until hemogram and neurologic symptoms improve or disappear; for maintenance give 100 μg intramuscularly once a week; or 250 to 500 μg by mouth every day.

Pellagra

Ataxia will occur only rarely in pellagra, but it may be an important manifestation when dermic symptoms are little marked or totally absent. If there are no other clues to more frequent diseases, check for hypertrophic red papillae of the tongue, redness and roughness of exposed parts of the skin, diarrhea, or other symptoms of more advanced avitaminosis, which will be almost diagnostic when present (atrophic tongue papillae, scarlet-red tongue, typical red-roughness of the skin on areas exposed to light or friction, particularly the dorsal side of the hands, abdominal distention, mental reactions with dullness or depression not rarely ending in demential syndromes, mouth movements as if sucking, and so on). In the South, doctors used to talk about the three diagnostic D's: dermopathy, diarrhea, and dementia.

Give a diet rich in calories, proteins, and vitamins, plus the basic therapy with nicotinamide. Demential reactions occasionally require permanent care.

> Nicotinamide, injectable in containers with 100 or 200 mg in each ml, to start therapy intravenously or intramuscularly by giving 100 to 500 mg a day, according to response and tolerance; resort to oral administration (tablets containing 50, 100, or 500 mg each), to give similar amounts, according to response and tolerance, until symptoms frankly improve or disappear.

Beri-beri

Beri-beri will cause ataxia as one of the symptoms of polyneuritis, the latter a condition usually present in this disease. When ataxia is present, other symptoms of a severe avitaminosis will also be present: tenderness, paresthesias, and even paralyses of the legs, thereafter spreading to the arms; mental confusion, aphonia, and weakness of the nervous abducens of the eye, possibly followed by a complete ophthalmoplegia; or a more severe clinical picture with biventricular heart failure with metabolic acidosis.

Thiamine is specific for treatment, in such a way that a positive effect noted in 1 or 2 days is almost a pathognomonic sign.

> Thiamine hydrochloride, containers for injection with 50 or 100 mg in each ml, to start by the intravenous or intramuscular route, giving 50 to 100 mg in severe cases or a lower dosage in milder ones; to follow with a daily maintenance schedule of 10 to 50 mg in tablets (each containing 5, 10, 15, 25, 50, or 100 mg) when the initial therapy controls symptoms.

Cerebral Ataxia

When ataxia is due to a brain disease, it is only one more symptom in the complex clinical picture, whether due to a stroke, a tumor, an infection, or other disease.

Cerebral arteriosclerosis: following forgetfulness of recent events, there is confusion together with behavioral changes and the possibility of ataxia, all usually ending in a thrombotic or an embolic accident.

Cerebral thrombosis: there is a slow onset not related to injury or exertion with attacks of aphasia, dizziness, paresis, and other neurological symptoms, including ataxia; if vessels of the *aortic arch* are involved, there will be intermittent claudication and different blood pressure when it is taken in both arms; and there will be more marked dizzy spells when the *subclavian steal syndrome* occurs; in *basilar artery* occlusion there will be weakness and numbness of limbs predisposing the patient to ataxia, and also dysarthria, dysphagia, ophthalmoplegia, and pupillary abnormalities; in *internal carotid occlusion* there are heterolateral alternate hemiparesis and blindness, together with difficult speech, diminished intelligence, behavioral changes, and final frank hemiplegia.

Cerebral embolism: there is the same symptomatology as in the above entry, but it is of a sudden onset.

Intracranial hemorrhage: when the stroke proceeds gradually, ataxia may be noted among the regular symptoms; in *subdural hematoma* there is a previous injury to the head followed by irritability and confusion, and ending in hemiplegia; in cases of *subarachnoid hemorrhage* there is a previous stressing activity, and among the elderly there may be a history of recurrent similar attacks; other hemorrhages will show the usual symptomatology, which can be consulted in other entries.

Radiologic, arteriographic, electroencephalographic, and other similar tests will greatly help in reaching a final diagnosis. For more details, see each item in the corresponding more specific entry.

For treatment, see also other entries, particularly those presented in the chapter devoted to unconsciousness.

Cerebellar Ataxia

Cerebellar ataxia is the classic "drunkard's gait," with markedly staggering steps of excessive amplitude, not influenced by walking in the dark or by closing the eyes (Romberg's sign is negative), as it is with patients suffering from tabes dorsalis. Movements are totally asinergic, the finger hesitating on its way to touch the nose, and so on. Alternate opposite movements are very difficult to perform (adiadochokinesia), muscles are hypotonic and usually show tremors, and there is nystagmus; the lack of pure auditory symptoms will help in differentiating cerebellar ataxia from labyrinthine ataxia, which has a very similar symptomatology. In short, cerebellar ataxia is accompanied by other symptoms and signs of a cerebellar nature. The cerebellar syndrome will be present in cases of cerebellar tumors (may also occur in some instance of tumors of the frontal lobe of the brain, because of compression), abscesses, hemorrhages, infections, injuries, congenital cerebellar disease, and others.

Cerebellar tumors: either primitive or metastasic, they present together the cerebellar syndrome and the syndrome of intracranial pressure; the not-too-rare angiomata may improve symptomatologically with advancing age and are accompanied by other angiomas (retina) and malformations (pancreas, kidneys).

Cerebellar abscess: the abscess may show a meager symptomatology; there may be the febrile syndrome and evidence of a suppurative lesion of the internal ear or the skull, or a general infection; the corresponding symptoms, when present, are localized headache, nystagmus of great amplitude, and mental dullness.

Cerebellar hemorrhage: the hemorrhage usually follows sclerosis of cerebellar arteries, giving a previous symptomatology of marked occipital headache and vertigo; the actual hemorrhage causes a stroke.

Cerebellar reaction to infections: this reaction may appear in the course of any infectious disease, to which symptoms are added others of a cerebellar nature.

Cerebellar injuries: when cerebellar symptoms follow an injury to the head, they are usually of a very bad prognosis.

Cerebellar poisoning: acute alcoholic intoxication is a true cerebellar syndrome; similarly, cerebellar symptoms may also occur in lead poisoning (with abdominal symptoms, asthenia, paleness, occasional palsies of extensor muscles ["wrist drop"], and increased basophilic stippling of erythrocytes).

Cerebellar hereditary ataxia: see next entry.

In some instances the diagnosis will be evident enough from the clinical point of view; but it usually needs the help of plain X-ray films, arteriographic studies, electroencephalographic records, spinal fluid examinations, and the like. In the case of an infection, its nature and the sensitivity of the germs to drugs must also be established.

Each etiologic factor will be treated accordingly; but surgery is usually the basic treatment in most instances, for which reason the action to follow will be discussed with specialists. If a vertiginous condition is the cause of ataxia, as not rarely occurs, some improvement may be obtained by the use of dimenhydrinate.

> Dimenhydrinate, tablets containing 50 mg each; give one every 4 to 6 hours, the dose to be adjusted to response and tolerance.

Cerebellar Hereditary Ataxia

There are two important clinical entities to be considered in this entry, namely, the Friedrich's hereditary ataxia (of little interest here because of its early onset in youth) and the Pierre Marie's ataxia, which starts later in life, with typical cerebellar ataxia (incoordinated wide steps), some evidence of spasticity, increased reflex response, lack of abnormalities, and not too rarely optic atrophy. Other cerebellar forms might be included here: Refsum's disease (with retinitis pigmentosa, sensory changes, and ichthyosis), Bassen-Kornzweig syndrome (similar to the former, but with scoliosis and steatorrhea), and ataxia telangiectasia (see next entry).

There is no known therapy for these disorders, which will be treated only symptomatically, when possible.

Ataxia Telangiectasia

This is also a congenital disease, but patients may reach a relatively advanced age before bleeding becomes a nuisance. Usually, telangiectasis is noted in face tissues, or in the nose or pharynx, in the form of capillary telangiectasia of varied shapes and color (reddish or bluish). In ataxia telangiectasia there is a basic disorder with very low levels of immunoglobulins, and the clinical picture presents increased susceptibility to infections (manifested as pulmonary or paranasal involvement), progressive cerebellar ataxia, and the characteristic telangiectasias; and a very frequent impairment of intelligence arises, which may cause mental retardation.

There is no therapy for the disease; but because infections are the principal risk for these patients, help will be given with human immune serum globulin, for prevention, and antibiotics or sulfas, for treatment of infections.

> Human immune serum globulin, for monthly injections following instructions from manufacturers (average of 100 to 150 mg for each kilo of body weight).

Ear Ataxia

When diseases of the ear directly or indirectly affect the labyrinth, there is always a reactive vertiginous condition and the subsequent ataxia. Check for otitis, labyrinthitis, or Ménière's disease.

> *Otitis:* the main symptoms refer to the ear itself (local pain, deafness, bulging eardrum which eventually ruptures), but there may be vertigo with ataxic gait.

> *Labyrinthitis:* there is intense vertigo with corresponding ataxia in walking, deafness, tinnitus, nausea, and a tendency to fall in a certain direction.

> *Ménière's disease:* there are intermittent attacks similar to labyrinthitis with profuse sweating, nystagmus, headache, all lasting for minutes or hours and recurring at variable intervals.

The treatment for otitis is that of the corresponding infection, plus myringotomy when advisable. For labyrinthitis, the corresponding anti-infective therapy will be given whenever known, plus drainage performed by a specialist; and in noninfective cases, rest and sedation (phenobarbital, chlorpheniramine, or chlorpromazine in the early stages of the disease). Ménière's disease is treated with dimenhydrinate, atropine, or diuretics, though surgery is frequently the last resource for treatment. For more details on these subjects, see corresponding entries in the section devoted to "Vertigo."

Radiculitis

Actually, this should be a very extensive entry because all forms of inflammation or injuries affecting the nerve roots or the nerves themselves belong here, that is, neuritis or polyneuritis due to several different etiologic factors. Since these subjects have been duly reviewed in other sections of this book, the reader is referred to those sections for more complete information.

SPEECH DISORDERS

Aphasia

This loss of power to understand or express words properly may occur in any of the following forms: *anarthria,* the inability to say or to use words properly; *agraphia,* the inability to write words adequately; *alexia,* the inability to understand the written word; or *word deafness,* in which the heard sound lacks any meaning for the sick person. The occurrence of aphasia indicates a lesion of the left side of the brain (right side for purely left-handed people), and is accompanied in the great majority of instances by hemiplegia of the right side (the left for left-handed people). In *ataxic* or *motor aphasia* there are usually mixed anarthria (which is the basic disorder) and agraphia; in *sensory* or *receptive aphasia* alexia and word deafness are the main troubles; and in *complete aphasia* the motor and receptive forms occur simultaneously.

> *Motor aphasia:* check for symptoms of cerebral hemorrhage: evidence of stroke, with hemiplegia or only prodromal symptoms before the full symptomatology of the stroke. Check also for cerebral arteriosclerosis, with slowly progressive symptoms ending in a slow stroke; or infective cerebral arteritis, with a very intense initial headache, usually due to syphilis; or cerebral thrombosis, also of a relatively slow onset in a patient with a previous thrombotic lesion in other parts of the body; or cerebral embolism, with a very acute onset of the stroke syndrome, which is almost always complete and severe; or injuries to the head (with immediate or delayed symptomatology), brain tumors (also a slowly progressive malady, with symptoms of cranial hypertension and focal symptoms), or any other lesion affecting the neighborhood of Broca's center.

> *Receptive and complete aphasias:* check for the same basic situations as reviewed in the above paragraph.

Among elderly people, aphasia may be the outstanding symptom when any of the above situations occur, but it will rarely be the only symptom; so if patients are carefully checked, other symptoms will also be present to help provide the correct diagnosis.

Since the above-mentioned diseases have been more extensively reviewed in the chapter devoted to "Unconsciousness" as well as in this chapter under the heading "Paresis and Paralysis," the reader is referred to those sections for more information. Here we will refer only to *mutism,* that is, inability or refusal to speak, which may occur in the following situations.

General paresia may occur in some cases of late syphilis, with memory loss, headaches, poor concentration, dysarthria, if not complete aphasia, tremors of fingers, lips, and tongue, and severe personality changes; that is, patients become irresponsible, confused, and slovenly, and have tremors and speech difficulties. The treatment consists of large doses (up to 20 million units) of a short-acting penicillin, for prolonged periods of time.

Schizophrenia presents mutism mainly in acute stages of marked negativism, when the patient becomes unusually autistic and socially withdrawn, has had a previous suspicious behavior deviation, and has taken stimulant drugs which may precipitate schizophrenic reactions. These patients should be hospitalized; they will be given haloperidol or chlorpromazine for the acute episode, and thereafter a long-acting injection of fluphenazine every 2 weeks; but it is best to put them under the care of a psychiatrist.

Depression, though rarely, may also provoke mutism or a marked lack of interest in talking with others; patients seem to be sad, hopeless, incapable of thinking or concentrating, and lose interest in their surroundings; a careful check for abuse of drugs or toxics must be made. Since antidepressants are not always advisable for these patients, it is best to put them under the care of a specialist.

Dysarthria

Strictly speaking, dysarthria is any imperfection in the spoken language; but considering the subject from the clinical point of view, we must add that in most instances the wrong articulation of sounds is accompanied by forced movements of the lips and tongue, and not rarely by gestures with the face and hands. Marked dysarthria is easily diagnosed; but diagnosis is not so easy in mild cases, when it becomes necessary to ask the patient to say words that are difficult to pronounce. Marked dysarthria is at times an outstanding symptom in the following cases.

Alcoholism: other symptoms are tremors of the tongue and of other muscles, ataxia, depression following an initial phase of irritability, alcoholic odor of the breath, and other common evidences of inebriation.

General paresis: symptoms are poor concentration, memory loss, headaches, tremors of lips, fingers, and tongue, severe personality changes, and dysarthria (slurred speech), which may end in complete aphasia.

Multiple sclerosis: syllables are enunciated separately (staccato speech) by patients, who also show attacks and relapses of symptoms corresponding to an extensive involvement of the central nervous system, with intention tremor, diverse forms of neuritis, spastic paralysis, nystagmus, or impaired vision.

Hereditary ataxia: other symptoms are incoordinated wide steps, some spasticity, increased reflex response, and, occasionally, optic atrophy.

Senile pseudobulbar syndrome: see next entry.

Facial paralysis: in addition to the evident symptoms of paralysis of the facial muscles, there may also be a typical dysarthria due to impairment of lip and tongue movements.

Paralysis of lips, tongue, or palate: whenever this occurs, as in the cases of bulbar paralysis of any kind, myasthenia, basilar meningitis, or brain tumors, there will be more or less marked speech disturbance.

Parkinson's disease: dysarthria may occur, but the essentials for diagnosis are tremor and rigidity.

Bradylalia: slow speech may be due to a brain tumor of the frontal lobe or to hypothyroidism (myxedema).

Tachylalia: rapid speech is usually due to conditions provoking mental irritability, but mainly hyperthyroidism.

Stuttering or stammering is not a true dysarthria, but it seems appropriate to point out here that it may be related to emotional conditions and perhaps also to hypothyroidism. Usually, stutterers improve with age.

For more detailed information on diagnosis and treatment the reader is referred to other entries in this book, where each of these diseases has been duly considered.

SLEEP DISORDERS

Sleep, the regularly occurring condition of rest for both the body and the mind, may be disturbed by abnormal wakefulness (insomnia), pathologically uncontrollable drowsiness (hypersomnia), sudden attacks of sleep that occur at more or less regular intervals (narcolepsy), or unnatural activity during the natural period of rest (somnambulism).

Insomnia

It is a well known, but frequently disregarded fact that people do not all need the same amount of sleep, and that only a few hours of restful sleep are enough for maintenance of good health. That is, care must be taken to evaluate the statements of many patients, who may unduly magnify minimal wakefulness. True insomnia is characterized by a lack of sufficient rest to allow recovery from the daily waste of energy, and occurs mainly in the following conditions.

Occasional insomnia: minimal causes may provoke insomnia, which causes once corrected will not interfere further with a natural sleep; check for a change of normal habits, stressing unusual conditions, excessive use of toxic drugs, including alcohol and caffeine, unusual temperature in the room, and so on.

Symptomatic insomnia: this insomnia is due to a distressing symptom, such as cough, itching, pain, fever, and the like; the diagnosis depends on the causative disease, which will be adequately treated.

Anxiety neurosis: the insomniac also has a feeling of apprehension, uncertainty, and fear; other symptoms are tension, restlessness, and not rarely hyperventilation. Give sedatives and minor tranquilizers.

Mania: insomnia is an outstanding symptom accompanied by an expansive emotional state, elation, excessive talkativeness, continuous flight of ideas, hyperirritability, and increased motor activity; these patients usually show alternating manic and depressive attacks. Haloperidol is an acceptable drug for their treatment.

Encephalitis: instead of the regular lethargy, insomnia may be present in cases of encephalitis, either initially or alternating periodically with it.

Late syphilis: among the central nervous system manifestations, insomnia may be one of the earlier symptoms, along with memory loss, poor concentration, tremors, dysarthria, and personality changes. The treatment is with large amounts (up to 20 million units a day) of short-acting penicillins.

Diabetic acidosis: it is worth noting that at times insomnia precedes for a few days the complete clinical picture of diabetic acidosis; that is, any known diabetic who suddenly becomes insomniac (and apparently mentally bright) should be carefully investigated for an impending acidotic crisis, and the metabolic condition corrected adequately.

Uremia: the clinical picture may be that of anxiety neurosis with a very severe insomnia; also, there may be a persistent insomnia with other symptoms of depression, not rarely occurring during the involutional years and perhaps diagnosed as depending on senility when the real cause is the hidden uremic condition; these insomniacs will not be bright but depressed, and may also present symptoms of weakness, dyspnea, itching, paresthesia, other symptoms of peripheral neuropathy, weight loss, diarrhea, thirst, and hypertension. There will be suspicion of chronic renal insufficiency when there is a previous history of glomerulonephritis, urinary tract infections, obstructive uropathies, gout, intoxication by drug abuse, hypercalcemia, or any other urinary problem. Laboratory reports are needed to confirm all this and follow the signs of anemia, azotemia, and acidosis; an adequate treatment may be of great benefit.

Post-climacterium syndrome: insomnia may be one of the important symptoms of the menopause.

Other causes of insomnia: check also for cirrhosis, heart failure, and indigestion.

To avoid unnecessary repetition, the reader is referred to other sections where these conditions have been reviewed in more detail.

Hypersomnia

Normally, a person who has not slept well will be sleepy, that is, will show hypersomnia. Abnormally, this will occur no matter how much that person has slept previously. Most cases of hypersomnia respond to the same causes that induce comatose states. When this occurs, the sequence usually is hypersomnia, first, then lethargy, and finally coma. The real need in cases of hypersomnia is to be on the alert for the establishment of early diagnosis in case of any of the following diseases.

Congestive heart failure: this disease may cause insomnia, but most frequently hypersomnia, together with dyspnea on exertion and paroxysmal dyspneic attacks during the night, cough, pulmonary congestion, or dependent edema and hepatomegaly. Treatment is based on rest, digitalis, and diuretics.

Arterial hypertension: this condition may also present hypersomnia, but it is not an important symptom, nor is it an early one.

Polycythemia: not well-recognized by many authors, hypersomnia is one of the outstanding symptoms in polycythemia, either secondary or polycythemia vera, and should be considered significant whenever it occurs together with a dusky redness of mucosae and skin (lips!), headache, itching (more after bathing), asthenia, finger pains, and an elevated count of erythrocytes. Treatment includes venesection, radiophosphorus, or chemotherapy.

Pickwickian syndrome: this is, practically, a combination of extreme obesity with polycythemia, thus presenting hypersomnia (though some patients may be insomniacs), cyanosis, and other symptoms of heart failure. Treatment to reduce weight may be effective, and the use of progesterone is said to help.

Intoxications with barbiturates, alcohol, or opium derivatives will start with hypersomnia, rapidly turning into coma whenever dosage has been unduly elevated. For more information, see under ''Coma.''

Uremia: the initial phase, presented in the previous entry on ''Insomnia,'' is followed by hypersomnia or may go directly into coma.

Brain tumors: hypersomnia may be a part of the syndrome of cerebral hypertension, q.v. in other entries of this book.

Diabetic acidosis: in this instance hypersomnia is merely the initial phase of the final coma.

Postprandial somnolence of elderly persons may indicate a gastrointestinal or hepatic disturbance.

Hypothyroidism: there are myxedematous patients whose main symptom is hypersomnia, the diagnosis depending on the blood levels of the thyroid hormones and the treatment depending on adequate hormonal adjustment.

Encephalitis: in these patients hypersomnia is among the characteristic symptoms, but it may follow an initial phase of insomnia. See other entries in this book for more complete information.

Post-seizure hypersomnia is characteristic of epileptic attacks.

Narcolepsy

Uncontrollable recurrent attacks of deep sleep characterize narcolepsy, which will even occur several times a day, usually on inappropriate occasions and lasting from a few minutes to several hours. It is more frequent among men, and in most instances this sort of sleep seems to be like a normal sleep; in some cases it is accompanied by other symptoms, such as muscle hypotonus, hallucinations at the start of the attack, or paralysis of most muscles at the end of the sleep.

Attacks of sleep may be controlled by drugs, but not so the associated symptoms that may also be present (hypotonia).

> Amphetamine sulfate, tablets containing 5 or 10 mg each, and long-acting capsules with 15 mg; adjust dosage for each individual patient (average, 10 mg to start; 10 to 20 mg, twice or three times a day), taking care not to interrupt normal sleep.

> Methylphenidate hydrochloride, tablets containing 5, 10, or 20 mg each; adjust dosage to each individual patient (average 5 to 10 mg, three or four times a day).

Somnambulism

Somnambulism may be defined as habitual walking while sleeping, during which situation the patient may perform different activities, such as dressing, drinking water, or eating, and even more complex acts, such as trips to different towns; but with the characteristic feature that no memories of any of these activities remain. The two main conditions related to somnambulism that are of interest in advanced ages are epilepsy and chronic alcoholism.

Epilepsy: the diagnosis is usually established. The occurrence of typical seizures, the residual injuries, and so on, will help in making a final evaluation of the condition. The treatment is that of epilepsy.

Chronic alcoholism: again, the diagnosis is usually known; but the typical clinical picture will give the final confirmation. Treatment is as for chronic alcoholism.

For more information on epilepsy and chronic alcoholism, the reader is referred to other entries in this book.

VI. COUGH, EXPECTORATION, HOARSENESS

COUGH

A sudden noisy expulsion of air from the lungs may be a cry of pain, a sneeze through the nose and mouth, or cough, all three well-known to everyone because of the peculiar sound corresponding to each one. Cough is provoked not only by foreign bodies or secretions in the respiratory tract, but also by irritation of the nerve paths involved in coughing. Cough is a very frequent symptom, but it is also a good guidepoint in the diagnosis of the following diseases.

Coughing "sine cause": cough is without an organic etiology, but due to a neurotic personality.

Pharyngeal cough: there is an irritative factor in the pharynx, usually a pharyngitis; but at times it is mainly noted while in bed and due to a long uvula.

Sinusal cough: the cough is also accompanied by local pain.

Laryngeal cough: there is also hoarseness in the great majority of instances; and this is the usual finding among smokers and alcoholics.

Laryngeal cancer: cough, hoarseness, or both may be among the initial symptoms of laryngeal cancer.

Common cold: cough is mainly accompanied by rhinorrhea, and perhaps a modest fever.

Influenza: this starts as a common cold, but soon malaise and pains with more marked fever point out a more serious disease.

Bronchitis: cough is the main symptom of all tracheobronchial diseases, first dry and then turning into productive cough; on auscultation, ronchi, râles, and other pulmonary sounds will be present.

Pneumonia: not all elderly persons will show the elevated temperature usually present in these cases, together with intense cough, sharp chest pain, and typical sputum.

Bronchopneumonia: there is a clinical picture similar to pneumonia, but less acute and with more scattered auscultatory and radiologic signs.

Pulmonary infarction: an acute onset occurs with cough, sputum tinged with blood, side pain, and dyspnea, usually in patients with a previous phlebothrombosis elsewhere in the body.

Pulmonary abscess: symptoms are similar to those of bronchopneumonia, but with a very offensive odor to the sputum.

Blastomycosis: there is an undefined bronchopneumonic infection ending in a more definite picture of pleurisy, the diagnosis depending on the finding of *Blastomyces* in the sputum.

Lung cancer: cough is perhaps the earliest symptom, but the diagnosis depends on X-ray studies.

Pulmonary tuberculosis: cough and febricula are the earlier symptoms; again, the diagnosis depends on X-ray and laboratory studies.

Atelectasis: cough is not an outstanding symptom, but it may occur with dyspnea, fever, cyanosis, tachycardia, and narrowing of the intercostal spaces.

Pleuritis: there is dry, usually painful cough, at times provoked by change of position, and evident on auscultation and in radiologic studies.

Pneumothorax: there is a sudden onset of cough, chest pain, dyspnea, and decreased chest motion with auscultatory and radiologic findings.

Emphysema: the condition is very frequent among elderly smokers, with cough, dyspnea, and hyperventilation of the lungs.

Esophageal diverticulosis: symptoms are a dry, almost continuous cough, and also dysphagia, bad breath, regurgitation of undigested food, and positive X-ray findings.

Mediastinal diseases: check for cancer, aneurism, enlarged lymph nodes, aortitis, and goiter.

Aortitis: cough may be a very early symptom when there is some inflammation peripherally (periaortitis); cough is dry and repetitive.

Heart disease: cough is a frequent symptom in valvular diseases, mainly of the mitral valve, and also in pericarditis; in advanced heart disease it becomes more marked because of pulmonary congestion and other causes.

Rickettsioses: cough will occur together with the different clinical changes.

Radiologic studies are basic to the evaluation of cough, together with a detailed auscultation of the chest and laboratory procedures to detect infections whenever they are the cause of the symptom. The help of specialists (ear-nose-throat specialist, neurologist, and so on) will be of value.

Cough "Sine Cause"

This is, of course, a diagnosis by exclusion. First, be sure there are no causes of coughing present; then, be assured of the neurotic personality of the patient. A clue may be given by the timing of the cough, that is, its occurrence during emotional states even of a very minor nature, with long pauses when the patient is alone or sleeping. Residual coughing from previous diseases may be included in this category.

Mild sedatives may control the situation; but if they fail, put the patient under the control of a psychiatrist.

Phenobarbital, 15 mg tablets; give 15 to 30 mg prior to emotional occurrences, or on a continuous basis.

Pharyngeal Cough

This is usually due to simple pharyngitis, with a dry and sore mucosa, malaise, fever, mucus, and cough. The diagnosis is relatively easy because of the localized symptoms. But the condition may also be a case of tonsillitis, when the inflammatory symptoms center at the tonsils, which become inflamed. In other diseases of the pharynx, cough is not a symptom of any importance. For a complete diagnosis, the cause should be sought by laboratory procedures, in order to use the specific treatment.

Use antibiotics only when the infection is severe enough, or there is a true risk of spreading infection. Otherwise, advise rest and local gargling or irrigations with nonirritating antiseptics.

Note: *A long or large uvula,* which can be seen on inspection, may cause coughing, particularly when resting in bed; advise change of position, or resort to surgery if the coughing interferes with a good night's rest.

Sinusal Cough

Cough may be present in both acute or chronic sinusitis whenever the postnasal discharge irritates the pharynx and surrounding areas. In acute sinusitis there are symptoms of the febrile syndrome; in all forms of sinusitis, there are local pain (less marked in chronic cases), nasal symptoms, and clouding of the diseased sinus as seen on transillumination or on X-ray films. Try in all instances to identify the causative germ.

Treatment consists of the use of the specific antibiotic or an ample-spectrum one, decongestants, and local heat. After the acute phase is over, discuss the procedure to follow with a specialist.

Phenylpropanolamine tablets, containing 25 mg each; give one or two tablets every 8 hours.

Laryngeal Cough

In either acute or chronic laryngitis a painful cough is usually present, but the characteristic symptom is hoarseness. With local edema there will also be stridor and dyspnea. The diagnosis is made by examination with the laryngoscope, and completed with the finding of the causative factor (infection or irritation). Check for an infective germ; or find out whether the patient is a heavy smoker or drinker, since coughing from these causes is extremely frequent among the elderly.

The treatment consists of voice rest, steam inhalation, use of the specific antibiotic, and avoidance of the irritant (smoking or drinking).

Laryngeal Cancer

Hoarseness is the most important symptom, but coughing might be an earlier one. Cancer of the larynx gives the same symptoms as any other laryngeal tumor; in addition to hoarseness and cough there are other signs such as sore throat, dyspnea, or other respiratory obstruction, dysphagia, or otalgia. It is best to ask the help of a laryngologist.

Treatment consists of irradiation or extirpation.

Common Cold

The common cold usually starts with coughing and sneezing. There is nasal discomfort, and malaise with little or no fever, soon followed by nasal discharge and pharyngo-laryngeal symptoms. The real problem is in identifying a common cold as the initial syndromic complex of a more serious disease, such as influenza and the like, which usually presents additional symptoms and is more disabling. The diagnosis rests on the lack of lung involvement and development of other symptoms.

There is no treatment for the common cold; only symptomatic help will be given, with rest and good hydration, and analgesics when needed. Phenylephrine (0.25% solution), three to five drops, may be instilled into each nostril.

Influenza

Efforts are being made to vaccinate all elderly people against "flu," which is a very important cause of mortality at this time of life. But even those who are vaccinated may have an attack caused by a different virus strain. The disease may start as a common cold, but follows a rapid course toward a more acute symptomatology, with elevated temperature and chills, acute malaise, and characteristic muscle and bone aches all over the body. All patients with these symptoms are to be very closely watched for the development of a complicating pneumonia. The laboratory will report leukopenia, and the virus may be isolated from throat washings (early stage) or by serum tests (acute phase and convalescence). The parainfluenza viruses provoke a disease identical with influenza on clinical grounds, the distinction being made only by laboratory tests (complement-fixation, hemagglutination-inhibition, and so forth). The adenoviruses may also cause syndromes with a similar clinical picture. Only appropriate laboratory tests will disclose the final diagnosis.

The severity of most of the symptoms makes help necessary, since they usually reach burdensome proportions. Only symptomatic treatment can be offered. Because of the presence of fever and headache, acetylsalicylic acid should be tried first. When patients start to cough, codeine should be added to the above medication, but preferably at a low dosage. Nasal obstruction which may help to cause insomnia or to increase the headache must be relieved. Extreme care will be taken at all times to prevent, or to start an early cure for, possible pneumonic complications.

> Acetylsalicylic acid, 600 mg, in tablets, every 4 hours, preferably with meals. If needed, give the medication more frequently, to obtain effective analgesic and antithermic results.

> Codeine, 15 to 30 mg, by mouth, every 4 to 6 hours.

> Phenylephrine, 0.1 or 0.5% solution; instill a few drops (or use a spray) into each nostril, every 4 or 5 hours.

Bronchitis

Bronchitis (a primary disorder or a complication) presents a clinical picture suggesting the diagnosis, which is established by auscultation, X-ray, and examination of the sputum. There are: productive cough, purulent sputum, coryza, and possibly other symptoms of the URI series, with sore throat, malaise, and pain. Fever varies from mild to high. On auscultation, there are musical ronchi, sibilant or sonorous râles, wheezing, and almost moist râles, particularly in dependent areas. Bronchopneumonia and pneumonia differ from bronchitis because of the more localized auscultatory signs and the greater severity of the pneumonia. Of course, one must watch for the possibility of a complicating disease.

Bed rest is imperative, as well as the interdiction of smoking. Fluids should be forced, to avoid dehydration by drinking no less than 3 or 4 liters, in 24 hours. Inhalation of mist or steam is beneficial, either of simple water or with an added teaspoonful of eucalyptol and compound tincture of benzoin. Other measures are needed, at times, for instance, acetylsalicylic acid, codeine, or bronchodilators. Whenever a bronchospasm is present, a bronchodilator is given, which is particularly true for asthmatic patients.

> Eucalyptol and compound benzoin tincture; add a teaspoonful to a liter of boiling water, for inhalation of vapor.

> Acetylsalicylic acid, 600 mg, in tablets, every 4 to 6 hours, preferably with meals.

> Codeine, 30 or 60 mg, by mouth, every 4 to 6 hours, as needed.

Ephedrine, 25 mg, by mouth or by subcutaneous or intramuscular injection, every 6 to 8 hours.

Aminophylline, 250 mg, suppository, every 6 hours if needed.

Treatment of the basic cause includes antibiotic therapy, particularly when symptoms show some severity. Culture and sensitivity are better obtained from gastric lavage or intratracheal techniques, to ensure giving the specific antibiotic. But because most cases are due to gram-negative germs, ampicillin is recommended for use at the start, since it also covers *H. influenzae*.

Ampicillin, 250 to 500 mg, every 4 to 6 hours, either by mouth, intramuscularly, or intravenously.

Pneumonia

The general clinical picture of pneumonia develops with symptoms of an upper respiratory infection, namely, pharyngitis, and bronchitis. Suddenly, fever rises with a shaking chill, a sharp pain appears in the affected side of the chest, and coughing is accompanied by an almost diagnostic sputum. A rapid, dyspneic, and painful respiration is the rule. There is profuse sweating: coughing becomes more painful; and symptoms from other systems are noted: delirium (particularly among alcoholics), convulsions, abdominal distress, distention, vomiting, diarrhea, hepatic signs, and, possibly, jaundice. The examination reveals râles, suppressed breath sounds, tubal respiration, pleural friction rub, tachycardia, cyanosis, and, finally, the characteristic X-ray picture. Pneumonia will be suspected in older patients with chest pain, cough, sputum, and auscultatory signs of consolidation, who may show acute chills and fever, usually not too high.

Pneumococcal pneumonia: there is the above-mentioned clinical picture with a bloody sputum at the start, which soon becomes the characteristic rusty color to end in a yellowish, mucopurulent excretion during resolution. There is lymphocytosis. Bacterial cultures give the final diagnosis.

Hemophilus influenzae pneumonia: the clinical signs are the common symptoms of pneumonia, but cyanosis is more marked, and the sputum is of an apple-green color and very tenacious. Laboratory reports will disclose the causative germ.

Viral pneumonia: this is a frequent disease, due to influenza and many other similar viruses, usually resulting in a relatively mild infection, but it may be very serious (some influenza strains). Pneumonic symptoms are not characteristic, ranging from those of a common cold to severe respiratory insufficiency, in many instances resembling a bronchopneumonia, with auscultatory or X-ray signs noted only in a few restricted areas of the lung. The sputum is mucopurulent, at times blood-streaked. Serologic tests may help to provide a specific diagnosis.

Streptococcal and staphylococcal pneumonia: these types are frequent among the elderly, being complications of a previous disease, as influenza or pharyngitis. Symptoms are always marked, the pharynx is inflamed, the tonsils are covered with exudate, and patients are severely ill. The sputum is abundant and of a salmon color. Final diagnosis is made by laboratory isolation of the causative organism.

Other forms of pneumonia: Klebsiella pneumonia shows a slower onset, but once established appears to be almost fulminant, with a viscid, cherry-red sputum, and consolidation rapidly spreading from lobe to lobe. *Rickettsial pneumonia* shows no typical clinical picture, nor is there one in *mycoplasmal pneumonia,* or in *fungal pneumonia.* Finally, in *aspiration pneumonia* there is the history of an accidental passage of a foreign body into the larynx and trachea, as in anesthesia, acute alcoholism, epilepsy, profuse vomiting, or mental retardation. A few other entities are diagnosed by laboratory means: *Pneumocystis carinii,* or *tularemia.*

The basic treatment is the same for all types of pneumonia, differing only in the etiological aspect: patients will be confined to bed, with good hydration, comfortable feeding, oxygen administration, and analgesics for pain, codeine preferred because it can also control coughing. The direct treatment of the causative agent should be managed as indicated for each causative factor.

Codeine, 60 mg, by mouth, every 4 to 6 hours, according to response and tolerance.

Pneumococcal pneumonia: penicillin, 300,000 units, by intramuscular injection, every 12 hours (i.v., if so needed).

Streptococcal and staphylococcal pneumonia: oxacillin, 2000 mg, by intramuscular injection, every 4 to 6 hours: either alone or with cephalothin, same schedule (for streptococcal pneumonia, penicillin may accomplish the same results).

H. influenzae pneumonia: ampicillin, 1000 mg, by intravenous injection, every 4 to 6 hours (can also be given by mouth).

Viral pneumonia: only symptomatic treatment can be offered.

Klebsiella pneumonia: check sensitivity, but start with cephalothin, 8000 to 12,000 mg in 24 hours, and gentamycin, 1 mg for each kilo of body weight, every 8 hours (other antibiotics may work as well, i.e., tetracyclines, and so on).

Fungal pneumonia: amphotericin B for most forms, initial dose of 0.25 mg for each kilo of body weight in 24 hours, to be given by intravenous infusion lasting from 2 to 6 hours; dosage increased every few days by 0.25 mg for each kilo of body weight in 24 hours until 1 mg is reached; always dissolved in 5% dextrose. *Actinomyces* infection responds to penicillin: and *Nocardia,* to sulfadiazine.

Rickettsial pneumonia (usually Q fever): treat with a tetracycline.

Aspiration pneumonia: apply endotracheal tube or bronchoscope for aspiration of foreign material, to wash the affected parts: give cortisone, particularly if there is suspicion of aspiration of gastric juice (vomiting); give oxygen and watch for septic complications.

P. carinii pneumonia: give pentamidine isethionate, 4 mg per kilo in 24 hours, by intramuscular injection.

Mycoplasmal pneumonia: give a tetracycline or erythromycin.

Tularemic pneumonia: treat with streptomycin, and add a tetracycline if there is no improvement.

Bronchopneumonia

This seems like a pneumonia starting at different foci at the same time, the onset gradual and insidious, with the symptoms and signs less marked than in pneumonia, less organized in a sequence, and ordinarily the final crisis lacking. Some older patients will not show symptoms or signs; the disease is merely a radiologic finding; in other cases, symptomatology may be severe or extended for long periods of time. Bronchopneumonia will be suspected when pneumonia signs intermix with symptoms of a previous infective disease: influenza, typhus, scarlet fever, smallpox, plague, typhoid fever, pneumotyphus, ornithosis, and others.

Depending on the nature of the infecting germ, the treatment will be carried out with the specific antibiotic, starting as soon as possible. The control of pain is merely a palliative measure, with little effect upon the disease. To obtain this symptomatic action, the physician will advise bed rest, oxygen administration, good hydration, and analgesics.

Pulmonary Infarction

The disease starts with a sudden onset of side pain, followed by dyspnea and cough with bloody sputum. Symptoms resemble those of pneumonia; and many mimic myocardial infarction, pleurisy, or pericarditis. The diagnosis is suggested when venous thrombosis is present elsewhere in the body, as in the legs. Small infarcted areas will show few symptoms; large infarctions cause much trouble; acute pain and dyspnea, cyanosis, and finally symptoms of shock. If an electrocardiogram is made (myocardial damage suspected), only signs of right ventricular strain will be found (cor pulmonale); but other signs are not uncommon, as S-T depression, or T inversion. It is to be noted that the location of pain may vary with the location of the pulmonary infarction: at the left lower lobe, the pain is precordial or retrosternal; pain may be referred to the shoulder, or the abdomen.

The first choice in the treatment of pulmonary infarction is morphine, or meperidine as an alternate. If cough is severe, codeine is a help. Rest and oxygen therapy are very important. Surgery will be discussed with specialists.

> Morphine, 5 mg by intravenous injection; or 10 or 15 mg by the subcutaneous route, to be repeated as needed.

> Meperidine, 50 mg, intramuscularly, repeated as needed and tolerated.

Lung Abscess

Most abscesses of the lung follow a previous aspiration pneumonia or some form of bronchial obstruction; after 10 to 14 days symptoms appear—fever with chills, chest pain and coughing, dry at first then followed by expectoration of foul smelling purulent sputum, sweating, and evidence of pulmonary consolidation. Hemoptysis and expectoration may occur in periodic outbursts. The X-ray findings are likely to show an initial dense shadow, followed by formation of a central radiolucency, perhaps with a fluid level. Bronchoscopy is advised in all instances, since cancer is a frequent cause of abscess. Other less frequent symptoms are anemia, weight loss, and malaise. Examination of the sputum is needed, preferably obtained by suction from the trachea; tubercle bacilli and pyogenic aerobes and anaerobes should be sought and studied.

Treat the disease vigorously with antibiotics in most cases. The specific antibiotic will be selected and intensive therapy continued for 1 or 2 months. Almost any germ may be causative, but the most frequently found are staphylococci, aerobic pyogens, or anaerobes. Drainage of secretions will be obtained either by the adequate position in bed or by bronchoscopic aspiration. It is best to consult a specialist in these cases, since surgery is often required.

Blastomycosis

There is mild fever together with pulmonary symptoms of cough, dyspnea, and chest pains. Watch for pleurisy, elevated temperature, chills, purulent sputum, and X-ray densities irregularly distributed in the lungs and involving the mediastinal lymph nodes. Dermatological symptoms may appear, such as verrucae covered with miliary pustules, which erode leaving a central atrophic scar. Bones and the central nervous system may also be involved.

Diagnosis depends on the finding of *Blastomyces dermatitidis* and the rise of the complement-fixing antibody titer.

No specific treatment is known, but amphotericin B should be tried and surgery performed whenever needed, and the patient followed for several years.

> Amphotericin B, 0.5 to 1 mg per kilo of body weight, suspended in 500 ml of 5% dextrose in distilled water (not saline because of precipitation!), to be administered in a 6-hour period by intravenous infusion. Decrease adverse reactions by giving antihistamines previously, but watch for chills, kidney damage, and thrombophlebitis. Use the drug for at least 1 or 2 months.

Lung Cancer

Cough is of paramount importance. Pain of a pleuritic type is a late symptom. Dyspnea may appear either early or late in the course of the disease. Other symptoms belong to the common symptomatology of cancer.

Surgery or chemotherapy will be considered as the possible basic treatment, whenever indicated. Other measures will be taken, according to circumstances.

As in all forms of advanced malignancies, morphine is the drug of choice for alleviation of pain.

> Morphine, 10 to 15 mg, by subcutaneous administration, repeated as needed.

Tuberculosis

The disease presents with some evening fever, of varying degree during the first stage, with cough, asthenia, weight loss, and sweating, particularly during the night. This phase is similar to influenza, but persists, along with a tendency for all symptoms to worsen. Auscultatory signs are minimal, if present at all. X-ray findings are often inconclusive and may be limited to mottled densities, usually in an apex of the lung.

Among the elderly, the stage of chronic tuberculosis is more frequent. It is progressive, following the primary complex or from reinfection, and characterized by one or more pneumonic foci in the upper pulmonary areas; in advanced cases, with caseous necrosis and subsequent cavitation. Auscultation may reveal the character of the fine râles heard at the upper part of the lung. The diagnosis is suspected when a clinical picture similar to the primary complex worsens in all of its aspects, including the X-ray findings. The sputum will show *Mycobacterium tuberculosis,* and skin tests will show tuberculin sensitivity to tine and mantoux tests.

Treatment: isolate those with positive sputum; advise bed rest, good nutrition, etc., and the use of at least two of the first-line antituberculosis drugs. For more details see other entries in this book.

For all previously untreated patients: isoniazid, 5 mg for each kilo of body weight a day, or more if the patient acetylates the drug rapidly, plus ethambutol or rifampin. Additional pyridoxin (50 mg t.i.d.) will help.

Previously treated patient: use drugs not yet prescribed for that patient.

Extensive lesions: use three drugs, such as isoniazid, streptomycin, and ethambutol or rifampin.

Atelectasis

The main symptomatology of acute pulmonary atelectasis consists of fever, cough, dyspnea, cyanosis, tachycardia, some sort of chest pain, wheezing, restricted chest expansion on respiration, and narrowing of the intercostal spaces. Shock is to be feared. The X-ray findings show displacement of the mediastinum and "ground glass" density of the collapsed lung. The disease has to be differentiated from pneumonia, or from pulmonary infarction. Cough may be the only symptom in tumoral, slowly developing atelectasis.

Treatment should be carried out in the hospital, preferably by a specialized team, to hyperventilate the lungs or aspirate the mucus.

Pleuritis

In *fibrinous pleurisy* there is a sudden side pain with fever and malaise, frequently very intense, and related to respiration and coughing. The pain may radiate to the neck, shoulder, or abdomen, according to the location of the pleurisy. A shallow tachypnea is almost the rule, as well as a friction rub heard on auscultation. Do not take for pleuritic the rub heard on auscultation of dehydrated patients. In pleurisy secondary to tuberculosis, pneumonia, pleurodynia, pericarditis, mediastinal diseases, rheumatic fever, uremia, polyarteritis, systemic lupus erythematosus, and perhaps others, the symptoms of the underlying disease will enrich the clinical picture. In *serofibrinous pleuritis* with pleural effusion, the clinical picture may either be abrupt or develop gradually with pleuritic pain, after a period of time. Depending on the amount of fluid, the symptoms will be less or more severe (from mild to severe dyspnea and circulatory embarrassment) and the physical findings less or more marked (interfering with the normal sounds heard on auscultation). The best aids to diagnosis are X-ray examination, and collection of pleural fluid for examination when it is present.

The causative disease has to be treated, primarily, and the pleurisy will resolve. Of course, pain has to be relieved with analgesics or strapping. In pleural effusion removal of fluid is mandatory.

Codeine, 30 to 60 mg by mouth, every 4 hours, or 30 mg by intramuscular injection, every 4 hours; shift to the oral route as soon as possible.

Meperidine, 50 to 100 mg by intramuscular injection, four to six times a day.

Morphine, 10 to 15 mg, by subcutaneous injection, repeated as needed.

Procaine, 10% solution, up to 5 ml, by injection, for paravertebral infiltration to block intercostal nerves, if previous measures fail.

Pneumothorax

In traumatic or secondary pneumothorax, the diagnosis is relatively obvious, but not so with a spontaneous pneumothorax. Most frequently, the onset is dramatic, as in myocardial infarction or acute abdomen, with sharp side pain, severe dyspnea, and dry cough. X-ray examination and the physical signs (diminished or absent respiratory sounds, hyperresonance, hyperinflation) confirm the diagnosis.

Though the pain may be considerable, its treatment is of little consequence while the intrapleural tension is present. The simplest measure to be taken is to give oxygen therapy; also a tracheal tube with suction will help clear the bronchi and expand the lung. As a last resort, surgery may be needed. So, hospitalize the patient, and request the help of specialists, as soon as possible.

Emphysema

Emphysema is a very frequent problem among elderly smokers who have had a previous chronic bronchitis, an etiologic approach that has already been discussed. The onset of the disease is slow, with cough and dyspnea. Cough is almost always productive, but it is extremely hard to eject the mucus, thus leaving the patient exhausted after each attack of coughing. The diagnosis depends on radiologic and auscultatory findings, headed by the triad "cough, dyspnea, and the barrel-shaped inspiratory condition of the chest." These symptoms are worsened by even minor respiratory infections. As the disease progresses, other symptoms are added, such as asthenia, wheezing, liver displaced downward, cyanotic nail beds and lips, and finally evidence of hypoxia, even acidosis, and cor pulmonale with peripheral edema. Auscultation will reveal shortened breath sounds, ronchi, wheezing, and particularly a characteristic prolonged expiratory phase. On palpation, decreased movements and hyperresonance of the thorax are noted. X-ray studies will confirm hyperinflation of the lungs. Ventilatory insufficiency is also confirmed by specialized studies. A secondary polycythemia is not rare.

When a state of acute or chronic respiratory failure with hypoxia and acidosis is reached, the patient should be treated in the hospital by a specialized team. Otherwise, the basic chronic bronchitis or any other mechanical causative condition will be actively treated. Bronchodilators and mucolytic agents will be judiciously administered. Anti-infective therapy will be carried out and oxygen administered. Corticoids may give additional help.

> Aminophylline, tablets containing 100 or 200 mg, injectables containing 25 or 250 mg in each ml; give 250 to 500 mg intravenously in acute cases, or 100 to 200 mg by mouth every 6 or 8 hours.

> Beclomethasone dipropionate; use by oral inhalation according to instruction from the manufacturer.

Esophageal Diverticulosis

Nocturnal cough, which is among the characteristic symptoms of esophageal diverticulosis, occurs together with dysphagia, bad breath, and regurgitation of food, undigested or only partially digested. There are also weight loss, peculiar gurgling sounds, and positive findings in X-ray studies. These symptoms are more marked in the case of pharyngo-esophageal diverticulosis, where there may be large swellings in the neck, with impairment of adequate eating. In cases of diverticulae occurring in lower areas of the esophagus, symptoms are less marked, at times totally absent; the diverticulae are only symptomatic when they enlarge (better noted among the elderly, for this reason), but in all instances they give positive results in X-ray studies. Care must be taken not to misdiagnose malignant tumors, for which reason the help of a specialist will be welcomed.

There is little to be done in cases of diverticulosis, except for the surgical excision of the pouch. This is the best procedure for diverticulae at both ends of the esophagus. Because of the scarce symptomatology and little discomfort caused by diverticulae in the middle areas of the organ, no surgical procedures are advised for them.

Mediastinal Cough

This cough is usually a marked symptom—dry, constant but not generally paroxysmal, emetic and very bothersome. It appears early with, or soon followed by, dyspnea (stridulous and at times with glottic spasm), angina-like pains, bitonal voice, diminished voice sounds, possible congestion of lung bases, and perhaps resulting in cor pulmonale; this clinical picture is more or less common to diseases of the trachea and bronchi, the corresponding pulmonary vessels, the recurrent laryngeal nerves and the cardiac plexus, local lymph nodes, tumors, cysts, aneurism, aortitis, substernal thyroid and other conditions.

Tracheitis and bronchitis: see the corresponding entry in this section.

Recurrent laryngeal nerves: when irritated by neighboring masses, they will cause cough, which may present a bitonal character.

Mediastinal masses: in addition to cough and possibly hoarseness, there may also be substernal, angina-like pain, dyspnea, stertorous respirations, dysphagia, superior vena caval syndrome (dilation of veins of the neck, face and thoracic wall), Horner's syndrome (miosis, palpebral ptosis, and enophthalmos), and X-ray confirmation of a tumor, cyst, or goiter.

Aneurism: cough is caused by aneurisms of either the aortic arch or the descending aorta, with symptoms as caused by mediastinal masses (see above), plus active pulsations seen on X-ray examination, plus erosion of the spinal bones in cases corresponding to the descending aorta.

Aortitis: see next entry.

Goiter: cough may be accompanied by other symptoms of thyroid dysfunction; the goiter moves with the trachea when swallowing, and is evidenced by means of radiographic studies.

Aortitis

Most cases are due to syphilis, and most are symptomless. Nevertheless, in some instances with somewhat marked periarteritis (periaortitis) there is a very early occurrence of a dry cough that cannot be related to any of the other common causes. Only at a later stage anginal pains may occur, spreading to the orifice of the coronary vessels, or other symptoms of left ventricular failure, as dilation of the aortic valves with the corresponding diastolic murmur. X-ray studies may indicate increased width, pulsation, and opacity of the artery.

Treatment: Bed rest, cardiotonics, or vasodilators may be indicated in particular cases; but in almost all instances an antisyphilitic treatment should be carried out with no delay.

Penicillin; give relatively large amounts of the antibiotic, and repeat treatment at regular intervals (6 to 12 months) for a few years.

Heart Diseases

A large number of patients with a cardiopathy are coughers, perhaps heavy coughers if they have valvular diseases, particularly mitral. This cough is dry, with short emission, and possibly with other symptoms of cardiac involvement, such as dyspnea. But also a large number of elderly patients with a more or less long-lasting cardiopathy will present a productive, bronchial cough because of a respiratory reaction. In short, do not forget that coughing might herald a yet undiagnosed cardiopathy. Check carefully for it.

The treatment is that of the cardiac disease, but at times some help with codeine will be given if coughing is too bothersome.

> Codeine, 15 or more mg, several times a day, as needed and tolerated.

Epidemic Typhus (Classic Form)

Malaise and headache are followed by a sudden rise of temperature with chills, an influenza-like aggregate of symptoms (cough, chest pain, auscultatory signs), and thereafter the characteristic *rash;* first, maculae in the axillae, which spread to the trunk, becoming papular; then to the limbs, and very rarely involving palms, soles, or face. These maculae have a tendency to become confluent and to be purpuric or frankly hemorrhagic, with large areas of the skin appearing discolored. Other symptoms are: conjunctivitis, flushed face, pneumonitis, or frank pneumonia. Hypotension and bradycardia may occur, and also symptoms of complications, such as renal or cardiac disorders. Only 5 to 12 days after the onset of the disease, a positive Weil-Felix reaction will appear. Serial serum-specific complement-fixation tests will help to differentiate the disease from the other rickettsial diseases.

Complete isolation and bed rest are mandatory. The body has to be cleansed of lice, the usual vectors, and regular hygienic measures will be rigidly observed. Give plenty of fluids, in small amounts, or even intravenous infusions if indicated. The diet should be high in protein and calories. For high fever sponge the patient with water or alcohol, but avoid giving acetylsalicylic acid. For headache, give codeine or meperidine. But the basic treatment will be with a tetracycline or chloramphenicol.

> Codeine, 30 or 60 mg by mouth, every 4 to 6 hours.

> Doxycycline, 100 mg by mouth, every 12 hours the first day; thereafter, 100 mg every 24 hours. In severe cases dissolve a vial of 100 mg in 10 ml of sterile water, which solute will be added to 200 or 2000 ml of saline or 5% dextrose to be given in one or two infusions, at the regular speed. Severe cases may require 200 mg a day (with special watchfulness for adverse reactions!).

> Chloramphenicol, 50 mg for each kilo of body weight in 24 hours, in
> divided doses every 6 hours, either by injection (i.v.) or by mouth.

Murine Typhus (Endemic Typhus)

This disease is similar to epidemic typhus, but the symptomatology is milder: the fever rises gradually, chills are not always present, and the rash appears only on the trunk and disappears rapidly. Specific *Rickettsia mooseri* (or *Rickettsia typhi*) antigens provoke a rise of complement-fixing antibodies, on which diagnosis entirely depends.

Most patients run a mild course, and treatment can often be only supportive. Give a tetracycline only if needed.

Rocky Mountain Spotted Fever

The initial clinical complex is almost identical with epidemic typhus, influenza, and other diseases: fever, chills, cough, sore throat, conjunctivitis, headache, body pains, hepato- and splenomegaly, jaundice, gangrene, delirium, stupor, or coma. The rash appears on *wrists* and ankles, spreading to the extremities and thereafter over the whole body, is macular, and becomes confluent and petechial. Assume the diagnosis, if the patient has been previously exposed to ticks. Serum tests will give the diagnosis.

Because of high mortality, treat immediately as stated above for endemic typhus.

Q Fever

Q fever starts with a rise in temperature, possibly chills, cough, headache, and muscle and abdominal pains. Pneumonitis, jaundice, and prostration may also be present. The diagnosis is given by the laboratory. Evidence of hepatitis may be found (increased SGPT, SGOT, or LDH, and so forth). The marked pulmonary infiltration noted in the X-ray films, with slight clinical evidence of such infiltration, is typically characteristic. The disease has to be differentiated from pneumonia and hepatitis.

As with other rickettsial diseases, the basic treatment is carried out with tetracyclines (chloramphenicol should not be used, since the mortality of Q fever is minimal).

> Doxycycline, 100 mg, by mouth, once a day, but the first three
> doses only 12 hours apart.

EXPECTORATION

Expectoration is the act of spitting out matter formed in and ejected from the lower and upper respiratory organs. This formed matter, the sputum, usually provokes cough to expedite the expulsion; that is, all the diseases reviewed in the above section on "Cough" will be considered here whenever they present a productive cough. It is a good habit to examine carefully the sputum of all patients, and to send a portion of the specimen to the laboratory for study. References to the diagnostic clues given by sputa are made alphabetically in the following lines.

Albuminoid Sputum

This is a yellowish, frothy sputum, usually produced in relatively large amounts in *acute pulmonary edema* (more or less rapid onset of cough, dyspnea, wheezing, râles heard on auscultation, pallor with cyanosis, sweating, and the possibility of heart disease), and occasionally *after thoracocentesis* with extraction of pleural fluid. In cases of typical *pulmonary edema* the sputum may also be of a serious character, pinkish or frankly bloody in color.

Bile in the Sputum

Sputum tinged with bile, so acquiring a green or yellowish color, may be secondary to *subphrenic abscess* which opens into the bronchial tree. The clinical evidence of febrile abdominal symptoms will corroborate the diagnosis.

Black Sputum

A very dark or frankly black sputum is mainly seen in cases of *anthracosis*, with symptoms of progressive, mild emphysema or lung fibrosis, and possible X-ray findings; in *coal miner's pneumoconiosis*, also with very little symptomatology, or at most a progressive fibrosis; and in *silicosis* if this disease is associated with anthracosis. There is also a dark, perhaps not so black, sputum in *chronic bronchitis* when it is complicated by pulmonary sclerosis; this sputum is usually scanty, sticky, and mucous or mucopurulent.

Blood in the Sputum

According to the definition, hemoptysis is the expectoration of blood or sputa tinged with blood. The main differentiation between hemoptysis and hematemesis results from the way the blood is expelled: by coughing in the first case, with nausea and vomiting in the second; also, the blood is usually bright red in hemoptysis and more or less digested (darker) in hematemesis. In epistaxis it is the nose that bleeds; and blood from the mouth tinges saliva but not true sputum. Most frequently, the diagnosis is not difficult.

Pulmonary tuberculosis: sputum contains small amounts of blood during the first stages of the disease, becoming more abundant later, but, fortunately, not enough to bleed the patient white, as happened in the past. There will be evidence of cough, evening febricula, asthenia, weight loss, X-ray findings, and detection of the *Mycobacterium* in the sputum. These patients will be put on absolute bed rest until the bleeding stops; isoniazid and a second (or even a third) drug will be given, using rifampin or ethambutol, preferably.

Lung cancer: cough or bloody sputa may be the first signs of bronchogenic carcinoma; there will be, localized persistent wheeze heard on auscultation; X-ray films may also be of early help in diagnosing the condition; and finally, the progress of the implacable stressing condition will make it unmistakable. An early diagnosis may allow a beneficial surgical removal; otherwise, chemotherapy will be necessary.

Lung infarction: not rarely a thick bloody sputum will be an early sign of infarction; not rarely, either, a more copious hemorrhage will appear; there are also a sudden dyspnea with anxiety, cough, anginal pains, and X-ray densities. Most patients will present a thrombophlebitis elsewhere in the body, particularly in the legs. Emergency treatment is better given in the hospital, with oxygen, anticoagulants, meperidine for pain, and vasodilators for shock; and the help of a specialized team for embolectomy.

Pneumonia: bloody sputum may occur: for more details see below, the entry devoted to "Pneumonic Sputum."

Pneumoconioses: in most instances the sputum may be tinged with blood. In *anthracosis* there are also signs of progressive, mild emphysema and lung fibrosis, with fine nodules or large densities seen in X-ray films. In *coal miner's pneumoconiosis,* which is a more severe form of anthraxosis due to the heaviest inhalation of coal particles, there is also little symptomatology, but an eventual evolution to fibrosis. In *silicosis,* symptoms start with dry cough and dyspnea; so bloody expectoration is not an early sign. In *asbestosis,* on the contrary, early productive cough and dyspnea open the clinical picture, and the X-ray films present a ground-glass appearance. In all these diseases the treatment is symptomatic; but efforts must be made to reduce exposure.

Tracheo-bronchitis: these infections of the trachea or the bronchi may occasionally cause bloody sputa; nevertheless, the symptoms very rarely differ from the typical picture of these conditions, except for the erosive lesions giving way to blood extravasation. Treat each case individually.

Bronchiectasis: the typical case shows productive cough with copious expectoration of purulent or blood-streaked sputa. On auscultation ronchi and râles are heard; and the bronchogram reveals the dilations. Treatment is best discussed with a specialized team, including a pneumologist and a surgeon.

Pulmonary echinococcosis: not rarely bloody sputa are early symptoms in hydatid cysts of the lungs, a situation that will require X-ray examination and positive complement-fixation and skin tests when it occurs in certain areas of the United States, mainly California, Utah, and Alaska, and also in northwestern Canada, countries in South America, and Australia, and around the Mediterranean Sea. Allergic manifestations plus eosinophilia are additional suggestive symptoms.

Lung abscess: bloody sputum may occur.

Actinomycosis, blastomycosis, coccidiosis: the clinical picture with hemoptoic sputa is very similar to that of pulmonary tuberculosis; cases with actinomycosis and blastomycosis may also show dermic lesions; but the diagnosis depends on the identification of the causative microorganism.

Besnier-Boeck syndrome may cause hemoptoic sputa when localized in the lungs.

Injuries: obvious diagnosis.

Cardiac diseases: check for valvular diseases, aneurisms, cor pulmonale and hypertension.

Copious Expectoration

The amount of expectoration, for the same disease, varies widely from person to person. Nevertheless, very large amounts are common in the following instances.

Bronchiectasis: this is discussed in the above entry, ''Blood in the Sputum''; the amount expectorated is usually very large, either purulent or tinged with blood; there are ronchi and râles on auscultation, and the bronchogram reveals the cystic dilations; treatment varies, depending on different factors which will be discussed with specialists.

Pulmonary edema: the condition is usually secondary to a known cardiac disease, but may be primitive (in this case as an early man ifestation of a previous latent cardiopathy). In most instances the first manifestation appears during night rest, starting with laryngeal tickling followed by intense dyspnea and chest oppression, cyanotic lips and pale skin, continuous coughing, moist râles and stertorous ronchi heard over almost all the pulmonary area, particularly in the bases, perhaps more marked on the bases, and expectoration of thick, pinkish, frothy sputum. Patients will be semi-seated in bed, oxygen will be given at high concentration with assisted respiration in most cases, blood will be trapped by tourniquets or drawn by venesection, and diuretics and cardiotonics will complete the procedure. Transfer these patients to the hospital as soon as possible, and request the help of a specialist.

Bronchitis: the disease may present bronchorrhea in some instances.

Cavitary syndrome: this is usually present in advanced cases of tuberculosis and echinococcosis, after rupture of the cyst, and in other possible instances.

Hemoptysis: not only hemoptoic sputa, but true hemorrhages of large amounts of blood may occur in most diseases mentioned under ''Blood in the Sputum,'' above. Special care, because of the risk involved, will be given to large hemoptysis in cases of *tuberculosis, pulmonary infarction, lung abscess,* those due to *injuries, tumoral lesions, rupture of blood vessels* into the bronchial tree, and the like.

Vomica: there are large amounts of pus expelled as a very large expectoration, usually owing to the opening of a purulent collection into the bronchial tree; the condition will be due to *pleural lesions, lung abscess, post infarction, mediastinal lesions,* or *subdiaphragmatic abscess,* or will be *parasitic* (hydatid cyst, amebic vomica, or others).

Dark Sputum

See ''Black Sputum,'' above.

Egg Yolk Sputum

This is a sputum tinged with a bright-yellow color due to bilirubin, noted in some cases of *jaundice.*

Fetid Sputum

A frank putrid odor is noted in cases of gangrenous reaction in the lung; and a very offensive odor, as well, in cases of *lung abscess, empyema,* or any other *suppurative lesion* within the respiratory system, particularly those occurring in some instances of *bronchiectasis.*

Globular Sputum

This name is given to spherical yellowish lumps seen in the last stages of *pulmonary tuberculosis,* rarely seen today.

Gray Sputum

In some cases of *tracheitis* there is a grayish, opalescent, gelatinous, mottled sputum arranged in globular form.

Green Sputum

Infections with *Pseudomonas aeruginosa* may cause a bluish-green sputum; but much more commonly these greenish sputa will be indicative of *jaundice* because of their being tinged with bile. The green sputum is also called sputum aeruginosum.

Hemoptysis

See "Blood in the Sputum," above.

Icteric Sputum

This designation applies to any of the sputa tinged in green, bluish-green, or yellow by biliary pigments in cases of *jaundice.*

Laboratory Reports

Normally, this is an extensive section in books devoted to bacteriology and other laboratory procedures. Here we wish to summarize the basic information on the subject.

Mycobacteria are still very important suspects in all forms of pulmonary diseases; their presence will only show that there is some sort of tuberculosis of the respiratory system, but with no prognostic implication in any case; naturally, when there is a strong clinical suspicion of tuberculosis, and there are not demonstrable positive findings, these tests have to be repeated with great care before a negative assertion can be made. Do not forget that in many instances it is best to check for infective microorganisms in stomach contents.

Pneumococci are to be checked for in all forms of clinical pneumonia, since finding more than expected will give the final diagnosis.

Hemophilus influenzae will give the diagnosis of this not too frequent clinical form of pneumonia.

Klebsiella pneumoniae is a germ that causes a form of clinical pneumonia not rare among the elderly or in hospitalized persons, particularly if there is a previous history of alcoholism or of a debilitating disease. It is very important to achieve prompt detection for an early antibiotic treatment.

Mycoplasma pneumoniae requires a complicated procedure for an accurate diagnosis. Check for it when the sputum is scanty, cough increases markedly, and there are some respiratory symptoms and a febrile complex.

Streptococci in large amounts will indicate the nature of any infective, suppurative process, such as pneumonia or abscess.

Staphylococci, by the same token, will give the clue to the nature of the causative infection.

Bacteroides may appear in chronic respiratory diseases or infective diseases spreading from the abdomen.

Pneumocystis carinii infects the lungs (pneumonia) in cases of leukemia or of patients under immunosuppressive drugs.

Anaerobes may be causal factors, or at least co-factors, in cases of hypostatic pneumonia, lung abscess, and other forms of respiratory diseases.

Other infective agents may also be found in sputa, such as spirochetae, fungi, echinococci, and even viruses and many others.

Erythrocytes are examined in all forms of hemorrhagic disease; see the entry "Blood in the Sputum," above.

Leukocytes will accompany all suppurative lesions; but when eosinophiles are increased, allergy will be suspected.

Epithelial cells usually accompany all forms of inflammation of the bronchial tree, pneumonia, bronchopneumonia, and chronic pulmonary diseases.

Cancer cells are frequently noted in cases of *malignancies.*

Charcot-Leyden crystals are seen in asthmatic patients, but may be present in common cases of *bronchitis.*

Curschmann's spirals are bright coiled mucinous fibrils that may appear in cases of bronchial *asthma.*

Elastic fibers may indicate destruction of lung tissue, as in abscess, cavitation, or gangrene.

Other foreign material may be present, such as the bronchial fragments of *chronic fibrinous* bronchitis, *diphtheritic* membranes, fragments of *echinococcus* cysts, or lumps of *cancer* tissue.

Moss-Agate Sputum

See "Gray Sputum," above.

Mucopurulent Sputum

Classically known as "sputum coctum," the dense mucopurulent sputum is made of opaque mucopus, of a yellowish or greenish color, of a nummular discoid form, usually immersed in fluid mucosities and saliva, where the sputa sediment when left for a while. These sputa are found in *bronchiectasis,* at the end of *acute bronchitis,* and in *pulmonary cavitation,* in which instance the sputa are copious, constituting a homogenous mass of a dark green color with some markings of blood in the bottom of the container. In cases of *chronic bronchitis accompanied by pulmonary sclerosis,* the mucopurulent sputum is scanty, also dense, and of a very dark color.

Mucous Sputum

This is the classic "sputum crudum." It may be whitish or with a light tint of green or yellow, usually mucous and slightly frothy, as noted in *acute bronchitis,* in cases of *bronchial reaction* during other diseases, and in some patients with *tuberculosis.* But there is also a more dense, sticky, and scanty mucous sputum frequently found in early stages of *bronchitis* and *laryngitis,* and in *asthma.*

Nummular Sputum

As implied by the name, it is like a round disk similar to a coin. Mucopurulent sputum is usually of a nummular shape.

Pneumonic Sputum

In many instances, a typical clinical picture of pneumonia can be ascribed to a certain etiological factor because of the characteristics of the sputum.

> *Pneumococcal pneumonia:* the aspect of the sputum varies with the stage of the disease; it starts as an initial bloody sputum, rapidly turns into the well-known rusty sputum because it becomes darker, frankly stained with blood or blood pigments, and finally becomes yellowish and purulent.

> *Klebsiella pneumonia:* the sputum is viscid and presents a cherry-red color.

> *Mycoplasmal pneumonia:* the sputum is frankly bloody.

Hemophylus influenzae pneumonia: there is a very tenacious sputum of an apple-green color.

Streptococcal pneumonia: the sputa are abundant, presenting a salmon color.

Staphylococcal pneumonia: the sputa are as in the above streptococcal pneumonia.

Viral pneumonia: there is not any particularity about the sputum, but it is mucopurulent and occasionally tinged with blood.

Other forms of pneumonia: these forms are currently identified by bacteriologic or serologic means.

Prune Juice Sputum

As the name implies, this sputum bears some resemblance to portions of prune juice, thus resulting in a dark reddish-brown color, tinged with blood in most instances, and appearing in cases of *pneumonia, gangrene, cancer,* and other similar diseases of the lungs.

Purulent Sputum

This is a mucopurulent sputum with little mucus and much pus, which is present in cases of very active pulmonary suppurative lesions including lung abscess, *tubercular cavitation, malignant cavitation, large bronchiectasis,* cavitation secondary to chronic (or acute) *bronchopulmonary diseases,* and *aspiration pneumonia,* and particularly among older people in *chronic inflammatory diseases* of the lung or the pleura, chronic bronchitis, recurrent pneumonia or bronchopneumonia, pneumoconioses, or chronic tuberculosis, and in *aneurism, mediastinal tumors, adenopathies,* or *foreign bodies.*

Red Sputum

See under "Blood in the Sputum," above.

Rusty Sputum

With regard to the color, rusty means reddish-brown or reddish-yellow; that is, the color of iron oxide or hydroxide when deposited as material from oxidation of iron upon the surface of an object made of iron. The typical rusty sputum seen in *pneumococcal pneumonia* is but a sputum tinged with blood, but which presents the characteristics of iron rust. It may also be seen in other pulmonary diseases, whenever a bloody sputum is produced. Actually, the rusty aspect comes from the oxidation of iron contained in hemoglobin.

Serous Sputum

Serous sputum is typical of *pulmonary edema:* abundant and frothy, fluid and pinkish, but at times frankly hematic; it is so abundant that there are patients who present it leaking from the mouth or even the nose.

Suppressed Expectoration

When a habitual cougher stops coughing, that event may refer to a bronchial paresis of central origin, which is, of course, a sign of bad prognosis. This may occur in severe cases of *pneumonia,* in pulmonary tuberculosis, and in other diseases as well.

Tissue Particles in Sputum

See under "Laboratory Reports," above.

Vomica

See under "Copious Expectoration," above.

White Sputum

This is just a mucopurulent, purulent, or serous sputum, q.v.

Yellowish, Frothy Sputum

See "Albuminoid Sputum," at the beginning of this section.

HOARSENESS

In English there is a sharp difference between aphonia (lack of audible voice) and hoarseness (a rough quality of the voice). This is not so in other languages, which have made aphonia a word almost identical with hoarseness, with aphonia being not only the absence of voice but also a more marked hoarseness. Here we shall include the myxedematous voice, which is not a true hoarseness, but because of its acoustic characteristics comes very close to it. Other diseases in which there is also a rough character of the voice are included.

Acute Laryngitis

Precisely speaking, hoarseness is the main symptom in acute laryngitis (also in chronic laryngitis). Its intensity may increase even to the stage of true aphonia. In most instances it is accompanied by unpleasant sensations in the larynx, such as tickling, dryness, and roughness, which causes a continuous need to clear the throat. Pain and cough may accompany these symptoms. In severe infections there will be a complete febrile syndrome, and perhaps also dyspnea, dysphagia, and stridor. Check in all instances for the usual causes of acute laryngitis: excessive use of the voice or inhalation of irritant fumes or dust, for primary laryngitis; or the later ulterior development of the true causative disease, such as a common cold, influenza, pneumonia, bronchitis, Vincent's angina, tonsillitis, pharyngitis, or sinusitis, in secondary laryngitis.

If it is secondary, treatment of the basic disease is the best procedure to follow. In primary laryngitis, advise absolute rest of the voice and steam inhalations with plain water (a few drops of eucalyptol or any similar substance could be added) for 20 or 30 minutes each time, repeated several times a day. Other adjunctive therapy may be added, such as throat anesthetic lozenges, bechics, and the like.

Allergy

Hoarseness is not a typical symptom of allergic diseases, but it may occur occasionally in some cases because of a reactional edematous swelling of the vocal cords. In the first place, we have to think of *angioneurotic edema,* in which case it is a very alarming symptom requiring prompt action to avoid dangerous consequences. In this instance, together with the increasing hoarseness running toward complete aphonia, other symptoms of the disease will be apparent: itching, urticarial wheals increasing in size to invade large amounts of skin, and respiratory wheezing. In *serum sickness* the occurrence of hoarseness is not so frequent, but it may occur at times; urticaria, skin rashes, and adenopathy may be the important symptoms to note, together with the extremely rapid clinical course of the reaction. Very rarely, if at all, hoarseness will be heard in other allergic pulmonary diseases. Finally, *hay fever* reactions may involve the pharynx and more rarely the larynx, with some hoarseness of the voice; but the principal symptoms are always those related to rhinitis and conjunctivitis.

The treatment is that of any allergic condition, namely, the use of desensitizing procedures, antihistaminic drugs, and corticoids as heroic measures (corticoids particularly being given in the case of angioneurotic edema or anaphylactic shock, in this case following the immediate administration of epinephrine).

Chronic Laryngitis

Together with acute pharyngitis, this is the main etiological factor in the production of hoarseness, which is its outstanding symptom. Chronic laryngitis may be the consequence of repeated attacks of the acute form, or may be due to a different causative factor. In any instance, hoarseness is accompanied by productive cough with a sticky sputum, a sensation of dryness, and occasional mild pain due to possible ulcerations. Local examination will reveal the corresponding inflammatory reaction. In cases of chronic pharyngitis check for some of the following factors.

Speaking: many speakers, because of the effort made for the emission of sound, develop a chronic pharyngitis, with hoarseness as the main symptom, with a typical increase of hoarseness during the evening; the diagnosis is made because of the profession.

Playboy hoarseness: many men who expend nights drinking, shouting, and stressing their bodies in crapulous activities will develop a hoarsening chronic laryngitis with characteristics similar to the foregoing one, q.v.

Smoking: heavy smokers will very rarely be free from hoarseness due to the corresponding chronic laryngitis caused by the continuous irritation of the air passages; symptoms will be similar to those stated above, q.v.

Exposure to fumes or dust: chronic exposure to fumes or dust because of one's profession or residence in areas with a polluted atmosphere will also cause chronic laryngitis, with the corresponding group of symptoms; in most of these cases there will also be symptoms of lung involvement (pneumoconioses).

Syphilitic laryngitis: this will occur in late syphilis, with hoarseness, modest dysphagia, attacks of coughing, occasional hemoptysis, local syphilitic lesions seen with the laryngoscope, and the history of a previous infection.

Laryngeal tuberculosis: in this case the most important symptom is not hoarseness but an extremely painful dysphagia whenever the posterior pharynx is involved; there are also other symptoms of pulmonary tuberculosis; tuberculous ulcers may be seen through the laryngoscope; check for the finding of mycobacteria from exudates, whenever available.

Residual laryngitis: there is the history of a previous acute laryngitis not totally resolved. Also, it may be due to residual pharyngitis, or concomitant sinusitis.

Naturally, the treatment of chronic laryngitis depends on the nature of the basic etiologic factor. If it is due to the professional use of the voice, retraining with the use of loudspeakers will be tried before a formal prohibition of public speaking. Stress hoarseness will require avoidance of the stressing conditions, in the same way that the prohibition of smoking is mandatory in the case of smoker's laryngitis. For the treatment of laryngitis due to exposure to fumes and dust, see the corresponding paragraphs on pneumoconioses. Both syphilitic and tuberculous laryngitis call for the use of the corresponding medical procedures. For residual laryngitis, as well as for the symptomatic treatment of hoarseness due to any form of chronic laryngitis, notable benefit will be obtained from voice rest, inhalations of water vapor (with or without a few drops of eucalyptol), throat anesthetic lozenges, and bechics.

Central Nervous System Reactions

In the absence of true laryngeal inflammation there may be some form of paresis or dysfunction of the vocal cords due to lesions of the central nervous system, particularly tumors and injuries. In the case of injuries there is the history of a previous accident. In the case of tumors there are progressive focal neurologic changes, perhaps with other evidence of intracranial hypertension, which together with hoarseness will indicate the site of the lesion.

To complete a diagnosis and for evaluation of treatment, a neurologist and a neurosurgeon should be consulted for advice.

Edema of the Larynx

Hoarseness, developing rapidly, is accompanied by dyspnea and anxiety occurring with other symptoms of angioneurotic edema, including stridor and cyanosis.

If treatment starts early in the course of the disease, the use of corticoids or antihistaminics will be enough. Nevertheless, corticoids should be spared as much as possible because once started they are usually to be administered for prolonged periods of time. In cases of alarming symptomatology, as impending shock, epinephrine is to be given.

1:1000 Sol. epinephrine, 0.5 cc, by subcutaneous injection.

Encephalitis

Hoarseness may be present in some patients with encephalitis, but the general clinical picture gives the diagnosis. Sore throat may be among the initial symptoms. Also, the involvement of nerve function could be among the causes of this hoarseness. In all instances the diagnosis depends on the study of the spinal fluid and a good neurological evaluation.

If there is a known infection, it will be adequately treated; otherwise, treatment is merely symtomatic.

Foreign Body in the Larynx

Swallowed foreign bodies may lodge in the pharynx, the esophagus, the larynx, or the bronchi. Large foreign bodies are easily found, but for small ones much time must be spent in many cases; and while the patient complains of discomfort, it is better to believe that the swallowed material is still there, particularly when there are cough and gagging, stridor, and some sort of dyspnea, even capable of causing asphyxia; or when secondary symptoms develop. These secondary symptoms may be fever, swelling, pain, and other instances of inflammatory reaction. With these developments it is likely that a foreign body is lodged in the larynx.

A sudden, very acute food-choking accident should be treated by wrapping the arms around the patient's waist, with one hand making a fist and the other strongly grasping it and pushing violenting between the navel and the ribs, as if pushing the offending morsel out from the esophagus, larynx, or pharynx. Otherwise, the procedure calls for the use of a laryngoscope and direct extraction; it is best to work with the patient kept in Trendelenburg's position, and to use either local or general anesthesia.

Mediastinal Lesions

Most of these lesions can cause hoarseness because of involvement of the recurrent laryngeal nerve. But this will be only one factor in the complex mediastinal syndrome, with substernal pain, dyspnea, cough, stridulous respiration, bitonal voice, diminished vesicular chest sounds and congestion of bases, some evidence of cor pulmonale, and so on. For more details see under "Mediastinal Cough," at the beginning of this chapter.

Meningitis

See above in this section, the entry on "Encephalitis."

Multiple Sclerosis

There would not be the protean clinical picture that actually exists without the presentation of hoarseness as a symptom. Hoarseness is considered with other, also more-or-less transient, motor and neurologic disturbances, particularly tremor, slurred speech, nystagmus, visual impairment, and a possible increase of gamma globulin in the spinal fluid. The disease starts in early adulthood, but older patients can be seen.

There is no specific treatment for multiple sclerosis, but tries will be given to corticoids, isoniazid, tolbutamide, procaine, cyanocobalamin, or any other treatment advised by specialists familiar with the disease.

Myasthenia Gravis

Actual hoarseness or merely a "different" voice may occur during the ups and downs of myasthenia gravis. Because of the trend to easy fatigability followed by paresis or frank paralysis, the voice will change gradually until it becomes almost inaudible. There will also be ptosis of the eyelids, strabismus, diplopia, and other similar symptomatology. The diagnosis is positive if there is an immediate response to the administration of neostigmine or edrophonium.

Critical situations, such as asphyxia or any other risky paralysis, will be treated with the immediate intramuscular injection of 1 mg of neostigmine (which will always be carried by the patient, to use in emergency situations). Maintenance treatment consists of the use of oral neostigmine, pyridostigmine, edrophonium, or other measures to be discussed with specialists. For more details on myasthenia gravis see the corresponding entry under the heading "Paresia and Paralysis" in the chapter devoted to "Neurological Symptoms."

Myxedema

In myxedema it is not true hoarseness that develops, but a muffled voice caused by the myxedematous infiltration of the vocal cords. It is very characteristic; once heard, it will always be recognized. But for this to happen, the myxedematous condition will be well developed, and other symptoms of hypothyroidism will be evident. The face will be puffy as in nephritis, with very dry, perhaps itchy skin all over the body, loss of hair, slow pulse and slow speech, hearing impairment, rheumatic pains, slow cerebration, asthenia, somnolence, intolerance to cold, decreased sexual activity, and constipation, that is, a general picture of life presented in slow motion. If tegumental myxedema is well developed, the diagnosis is self-evident. The presence of a goiter may call attention to hypothyroidism, as well as a previous thyroidectomy. Overweight is a typical condition. Dubious cases will be solved by measuring thyroid hormones in the blood, T_3 and T_4, which will be decreased, below 25 and 5 μg %, respectively. The thyroid stimulant hormone of the hypophysis is increased in blood. It is very important to recall that many myxedematous patients will present a very scarce symptomatology.

Thyroid extracts or synthetic thyroid preparations are specific for the treatment of hypothyroidism. No matter what preparation is used, each patient will require a specific dosage, neither more nor less, which dosage has to be determined by personal adjustment, considering both symptomatology and laboratory findings. The start will always be with the smallest amount for that person, increasing by small steps until hypothyroid symptoms vanish; thereafter, any increase of pulse of 10 beats above the normal rhythm will indicate that the thyroid dosage is exceeding the adequate amount. Of course, it will be unwise to wait for the appearance of hyperthyroid symptoms. Do not forget that older persons may be sensitive to the administration of thyroid preparations, no matter how low their glandular activity is.

Thyroid extract (marketed as thyroglobulin), tablets containing 16, 32, 65, 100, 130, 200, or 325 mg each, to start by giving about 16 or 32 mg a day for at least 7 days, and increasing by 16 mg every week thereafter, until an acceptable control of symptoms is achieved; maintenance dosage is usually established between 100 and 200 mg a day.

Levo-triiodothyronine (liothyronine), 5, 25, or 50 μg per tablet, starting with 5 μg a day, for a rapid control of undesirable symptoms.

Levothyroxine, tablets with 0.025, 0.05, 0.1, 0.15, 0.2, 0.3, or 0.5 mg each, starting with 25 μg (0.025 mg) a day, to reach a maintenance dose of about 0.15 to 0.3 mg a day.

Paralysis of the Palate

Again, this is not true hoarseness, but a nasal voice with distorted consonant sounds. Additional symptoms are the expulsion of liquids and food from the nose and a bothersome dysphagia. Direct examination of the mouth will show the flaccid soft palate. It can be due to the following causes.

Diphtheric paralysis: this is rare among the elderly because the disease is not frequent at this time of life; it appears together with the membranaceous angina or any other form of the infection.

Botulism: the nasal hoarseness may be the first symptom; there are other paralytic symptoms, particularly of the eyes (diplopia), but also dysphagia, dry mouth, and a progressive weakness of all muscles; check for the toxin in the serum or the food.

Infective diseases of the palate: paralysis may occur in any severe disease of this kind, namely, typhoid fever, meningitis, rickettsioses, and the like.

Bulbar palsy: this disease is frequently associated with amyotrophic lateral sclerosis, with spastic weakness of the trunk and limbs, changes of the tongue, dysphagia, and a final respiratory paralysis.

Amyotrophic lateral sclerosis: see the above entry.

Myasthenia gravis: see under "Myasthenia Gravis," in the above lines.

Senile pseudobulbar syndrome: this follows attacks of "little strokes" in arteriosclerotic patients, with progressive weakness of the legs, a gait with little steps, possibility of parkinsonian symptoms, explosive attacks of laughter or weeping, expulsion of liquids and food through the nose, and not only the special resonance of the voice but also accentuated distortion of consonant sounds.

Polyneuritis: such hoarseness is rare, but may occur in cases of alcohol or lead intoxication.

The treatment of this condition depends on the nature of the etiological factor. Each individual disease will be treated by itself.

Recurrent Nerve Lesions

Most frequently, when the recurrent nerves are affected there is an alteration of the emission of the voice, which becomes hoarse and presents a bitonal character. When these patients cough, there is also a bitonal coughing. The nerve is affected in a large number of patients suffering from the following diseases.

Tracheitis and tracheobronchitis: with cough and other symptoms of an upper respiratory infection.

Tumoral masses in the mediastinum: with angina-like pain, dyspnea, stertorous respirations, dysphagia, and other symptoms of compression of neighboring structures; X-ray studies are confirmatory.

Aortic aneurism: of the arch or the descending aorta; symptoms as for any other tumoral mass (see above) plus active contractions and erosion of bones seen in X-ray studies.

Aortitis: which gives symptoms only when there is some periarteritis also present (hoarseness, dry cough, anginal pains, or other symptoms of left ventricular failure).

Goiter: mostly if substernal; will behave like any other tumoral mass.

Tabes dorsalis: see next entry.

Multiple sclerosis: see corresponding entry in this section.

Polyneuritis: either toxic or infective.

Each causative disease will be treated as usual.

Tabes Dorsalis

In this instance hoarseness is due to nerve impairment, and together with it there will be a loss of stability in the dark, lack of perception of vibrations, hypotonus and hyporeflexia of muscle function, diversity of paresthesias, including analgesia of some areas of the skin, occurrence of sudden very sharp pains of the muscles, particularly of the legs, pupillary reaction that is poor to light and adequate to accommodation, as well as visceral crises of pain, painless ulcers, and other symptoms, all confirmed by positivity of reactions to syphilis in blood and spinal fluid.

Basic treatment is with aqueous crystalline penicillin G, or an alternate in case of absolute intolerance. Dosages are to be elevated, and courses repeated as needed, according to control tests of the spinal fluid repeated about every 3 months.

Penicillin; give up to 20 million units a day for 10 to 20 days, repeating these courses for as long as needed.

Traumatic Hoarseness

Any injury affecting the vocal cords or their innervation will be the cause of more or less marked hoarseness, depending on the intensity of the provoked lesion. In most instances the diagnosis will be obvious because of the history of the previous accident. Lesions caused by foreign bodies should be included in this category.

Following trauma, care will be exerted to avoid a resulting infection; so lesions are to be cleansed and disinfected, and anti-infective therapy given whenever necessary. Efforts to minimize subsequent inflammation will be carried out, with soothing medication, vaporizations, and the like. In the last instance, surgery may be advisable; so a surgeon should be consulted.

Tumors of the Larynx

Among the elderly, tumors are very frequent, especially among those with hoarseness; hence, the assumption is that a tumor is developing in the larynx, either a benign or a malignant new growth. Hoarseness is the primary symptom in these cases of tumoral lesions. Cough, which may be dry, productive, or frankly hemoptoic, is also a very important symptom. The clinical picture in completed with sore throat, which may cause some pain referred to the ear, or may cause a "sticking" sensation locally, a more or less marked dysphagia, and possibly a respiratory obstruction. The diagnosis is completed with a direct laryngological examination, which will reveal either an ulceration or a swelling; but in a very large number of cases a biopsy is needed to determine the nature of the tumor.

> *Malignant tumors:* hoarseness may lead to complete aphonia; frequently there is marked dysphagia; and unilaterality of the lesion is an important sign.

> *Benign tumors:* these tumors show no specific symptom, and the hoarseness may vary in tone.

Whenever a diagnosis of tumor of the larynx is made, or there is the need of confirmation, the patient must be sent to a specialist, who will take care of not only establishing the final estimate of the nature of the disease but also its treatment in case it is a tumor. Make the diagnosis by biopsy if necessary, and then carry out the proper treatment if it is a tumor.

VII. DYSPNEA

If dyspnea is, according to definition, a difficult or labored form of respiration, any abnormal respiratory rhythm has to be considered a particular type of dyspnea because the physiologic pattern is already broken. Following this concept, the frequent deviations from the regular respiratory physiology will be reviewed here, listed in alphabetical order.

BIOT'S RHYTHM

Following four, five, or six respiratory movements of identical depth there is a period of apnea of variable duration. This type of respiration usually is associated with cranial hypertension, but is also very frequent in meningitis (it was also called meningitic respiration), and may be seen in Addison's disease.

Meningitis

In most forms of meningitis the symptoms are often the same, except for the slower onset in tuberculous meningitis. After an initial febrile attack not too characteristic of any particular disease, there is a relatively rapid change consisting of fever (some elderly persons not reaching high temperatures), often accompanied by chills, headache, and the first true symptoms from the nervous system, namely, confusion, delirium, and not rarely convulsions. There are diffuse pains all over the body, nausea, and vomiting; and a final shock or comatose stage. With Biot's, the respiration is better noted during coma. Stiffness of the neck and abnormal reflexes (Brudzinski, Kernig, Marañon) will strengthen the suspicion of meningitis, which will be confirmed with the examination of the spinal fluid: elevated pressure, cloudy aspect of a purulent fluid, increased protein content, and lowered glucose. Bacteriological studies will substantiate the nature of the infection, that is, meningococcal, pneumococcal, staphylococcal, streptococcal, tuberculous, or whatever other germ is involved.

The treatment will vary according to the causative germ. Aqueous penicillin G is the choice for meningococcus, pneumococcus, and streptococcus; nafcillin is used for staphylococcus. Tuberculous meningitis will be treated with at least three drugs, namely, isoniazid, rifampin, and ethambutol. Care for annoying symptoms is a part of the treatment, namely, hypovolemic shock, cranial hypertension, circulatory hypotension, and intravascular clotting.

> Penicillin G, in large amounts, even up to 20 million units a day, if tolerated and needed, by intravenous drip, until the temperature is normal for at least 5 days.

> Nafcillin, to be used if the germ is not sensitive to penicillin, injecting large amounts intravenously, up to 10 or 12 g a day, if tolerated.

> Isoniazid; give about 300 mg in 24 hours, by mouth.

> Rifampin; give 600 mg a day.

> Ethambutol; give 15 mg for each kilo of body weight every 24 hours. Treatment to be continued for about 2 years.

Cranial Hypertension

There is an intense headache, projectile vomiting without nausea, papilledema, and final coma. In addition, there may be bradycardia, sleepiness, ocular palsies with diplopia, dizziness, or jacksonian seizures, and abnormal respiration. This condition can be due to: a brain tumor, with additional symptoms according to the location of the tumor; a brain cyst, also with symptoms according to location; cerebral abscess, with additional symptoms due to the infection; or pure arterial hypertension (with vomiting, headache, and papilledema).

Cranial hypertension is usually relieved by the use of mannitol, urea, invert sugar, or glucose solutions injected intravenously.

> Mannitol, 10% solution; give by intravenous drip.

Addison's Disease

The Biot's respiration will be present during an addisonian shock, when the patient, generally with a diagnosis established, presents symptoms of dehydration, hypotension, abdominal pain, vomiting, diarrhea, and fever. If the diagnosis has not been established, the presence of marked hyperpigmentation (skin, pressure sites, creases, mucosae), sparse body hair, and small heart will alert the physician to the possibility of addisonism. Laboratory reports will confirm the diagnosis, particularly when showing very low figures for cortisol in blood and urine.

Hospitalize these patients to treat shock, with emphasis on the administration of intravenous plasma and fluids with sodium, dopamine, antibiotics, and hydrocortisone.

For more details see the corresponding entry in the section devoted to "Shock."

BRADYPNEA

The name implies the slowness of respiration. It may be a pure slow respiration, but rhythmic; or a respiration not only with less than 12 movements every minute but also accompanied by some other irregularity. It is also seen in cranial hypertension, as well as in strokes, shock, diabetes, uremia, and intoxications with alcohol, barbiturates, and opium.

Cranial Hypertension

Instead of the Biot's respiration there may be a simple bradypnea accompanying the intense headache, projectile vomiting without nausea, papilledema, and final coma. Treatment will be carried out with mannitol, glucose, urea, or other similar solution injected intravenously. For more details see other entries in this chapter and in the chapter on "Neurological Symptoms."

Stroke

Unconsciousness and the following paralysis are the main traits for the diagnosis of a stroke. Patients are as in a deep sleep; respirations are stertorous and most frequently abnormal, in the sense of bradypnea or of Cheyne-Stokes' respiration. Other symptoms may be: previous headache, dizziness, nausea or vomiting, and transient weakness or paresthesia on one side of the body; thereafter there will be noted a flushed face, bradycardia, hypertension (not always), complete relaxation of all muscles of one side of the body (hemiplegia), lack of reflexes, and a positive Babinski sign. The spinal fluid is frequently bloody and with an elevated pressure. Specialized radiographic studies will complete the diagnostic procedure. Additional symptoms depend on the involved arteries.

Subdural hematoma: almost immediately follows an injury to the head; but if it is delayed, there are irritability and mental confusion, with the usual symptoms of a stroke. An electroencephalogram will help the diagnosis. Surgery is the best approach.

Subarachnoid hemorrhage: may follow any type of exertion, or may start abruptly as a simple stroke; there is neck stiffness, and not rarely convulsions and fever. The spinal fluid is under elevated pressure. Older patients may have a history of recurrent similar attacks. Meningeal signs are positive. If symptoms improve after a spinal tap is performed, it will be repeated until bleeding stops. Otherwise, use aminocaproic acid, or resort to surgical procedures.

Intracerebral hemorrhage: is of sudden onset with headache, hemiplegia, and coma, with a clinical picture rich in neurological manifestations. Also, exertion may precede it. A neurosurgeon will help in deciding on further treatment.

Internal carotid occlusion: starts with hemiparesis, ending in complete hemiplegia on the side opposite the lesion, and blindness of the same eye; there are also speech disturbances, emotional upsets, and lowering of cerebration. Not always, but not rarely either, there is bradypnea. The final diagnosis depends on arteriographic studies. Treatment calls for anticoagulation (not to the severely hypertensive), and for surgery in selected cases.

Cerebral thrombosis: follows a gradually progressive clinical course unrelated to trauma or exertion. Most patients will present other symptoms of advanced arteriosclerosis. Perform arteriographic studies. Anticoagulant therapy is a relatively poor help; surgery will be decided on by a neurosurgeon. Rehabilitation also depends on specialized attention.

Cerebral embolism: occurs with a fulminant development of a hopeless-looking stroke syndrome, even though a few patients will present a rapid apparent recovery. Among the elderly, many have had previous coronary thrombosis of the carotid, and other thrombotic lesions in the abdomen, limbs, and so forth. Consult a neurosurgeon about the advisability of surgery.

Basilar artery occlusion: presents neurological symptoms of mostly intermittent bradypnea, confusion, dizziness, impaired speech and vision, with lethal results as soon as it becomes a complete occlusion. Surgery is the only therapy, whenever applicable.

Arteriosclerosis and atherosclerosis: will show some circulatory deficit in the brain, coronaries, extremities, kidney, or the terminal aorta. This is a disease very frequently found in advanced age. Therapy consists of prophylaxis against the disease, early prelesional treatment, and treatment of the established disease to stop the progress of atherogenesis, to avoid thrombosis, and to deal with possible accidents.

Temporal arteritis: will present headache, other pains, and local tenderness. The disease responds well to corticoids.

Arterial hypertension: will cause bradypnea only in a few patients, only if the disease is severe or comes close to a stroke.

Other diseases causing stroke (that is, a stroke or a strokelike condition, such as new growths within the skull): epilepsy, migraine, mitral stenosis, polycythemia, thrombocytopenic purpura, leukemia, meningitis, or encephalitis, all of which predispose to stroke.

Bradypnea will occur with the foregoing diseases only if the clinical picture shows great clinical severity, or when they reach the condition of a stroke syndrome, when the abnormal respiration may be one of the accompanying symptoms of the stroke itself. In each particular instance the treatment will depend on the basic problem, and almost always the advice of a neurosurgeon will be needed.

Shock

As stated in more detail under the heading "Shock" in the chapter on "Unconsciousness" (q.v.), this condition is characterized by a profound depression of circulatory and nervous function, resulting in marked dyspnea, arterial hypotension, weak tachycardic pulse, pale and clammy skin, and more or less marked loss of consciousness. This situation may be due to loss of fluid, hemorrhage, burns, vomiting, diarrhea, surgery, or toxemia, sepsis, diabetes, cancer, pneumonia, or other causes.

Specific treatment will be given to each variety of shock. Patients will rest in bed with the legs only slightly elevated, the respiration will be assisted whenever necessary, the body will be kept at due temperature, pain will be controlled whenever present, and blood volume will be properly controlled with blood expanders or blood transfusions, together with dopamine or levarterenol. Mannitol is reserved for suspected intracranial hypertension.

Hypoglycemia

Paroxysmal dyspnea or any other form of dyspnea may occur during hypoglycemic coma, but this symptom will be obscured by marked tremors, intense perspiration, flushed face, and the loss of consciousness. Blood glucose below 40 mg% and rapid recovery after glucose administration will substantiate the diagnosis of hypoglycemia.

> Glucose, 25% solution, for intravenous administration; give a total amount of 10 to 20 g.

Uremia

It has been said that the Cheyne-Stokes' rhythm is most consistent with a uremic state. Nevertheless, other abnormal types of breathing may also be present, bradypnea being a frequent one. Older persons with uremia are usually cachectic, markedly asthenic, and present skin itching and paleness, gastrointestinal upsets, increased ammonia odor of the breath, miosis, hypertension, and other suggestive symptoms. There is a previous disease in the majority of cases, namely, glomerulonephritis, with proteinuria, hematuria, and casts, or nephrosclerosis, with marked hypertension, or pyelonephritis, with persistent bacteriuria.

Treatment will be addressed to each individual disease. Proteins will be restricted in the diet, with the addition of amino acids or vitamins whenever needed. Patients will receive due amounts of sodium, calcium, phosphate, and potassium. But the advantage of transplants or dialysis will be discussed with specialists in the field.

Intoxications

In acute or chronic intoxications there is frequently some form of dyspnea (bradypnea) present. The symptoms, of course, will vary according to the intoxicant.

Alcohol: not too deep coma, alcoholic breath, red face and eyes, mydriasis, noisy respirations and perhaps other symptoms of hypoglycemia.

Barbiturates: usually due to an attempted suicide; respirations not only slow but shallow, mydriatic non-reactive pupils, and symptoms of circulatory collapse.

Opium derivatives: initial nervous stimulation followed soon by depression, miosis, bradypnea or Cheyne-Stokes' rhythm, muscle relaxation, low temperature, low blood pressure, and final shock or coma.

Carbon dioxide: dyspnea with palpitation, extreme weakness of muscles, red throat, and an initial hypertension followed by hypotension as the poisoning progresses.

Carbon monoxide: also stertorous dyspnea, full bounding pulse, and changed skin color; following suicide attempts.

Laboratory reports will disclose alcohol over 2000 mg% in the blood, the presence of barbiturates in urine, or the other abnormal products.

In each particular instance the treatment will be directed to eliminate as much poison as possible, control unpleasant or dangerous symptoms, and assist respiration whenever needed. For more details see individual entries in previous sections of the book.

CARDIAC DYSPNEA

It is so named because it is due to cardiac diseases that impair proper tissue oxygenation. It is almost always due to a primary or secondary heart failure, the latter due to valvular diseases, coronary insufficiency, hypertension, or the causative factor for paroxysmic dyspnea.

Cardiac Failure

Dyspnea, graphically called "air hunger," is one of the outstanding symptoms of heart insufficiency, no matter that there are patients who specifically complain of fatigue or tiredness on exertion. In this particular case both dyspnea and fatigue go together because the tiredness of the muscles depends on the lack of oxygen, that is, insufficient oxygen intake which has to be compensated with rest and increased respiratory attempts to inhale oxygen. The complete clinical picture of cardiac failure consists also of cough, fatigue, cardiac enlargement, gallop rhythm, elevated venous pressure, pulmonary venous congestion, dependent edema and even ascites, and a tender hepatomegaly. The symptoms corresponding to right ventricular failure are mainly those of dependent edema, hepatomegaly, and elevated venous pressure. The other symptoms are mainly due to left ventricular failure. Regarding dyspnea, it will be correct to state that it may be a pure dyspnea, present at all times, day and night; or it may be an exertional dyspnea, mainly noted after unusual exercise, or when even slight muscle efforts are made; or it may be orthopnea, when the patient cannot be comfortable in bed because of actual suffocation (these patients sleep sitting in chairs); or it may be paroxysmal dyspnea, usually accompanied by elevated blood pressure, aortic insufficiency, or myocardial infarction. The onset is mostly gradual, with increasing dyspnea and dependent edema (noted on pressure at the ankles); or it may be somewhat abrupt when precipitated by an intercurrent disease or an unusually stressing condition. With the progress of the disease the disability of the patient also progresses. In X-ray studies the heart appears enlarged. An underlying cause will be determined whenever possible: myocarditis due to rheumatic fever or other infectious disease, valvular diseases, particularly aortic insufficiency, endocarditis, hypothyroidism, hyperthyroidism, chronic pulmonary diseases, or any other occurrence imposing strenuous conditions on the heart.

Treatment includes: general hygiene, with rest and diet; cardiotonics, principally digitalis; diuretics; and surgical procedures (paracentesis, dialysis), as advisable. Elderly persons on rest will be carefully watched to avoid decubitus ulcers or leg phlebitis (by change of position or water mattress, active or passive exercises). Also, cardiotonics will be prescribed according to individual tolerance, since the elderly require smaller doses.

Digoxin, 0.25 or 0.5 mg in each tablet; start with 2 mg, rarely more, in 24 hours in four divided doses every 6 hours; but after the second day a maintenance dose of 0.25 or 0.5 mg will be prescribed; of course, in all instances tolerance and response are to be carefully checked. For other ways of digitalizing the patient, it will be better to consult a cardiologist.

Chlorothiazide, tablets containing 250 or 500 mg each; give 500 but rarely more than 750 or 1000 mg in 24 hours, in divided doses, according to tolerance (check for potassium depletion).

Valvular Diseases

Any valvular disease may cause dyspnea as soon as it causes heart failure. The symptoms are, naturally, those corresponding to congestive heart failure, plus those corresponding to the involved valve.

Mitral stenosis: dyspnea due to fibrillation; there may also be orthopnea, tachypnea, or paroxysmal dyspnea; hemoptysis may occur. In the apex a presystolic murmur is heard and also an intense first sound with an enlarged left atrium.

Mitral insufficiency: scarce symptomatology; slowly progressive clinical course; diastolic murmur at the apex. which spreads to the axilla; enlarged left atrium and ventricle.

Aortic stenosis: exertional dyspnea; systolic murmur at the second interspace at the right side; concentric hypertrophy of the left ventricle.

Aortic insufficiency: not too rare among the elderly, exertional or paroxysmal dyspnea; diastolic murmur over the second interspace on the left side; enlarged left ventricle.

Tricuspid lesions: murmurs heard over the left sternal border; enlarged right atrium (stenosis) or atrium and ventricle (insufficiency).

Age is against surgery for a large number of patients, but the desirability of the procedure will be evaluated by specialists. Otherwise, the treatment is mainly that for heart failure, with cardiotonics and similar drugs.

Coronary Dyspnea

In cases of coronary insufficiency the symptom to which the most attention is given is pain; but a number of patients will also complain of dyspnea increased by exertion, dizziness, faintness, sweating, and palpitations. The diagnosis is not always easy.

For more details see entries on angina.

Hypertension

Dyspnea is only a secondary sympton in arterial hypertension, felt only when heart failure begins. Symptoms due to hypertension itself do not start for many years, becoming apparent when the heart cannot provide adequate oxygenation to body tissues. First symptoms are vague, mostly related to asthenia, palpitations, or other anxiety evidence. When heart failure is apparent, there is most commonly paroxysmal dyspnea, but there is also exertional dyspnea. In essential hypertension (hyperpiesia) no causative factors are found. In *secondary hypertension* there will be evidence of impairment of the endocrines (pheochromocytoma), and of the kidney (renal arteries insufficiency, glomerulonephritis, and so on), intracranial hypertension, lupus erythematosus, polyarteritis nodosa, and so forth. The diagnosis is made by taking the blood pressure. Retinal changes depend on the severity of the disease, narrowing of the arteries, or production of exudates. The severity of the disease depends on the involvement of the brain, the circulatory system, and the renal function.

First treatment approach will be the use of diuretics, to which a large number of patients will respond; a second line of treatment will be with diuretics plus methyldopa or apresoline; and, finally, all these drugs will be given concomitantly.

> *Diastolic 90–110:* give hydrochlorothiazide or chlorothiazide to start; may be complemented with reserpine or methyldopa.

> *Diastolic 110–130:* give the diuretic, as above, but together with methyldopa; may complement it with hydralazine or guanethidine.

> *Diastolic 130–150:* give the diuretic, as above, but with guanethidine; may complement with methyldopa.

> *Diastolic over 150:* give the diuretic together with methyldopa and guanethidine; may supplement with hydralazine.

The above suggestions are only tentative; each individual patient will be treated according to particular response and tolerance to medications. By the way, there are other schedules well praised by specialists.

> Hydrochlorothiazide, tablets containing 25, 50, or 100 mg each; give 25 or 50 mg every 12 hours.

> Methyldopa, tablets containing 125, 250, or 500 mg each; give 250 mg every 12 hours; but may increase dosage to close to 500 mg

every 6 hours if there is no satisfactory response and the tolerance is good; or also use these higher doses in severe cases.

Guanethidine, tablets containing 10 or 25 mg each; give 10 mg up to once every 6 hours; dosage may be increased to 25 or more mg every 6 hours, according to response and tolerance.

Reserpine, tablets containing 0.1, 0.25, or 1 mg each; give about 0.25 mg a day.

Hydralazine, tablets containing 10, 25, or 100 mg each; give 25 mg every 12 hours; may increase to 50 mg every 8 hours, or according to response and tolerance.

Paroxysmal Dyspnea

This subject will be discussed in some detail in a section, below, entirely devoted to the subject.

CHEYNE-STOKES RHYTHM

After a period of apnea of variable duration, respirations start with little intensity, but increasing gradually to a maximal depth, from whence they decrease again gradually to another apneic period. This pattern seems to be almost typical of uremic coma, but it is also frequent in meningitis, intoxication with opium, hypoxia and anoxia, heart failure (hyposystolia), and stroke. The Pickwickian syndrome (see under "Restrictive Dyspnea") presents this type of respiration.

Stroke

During the deep sleep of patients in stroke, respirations are stertorous and usually abnormal, with the Cheyne-Stokes rhythm, or with a simple bradypnea. The diagnosis results from the occurrence of this comatose state together with hemiplegia and abnormal reflexes. To avoid repetition, the reader is referred to the entry "Stroke" in this chapter, under the heading "Bradypnea." Other entries may also help (q.v.).

Cardiac Failure

In heart failure dyspnea is one of the diagnostic symptoms; it may present a common trait of simple difficulty ("air hunger") or a more complex Cheyne-Stokes respiration. Other dyspneic forms may also occur in this instance, namely, orthopnea, paroxysmal dyspnea, and rest dyspnea, which will always be kept in mind by the physician making a diagnosis. Nevertheless, in the section headed "Cardiac Dyspnea" there is more information about this subject, to which the reader is referred.

Uremia

Cheyne-Stokes respiration has been considered almost typical of uremic coma. This is not always so; thus some modern books do not mention dyspnea among the uremic symptoms even during the lethargic or comatose stages. Nevertheless, it is an important symptom to note during coma, particularly if the patient is not known to be suffering a renal disease. During the precomatose stage exertion or paroxysmal dyspnea may be present if there are respiratory implications or hypertension. The uremic condition may develop gradually following a chronic renal disease, or may be acute. In chronic uremia there are unspecific symptoms from almost all organs and systems of the body; of some particular diagnostic interest are a rapid weight loss with marked reduction in size of muscles in generalized edema, paresthesias and neuralgias, itching, and other symptoms that are substantiated by laboratory findings of protein and casts in the urine, elevated blood urea nitrogen, and creatinine. The comatose stage will show unconsciousness, difficult respiration, ammoniacal odor to the breath, miosis, paleness, oliguria or anuria, hypothermia (hyper- in a few cases, when there is marked dehydration), and the laboratory evidence of the condition (blood urea nitrogen on the increase, elevated creatinine and potassium in blood, with decreased amounts of sodium). In chronic uremia the clinical course worsens in acute renal failure. After the oliguric stage there comes a diuretic phase, pointing toward a more or less complete recovery. The basic disease causing the uremic stage has to be determined.

> *Acute renal failure:* check for toxic agents such as antibiotics, sulfonamides, or other poisons; infectious diseases, particularly septicemia; severe injuries of all kinds, including surgery; tissue destruction, as in infarcts or burns; dehydration; or blood transfusions.

> *Uropathies:* check for glomerulonephritis, renal sclerosis, tuberculosis of the kidneys, other infections of the kidneys, pyelonephritis, obstructive nephropathy, renal vascular disease, amyloid kidney, nephrotic syndrome, chronic radiation nephritis, or any other similar disease.

> *Extrarenal uremia:* check for pyloric stenosis, intestinal obstruction, cirrhosis, and other causes also included in the paragraph above on acute renal failure (q.v.)

The confirmation of the uremic condition in any of the above diseases rests on laboratory findings, as already stated—the "triple A": azotemia, anemia, and acidosis.

During the preuremic stage, in chronic renal insufficiency, all curable causative diseases will be treated as such, and the results will usually be excellent. In all other instances order a diet with no more than 0.5 g of protein for each kilo of body weight in 24 hours or a protective mixture of essential amino acids, but adequate in calories and vitamins. Fluid intake depends on fluid output, considering the presence or absence of edema. Measures to be considered are: sodium supplementation; potassium restriction or supplementation; calcium for hypocalcemic tetany and vitamin D for osteomalacia; symptomatic approach for whatever disabling symptom may occur; and surgery (transplant or dialysis). In acute renal failure treat both shock and the causative basic problem. Dialysis will be advised in all severe cases, even during the preuremic stage. During the first oliguric stage reduce fluid intake to a minimum (about 400 ml a day, plus basic fluid losses); protein, to zero; glucose to 100 or 200 g a day; and fat to as low as possible, better none. Electrolyte balance has to be brought as close as possible to normal, preferably to normal. During the diuretic stage keep both water and electrolyte metabolism within normal limits.

Diabetes

During the regular clinical course of diabetes mellitus respiration is usually normal, except for those patients with cardiorespiratory involvement, or renal impairment, when a dyspneic state may be present. Otherwise, dyspnea will not be present until a diabetic coma occurs, when the Cheyne-Stokes or the Kussmaul respiration takes place. The latter is perhaps more frequent among diabetics, but either may occur. With known diabetics the diagnosis of coma is easy, but this is not so when we are facing a comatose patient with no information about the preceding condition; then the diagnosis depends on the diagnosis of unconsciousness (q.v.).

Diabetic coma requires emergency treatment following the established rules, which have been summarized under the heading "Coma" in the chapter on "Unconsciousness."

Hypoglycemia

In hypoglycemic coma, with blood glucose below 40 mg%, some sort of paroxysmal dyspnea, perhaps Cheyne-Stokes respiration, may be present but it will be inconspicuous among other prevalent symptoms, as increased perspiration, marked tremors, flushed face, and unconsciousness. The low glucose figures and the rapid improvement of symptoms after the administration of glucose will give the final diagnosis.

Glucose, 25% solution, for intravenous administration, to give a total of 10 to 20 g of glucose.

Hypoxia and Anoxia

Deficient oxygenation of tissues is responsible for most of the symptoms of cardiac failure; but there are several other causes of interference with proper oxygenation, a condition that results in dyspnea which may be Cheyne-Stokes or tachypneic, tachycardia, headache, and cyanosis of the bed of the nails, lips, or large areas of the body, the last either early or late in appearance. In acute cases, for instance, when moving to places at higher altitude, there may be insomnia and delirium. Announcing the final state of anoxia, there may be other symptoms, such as convulsions or muscle twitching, and unconsciousness.

Anemia: shows paleness, asthenia, vertigo, irritability, tinnitus, and oligemia found in the hemogram.

Deficient blood circulation: occurs in cardiac failure, embolic or thrombotic conditions, and chock.

Deficient oxygenation of the air: occurs when the patient goes to places located at higher altitudes or where there is not a proper replenishment of the air, as in caves, closed rooms, or where there is an excess of inert gases.

Airway obstruction: as caused by foreign bodies, emphysema, asthma, edema, pneumonia, or other respiratory diseases which do not entirely obstruct the airway but do so partially.

Poisoning: caused by alcohol, barbiturates, and other similar agents; has been reviewed in this chapter.

Laboratory confirmation of hypoxia can be obtained by measuring oxygen saturation of the blood, and also the carbon dioxide combining power of the plasma.

Remember that even with good treatment, particularly in acute conditions, symptoms will not recede in less than 1 or 2 days—headache, gastrointestinal upsets, or lethargy. Therapy consists of the administration of oxygen and assisted respiration, if so needed; but the basic procedure is to treat the causative factor, whatever it is. Respiratory stimulants may help. Avoid nervous depressants, as morphine, as much as possible.

Meningitis

Biot's respiration is more frequently found in meningitis, but there are also cases which present the typical Cheyne-Stokes rhythm; otherwise, there is not any basic respiratory difference in symptomatology among these patients. This topic has been reviewed in some detail at the beginning of this chapter (q.v.).

Opium Intoxication

Either Cheyne-Stokes respiration or only a form of bradypnea may be noted in cases of intoxication with opium derivatives, when the symptoms consist of initial nervous stimulation soon followed by a state of depression, with miosis, muscle relaxation, low temperature, low blood pressure, and a final state of shock and coma, in which the pupils become mydriatic. These patients are often addicts, who may show the scars of such a habit: erosion of mucous membranes and punctures from injections. Diagnosis of accidental intoxication depends on the history or the finding of containers.

Avoid as much as possible the absorption of any remaining amount of the offending substance: use copious lavages, tourniquet, and so forth. Control respiratory depression with levallorphan or nalorphine and assisted respiration. Beware of hypostatic pneumonia (change position).

> Levallorphan, 1 mg in each ml, in 1- or 10-ml contianers; give 0.02 mg for each kilo of body weight, intravenously. Repeat in 15 minutes if needed and tolerated.

EXERTIONAL DYSPNEA

When dyspnea becomes apparent following exertion or even a little more stressing activity than usual, it is called exertional dyspnea. It may reveal initial stages of any of the common causes of dyspnea, particularly the first phases of cardiac diseases. But it also becomes apparent in cases of extreme asthenia, Addison's disease, anemia, hemorrhage, restricted or obstructed respiration, or pulmonary fibrosis.

Cardiac Diseases

The reader is referred to the section headed "Cardiac Dysnpnea" in this chapter.

Addison's Disease

Because extreme asthenia is the main symptom in this disease, the patient will easily become dyspneic even when minimally stressing the muscular performance. If the diagnosis is not yet known, it will be suspected as soon as there is marked hyperpigmentation of the skin and muscosae, especially pressure sites and creases, with scarce hair on the body surface, small heart, and hypotension. The laboratory reports will show very low figures for cortisol in blood and urine. Addisonian crises are noted by abdominal pain, vomiting, diarrhea, fever, and symptoms of dehydration.

A patient in shock or impending shock must be hospitalized immediately for the administration of intravenous plasma and fluids with sodium, dopamine, antibiotics, and hydrocortisone. Those in the chronic stage will be treated with cortisone or hydrocortisone, and perhaps additional amounts of sodium.

Cortisone, tablets containing 25 mg each; give half a tablet every 8 hours, adjusting to needs and tolerance.

Restrictive or Obstructive Dyspnea

See the corresponding sections later in this chapter.

Anemia

Anemic patients will show pale skin and mucosae, generally accompanied by asthenia, tachycardia, dizziness, and evident exertional dyspnea. Hemograms and bone marrow biopsies will establish the diagnosis. This diagnosis is easy in most instances, but the etiological diagnosis may be a problem.

Blood loss: it is either an evident or occult loss; it causes iron deficiency anemia, with low levels of iron in the blood and elevated total iron-binding capacity; there is no hemosiderin in the marrow.

Pernicious anemia: additional symptoms are smooth, sore tongue, gastrointestinal symptoms, and paresthesias; there are large oval erythrocytes, neutrophils appear hypersegmented, and the bone marrow is megaloblastic.

Hemolytic anemia: there is splenomegaly, the Coombs test is positive in most cases, and there is reticulocytosis.

Aplastic anemia: there are purpuric symptoms and bleeding; blood cells are scanty, and the bone marrow is largely replaced by fat.

Paroxysmal nocturnal hemoglobinuria: there is mild hepatosplenomegaly, as well as scanty red and white cells and platelets; bone marrow is generally hyperactive.

Secondary anemias: Symptoms of the primary disease are prominent in most instances (cancer, cirrhosis, uremia, and so on.

The treatment of anemia depends on the type. For iron deficiency, ferrous sulfate is generally given. Pernicious anemia is treated with cyanocobalamin (folic acid only for folic acid deficiency anemia). For hemolytic anemias, corticoids are beneficial in most cases; but also transfusions and other surgical means will be evaluated. For aplastic anemia, transfusions and androgenic steroids are given. Paroxysmal nocturnal hemoglobinuria usually requires transfusions. Secondary anemias may require transfusions, but the treatment depends on the basic cause.

Ferrous sulfate, tablets containing 100 mg each; give about 300 mg a day, according to response and tolerance.

Cyanocobalamin, injectable; give 0.5 mg once a week or once a month, according to response and tolerance. Many patients will respond to 0.1 mg a month. Intramuscular injection.

Prednisolone, tablets; give high dosage until hemograms come close to normality (up to 20 mg, even four times a day); thereafter, reduce dosage gradually, according to response.

Testosterone enanthate, for intramuscular injection; give about 300 mg for each kilo of body weight, twice a week.

Hemorrhage

An acute, massive hemorrhage will combine symptoms of acute anemia and anoxia; chronic bleeding will cause iron deficiency anemia, q.v., above.

Treatment will consist of transfusions and surgery.

Pulmonary Fibrosis

Pulmonary fibrosis may be due to systemic diseases, exposure to toxic substances, inhaled or swallowed, or an unknown cause. Exertional dyspnea is progressive and is accompanied by cough, clubbing of the fingers, some pulmonary sounds (râles), and finally symptoms of developing cor pulmonale. The diagnosis may be given by X-ray films showing initial ''ground-glass'' opacities progressing to marked fibrotic changes. Check for the causative disease.

Treatment is carried out with large doses of corticoids. Also treat the basic causative disease.

Prednisone, tablets; give up to 20 mg, even four times a day; decrease dosage as soon as improvement is noted; and discontinue as allowed by the evolution of the disease.

EXPIRATORY DYSPNEA

Typically, the expiratory phase of respiration appears prolonged in emphysema. Similarly, in bronchial asthma, in spite of the contracture of bronchioalveolar musculature, the expiratory phase is also prolonged. These are the two diseases that will be reviewed here.

Asthma

The diagnosis is almost obvious from repeated attacks of dyspnea with wheezing, cough, and expulsion of a sticky mucoid sputum. On auscultation, the expiratory phase of respiration is prolonged, at the same time that musical râles and wheezing are also heard. Prolonged attacks constitute status asthmaticus. Long-lasting asthma may lead to cor pulmonale, emphysema, atelectasis, and other complications. The finding of specific allergen causing the allergic response may be the key to relief, through desensitization.

The acute attack is treated with epinephrine or aminophylline. Other drugs may also be used, particularly corticoids, when there is a poor response. A patient in status asthmaticus has to be hospitalized, and treated with aminophylline and corticoids. For chronic conditions, try drugs such as aminophylline, ephedrine, terbutaline, or beclomethasone.

> Epinephrine, 1:1000 solution; give 0.5 mg (0.5 ml) or less, repeating every 1 or 2 hours. Subcutaneous injection.

> Aminophylline, ampoules containing 250 or 500 mg each; give 250 mg by intravenous injection, being careful to procede very slowly.

> Prednisone or prednisolone; give up to 60 mg a day, in divided doses, the first accompanied by the intravenous injection of 100 mg or even more of hydrocortisone, to start prompt action.

> Ephedrine, capusles or tablets containing about 25 or 50 mg (a little less when weight is expressed in grains).

> Terbutaline, tablets containing 2.5 or 5 mg each; give up to 5 mg, three times a day (try to give 2.5 mg each time).

> Beclomethasone, for oral inhalation through the oral adapter provided by the manufacturer; give only in chronic conditions. If patient is on corticoid therapy, this should be discontinued, as usual, at a very slow pace! Give beclomethasone, two inhalations, three or four times a day; *never* more than 20 inhalations a day.

Pulmonary Emphysema

This is a relatively common disease of men in older years, particularly heavy smokers, members of a family of emphysematous inheritance, or those with known chronic pulmonary diseases. The disease is heralded by progressive exertional dyspnea and cough, initially dry, but rapidly becoming productive with a whitish mucous sputum. Dyspnea becomes worse as the disease progresses, thus turning into rest dyspnea and orthopnea. The resultant hypoxia may cause asthenia, weight loss, and even lethargy; and in more severe cases cyanosis, tremors, headache, miosis with papilledema, and some sensorial changes. Wheezing is common, and coughing efforts are not always successful in cleansing the lungs. The chest stays fixed in the inspiratory position ("barrel-shaped chest"), the respiratory movements depending mostly on accessory musculature. On auscultation wheezing and prolonged expiratory sounds are heard. Other symptoms are less characteristic, but may be present. On X-ray examination clear hyperinflated lungs are diagnostic. Other evidence of hypoxia will be obtained. Older patients will especially avoid complications, in the first place those infective in nature. Also, older patients may present the so-called senile lung or senile emphysema, with decreased mobility of the thorax (fixed in the inspiratory position), decreased lung size, abdominal respiration, and very little further symptomatology.

Keep patients ambulant as much as possible; check infection, even in cases of little impairment; relieve bronchospasm (as for asthma, in the foregoing entry); treat hypoxia and cardiac failure when present; and resort to corticoid therapy in severe cases, but with due care.

INSPIRATORY DYSPNEA

Inspiratory dyspnea may be due to obstruction or restriction of the physiologic respiratory movements. To avoid repetition, we refer the reader to the sections on "Obstructive Dyspnea" and "Restrictive Dyspnea," below.

KUSSMAUL'S RHYTHM

In Kussmaul respiration the rhythm is totally irregular, deep and shallow movements being intermixed without any special pattern. At first it was ascribed to impending diabetic coma; but other forms of metabolic acidosis may also cause the same respiratory arrythmia.

Diabetic Coma

Diabetics may go into coma, but it will not always be the ketoacidotic diabetic coma. Be very careful that the type of coma is clearly distinguished. Let us note here that the pure ketoacidotic coma is very frequently accompanied by the Kussmaul respiration. Coma types are summarized here.

Injury-caused coma: there is an obvious history of a previous accident and a lack of ketoacidosis in traumatic cases.

Hypoglycemic coma: there is inadequate timing for feeding and antidiabetic therapy; profuse perspiration; low glycemia.

Uremic coma: there is probably Cheyne-Stokes respiration; also, ammoniacal odor of the breath, and azotemia.

Lactic acidosis: see next entry, on "Metabolic Acidosis."

Others: coma may also be due to encephalitis, infections, hemorrhages, epilepsy, endocrinological diseases, cranial hypotension, poisoning, physical agents, bradycardia, and so forth.

The initial stage of diabetic coma may show weakness, vomiting, excessive thirst and urination, symptoms of dehydration, and very dry skin; symptoms steadily worsen to reach the final stage of unconsciousness, deep or shallow respirations mixing irregularly; there are hypotonic muscles, forceful pulsations, possible mydriasis, and the laboratory findings of elevated glycemia, glycosuria, ketonemia, and ketonuria.

Transfer the comatose patient to the hospital immediately to be monitored for vital signs and given intravenous fluids and medication. With the normal saline solution (1 liter the first hour and 300 to 500 ml an hour thereafter), give insulin at a rate of 5 to 10 units an hour (alternate schedules are also advised). With marked acidosis, give the same amounts of hypotonic saline with sodium bicarbonate (one or two 50-ml ampoules of 45 mEq each). Three or four hours after starting the treatment, give 40 mEq of potassium every hour. Treat vigorously any other disease. Note that glycemias above 500 mg% require 0.45% saline solutions; and that when the glucose level falls below 250 mg%, it is better to use 5% glucose solution and to cut insulin administration to one half of the initial dosage. If ketone bodies are not elevated, start with hypotonic saline and give 4 or more liters the first hour, to obtain the correct amount of urine output (no less than 50 ml an hour); potassium may be given at the start, but dosage will be no more than 20 mEq an hour; and insulin therapy may start intravenously with 15 units plus the subcutaneous injection of about 20 units, this later form to be continued in the same amount every 4 hours.

Regular insulin, 100-unit vials (100 units in each ml).

Potassium phosphate, 40 mEq in each 20-ml ampoule.

Metabolic Acidosis

Respiratory dysrhythmia may be conspicuous or not in cases of metabolic acidosis. As stated in the foregoing entry on diabetic coma, Kussmaul's respiration is usually noted. When the full clinical picture is well established, the respiratory pattern is of little diagnostic interest; but it may be a help when it occurs in early phases of the acidotic condition.

Water loss: may occur with diarrhea, enteric fistula, starvation, and renal insufficiency.

Lactic acidosis: is noted in diabetics treated with phenformin (or not), in vascular shock, and in other conditions that increase the lactic acid content of blood (0.6 to 1.8 mEq in each liter).

Intoxications: with salicylate, methyl alcohol, or ammonium chloride.

In these cases the Kussmaul's rhythm may be present, but more frequently there will be a simple hyperpnea of the tachypnea type. In these cases the breath will present a fruity or acetone odor. Coma is the final stage. Laboratory reports will show a very acid urine (with normal kidneys). The blood pH will be below 7.35, and other abnormalities may also be reported.

The basic treatment will be addressed to the causative factor. The acidosis itself may be corrected with sodium bicarbonate intravenously. Lactic acidosis is also treated with sodium bicarbonate.

Neurogenic Dyspnea

There is not any distinctive characteristic for neurogenic dyspnea, since it is clinically present in any modality of the forms discussed in this chapter. Here we merely wish to remind the reader that dyspnea due to neurogenic insult may be reactive to injuries, strokes, brain tumors, encephalitis, or any other disease that may disturb the respiratory function.

Injuries

Cranial injuries causing either shock or stroke can bring on dyspnea, which may be a simple difficult respiration or an abnormal respiration of the Cheyne-Stokes rhythm or possibly dyspnea accompanied by stertorous sounds. The face will be flushed; there will be bradycardia, with full pulse, normal or elevated blood pressure, and some paresia or paralysis in the case of stroke. In shock, the blood pressure will be low and the pulse weak and rapid. Check for symptoms of intracerebral hemorrhage, such as angiographic findings; extradural hemorrhage, with transient unconsciousness, gradually developing intracranial hyperpressure, and X-ray evidence of fracture (crossing the middle meningeal groove); subarachnoid hemorrhage, with stiff neck and fresh blood in the spinal fluid; or subdural hematoma, with gradual progress of weakness on one side of the body and other symptoms.

The treatment includes emergency treatment for shock with adequate nursing care and administration of blood or plasma, dopamine, mannitol, and antibiotics. These patients are to be hospitalized and the help of a surgeon requested.

Stroke

There is no need to repeat here what was discussed in some detail earlier in this chapter, under the heading ''Bradypnea,'' and in the chapter devoted to ''Unconsciousness'' (q.v.).

Brain Tumor

Symptoms of brain tumor begin with headache, projectile vomiting, personality changes, papilledema, and other neurological symptoms that occur as the spinal fluid pressure increases. Dyspnea may be one of the indicative symptoms, but it is not a characteristic one. The location of the tumor or cyst will cause additional symptomatology.

Temporal lobe: there are seizures, visual field defect, and aphasia if the left side is involved.

Frontal lobe: symptoms are as above, plus anosmia and more marked personality changes.

Parietal lobe: there is a similar picture, plus focal seizures, hemiparesis, and hyperreflexia.

Occipital lobe: visual changes predominate.

Cerebellar: disturbances of coordination and equilibrium predominate.

Radiologic studies are needed for completion of the diagnosis. The procedure to follow is to be discussed with a neurosurgeon.

Encephalitis

Symptoms are not too different from those of meningitis. In very acute cases shock is the first clinical evidence of the disease. Patients present variable fever, more frequently among older people. Symptoms to be expected are: backache, headache, stiff neck, malaise, insomnia, vomiting, convulsions, myoclonus, tremors, ocular paralysis (or other forms of paralysis), hemiplegia, and final shock or coma. In the case of St. Louis encephalitis the symptoms are typically mild; in Eastern encephalitis, they are very severe; other strains may be of intermediate severity. There are, usually, exaggerated deep tendon reflexes, and diminished or absent superficial reflexes. The spinal fluid will show increased pressure and proteins, and the causal organism may be recovered.

Provide good hospital care; if the specific anti-infective drug is known, give it, and treat symptoms as they arise; corticoids may help for headache and convulsions; analgesics may be tried; cranial hypertension may respond to mannitol; phenobarbital may control convulsions. For more details see other entries in this book.

Meningitis

Elderly patients usually start meningitis with paralysis of limbs and the face after a period of vague symptomatology. At this time, contracted pupils will be noted, and a very rapid course to lethargy and loss of consciousness. A backache and stiffness of the neck are important symptoms. The examination of the spinal fluid will follow immediately, for a positive diagnosis: increased pressure, increased number of cells, increased proteins, decreased glucose, and isolation of the causal organism.

Give good hospital care, particularly maintenance of water and electrolyte balance; give the specific anti-infective drug as soon as possible, but start immmediately with ampicillin, methicillin, kanamycin, or polymyxin B, according to the infective germ. Corticoids may help for pain. Normalize blood pressure and volume with electrolyte solutions and isoproterenol.

OBSTRUCTIVE DYSPNEA

Whenever there is an obstacle to the free entrance of air into the lungs causing difficulties in respiration, obstructive dyspnea will take place. Obstruction may be caused by a foreign body, by external masses pressing on airways, or by pulmonary obstacles, as in spasm of the alveolar muscles from asthma or air stagnation as in emphysema.

Foreign Bodies

Swallowing a foreign body that obstructs respiration usually happens during mealtime, or to those who wear prosthetic appliances in the mouth, or who chew candies, and gum. The morsel or piece may go to the pharynx, the esophagus, or the larynx, choking the patient. This is a sudden accident, and the diagnosis is easy. If it impacts above the crycopharyngeus, the patient will refer to it as being on one side of the throat; below, as being centrally impacted. If needed, and there is time, check with a laryngoscope. When it is impacted in the larynx, violent coughing and suffocation are the outstanding dangers.

Emergency treatment is needed. If the foreign body cannot be dislodged with the fingers (which is the easiest way, provided that it is not pushed farther into the larynx or esophagus), try to wrap your arms around the patient's waist, making a fist with one hand and holding it firmly with the other to press violently on the epigastric area as if intending (in fact, intending), to push it out from below; this operation may be repeated several times; and it has been admitted that even if it ruptures the stomach (which has happened), this second accident is preferable to the death of the patient. Otherwise, emergency tracheostomy will be performed.

Asthma

In listening to the asthmatic chest it appears that the expiratory phase is longer, even though the spasm of the bronchioles impedes both inspiration and expiration. Repeated attacks of dyspnea with wheezing, cough, and expulsion of a sticky mucoid sputum will give the diagnosis.

If the specific allergen is found, desensitization will be attempted as the final goal of treatment; but the attack must be relieved rapidly with epinephrine or aminophylline. Status asthmaticus (continuous attacks) is treated with aminophylline and corticoids in the hospital. For more details see other entries.

> Epinephrine, 1:1000 solution, give 0.5 mg (0.5 ml) or less by subcutaneous injection. Repeat every 1 or 2 hours.

Pulmonary Emphysema

This is very common among the elderly, particularly if they are heavy smokers or carriers of a chronic pulmonary disease. Symptoms start with progressive exertional dyspnea and dry cough, but they soon become worse, the dyspnea being noted even at rest and causing orthopnea; the cough turns productive with a whitish mucoid sputum. Other symptoms of hypoxia appear. The chest becomes fixed in the inspiratory position ("barrel-shaped chest"); resulting symptoms are cyanosis, tremors, and others. The X-ray picture will substantiate the diagnosis. In senile emphysema or senile lung, the result will be decreased lung size and abdominal respiration, but very few other symptoms.

Keep the patient ambulant, check infections, relieve bronchospasm, control hypoxia and heart failure, and resort to corticoid therapy, with due care, in severe cases. For more information, see other entries.

Masses Obstructing Airways

In the great majority of instances the symptoms develop gradually, and dyspnea is mostly obscured owing to the greater importance of other symptoms.

> *Goiter:* the diagnosis is helped by finding an enlarged thyroid gland. This is not so in cases of substernal goiter, which may be suspected to exist when there is some impairment of blood circulation in the neck; it will be confirmed by X-ray examination.

> *Thyroid cancer:* the medical procedure is the same as with goiter.

> *Mediastinal diseases:* the superior mediastinal syndrome is characterized by cyanosis, edema of the face and neck, and progressive dypsnea. It results from enlargement of lymph nodes, as in Hodgkin's disease, or of other structures located in the area.

Every effort will be made to achieve accurate diagnosis of these diseases; but rarely will the pressing reason be the dyspnea itself.

Treatment varies according to the causative factor, surgery or radiotherapy for most of the patients. Rarely will it be necessary to treat only the dyspnea.

Restrictive Dyspnea

See the corresponding section in the following pages.

ORTHOPNEA

Orthopnea means that the patient can breathe only in the upright position. This is one of the characteristic symptoms of severe heart failure, when the patient has to sleep in a chair, in a sitting position, because it is impossible to tolerate clinostatic rest.

Heart Failure

This subject has been reviewed in some detail under the heading "Cardiac Dyspnea."

PAROXYSMAL DYSPNEA

As implied by the name, this type of dyspnea occurs in attacks of temporary shortness of breath. It can be seen in heart failure, diseases of the aortic valve, coronaritis, myocarditis, aortitis—in short, whenever the left ventricle or the coronaries are involved.

Heart Failure

The patient is known to be a cardiac patient when he develops paroxysmal attacks of dyspnea. The well-known "air hunger" access follows an extra effort, or an emotion, or occurs during sleep without any apparent cause. A very intense anxiety is characteristic, accompanied by chest oppression or angina-like distress, and by a mild symptomatology of dependent pulmonary edema, with perhaps bronchial symptoms as well. In a way, these attacks bear some similarity to an asthmatic attack, the diagnosis becoming extremely difficult when they occur in patients also suffering from bronchial asthma. Nevertheless, among elderly patients who did not have a previous asthmatic condition, if such a crisis takes place, the most probable diagnosis is that of paroxysmal nocturnal dyspnea. On the other hand, if epinephrine is given to the patient, it will be effective only for true asthmatic cases and not for "cardiac asthma," which may even worsen; these patients will respond very well to cardiotonic therapy. For more details on cardiac failure, see the corresponding entry under "Cardiac Dyspnea," earlier in this chapter.

Valvular Diseases

When any valvular disease causes heart failure, it may induce attacks of paroxysmal dyspnea as described in the paragraph above; but mainly be on the alert for aortic valve lesions. In addition to the regular heart failure symptomatology, there will be the following symptoms and signs in each particular case.

Aortic stenosis: may also show exertional dyspnea; systolic murmur in second right interspace; concentric hypertrophy of the left ventricle.

Aortic insufficiency: is frequent among the elderly; also may show exertional dyspnea; diastolic murmur in second left interspace; enlarged left ventricle.

Mitral stenosis: may also show orthopnea or tachypnea; hemoptysis may occur; presystolic murmur at apex; enlarged left atrium.

Mitral insufficiency: follows a slowly progressive course; diastolic murmur at apex spreading to axilla; enlarged left atrium and ventricle.

Tricuspid lesions: show murmurs on the left sternal border; enlarged right atrium in stenosis; enlarged right atrium and ventricle in insufficiency.

Valve replacement is the best treatment, but the elderly are not good subjects for the procedure, which should be evaluated by specialists. Mainly treat heart failure with cardiotonics and similar drugs.

Coronary Diseases

Narrowing of the coronary arteries will cause the corresponding clinical picture of angina pectoris, even reaching the complete closing that occurs in myocardial infarction. The symptoms consist almost exclusively of substernal pain or oppression, of short duration in the case of typical angina, or intermediate duration in acute coronary insufficiency, and long-lasting pain together with anxiety and fear of death in myocardial infarction. Paroxysmal dyspnea will be present only in a few cases, and will be an alerting sign, but not a conclusive diagnostic element. For more details see other entries on angina.

Aortitis

Usually due to a syphilitic infection, symptoms of aortitis will be lacking almost until some dilation takes place. In this instance dyspnea will be due to extrinsic pressure over the airways, causing some mediastinal syndrome:

progressive dyspnea, with occasional and not too frequent paroxysmal dyspnea; cyanosis, edema of the face and neck; possible stridor and cough; dysphagia or hoarseness. X-ray may help the diagnosis, but at times angiography is needed.

Surgery, whenever feasible for the elderly patient, will be the treatment of choice and as such discussed with specialists. Treat the syphilis, as well.

Myocarditis

Primary myocardial disease or secondary myocarditis will present the particular symptoms due to heart involvement plus the symptoms due to the causative factor. Intrinsic symptomatology will show dyspnea with occasional incidence of paroxysmal dyspnea, severe asthenia even leading to a syncopal condition, dizziness, nausea, and chest pain, all of these symptoms running a more or less acute course. X-ray may show an enlarged left ventricle, congestion of pulmonary veins, and other evidence of left ventricular failure. Electrocardiograms will show conduction defects (blocks), low voltage QRS, and flat or inverted T waves. Serial electrocardiograms are helpful in cases of infectious diseases of any kind. Myocardial damage will be suspected in cases of alcoholism, thiamine deficiency (beri-beri), amyloidosis, sarcoidosis, scleroderma, and others.

The treatment is unspecific, and will vary according to the type of inducing factor and the myocardial response. It will be discussed with specialists.

PULMONARY DYSPNEA

Whenever any part of the bronchopulmonary area is damaged, dyspnea and cyanosis are prone to occur. Dyspnea comes first, but in the long run cyanosis may be more marked because the lungs try to accommodate to the new condition. Exertional, expiratory, inspiratory, obstructive, paroxysmal, rest, and restrictive forms of dyspnea, or tachypnea and orthopnea may occur as a result of respiratory diseases, and thus are considered as pulmonary dyspnea. Here only the more specific respiratory diseases causative of pulmonary dyspnea will be considered, namely, asthma, emphysema, pneumonia, bronchopneumonia, lung infarction, pulmonary edema, atelectasis, pneumothorax, lung cancer, and pleuritis.

Asthma

This disease has already been discussed several times in this volume. It will be enough to remind the reader that the repeated attacks of paroxysmal difficulties in breathing, together with wheezing, cough, and expulsion of a sticky mucous sputum, and the hearing on auscultation of prolonged expiratory râles and wheezing, will point out the exact diagnosis. Long-lasting cases may present status asthmaticus (subintrant attacks), cor pulmonale, emphysema, atelectasis, or other complications. Find the causative allergen whenever possible.

The acute attack is treated with epinephrine or aminophylline (other drugs, including corticoids, may be used when the response is poor). For status asthmaticus, hospitalize the patient, and treat with aminophylline and corticoids. Other drugs may also be used, and the patient desensitized whenever the allergen is known.

> Epinephrine, 1:1000 solution; give subcutaneously 0.5 mg (0.5 ml) or less, repeating every 1 to 3 hours, as needed and tolerated.

> Aminophylline, ampoules of 250 or 500 mg each; give 250 mg intravenously and very slowly.

Emphysema

A very frequent condition among aged people, smokers, and carriers of chronic pulmonary diseases, it starts with progressive dyspnea and dry cough. Soon it becomes productive of a whitish mucous sputum, the condition worsening to rest dyspnea and orthopnea. Other symptoms are: cyanosis, asthenia, tremors, headache, miosis, papilledema, some sensorial changes, weight loss, and lethargy. Wheezing is common, and cough does not always adequately cleanse the lungs. The chest is fixed in the inspiratory position, respiratory movements are mostly abdominal, and wheezing and prolonged expiratory sounds are heard on auscultation. X-ray studies confirm the diagnosis. Senile emphysema (senile lung) gives little symptomatology. Protect the elderly against complications.

Keep patients ambulant, relieve bronchospasm, treat hypoxia and cardiac failure whenever present, prevent infections, and resort to corticoid therapy, with due care in severe cases.

Pneumonia

In previous chapters (q.v.), pneumonia has been discussed in some detail. Here only a brief summary is given. The sudden shaking chill and stabbing sharp chest pain are the main symptoms in pneumonia; but keep in mind that older persons may have little pain and a not-too-elevated temperature. Tachypnea and tachycardia may be the opening symptoms for these patients, but for most of them the general condition deteriorates very rapidly; when there is a previous disease, its symptoms worsen, and the patient becomes confused and intensely weak. Other signs are: dehydration, abdominal distention, appendicitis-like symptoms, and cough with the production of a sputum that may be diagnostic. Pneumonia types and their sputa are as follows:

Pneumococcal pneumonia, with a pinkish purulent sputum that turns rusty and then yellowish.

Klebsiella pneumonia, with reddish, sticky, mucoid sputum.

H. influenzae pneumonia, with apple-green, bloody, sticky sputum.

Viral pneumonia, with scanty, mucopurulent sputum.

Streptococcal or staphylococcal pneumonia, with an abundant sputum of a salmon color.

Other forms of pneumonia are: aspiration pneumonia (history of passage of a foreign body), fungal pneumonia, rickettsial pneumonia, or pneumonias due to infection with *Pneumocystis carinii,* tularemia, etc. The clinical diagnosis is confirmed by radiologic studies and laboratory identification of the causative germ.

Patients will be kept in bed, with good general care; symptoms will be alleviated as they arise, the basic infection being treated accordingly; pneumococcal pneumonia, with penicillin; klebsiella pneumonia, with cephalothin and gentamycin; *H. influenzae* pneumonia, with ampicillin; streptococcal and staphylococcal pneumonia, with oxacillin, either alone or with cephalothin; fungal pneumonia, with amphotericin B; actinomyces pneumonia, with penicillin; nocardia pneumonia, with sulfadiazine; *P. carinii* pneumonia, with pentamidine isethionate; mycoplasmal pneumonia, with erythromycin or a tetracycline; rickettsial pneumonia, with a tetracycline; tularemic pneumonia, with streptomycin plus a tetracycline if there is no improvement; and aspiration pneumonia (so frequent among the elderly), with aspiration, washings, assisted respiration, cortisone, and a constant watch for septic complications. Terminal pneumonia has to be aggressively treated with specific antibiotic therapy.

Bronchopneumonia

There is a gradual onset of symptoms, mostly following a previously established disease (influenza, typhoid fever). The symptoms are similar to those of pneumonia (which see, in the immediately preceding entry), but less marked. X-ray studies will give the only positive diagnosis of the disease.

Treatment is as for pneumonia (q.v.).

Lung Infarction

There is a sudden onset of dyspnea with a rise in temperature, substernal pain, and anxiety. Cough with hemoptoic sputum is almost characteristic; and a previous history of thrombophlebitis helps to confirm the diagnosis, which is finally established by X-ray studies. On auscultation there are râles, friction rub sounds, signs of pleural effusion, and other evidence of lung damage. At a later stage, there is heart failure, and, not rarely, shock.

Emergency treatment is needed in consultation with a surgeon, to evaluate the need for an embolectomy. Send the patient to a cardiopulmonary unit as soon as possible, but start oxygen therapy (100% by mask) immediately, with meperidine for pain, levarterenol for shock, and anticoagulants.

Meperidine, 50 to 100 mg, by subcutaneous injection.

Levarterenol, 2 mg in 5% glucose solution by intravenous drip.

Heparin, up to 10,000 units, every 6 hours, by subcutaneous injection, checking clotting time.

Warfarin, 20 to 30 mg by mouth, starting at the same time with heparin, and adjusting dosage according to prothrombin time.

Pulmonary Edema

Pulmonary edema may start at a relatively slow pace, but usually it is sudden in onset and poses an immediate emergent situation, mostly related to cardiac failure. It may occur in cardiac patients, those with hypertension, pulmonary embolism, strenous physical activity, excursionists at high altitudes, inhalation of fumes or other toxic substances, and injuries to the head. Cough with some wheezing may open the clinical picture, rapidly followed by dyspnea with tachypnea and orthopnea, oppression in the chest, a frothy sputum leaking from the mouth (and the nose), cyanosis with pallor, and sweating. On auscultation, râles are heard, initially in dependent parts of the lung, rapidly extending over all the chest. At times, during paroxysmal dyspnea attacks, some edema may develop. Mild attacks may occur in patients with mitral stenosis. Do not mistake pulmonary edema for pulmonary infarction or an asthmatic attack.

An acute pulmonary edema is an alarming situation for both the patient and the physician. Keep calm and try to calm the patient; to allay anxiety and dyspnea, give meperidine. A sitting position is best, with quiet, relaxation, and administration of oxygen or even assisted respiration if there is any evidence of left heart failure. In very acute cases with secretions in the upper airway, suction will be applied or a tracheostomy performed, if necessary. A diuretic given intravenously is a good help. For more rapid relief, a phlebotomy may be performed (draw no more than 250 ml of blood); or instead, application of intermittent positive pressure breathing. The etiologic factor will be treated, also.

Meperidine, 50 mg, by intravenous injection.

Furosemide, 10 mg in each ml, in containers of 2 or 10 ml each; give by slow intravenous injection from 20 to 40 mg (according to patient's weight), repeating the dose 90 minutes later, if necessary.

Atelectasis

Dyspnea, fever, cyanosis, tachycardia, some sort of chest pain, cough, wheezing, restricted expansion of the chest during respiration, narrowing of the intercostal spaces, and X-ray findings will point out the pulmonary atelectasis. Care will be taken to differentiate it from infarction or pneumonia.

Send the patient immediately to the hospital, under the care of a specialized team.

Pneumothorax

Older persons may show a very scarce symptomatology when pneumothorax occurs. Nevertheless, dyspnea of sudden occurrence is rarely absent. This respiratory difficulty is due not only to the restriction of pulmonary surface but also to the usually present pain on the affected side, which increases with effort, including respiration. The pain may be referred to the shoulder or the arm of the corresponding side. Physical examination will reveal diminished respiratory movements, hyperresonance of the chest, decreased sound of the voice and breath noted on auscultation, and some evidence of a shifting mediastinum away from the affected side. When the trapped air increases with respirations, the valve effect will soon increase intrathoracic pressure and provoke cyanosis, leading to shock by tension pneumothorax. On X-ray examination an enlarged pleural space with retraction of the lung will be diagnostic. Check for the possibility of a causative disease, first tuberculosis, but also abscess, bullous emphysema, or some other pulmonary disease.

Treat with bed rest, control of pain and cough, and aspiration of the trapped air if there is dyspnea or the space is large. Aspiration with an intercostal catheter, water trap, and suction pump, continued for 24 hours after complete lung re-expansion, may be needed when air leakage is continuous. For tension pneumothorax, aspiration of air is an emergent need, to be done with a trocar or a needle (large opening and short bevel) with good care not to injure the re-expanding lung; thereafter, use an intercostal catheter for the chronic condition.

Lung Cancer

This disease is more frequent among the elderly than at earlier ages. The onset is usually gradual, starting with cough or hemoptysis. A localized wheezing may also occur. The clinical picture may resemble a different respiratory disease (pneumonia, pleurisy, atelectasis, abscess), or the symptoms of a concomitant problem may obscure those of cancer. The final diagnosis usually depends on the finding of characteristic shadows on the

X-ray films. Metastasis may be the first symptomatic sign of bronchogenic carcinoma; and always be on the alert for this malignancy when there is evidence of an unusual case of myasthenia gravis, carcinoid syndrome, Pancoast's syndrome, Cushing's syndrome, and so forth. Other helps for diagnosis, besides X-ray studies, are cytologic evaluation of the sputum, bronchoscopy, biopsy of neck lymph nodes, and other resources better performed by specialists.

Surgery at an early stage offers the only possibility for cure. Otherwise, use chemotherapy and radiotherapy.

Pleuritis

Because of the inspiratory pain (which is quite characteristic in pleuritis) some dyspnea may take place, but this sign will be more evident when due to large effusions (restrictive dyspnea). On auscultation a friction rub will be heard (fibrinous pleurisy) or the auscultatory sounds corresponding to pleural effusions. Efforts will be made to find a causative disease. X-ray studies can substantiate the diagnosis; examination of pleural fluid may also be of help in determining the etiological factor, e.g., tuberculosis or cancer.

Treat the basic cause, if known. Aspiration of fluid must be done carefully.

REST DYSPNEA

Dyspnea at rest merely indicates a severe condition or a poor tolerance to hypoxia. Any of the dyspneic forms reviewed in the foregoing lines may end in dyspnea at rest; the diseases most frequently present center on the heart, those which cause cardiac dyspnea but also the debility of Addison's disease. See the corresponding entries in this same chapter.

RESTRICTIVE DYSPNEA

Also called "expansional dyspnea," restrictive dyspnea occurs when there is some difficulty opposed to the normal expansion of the chest for inspiratory movements. This restriction may be due to difficulties arising from the chest walls (including the diaphragm) or the lungs themselves. This will occur with chest deformities, pulmonary fibrosis, and the Pickwickian syndrome, but also other pulmonary diseases, such as emphysema, pulmonary edema, and paralysis of the diaphragm. Other diseases not properly causing a pure restriction of respiratory movements should be included, such as pulmonary infarction, lung abscess and cancer, atelectasis, pneumonia, pneumothorax, pleurisy with effusion, and empyema. There is no need to review all these diseases again; see other entries in this book for more information.

Chest Deformities

These deformities are evident on inspection; most of them are congenital in nature, but some may be residuals of surgery or accidents. Among the elderly, rheumatic deformity of the spine is the main abnormality to be noted; there may also be other forms of scoliosis, kyphoscoliosis, and abnormal rib cage. Some patients will be referred to an orthopedic surgeon for correction, if the respiratory impairment reaches unacceptable levels.

Pulmonary Fibrosis

Systemic diseases, toxic substances, local suppuration, and other, unknown causes may give origin to pulmonary fibrosis, usually with symptoms of progressive exertional dyspnea, cough, clubbing of the fingers, râles, and a final cor pulmonale. X-ray films will show the initial ''ground-glass'' opacities and final marked fibrotic changes. Check for tuberculosis, pneumonia, pulmonary infarction, pleuritis, chronic bronchitis, silicosis, the pneumoconioses, or other chronic lung affections.

The basic disease will be treated; but for fibrosis itself, treatment usually requires large amounts of corticoids.

> Prednisone, tablets; give up to 20 mg, even four times a day; decrease dosage as soon as improvement is noted; discontinue it as allowed by the course of the disease.

Pickwickian Syndrome

This is only an example of extreme obesity with marked hypoventilation, which in the absence of a clearly proven primary cardiac or pulmonary disease presents a syndrome with dyspnea of the Cheyne-Stokes type, lethargy (some may present insomnia), cyanosis, and very large protruding abdomen; on examination, other symptoms are noted, of hypoxia, respiratory acidosis, hypercapnia, polycythemia, and right ventricular hypertrophy, with other evidence of heart failure. In short, this is the big-bellied, lethargic, and cyanotic patient.

Diet reduction is the best treatment: determine the basic metabolic need of each individual, then give that patient 500 calories less than he needs, and there will be a loss of about 500 g a week; but take care to re-evaluate periodically the basic caloric needs of the patient. Use of progesterone has been advised to help ventilation.

> Progesterone, injectable in oil suspension; give 25 mg or less every other day, according to tolerance and response.

Paralysis of the Diaphragm

The phrenic nerve may be paralyzed bilaterally in cases of infective diseases (polio, diphtheria), or infection occurring in the region: peritonitis, pleuritis, mediastinic infections, or those following injuries. When this occurs, there are no diaphragmatic movements, and such symptoms will arise as exertional dyspnea, lack of expulsive power during defecation, and shorter expiratory movements. On radioscopic examination no diaphragmatic movements are noted.

Treat the basic causative condition.

Emphysema

This very common disease of older people has already been discussed twice in this chapter. It usually occurs in smokers or carriers of chronic pulmonary diseases. Symptoms include a slow progress of dyspnea and dry cough, which will typically become productive, with a whitish mucoid sputum. The dyspneic state worsens to reach dyspnea at rest and orthopnea. Other symptoms are: asthenia, weight loss, lethargy, cyanosis, tremors, headache, miosis, papilledema, some sensorial changes, wheezing, with the chest fixed in the inspiratory position (''barrel-shaped chest''), and prolonged expiratory sounds on auscultation. The clear hyperinflated lungs seen in X-ray pictures are almost diagnostic. Watch the elderly to avoid complications. In senile lung or senile emphysema the anatomical changes are very similar, but there is little symptomatology.

Ambulant patients do better, as activity prevents developing infections; relieve bronchospasm (as for asthma); treat hypoxia and cardiac failure when present. With due care, use corticoids in severe cases.

Pulmonary Edema

A grave situation occurs in the great majority of cases, presenting cough, wheezing, rapidly developing dyspnea (with tachypnea and orthopnea), oppression of the chest, frothy leaking sputum, cyanosis with pallor, sweating, and on auscultation râles, first at the bases but rapidly spreading over the whole field. This may occur in cardiac patients or those with injured pulmonary surfaces. For more details, see under ''Pulmonary Dyspnea,'' in this chapter.

The patient will stay in a sitting position; if he is too anxious or dyspneic, give meperidine (50 mg, intravenously); apply suction or perform a tracheostomy if secretions are abundant in the upper passages; perform a phlebotomy, or apply rotating tourniquets, or use intermittent positive pressure breathing; and give a diuretic intravenously: furosemide, 20 to 40 mg, slowly by vein. For more details, see under ''Pulmonary Dyspnea,'' in this chapter.

SIGHING DYPSNEA

This form of dyspnea is characterized by long, deep, audible (not wheezing) breaths, as if expressing sorrow or anxiety, the depth of respirations increasing, but not so the overall rate. Sighing dyspnea rarely is linked to organic diseases; mostly, it is due to neurotic conditions, emotional upsets, or vagotonic reactions. Nevertheless, some asthmatic patients or others with mild acidotic conditions may present this sighing dyspnea.

If there are vagotonic reactions, an asthmatic state, mild acidosis, or emotional circumstances, try to allay the tension of the patient, even by using some tranquilizers, if necessary.

TACHYPNEA

Rapid respirations may accompany any other type of dyspnea, such as cardiac, exertional, expiratory or inspiratory, neurogenic, obstructive, paroxysmal, pulmonary, rest, or restrictive dyspnea, or orthopnea.

In addition to the aforementioned circumstances, tachypnea may be a "normal" way for respiration among some people, perhaps more frequently noted among the elderly; naturally, this condition will be exaggerated following even mild forms of exercise or stress. Most people living in cities located at high altitudes present some sort of tachypnea. Also, divers in deep waters become more conscious of their breathing. Hyperthyroid patients always present tachypnea, but they do not complain of "air hunger." Tachypnea is a part of the febrile syndrome, and a normal reaction to stress.

Hyperthyroidism

More females than males are affected by hyperthyroidism, and though a fully developed clinical picture may be diagnosed very easily, diagnosis will not be so easy with milder, incomplete forms, particularly for older people.

Most patients will present a goiter, but it may atrophy at this time of life. Also, most patients will present tachycardia, which together with the goiter is one of the characteristic signs of hyperthyroidism; but many older persons will show instead auricular fibrillation with a complete arrhythmia. Sweating may be worse, also, at this age, particularly among women; almost all hyperthyroid patients will present a moist, wet skin, but some will perspire profusely. More cases than in earlier years will be seen with insomnia, skin hyperpigmentation, ophthalmoplegia, and hyperacusia. Those living in relatively temperate zones will present an unusual incidence of diarrhea as a tendency. Otherwise, the rest of the clinical picture should be typical: tachycardia, with possible palpitation, goiter, exophthalmos, fixed look with wide open eyes, nervousness causing quickness in all sorts of motion and speech, moist and heat-intolerant skin, tremor (may be more easily noted on a trembling paper placed over the extended hand), weight loss in spite of increased appetite, asthenia, and elevated basal metabolism, now rarely checked and superseded by the new tests of thyroid function, such as protein-bound iodine. Results are abnormal if they exceed: 4 to 8 μg per 100 ml blood, for free thyroxine; 1.4 to 3.5 nanograms (ng) per 100 ml of blood, tetraiodothyroxine, or T_4; 5 to 14 μg per 100 ml of blood, triiodothyroxine; 60 to 190 ng per 1 ml of blood, the radioiodine uptake of the gland; and so on.

Surgery is a good treatment in many instances, but must be carefully evaluated for practicality when dealing with patients of advanced age. Otherwise, thyroid-suppressing agents will be used, such as propyl-thiouracil, which seems to be the preferred method. When these agents are used with the elderly, more care for untoward reactions will be carried out (agranulocytosis, in the first place). Also, the administration of radioactive iodine has some advocates. The worse complications are malignant exophthalmos, cardiac failure, and thyroid storm.

Fever

As soon as the febrile symptom is of some intensity, increasing tachycardia and tachypnea will appear. In all instances, the diagnosis will depend on the evaluation of the entire clinical picture, and the reader is referred to the chapter that follows, entirely devoted to "Fever."

Stress

Any unusual activity or stress will increase in a physiological way the speed of respiration, thus provoking tachypnea. Self-defense will put a halt to this unusual expenditure of energy. No treatment is needed, unless there is a reactional heart failure or respiratory distress, when the help of oxygen administered by mask is advisable.

High Altitude

The complete syndrome of high altitude sickness includes tachypnea, or other form of exertional dyspnea, tachycardia, headache, anorexia, and insomnia; as it increases, add cyanosis, pulmonary edema, muscular twitching, and even delirium, usually of a euphoric type, and convulsions; and in a severe attack there will be unconsciousness and possibly death. A similar syndrome will occur when the patient stays in places with poor oxygenation, as caves, closed rooms, or an atmosphere of inert gases. Laboratory evidence of hypoxia will be given by the evaluation of blood oxygen saturation and CO_2 saturation.

Therapy consists of the administration of oxygen plus assisted respiration if needed. Respiratory stimulants may be of some help. Rest is also essential;

and resumption of activities will be at a slow pace because in almost all instances total recovery will take at least 1 or 2 whole days.

VIII. FEVER

Most febrile diseases are infective in nature; but metabolic, ecologic, hormonal, or neurologic disorders may also induce hyperthermia. The number of diseases included in this category is very large; so it was imperative that we summarize them, to the extent of giving basic help in planning a final diagnosis in each particular instance. More complete information will be found in other sections of this volume, under such headings as "Pain," "Cough," "Nausea and Vomiting," or whatever other symptom considered here may be of interest; or see our book on *Fever: From Symptom to Treatment,* in which practically all prevalent febrile diseases have been included.

Always remember that among the elderly the following points are of considerable importance:

1. Most diseases are chronic and multiple.
2. Symptoms are milder; with respect to fever, very high temperatures will be noted only in rare instances.
3. Symptoms may be unspecific or even absent.
4. Drug tolerance is lower, particularly if there is kidney insufficiency.
5. Some diseases will hardly be found at older ages (e.g., measles).
6. Tuberculosis, influenza, and pneumonia must always be considered a possibility.

To make diagnostic efforts easier, a second prevalent symptom or group of symptoms has been added, but we have tried not to duplicate entries discussed in a previous section. For this purpose, we have included sections on chills, pain, and respiratory, dermatological, gastrointestinal, neurological, and "other" symptoms, as well as febricula.

CHILLS

A chill is merely a shivering or a shaking, that is, an involuntary contraction of voluntary muscles accompanied by a sensation of cold. Chills may be mild, with little tremors, or very intense, even enough to shake the bed.

Pneumonia may start with a shaking chill, "stabbing" pain in the chest, cough, rust-colored sputum, and the symptoms characteristic of a particular variety of pneumonia. The diagnosis will be established by physical examination, X-ray, and laboratory identification of the causal organism. Treat with the corresponding antibiotic.

Psittacosis is an almost typical pneumonia, but with more marked abdominal distress, cyanosis, and the presence of rose spots, all occurring in a patient previously exposed to birds. Use a tetracycline and control cough.

Influenza, together with pneumonia, is one of the most frequent occurrences in this age group, showing muscle aches, weakness, and leukopenia. Provide only symptomatic treatment.

Para-influenza cannot be distinguished on clinical grounds, but only by laboratory means.

Legionnaires' disease is a pneumonia with some epidemic characteristics. The causative germ may be isolated for diagnosis. Treat with erythromycin.

Acute bronchitis may simulate a complication of influenza, but no more than auscultatory signs will be found, and the examination of an X-ray film and the sputum will clarify the situation. Treat it symptomatically, and give ampicillin if needed.

Scarlet fever shows marked sore throat followed by a generalized erythematous rash, pallor around the mouth, and the finding of the streptococcus on culture. Use penicillin.

Tularemia is suggested by a history of exposure to rabbits or other rodents (in laboratory workers). It begins as a fast-developing infection centering in the regional lymph glands at the point of infection—the skin, eye, lung, or gastrointestinal tract. The treatment of choice includes streptomycin, alone or with a tetracycline or chloramphenicol.

Coccidioidomycosis has many forms, acute and chronic, the first with chills (acute respiratory type) in patients having been exposed to dust or dry agricultural products from endemic areas. The symptoms may be those of pneumonia or erythema nodosum (desert rheumatism). A try will be given to amphotericin B (with heparin).

Tonsillitis and pharyngitis show enlarged, red tonsils and sore throat, with chills when the infection is severe. Penicillin is the best drug to give.

Agranulocytosis presents a maculopapular skin rash and sore throat, and is diagnosed by the characteristic lack of granulocytes in blood smears. There might be a history of the use of certain drugs. Start with carbenicillin and cephalothin, but try to find the specific antibiotic.

Lung abscess is suggested by a respiratory syndrome following a previous pulmonary disease, and confirmed by X-ray, with a slow start and signs of lung consolidation or nodules with suppuration. Drain secretion, and use the specific antibiotic.

Blastomycosis starts with poor symptomatology, but turns into a more serious pleurisy, with fever, chills, purulent sputum, and X-ray opacities; it will be confirmed by laboratory procedures. Treat with amphotericin B.

Toxoplasmosis presents a pneumonitis accompanied by a maculopapular rash and the infecting parasites in the blood smear. Give pyrimethamine plus trisulfapyridine.

Epidemic typhus will show an initial influenza-like syndrome, usually more severe, with excruciating headache. Soon macules (possibly purpuric) will be seen, first in the axillae and then spreading over the body, except for the face, palms, and soles, occasionally turning into papulae. Drugs of choice are doxycycline and chloramphenicol. The Weil-Felix reaction and the complement-fixation tests will indicate the diagnosis.

Murine typhus is similar to the epidemic type, but milder. Usually the fever increases gradually, the rash appearing only on the trunk, and the disease runs a rapid course. The diagnosis depends on the complement-fixation tests.

In *Rocky Mountain spotted fever* there may be an anamnesis of a previous bite by ticks. It starts with typhus-like syndrome, and the macular rash may become petechial, starting on wrists and ankles. The diagnosis also may be solved by the complement-fixation test. Give a tetracycline or chloramphenicol at the earliest possible time.

In *Q fever* the upper respiratory typhus-like syndrome has to be differentiated from pneumonia and hepatitis, but usually there is only a laboratory diagnosis. Treat with tetracycline or chloramphenicol.

Rickettsialpox also presents pains; there is a widespread maculopapular rash, becoming vesicular and resembling varicella, with a tendency to leukopenia and a characteristic complement-fixation test.

Dengue fever is characterized by severe pains in the extremities and the remission of fever, with profuse sweating, before the appearance of a scarlatiniform maculopapular rash, which starts on the dorsum of the hands and feet; there are leukopenia and an increase of serum antibodies, and the virus can be isolated. Only supportive treatment can be offered.

Herpes simplex presents a rash that may consist of isolated vesicles or clusters of burning vesicles on the face, the mouth, the genitals, or, rarely on other sites; there is adenitis, and the virus may be isolated. Provide local treatment. Do not use corticoids!

Herpes zoster is similar to herpes simplex, but the lesions provoke pain, are noted only on one side of the body, and follow the path of distribution of a nerve (cranial, intercostal, and so on). Corticoids will afford good help.

Typhoid fever shows a gradual increase in temperature during the first week, usually together with gastrointestinal symptoms—constipation, distention and pain, or pea-soup diarrhea, a maculopapular rash that fades on pressure, stupor, and positive laboratory findings. Drugs of choice are chloramphenicol or ampicillin.

In *rat-bite fever* there is a history of having been bitten by a rodent; the local lesion swells, is painful, and becomes a purplish color; it may ulcerate, and is followed by lymphadenitis and a maculopapular rash; the fever is undulant in character. Penicillin is active against all strains; tetracyclines, against *Streptobacillus moniliformis;* and streptomycin, against *Spirillum minus*.

Relapsing fever follows (if untreated) a course of up to 10 relapses, each one lasting about 1 week. The patient may recall bites by ticks or lice, and complain of generalized aches; early in the course of the disease a rash appears on the trunk and extremities, starting as an erythema and developing pink-rose spots; both liver and spleen are enlarged. Try a tetracycline, penicillin, or chloramphenicol.

Leptospirosis presents the fever syndrome with pain, a purpuric rash, and jaundice, and gives the corresponding laboratory tests. Start an early treatment with tetracycline.

Yellow fever also presents jaundice, with black vomit, albuminuria, and an acute fever syndrome; there is leukopenia, and the virus can be isolated. Give supportive treatment.

Spirochetosis icherohemorrhagica presents a sudden onset with abdominal and muscular pains, severe headache, vomiting, conjunctivitis, hepatomegaly with jaundice (the fifth day), and possibly purpura, nephritis, or meningeal irritation. Treat immediately with tetracyclines or penicillin.

Cellulitis may present superficial or deep symptoms: superficially, the skin is swollen, red, warm, and painful to touch, usually following a previous local infection, and the erythematous area is not sharply demarcated; deep cellulitis presents local discomfort, pain on pressure and crepitation if there is gas (anaerobic infection), leukocytosis, and an elevated erythrocyte sedimentation rate. Use a penicillase-resistant penicillin.

In *erysipelas* the rash spreads continuously from a bright red spot (nose, mouth, a fissure), creating a red, swollen, sharply demarcated area (there is a border), at times with vesicles or bullae; also, there are leukocytosis and an elevated erythrocyte sedimentation rate. Treat with penicillin.

Sunburn is characterized by an erythematous rash that follows exposure to sunlight (summer, beach), usually with vesicles that appear on the exposed areas. Use local wet, cool dressings.

Trichinosis may start with a fever syndrome, edema of the eyelids, urticaria, sweating, subungual hemorrhages, muscle pains, especially in the chest, and mild gastrointestinal symptoms. Find out if the patient has eaten pork, raw or underdone. Blood smears showing eosinophilia and leukocytosis will help the diagnosis. Give corticoids and thiabendazole, with or without pyrvinium pamoate.

Filariasis shows lymphangitis and adenitis, but other organs might be involved; the laboratory will report eosinophilia, positive skin tests, and the presence of microfilariae in the blood. Poor results are obtained with diethylcarbamazine.

Lymphogranuloma venereum is a venereal disease with the fever syndrome following local unilateral lesion, which causes the development of a cluster of lymph nodes adherent to the skin, which become suppurative. The Frei reaction and the complement-fixation test will give the final diagnosis. Tetracyclines are the drugs of choice.

Phlebitis is not a rare disease; a superficial, inflamed vein appears, together with the usual febrile syndrome. If the vein is a deep one, it is not felt beneath the skin, but there will be, nevertheless, turgor and cyanosis, and the patient will complain of heaviness and pain. Anticoagulants may be considered.

Abscess will give special symptoms, not always together with fever and chills, but these symptoms may occur. Try to use the specific antibiotic.

Glanders (farcy) follows a history of exposure to horses; the onset is sudden; at the site of the infection a painful ulcer appears, and the laboratory gives the final diagnosis. Use antibiotic or sulfa therapy; in severe cases use a combination of two drugs.

Variola presents body pains along the spine and in the muscles, with a characteristic rash, one crop only of macules, changing to papules, umbilicated vesicles, and, finally, pustules, which are all at the same stage of evolution; the rash starts on the face and head and includes the palms and soles. Treatment is symptomatic.

Cholecystitis exhibits a more localized symptomatology: sudden pain in the right hypochondrium or closer to the epigastrium, with fever, possibly chills, and pain on pressure, with tense muscles. Use anticholinergics and antibiotics.

Pyogenic hepatic abscess starts abruptly with fever, at times with chills, pain, and jaundice. Use kanamycin, and drain it if necessary.

Calculi in the urinary tract will present fever and chills if there is also infection; the pain is noted on the corresponding flank, usually reaching excruciating proportions. Use septra or bactrim for these cases; control pain with morphine.

Pyelitis and pyelonephritis present a sudden onset with fever, chills, headache, and nausea, with frequency, urgency, and burning on urination with pyuria and costovertebral pain on pressure. Use septra or bactrim.

Cystitis gives suprapubic pain and a history of some sort of obstruction in the urinary tract. Mandelamine, septra, or bactrim may be used.

Otitis media accompanies an upper infection and gives pain in the ear, fever, a sensation of pressure and deafness, and the positive signs noted on otoscopic examination. Use the specific antibiotic or ampicillin.

Lymphangitis shows inflammation and pain along the lymphatic channels, mostly with enlarged tender lymph glands, fever, and chills. Penicillin is the first choice; nafcillin or methicillin may also be used.

In *Sinusitis* the nares are congested, with purulent discharge from the nose; the frontal or maxillary sinus regions are tender on pressure, headache and other symptoms from the neighboring organs are present, as are fever and chills. Doxycycline may help; also use phenylephrine.

Gout is suggested by a sudden attack of excruciating pain in a joint of the foot, ankle, or knee, which becomes swollen and very tender, with the skin tense, bright red, and warm. Colchicine is the first choice; phenylbutazone may also be used.

Peritonitis induces abdominal pain so intense that the patient prefers to lie on his back, legs flexed on his abdomen, with shallow respirations and avoidance of unnecessary movement. The etiologic factor to check may be: post-surgery, trauma, infective disease, or local pelvic or abdominal disease, the last the most frequently found. Start treatment with kanamycin or gentamycin.

Acute suppurative gastritis is suspected if symptoms similar to those of peritonitis are abrupt in onset, with vomiting and severe diarrhea. Start treatment with kanamycin or gentamycin, and call a surgeon.

Appendicitis presents fever and chills in complicated cases; the main symptomatology is pain in the right iliac region and gastrointestinal disorders. Surgery is to be done as soon as possible. Start with colistin, ampicillin, or gentamycin.

Diverticulitis shows a clinical picture very similar to that of appendicitis, but it may be on the left side, also with fever, chills, nausea, abdominal distention, and constipation or diarrhea; pain is in the left iliac region. Care is as for appendicitis, q.v.

Acute gastritis presents anorexia, nausea, diarrhea, intestinal colic, and a febrile syndrome, possibly with chills; gastric rest is basic. Inject codeine or meperidine, if needed.

Meningitis appears with abrupt symptomatology: fever, chills, headache, vomiting, possibly convulsions, a special high-pitched meningeal cry, and nasal itching; also, irritability, bradycardia, abnormal reflexes, and the characteristic rigidity of the neck. The causative factor has to be found, for a better treatment with the adequate antibiotic.

Encephalitis symptoms resemble those of influenza; but soon there appear tremors, muscle spasms, changes in reflexes and behavior, paresis, sialorrhea, and the very important symptom—diplopia. Use the specific antibiotic.

In *malaria* the sequence chill–fever–sweating (a very *severe* chill with general shivering, chattering teeth, and difficult speech; elevated fever; and drenching sweat), repeated at predictable intervals, is almost diagnostic. The variety of the infecting plasmodium must be established for final adequate treatment.

Plague presents a rapid onset with hyperthermic chills, possible headache, tachycardia, hypotension, enlarged lymph nodes, and rapid deterioration. Streptomycin is the drug of choice.

Septicemia or bacteremia presents septic fever with chills, tachycardia, weak pulse, mild splenomegaly, and purpuric or petechial skin eruptions, and other symptoms of the initial disease; but the patient must be watched for secondary complications, such as endocarditis, myocarditis, pericarditis (check the heart daily), bronchopneumonia, pulmonary abscess, meningitis, or glomerulonephritis. Treat with the adequate antibiotic.

Acute bacterial endocarditis may show a similar febrile picture, but patients may tell about previous heart disease, and there are suggestive signs found on auscultation of the heart; embolic phenomena, as petechia, are important to note. The specific antibiotic must be used.

Septic shock occurs in the course of an infective disease, the symptomatology of which worsens with addition of peripheral vasodilation with hypotension and very weak pulse, pallor, sweats, superficial respiration, anoxia, asthenia, lassitude, immobility or irritability, and delirium. Treat shock.

Hemolytic anemia crisis is to be suspected from an abrupt onset of fever, chills, malaise, nausea, vomiting, pain in the back or abdomen, pallor, jaundice, tachycardia, weakness, splenomegaly, and dark urine. Treatment includes blood transfusion, sodium bicarbonate, and elimination of the causative factor.

Paroxysmal hemoglobinuria has similar symptoms, with constant hemoglobinemia and hemoglobinuria. Provide transfusions and symptomatic treatment. *Transfusion reaction* will be easily diagnosed because during or following a blood transfusion there appear fever, chills, and pain in the vein, chest, back or abdomen; there are also hemoglobinemia, hemoglobinuria, headache, and anxiety. Stop transfusion immediately at the first symptom; warm the patient; give mannitol; treat kidney damage.

PAIN

Several of the diseases that present an outstanding painful symptomatology together with chills were dealt with in the foregoing section on "Chills." Here we include only those diseases that may present pain but not chills. Like other symptoms, pain may not reach severe proportions among the elderly; nevertheless, some will exaggerate this symptom, and thus may induce a false estimate of it.

In *myocardial infarction* fever is not always accompanied by chills; many older persons feel little substernal pain; there is mostly apprehension and fear of death; diagnosis mainly depends on electrocardiograms; there are also leukocytosis and elevated SGOT and LDH in blood. Keep patients in bed, use anticoagulants and treat complications as they arise.

The *common cold* should not be mistaken for more severe diseases in spite of the nonspecific syndrome of headache, mild fever, coughing, sneezing, and general malaise. Treat symptomatically, with rest and acetylsalicylic acid.

AFRI (or acute febrile respiratory illness) shows a symptomatology similar to that of influenza but occurs only during the cold months. Treat symptomatically.

In *herpangina* the diagnosis is made by finding, in addition to headache and fever, the characteristic herpetic stomatitis, a papulovesicular rash on the tonsils, spreading in the form of large lesions to the rest of the mouth. Give symptomatic help.

Pharyngoconjunctival fever is suggested by fever, pharyngitis, and conjunctivitis among campers or swimmers in lakes or pools during the summer season. Give symptomatic treatment.

Pulmonary infarction presents sudden chest pain, with fever, dyspnea, and anxiety, symptoms of heart failure, cough (may be hemoptoic), and râles on auscultation; diagnosis is very difficult at times. Treat with anticoagulants, morphine, and levarterenol.

Epidemic pleurodynia shows headache, sore throat, and pain in the muscles of the intercostal area with no auscultatory signs of pleuritis. Provide symptomatic treatment.

Poliomyelitis is very rare among the elderly; usually little clinical information is obtained during the first stage—headache, sore throat, fever, vomiting, and malaise. The later occurrence of flaccid paralysis of leg muscles or of muscles innervated by cranial nerves, as shown by difficult swallowing, regurgitation, and nasal voice, will provide important diagnostic clues. It will be treated in hospital by specialized teams.

Aseptic meningitis is diagnosed by the failure to find easily any specific causal virus or larger germ, in cases of suspected meningitis. Only symptomatic help is available.

Colorado tick fever patients come from or live in the western states and usually appear from March to August with symptoms of headache, muscle pains, fever, and a rash, all subsiding to reappear after 2 or 3 days. Use salicylates and coal-tar derivatives.

Brucellosis begins with headache, fever, joint pains, sweating, and gastrointestinal upsets. Lymphadenopathy and splenomegaly are characteristic. The symptomatology, particularly the fever, is of the undulant type. Check laboratory reports, and treat with tetracyclines.

Syphilis in the secondary stage shows headache and slight fever with a typical rash. Cerebral syphilis manifests itself with severe headache and fever. The diagnosis depends on the history and laboratory findings. Penicillin is the drug of choice for treatment.

Intracranial abscess will be suggested by the combination of a previous known infection with symptoms of intracranial pressure. Check the spinal fluid, and use an adequate antibiotic.

Iritis and iridocyclitis will be suspected when there are outstanding ocular symptoms with edema of the upper eyelid, lacrimation, photophobia, pain, miosis, enlarged corneal vessels, swelling of the iris, or cloudiness of the intraocular fluids. Pupils will be dilated with atropine; use corticoids locally and the specific antibiotic as soon as possible.

Pain in the Face

Ophthalmic herpes zoster is characterized by pain along branches of the ophthalmic nerve, with vesicles at the same site; *erysipelas,* by the red rash with elevated borders, usually around the mouth or the nose; and *sinusitis,* by local pain at the site of a sinus exaggerated by certain movements of the head, possible purulent discharge, and evidence of the disturbance as checked by transillumination.

Pain in the Mouth

Dentoalveolar abscess showed a previous suppurative pulpitis; the gum is locally inflamed, and edema extends to the face. *Gangrenous stomatitis* is a more severe disease, showing a grayish slough of the buccal mucosa—which swells and turns red and finally black—together with marked tissue destruction; pain is not as severe as the damage; there is an intolerable fetor. *Vincent's angina* starts as a common tonsillitis, with redness and swelling, but ulcerates and ends in necrotic tissue. *Tonsillitis* or *pharyngitis* presents pain increased by swallowing, local swelling and redness, and some exudate, at times. *Herpangina* presents a tonsillitis with local vesicular eruption. *Scarlet fever* presents a severe tonsillitis or pharyngitis, but the characteristic scarlet rash makes the diagnosis. In *infectious mononucleosis* sore throat is not accompanied by evident signs of tonsillitis, but by enlarged lymph glands, particularly of the neck. *Peritonsillar* and *retropharyngeal abscesses* are noted by fluctuation in the affected areas, together with pain increased on swallowing.

Pain in the Eye

Conjunctivitis may occur in local disease, iritis, iridocyclitis or general infections of the type of the common cold, AFRI, pharyngoconjunctival fever, coccidioidomycosis, or leptospirosis. *Iritis* symptoms are congestion of the blood vessels around the cornea, miosis, swelling and change of color of the iris, and edema of the upper eyelid. *Iridocyclitis* symptoms are as in iritis but more severe; the aqueous humor in the anterior chamber is clouded and shows precipitates. *Endophthalmitis, panophthalmitis,* and *orbital cellulitis* cause notable deterioration of the patient presenting ocular symptoms, as chemosis and production of pus, suppuration limited to the retina and the uveal tract at first, then spreading to the whole eye, then finally located in the orbit.

Pain in the Ear

Herpes zoster occurs with ear pain from the geniculate ganglion and the facial nerve, which nerve paths give rise to pain and vesicles. *Otitis media* follows infections of the nasopharynx; there are fullness of the ear, deafness with tinnitus, and swelling and redness of the eardrum. *Mastoiditis* presents pain, increased by pressure, and edema over the mastoid area.

Pain in the Spine

In *variola* patients appear very ill; the rash practically determines the diagnosis. In *meningitis* stiff neck is suggestive of the disease, strongly backed by other neurological signs and symptoms centering in the central nervous system. *Encephalitis* symptoms are more centered in the brain itself and may present varied combinations. In these two involvements, meningitis and encephalitis, the diagnosis depends largely on the examination of the spinal fluid. In *influenza and para-influenza* an acute respiratory or abdominal condition is accompanied by aches of many muscles and extreme weakness. *Acute adenovirus diseases* present an almost identical symptomatology, with "flu," to be distinguished only by virus isolation studies: the acute febrile respiratory illness (AFRI) is more frequent among children; acute respiratory disease (ARD), among the military; pharyngoconjunctival fever, among swimmers. *Myelitis* symptoms are paresthesias, tingling, hesitation in walking, and finally paralysis. *Rickettsial diseases (typhus, Rocky Mountain spotted fever, Q fever, and trench fever)* present pains along the spine and in the legs, but headache is frequently the most prominent complaint. *Spinal epidural abscess* causes pain in the back, aggravated by motion, fever, paresthesia, or paresis. *Trichinosis* presents pain in the back and in most large muscles, edema of the eyelids, diarrhea, fever, and extreme eosinophilia. *Tuberculosis* of the mediastinum is suggested by the "mediastinal syndrome" of rachialgia, interscapular pain (worse on lying in bed), dysphagia, and Horner's syndrome, plus other evidence of tuberculosis, such as fever and auscultatory chest signs. *Pancreatitis* presents agonizing pain largely centered at the left side of the epigastrium.

Pain in the Thorax

In *myocardial infarction* a sudden retrosternal oppression or pain strikes with apprehension and fear. In *acute pericarditis* there is also acute retrosternal pain, increased by certain positions or movements, as well as shallow, rapid respiration, anxiety and weakness, and the characteristic friction rub, heard during the complete cardiac cycle. *Pneumonia* presents a stabbing, sharp pain on one side, intensified by motion with a sudden onset of fever, typical of an acute infection, a productive cough, chills, and prostration. In *bronchopneumonia* the clinical picture is similar to that of pneumonia, but with a gradual onset and milder symptoms; it frequently follows a previous infective disease. *Pharyngoconjunctival fever* is a "bad cold" that develops in summer among those in camps and those who swim in pools. *Pulmonary infarction* is a severe disease with an abrupt rise in temperature, substernal pain of varying intensity, dyspnea, and anxiety. *Pleuritis* resembles pneumonia, but the pain disappears on holding the breath or splinting the sides with adhesive, which also diminishes the pleuritic friction rub. *Epidemic pleurodynia* shows sore throat, fever, headache, malaise, and muscle pain in the intercostal area; there is no auscultatory evidence of pleuritis. *Subdiaphragmatic abscess* presents pain in the lower part of the chest, radiating to the shoulder and showing elevation and immobility of the corresponding diaphragm. *Hepatic abscess,* with a similar symptomatology, is often caused by amebic infections. *Cholecystitis* has a history of biliary colic.

Pain in the Abdomen

In *appendicitis* there is an acute continuous pain of a colicky nature, aggravated by pressure over the right iliac fossa, usually accompanied by local muscle spasm and increasing leukocytosis. In *acute pancreatitis* pain is located at the left side of the epigastrium, constant and very severe, exaggerated by certain positions (lying supine) and by local pressure, and accompanied by local muscle rigidity; the patient may appear critically ill or even in shock. In *typhoid fever* little pain is felt, but it may be severe in cases of perforation; there is a gradual onset with fever, moderate headache, gastrointestinal discomfort, stupor, and bradycardia, and, in some instances, the characteristic rash on the abdomen and thorax. In *pyelitis and pyelonephritis* pain is referred to the bladder, or felt on urination; there are pyuria, a febrile syndrome, and also pain referred to the back. *Perirenal abscess* and *carbuncle* present a sudden onset of fever, chills, prostration, nausea, vomiting, and pain with tenderness in the costovertebral angle. *Renal colic* presents an excruciating pain from the corresponding costovertebral area to the abdominal flank, and to the genitourinary organs, accompanied by fever, chills, and vomiting. *Tuberculosis* of the urinary organs shows a dull pain in the corresponding costovertebral region and abdominal flank, with frequency and terminal painful dysuria. *Salpingitis* presents pain in the iliac fossa, more frequently the right, with fever and sometimes peritoneal reaction. *Abdominal tuberculosis* occurs in patients with a previous history of tuberculosis, with crampy abdominal pains and diarrhea, with a constant sensation of discomfort in tuberculosis of the intestines, and with tenderness, ascites, and cachexia in tuberculosis of the peritoneum. *Peritonitis* almost always follows an antecedent disease; there is an agonizing, constant pain in the abdomen, exaggerated by motion; the legs are flexed, and the face is pale with an anxious expression (hippocratic facies). *Perigastritis* follows a peptic or duodenal ulcer, and is noted by an epigastric mass and febricula. *Cholecystitis* presents fever, dyspepsia, and vague aches in the right flank; a history of colic if there is lithiasis; and Murphy's sign (pain on pressure increased by deep inspiration, at the right hypochondrium). *Liver abscess* presents a combination of digestive and fever symptoms; pain in the right hypochondrium, radiating to the shoulder and increased with movement; hepatomegaly and hepatalgia. *Hepatitis* starts like a case of abdominal influenza with weakness, fever, hepatalgia, and other abdominal discomfort; soon jaundice is noted; serum hepatitis follows a blood transfusion, and infectious hepatitis behaves like a contagious disease. *Subdiaphragmatic abscesses* follow abdominal surgery, perforation, or an infective disease of the digestive system; there is pain in the upper abdomen and lower chest radiating to the corresponding shoulder, the pain increasing under local pressure. *Crohn's disease* is a regional enteritis showing fever, crampy pains, diarrhea, weight loss, and a mass located in the right iliac fossa. *Diverticulitis* mimics an attack of appendicitis located in the left iliac fossa.

Pain in the Limbs

Rheumatic fever symptoms are pain in the large joints and possibly cardiac murmurs. *Rheumatic pains* may be due to arthritis, with swollen, tender joints, or stiffness; or to rheumatoid arthritis, in which fever is a very minor symptom or does not exist at all. *Coccidioidomycosis*, or "desert rheumatism," starts with an acute pneumonic picture followed by arthritis, conjunctivitis, and erythema nodosum. *Influenza and para-influenza* present an acute picture of a respiratory or abdominal infection, with general muscle aches. *Dengue*, or "breakbone fever," shows headache, muscle and joint pains, fever, and a rash. *Trichinosis* presents pain over all muscles, but there is also edema of the eyelids. *Osteomyelitis* symptoms are fever and localized pain, tenderness, and swelling. *Tuberculosis* of bones follows other infections (lungs), and starts with limitation of motion. *Phlebitis* shows signs of venous obstruction, edema, local hyperthermia, fever, tachycardia, and local tenderness along the vein; with leukocytosis and more severe symptomatology in thrombophlebitis than in phlebothrombosis. *Gangrene* may be dry or moist; there are necrosed tissues and a picture of severe infection. In *gout* the great toe is most frequently affected, with extremely intense pain, local swelling, redness, and shining of the distended skin. *Colorado tick fever* patients come from the West, in March to August, presenting a general infection with muscle pains; they will have a remission and then a relapse of all symptoms. *Brucellosis* pains occur together with gastrointestinal symptoms, sweating, enlargement of lymph nodes, and a characteristically undulant fever. *Relapsing fever* also is found in western patients who were bitten by lice or ticks; there are pains and a rash, and a remission followed by a relapse. *Leptospirosis* presents a similar infective picture together with a conjunctival effusion, remission, and relapse.

Other Pains

Cystitis does not always occur with fever, but there are always hypogastric discomfort, urgent urination, and a persistent sensation of bladder fullness. Be on the alert for *prostatitis* when there are perineal pain and a feeling of pressure, together with symptoms of cystitis; this is a very frequent complaint among the elderly. *Urethritis* presents burning on urination and urethral discharge of pus. In *bartholinitis* there is a painful nodule in the inferior portion of one of the labia minora. *Lymphogranuloma venereum* shows a combination of joint or abdominal pains, headache, fever, with chills, conjunctivitis, splenomegaly, marked enlargement of the inguinal glands, and exaggerated edema of the sex organs. *Orchitis* and *orchoepididymitis* show epididymitis followed by fever and swelling of the scrotum. In *carbuncle* there are several openings draining pus, cellulitis extending to the surrounding tissues, and frank elevation of the tumorous mass above the skin level. *Cellulitis* presents fever, with regional inflammation, induration, swelling, pain, and lymphangitis. *Abscesses* show local symptomatology, depending on the site of the infection, together with the symptoms of a general infection: *intracranial,* with evidence of intracranial pressure; *dentoalveolar, peritonsillar,* and *retropharyngeal,* with local fluctuation; *epidural,* with painful motion of the spine; *hepatic,* with pain in the right side of the epigastrium; *subdiaphragmatic,* with radiologic evidence; and *perirenal,* with pain in the corresponding costovertebal angle. In *herpes zoster* there are vesiculation and pain along the path of a nerve. *Herpes simplex* shows the same symptoms, but less pain and with no relation to the path of nerves. *Erythema nodosum* presents tender, red nodules, which turn bluish and brown, located on the anterior aspect of the legs. *Erythema multiforme* presents symmetrical concentric rings on the distal half of the limbs; also bullae on the mucous membranes in severe cases.

RESPIRATORY SYMPTOMS

Rhinitis symptoms are sneezing and mucous nasal discharge, minor febricula, or no fever at all, and some itching, mostly in allergic patients; there may be nasal obstruction; a hyperemic mucosa is seen through the rhinoscope; watch for the possibility that rhinitis might be the starting point of a general infectious disease (influenza, sinusitis, glanders); help with nasal decongestants, and treat the basic disease.

Tracheobronchitis: most common colds starting with a rhinopharyngitis end in a tracheobronchitis; symptoms are low fever, rhinitis, pharyngitis, soreness and hoarseness, productive sputum, and, on auscultation, ronchi. Keep patients in bed; give symptomatic help; and basic treatment whenever known and needed.

Diphtheria shows a grayish, tenaciously adherent pharyngeal pseudomembrane which bleeds when detached, and there is a surrounding erythema and edema; neck nodes may enlarge; watch for myocarditis, neuritis, or a strabismus; bacterial cultures give the diagnosis. Treat with antitoxin and penicillin (or an alternate).

Rheumatic fever may start with a streptococcal pharyngitis, with sore throat followed by articular pains and complicated by cardiac murmurs and failure; other symptoms may occur, as chorea or dermatological symptoms. The diagnosis depends on summing up a few of these symptomatic complexes. Treat with penicillin and salicylates.

Acute leukemia presents a sudden onset with sore throat and fever; there may be evidence of infection in the mouth or the lungs, articular pains (do not mistake for rheumatic fever!), bleeding under the skin, adenopathy, and possible hepato- or splenomegaly; the hemogram will give the diagnosis. Acute lymphocytic leukemia is treated with vincristine and prednisone; myelocytic leukemia, with cytoxan, oncovin, Ara-C and prednisone, or an alternate schedule.

In *Vincent's angina* the onset is rapid, with fever and painful pharyngitis; bleeding gums, and the rest of the oral mucosa; extremely offensive oral fetor; difficult speech and swallowing; neck adenopathy. It is best to treat it with mouthwashes of peroxide, followed by diluted Fowler's solution; use antibiotics only in severe cases.

Monocytic angina is rarely seen; symptoms are hyperpyrexia, tonsillar and peritonsillar congestion, pseudomembranous or pultaceous appearance, adenopathy, and possible splenomegaly; the hemogram will give the diagnosis; do not mistake it for Vincent's angina, which has more extensive lesions. Treat symptomatically, and watch for complications such as ruptured spleen, hepatitis, encephalitis, or myocarditis.

In *atelectasis,* fever, dyspnea, cyanosis, tachycardia, chest pain, wheezing, cough, restricted chest expansion on respiration, narrowing of the intercostal spaces, and X-ray findings will give the diagnosis. Ask for specialized help.

Pneumoconioses present a general syndrome of chronic cough, mild fever, diffuse pulmonary fibrosis, granulomatotic or allergic reaction, and X-ray findings. Individual symptomatology: *berylliosis,* from exposure to fluorescent light powders—minute nodules, diffuse reticular markings on skin, no adenopathy; *silicosis,* from exposure to silica (mining, drilling, sand)—hilar adenopathy with peripherally calcified nodes, fibrosis, radiolucency; *siderosis,* from exposure to metallic debris—small discrete round shadows all over the lungs; *coal miner's pneumoconiosis*—fine discrete nodulations or denser shadows; *asbestosis,* from exposure to magnesium silicate or asbestos—thick calcified pleura, fine reticular markings in lower lung fields; *bauxite pneumoconiosis,* from exposure to aluminum ore— fibrosis with emphysema and adenopathy; *byssinosis,* from exposure to cotton dust—no characteristic clinical picture; *bagassosis,* from exposure to moldy hay or bagass—a diffuse interstitial granulomatosis; and *bronchiolitis obliterans,* from exposure to oxides of nitrogen—diffuse miliary lesions. There is no treatment for the pneumoconioses; give symptomatic care; and give corticoids, which may benefit many patients. Restrict exposure to noxious agent.

Laryngitis presents hoarseness as the main symptom; local pain, increased with cough and talking; more or less marked fever; productive cough, dyspnea, and stridor in case of local edema; laryngoscopic diagnosis. Advise voice rest, control cough and infection, give corticoids in cases with edema, and perform a tracheostomy if there is a threatening obstruction.

Actinomycosis shows fever, chest pain, productive cough, dyspnea, marked asthenia, dysphagia, night sweats, weight loss, and multiple infected sinuses formed from abscessed foci secreting "sulfur granules," where the *Actinomyces* may be found for diagnosis. Penicillin is the drug of choice.

Pleuritis presents an abrupt onset with fever, chest pain, tachypnea, dry coughing, and pleural friction rub on auscultation; symptoms vary with effusion; X-ray may help for the final diagnosis. Treat symptomatically.

Tuberculosis: check all elderly patients carefully for tuberculosis; there may be suspicious complaints and evening febricula or frank fever, cough, asthenia, weight loss, and night sweats. There may be an initial stage similar to influenza, but which will be more prolonged while symptoms worsen. Erythema nodosum may occur at this time. Auscultatory and radiologic signs are minimal at this stage. The chronic stage shows one or more pneumonic foci in the upper lung areas, in advanced cases with caseous necrosis and subsequent cavitation. Auscultation will be informative, but the diagnosis depends on adequate X-ray findings plus laboratory reports of germs in the sputum, and skin tests reactive to tuberculin. Treatment will start with at least two of the major antituberculous drugs, such as isoniazid and streptomycin.

DERMATOLOGICAL SYMPTOMS

Malaria symptoms are: fever only in severe cases, very small maculopapules that rapidly turn into small vesicles noted on skin areas exposed to sun or heat during summertime or in hot weather, and burning and itching. Treat with a cooling antipruritic lotion.

Secondary syphilis appears 6 to 8 weeks after the chancre, with low fever, sore throat, generalized adenopathy, malaise, and dermic lesions of varied characteristics (pustules, nodules, etc.) Lesions are moist and rich in treponemas, and very contagious. Penicillin or an alternate is the treatment of choice.

Dermatomyositis is not a frequent disease; it starts abruptly with an erythematous rash, fever, swollen painful muscles, prostration, asthenia, vasomotor disturbances in the hands, purplish periorbital edema, other edematous ,areas of the skin, desquamation, and symptoms from other systems—gastrointestinal, pleural, cardiac, or lymphatic; a suggestive aid for diagnosis is the scleroderma-like changes of the skin; check for malignancies. Treat with corticoids.

Erythema nodosum presents red, tender nodules in an area of erythema, usually on the pretibial area. Treat with a tetracycline; but check for an accompanying disease, which may be: tuberculosis, syphilis, streptococcal infection, meningococcal infection, cat's scratch fever, rheumatic fever, ulcerative colitis, fungal infection, endocarditis, leukemia, sarcoidoisis, or the use of certain drugs.

In *erythema multiforme* the erythematous lesions show a target-type pattern with concentric rings, and are usually noted on hands, feet, and mucous membranes; there are fever, malaise, and articular pain; when lesions are widely distributed they constitute the Stevens-Johnson syndrome. Give symptomatic treatment; corticoids may be used.

In *cat's scratch fever* a vesicle appears at the scratch site, and a suppurative adenopathy develops, with fever but no lymphangitis. Removal of a large nodule may give some relief. Try a tetracycline.

In *anthrax* a relatively large papule vesiculates, presenting a purplish or black center and surrounded by erythematous skin filled with small vesicles; the dark center ulcerates and develops a necrotic eschar, and all symptoms worsen; the laboratory will recover the causative germ. Treat mild cases with a tetracycline, and more severe ones with penicillin.

Carbuncle is an aggregate of several furuncles, with multiple draining openings, fever, and malaise. This lesion may appear anywhere on the body, but most frequently on the nape of the neck. Do not overmanipulate the lesion; give erythromycin or methicillin.

In *systemic lupus erythematosus (SLE)* ulcers may occur in the mouth, but the diagnosis requires an aggregate of three or more of the following symptoms: butterfly rash, discoid lupus, Raynaud's phenomenon, alopecia, photosensitivity, oral ulcers, arthritis, lupus erythematosus cells, false positive tests for syphilis, proteinuria with cell casts, serositis, central nervous symptoms or blood changes. Treat with corticoids or with ACTH.

Wegener's granulomatosis is a very severe disease with symptoms of a serious sinusitis; ulceration with progressive destruction of the nasal septum and necrosis of the skin caused by inflammatory lesions in the extensor muscular surfaces; more or less marked pulmonary involvement; heart failure; renal insufficiency, which may be terminal; and other less frequent symptoms, such as. exophthalmos, chemosis, papillitis, carditis, articular pains, prostatitis, and parotitis. Acceptable results are obtained with methotrexate.

Histoplasmosis symptoms are fever, dyspnea, cough, prostration, loss of weight, hepato- and splenomegaly, possibly diarrhea, and ulcers in the pharynx and nose in the usually fatal case; the diagnosis depends on serology, skin tests, and the finding of the offending histoplasma. Give sulfadiazine for mild cases, amphothericin B for others.

Leishmaniasis, in its cutaneous form, will show a low fever, if any; the previous bite from a sandfly swells and ulcerates, and the Leishman-

Donovan bodies are recovered from the pus. Treat with antimony sodium gluconate or ethylstibamine.

Hepatitis is characterized by: jaundice, from conjunctival subicterus to marked discoloration of the whole body following worsening of a previous clinical picture with fever, upper respiratory and gastrointestinal symptoms, urticarial rash, and articular pain; a relatively abrupt onset in infectious hepatitis (serum A) and more marked dermic and articular symptoms in serum hepatitis (serum B); a variable clinical picture from mild symptoms to severe hepatic coma, hyperbilirubinemia, elevated SGOT (over 40 u) SGPT (over 45 u), and LDH (over 200 mu), and the presence of Australian antigen for serum hepatitis (serum B). Advise prednisone in large doses for the severely ill; otherwise, a complete diet with small feedings.

Cholangitis shows jaundice, fever with chills, pain at the upper right quadrant of the abdomen, and tenderness on pressure over the gall bladder. Give meperidine for the acute pain, and a tetracycline for infection; and consult a surgeon.

Endocarditis lenta presents bleeding areas (skin, mucosae, retina, beneath the nails, epistaxis), fever with chilly sensations, indefinite aches, malaise, night sweats, possible embolism (brain or elsewhere), and heart murmurs; avoid the infection in those operated on in the urogenital system; blood cultures are usually positive during the first week; do not mistake it for rheumatic fever or similar diseases. Treat with the specific antibiotic (large doses for resistant microorganisms).

Polyarteritis nodosa symptoms include dermic manifestations, as purpura, erythema, urticaria, subcutaneous nodules, or edema; fever; pain in the abdomen, loins, muscles, and joints; hypertension; and wide disparate involvement of organs and systems. Diagnosis is made only by biopsy findings. Give supportive treatment; corticoids may help a little.

Sarcoidosis presents multiple nodules all over the body, with fever, arthralgias, skin lesions (erythema nodosum, plaques, papules), hepatomegaly, uveitis, and symptoms depending on the location of lesions; there may be diabetes insipidus or heart or respiratory symptoms; diagnosis depends on biopsy and the positivity of the Kveim test. Treat with corticoids and hydroxychloroquine.

In *Hodgkin's disease* fever, adenopathy, itching, and sweating are the main clues to diagnosis (neck nodes may appear first); a biopsy of a node will give the final diagnosis. Consult a specialist for treatment.

Drug hyperpyrexia is most likely to occur in debilitated people; it starts with headache, dizziness, nausea, visual disturbances, and convulsions, followed by a sudden loss of consciousness, hyperpyrexia, arrhythmic tachycardia, and dryness of the skin, which appears flushed and hot; there is a previous history of using phenothiazines, haloperidol, benztropine mesylate, chlorprothixene, doxepin, imipramine, amitryptyline, biperidin, or antihistaminics. Discontinue the offending drug, rehydrate the patient, maintain electrolyte balance, lower the body temperature carefully, prevent seizures, and use anticoagulants.

Drug rash presents a less "showy" symptomatology than that of drug hyperpyrexia: fever and urticarial or other skin manifestations, muscular and joint pains, and the previous use of an offending drug. Discontinue this drug; use antihistaminics for milder reactions and corticoids for more severe or longer-lasting changes.

Serum disease appears a few days after the use of serum, when some sort of allergic symptoms may develop; symptoms may be similar to those of drug rash (q.v., immediately above); skin tests may be made. For milder reactions use antihistaminics or corticoids; if anaphylactic shock threatens, use epinephrine intramuscularly or intravenously.

GASTROINTESTINAL SYMPTOMS

Dentoalveolar abscess presents local gingival inflammation, with edema spreading to the surrounding facial structures, and local pain; there may be a history of pulpitis. Give penicillin, and send the patient to the dentist.

Peritonsillar abscess (*quinsy*) symptoms are: pus around the tonsils or in the wall of the nasopharynx; fever and pain on the affected side; dyspnea, cough, hoarseness, stiff neck and jaw. Drain the pus and use soothing mouthwashes; it is best to request the help of a specialist.

Gangrenous stomatitis (*noma*) shows a grayish slough of the oral mucosa, which turns red and thereafter black, usually starting in the gum or cheek opposite the first molar; intolerable fetor; red edema spreading to the face and eyelids; perforation of the cheek if the disease is allowed to progress uncontrolled. In contrast, general symptomatology is of a mild nature. Check for a complicating disease (diabetes, pellagra, leukemia, pernicious anemia, an infective disease). Treat the complicating disease aggressively, cleanse the mouth locally, and use penicillin, if it is indicated.

In *amebic liver abscess* the main features are the previous amebic dysentery followed by evidence of liver damage with local discomfort and pain, occasional mild jaundice, sweating, weight loss, and a tender hepatomegaly. Try metromidazole first; alternate emetine, chloroquine and diiodohydroxyquin.

In *pancreatitis* there are nausea and vomiting, but the outstanding symptom is epigastric pain, somewhat shifted to the left, with fever and disabling malaise, the patient looking very ill. Use the specific antibiotic, but start treatment immediately with tetracycline, kanamycin, gentamycin, or ampicillin.

In *cholera* there are nausea and vomiting, but the main symptom is the very profuse watery diarrhea with thirst, oliguria, and other evidence of dehydration. Start a food infusion schedule immediately, and give a tetracycline.

In *gastroenteritis*, fever, vomiting, diarrhea, and abdominal pains that follow an excess of eating or drinking (or the use of a noxious substance) will give the diagnostic orientation; there are abdominal borborygmi, tenderness on palpation, distended walls, and no muscle rigidity; subsidence of symptoms occurs in 24 or 48 hours. Watch for acidosis (with severe diarrhea) or alkalosis (with severe vomiting). Give a rest to the digestive system; treat dehydration, acidosis, alkalosis; check vomiting (prochlorperazine) or diarrhea (belladonna or paregoric).

Enterocolitis starts abruptly with fever and diarrhea, usually in hospitalized patients; in *staphylococcal enterocolitis,* with abdominal distention, ileus, hypotension, and an abundant staphylococcal flora in the stools; in *pseudomembranous enterocolitis,* with more severe symptoms, profuse watery and usually bloody diarrhea with necrotic odor, tachycardia, and symptoms similar to the above-mentioned type, but with the stools presenting not only the same flora but also leukocytes and debris of the pseudomembrane. Immediately discontinue the antibiotic in use, and check for sensitivity, to determine the specific one to administer; give corticoids to the severely ill; give cephalothin until the specific antibiotic is known.

Ileitis is usually noted in patients with regional enteritis, with steady or colicky remittent pain in the lower right quadrant or around the umbilicus with diarrhea and fever. Other symptoms are: anorexia and flatulence, aggravation by milk and irritant foods, loss of weight, tenderness at the site of pain, occult blood in stools, ulcerations of intestines, and rigidity of the abdominal wall. Complications are obstruction, fistulas, perforation, malabsorption, and asthenia. Treat with rest, and a high-calorie, high-vitamin diet; avoid roughage; check diarrhea and dehydration; use corticoids, ampicillin, or a tetracycline.

Crohn's disease symptoms are fever, crampy pain, and diarrhea; discomfort in the right iliac fossa; malnutrition and loss of weight; not too rarely a mass in the same iliac fossa; arthritis, erythema nodosum, or other dermic manifestations, and fistulas in the anorectal area; incomplete intestinal obstruction; tenderness and rigidity on palpation. Radiologic studies give the final diagnosis. Treatment is as for ileitis (q.v., above), and give azathioprine; request the help of a surgeon.

In *subdiaphragmatic abscess* there is a history of surgery or a localized abdominal infection; the pain is ill defined but perhaps more marked at the hypochondrium; other symptoms are mild or spiking fever, gas collection, and openings into nearby organs; X-ray films show elevation and diminished mobility of the corresponding hemidiaphragm. Treatment is surgical, but start with kanamycin or gentamycin.

In *perigastritis* there are: febricula in a patient with a history of peptic ulcer; articular pains; asthenia; anemia; local epigastric pain, a mass noted on palpation, at times hard enough to suggest a neoplasm. Final diagnosis depends on X-ray studies or surgery. Try conservative treatment with kanamycin or gentamycin, but consult a surgeon in all instances.

Perirenal abscess and carbuncle presents a sudden onset of fever, chills, prostration, nausea and vomiting (often simulating an acute abdomen); there is pain in the corresponding costovertebral angle, with tenderness on palpation; diagnosis is confirmed by X-ray studies. Treat with trimethoprim plus sulfamethoxazole, but preferably with specific antibiotic therapy.

In *actinomycosis* of the ileocecal area there are colicky pains, diarrhea, and the possible involvement of other organs; the "sulfur granules" will help in the diagnosis. Give penicillin in high and prolonged doses.

Kala-azar shows progressive hepatomegaly; characteristic splenomegaly; irregular hyperpyrexia; darkened forehead and hands, hypopigmented nodules simulating a leprosy, patchy erythema on the face; progress toward marasmus; anemia, leukopenia, and Leishman-Donovan bodies. Treat with antimonials or ethylstibamine (checking with the Infectious Disease Center, U.S. Dept. of Public Health Service, Center for Disease Control, Atlanta, Georgia.)

NERVOUS SYSTEM SYMPTOMS

Anaphylactic shock presents an extremely rapid sequence of symptoms, of which fever is a minor one. Following the administration of an offending substance (usually by injection, or insect sting) there are apprehension, agitation, cyanosis, tachycardia, a choking sensation, throbbing in the ears, paresthesias, itching, sneezing, coughing, wheezing, incontinence and evidence of vascular collapse, laryngeal edema or bronchospasm; shock and convulsions; possible death within 10 minutes of starting the accident. Immediately administer epinephrine, 1 mg, or 1 cc of 1:1000 solution.

Sleeping sickness: in the *rapid Rhodesian* trypanosomiasis there are irregular fever, tachycardia, headache, personality changes, skin rashes, anorexia, tremors, disturbances of speech and gait, and possible myocarditis; in the *slow Cambian* trypanosomiasis, similar symptoms but with splenomegaly and adenopathies. The final diagnosis depends on laboratory findings. For treatment, check with the Center for Disease Control in Atlanta, Georgia.

Heatstroke and sunstroke: persons debilitated by age may react more easily to elevated temperatures; symptoms are headache, dizziness, nausea, visual disturbances or convulsions, all followed by a sudden loss of consciousness, very intense hyperpyrexia, arrhythmic tachycardia, dryness of the skin, which appears flushed and hot, and hypotension. After sunstroke, bullae are likely to develop. Once one has had this reaction, a repetition is easier. Progressive cooling, massage, and symptomatic help are proper treatment.

Tetanus symptoms are: convulsions, cyanosis, glottic spasms following the characteristic onset of stiffness of the jaw and other muscles, fever, dysphagia, irritability, marked hyperreflexia, and history of a previous wound. Give tetanus immune globulin with penicillin, and chlorpromazine and phenobarbital.

Rabies follows a previous bite by an infected animal; there are very intense painful spasms of pharynx and larynx, and a final stage with general paralysis, exhaustion, and asphyxia. The only hope for cure is the prophylactic vaccination.

Dehydration is water depletion casued by vomiting, diarrhea, excessive perspiration, or little water intake. Symptoms include: skin without turgor, dry tongue and conjunctivae, postural hypotension, and, as the condition progresses, weakness, lethargy, oliguria, confusion, and final shock. Check at all times for renal and adrenal dysfunction. Give extra amounts of water and sodium, by mouth in milder cases, or by intravenous drip.

OTHER SYMPTOMS

Cytomegalic inclusion virus presents a fever of sudden onset, malaise, arthralgia, myalgia, hepatomegaly, and generalized adenopathy; it may follow massive transfusions, and is diagnosed by isolation of the virus from urine or other materials, and by specific complement-fixing antibodies. Try corticoids or antiviral therapy.

Conjunctivitis is evidenced by discomfort in the eye and conjunctival redness; check for a causative disease, which is usually present (iritis, iridocyclitis, common cold, adenovirus infection, coccidioidomycosis, leptospirosis); differentiate from glaucoma and iritis; check for the causative microorganism, and treat specifically.

In *endophthalmitis and panophthalmitis* the eye presents very severe pain, rapidly followed by loss of vision, marked congestion of blood vessels, chemosis, production of pus (limited to the retina and uveal tract in endophthalmitis; involving the whole eye in panophthalmitis); there is elevated temperature, and general deterioration; an early diagnosis is needed to avoid destruction of the affected eye; check for the causative microorganism. Use specific antibiotherapy (a broad-spectrum one until the specific one is found), relieve pain, and call an ophthalmologist.

Orbital cellulitis is similar to the above condition (q.v.), but the pain is referred to the orbit rather than the eye; there are restricted mobility of the eye, exophthalmos, edema of eyelids and conjunctivae, and history of a previous infection. Treat with the specific antibiotic. (See the immediately preceding entry.)

Mastoiditis presents pain at the mastoid area; there may be pain in the ear, with or without local edema, and there may be a purulent discharge from the ear canal; pressure over the mastoid area increases pain. Treat with the specific antibiotic, check pain, and consult a specialist.

Acute pericarditis shows substernal pain, with fever and chills at times; the pain may increase with some positions and be relieved by others; the disease is not to be mistaken for myocardial infarction; there are also tachypnea, shallow respirations, cough, anxiety, weakness, and friction rub heard during the complete heart cycle; diagnosis is based on pain and friction rub, and confirmed by electrocardiography. Treat the causative infective disease; use corticoids; check pain; pericardiocentesis is to be performed if pressure increases; it is best to have the help of a specialist.

In *osteomyelitis* there are fever, pain in the affected bone, tenderness, redness, and swelling; fluctuation may be present; motion is restricted; diagnosis is given by radiology. Use the specific antibiotic (alternates are oxacillin, nafcillin, or methicillin), check pain, and evaluate surgery together with a specialist.

Prostatitis is very frequent among the elderly; there are fever, hypogastric and perineal pain, sensation of pressure, abnormal micturition, and general symptoms, including those of cystitis (frequent and urgent urination of even a few drops). Use antispasmodics, but the specific antibiotic is essential (use alternates of the combination of trimethoprim and sulfamethoxazole).

Orchitis and epididymitis: epididymitis is most frequently the first step, which may follow a previous prostatitis; there are soreness or frank pain in the spermatic cord, tenderness on touch, fever, swelling of the scrotum, and redness of the skin. Support the scrotum; advise bed rest, cold compresses, antibiotic therapy (penicillin or gentamycin), and drainage, better done by a urologist.

Urethritis symptoms are: swelling and redness of the meatus, discharge of pus (thick and yellowish in cases of gonorrhea), burning on urination, and mild fever. Use the specific antibiotic (start with penicillin or ampicillin).

Bartholinitis symptoms are: a painful nodule in the inferior portion of one of the labia minora, fluctuation when the gland is occluded, tenderness and dyspareunia, and mild fever; do not misdiagnose as cancer (harder touch). Always check with a gynecologist, since surgery depends on individual conditions, but start soon with antibiotherapy.

Metritis shows hypogastric or pelvic pain, from moderate to severe; muscle rigidity and abdominal distension; nausea and vomiting; fever with tachycardia; prostration; tenderness on pressure; and a more or less fixed painful uterus. Assume there is a pelvic abscess if increased induration is followed by fluctuation, fever and pain do not abate, and there is rectal pressure. Treatment includes bed rest, antibiotic therapy, and local care; consult a gynecologist.

Salpingitis must not be misdiagnosed as appendicitis or diverticulitis; the onset is more rapid and there is a tendency to improvement. Pain is perhaps more localized at the start; other symptoms are less marked muscle rigidity, flushed face, low back pain, no rebound pain, and the vaginal examination showing bilateral pain and possibly enlarged tubes. Treat as for metritis (see above entry).

Adrenal hemorrhage follows prolonged stress, severe trauma or surgery (general or to the adrenals), severe infection, or sudden withdrawal of cortisone therapy, or occurs in clot-inhibiting disease or in cases of chronic adrenal insufficiency; there will be high fever, hypotension, petechiae, hypoglycemia, hyponatremia, and other evidence of dehydration, as well as headache, asthenia, vomiting, and diarrhea; diagnosis is backed by hypoglycemia, hyponatremia, hyperkalemia, and elevated blood urea nitrogen, and by decreased corticol in the blood (below 5 μg) and urine (below 20 μg). Treat shock; use hydrocortisone; but do not overtreat.

Hyperthyroid storm may occur in hyperthyroid patients subject to surgery, intercurrent infections, or exaggerated emotional stress, with hyperpyrexia, extremely rapid tachycardia and exacerbation of hyperthyroid symptoms. Because of the seriousness of the reaction, hospitalize patients as soon as possible, give large amounts of intravenous infusions, reduce fever, and use iodides, propylthiouracil, propranolol, and corticoids.

FEBRICULA

The elevation of temperature is very mild, the temperature not surpassing 38°C (100.4°F) and usually between 37.2°C and 37.6°C, taken orally. It is very important to remember at all times that elderly persons may present very serious diseases with only modest elevations of temperature. In other words, when dealing with these patients, any elevation of temperature, no matter how mild, will be considered to be fever. This is the most conservative approach. Nevertheless, the following diseases are most frequently accompanied by only febricula (at times, fever may be high);

> Diseases with prevalent *respiratory symptoms,* such as the common cold, bronchitis, pneumoconioses, lung abscess, lung cancer, pharyngeal abscess, and, most important of all, tuberculosis.

> Diseases with prevalent *gastrointestinal symptoms,* such as Crohn's disease, appendicitis, diverticulitis, liver abscess, and gastrointestinal abscess.

> Diseases with prevalent *genitourinary symptoms,* such as renal tuberculosis, genital tuberculosis, and genitourinary abscess.

> Diseases with prevalent *dermatological symptoms,* such as angioneurotic edema and erysipelas.

Other symptoms will characterize sinusitis, rheumatoid arthritis, tetanus, toxoplasmosis, kala-azar, sarcoidosis, or any other fever!

IX. HYPERTENSION AND HYPOTENSION

HYPERTENSION

Hypertensive Syndrome

Normal blood pressure after age 60 may be estimated to be at the higher limits of the accepted average of:

Diastolic blood pressure	60 to 90 mm Hg
Systolic blood pressure	90 to 140 mm Hg

Some authors accept an upper diastolic limit of 95 mm Hg; but with this pressure it would be highly advisable to recheck it at least every 6 to (at most) 12 months. What there is no doubt of is that anyone with a diastolic pressure over 105 mm Hg does require immediate treatment. Below 105 mm Hg diastolic, treatment will be given considering individual risks.

The hypertensive syndrome may be—and actually is many times—entirely silent; it will be detected only when the blood pressure is taken with the sphygmomanometer. When there are symptoms, they may be as follows: headache, mainly in the morning, but occurring at any time; palpitations; asthenia; tinnitus or lightheadedness. In longstanding, more severe cases, symptoms depend on deterioration of organs and systems, such as cardiovascular and renal involvement, brain and retinal changes, and others.

Essential Hypertension

The elevated blood pressure is generally associated with generalized arteriolar vasoconstriction, but no other changes are noted, at least in the earlier stages; though later on in the course of the disease there will be cardiac hypertrophy and some symptoms will appear, such as asthenia, dizziness, nervousness, and headaches. Of course, in time, all other forms of deterioration will take place: narrowing of the retinal arteries, or production of retinal exudates; coronary insufficiency; cerebral vasoconstriction or edema; diminished renal function, with polyuria, nocturia, and possible urine abnormalities.

Treatment will depend mostly on the blood pressure readings. Patients with a *diastolic below 105 mm Hg* may go without medication, except in the case of systolic readings over 160, heavy smokers, diabetics, or persons who show heart hypertrophy, hypercholesterolemia, hypertriglyceridemia, or are males, or present a family history of frequent complications from hypertension; in these cases start with a thiazide diuretic (hydrochlorothiazide, chlorthalidone), or give spironolactone or trimaterene (these alone or with the thiazide) if hypokalemia is suspected or actually develops. Do not forget that digitalis toxicity increases when digitalis is used with a diuretic, precisely because of hypokalemia. Patients with a *diastolic between 105 and 130 mm Hg* will be treated initially with a diuretic, as above; but if there is no adequate response, a second drug will be added, such as propranolol, methyldopa, or reserpine, small dosages at the start, to be increased gradually. Patients with a *diastolic over 130 mm Hg* require any of the above schedules plus an additional hydralazide, but with care in anginal patients, and guanethidine (instead of or together with the hydralazine) as a last step. In all instances try to reduce dosage when good results are achieved; and try to find the cause of the failure when the desired response is not achieved. (disobedience; excessive sodium intake; use of additional drugs with vasoconstrictor effect, such as those for colds).

Hydrochlorothiazide, to give 50 to 100 mg a day.

Spironolactone, to give 50 to 100 mg a day.

Propranolol hydrochloride; give 40 mg a day to start, increasing to 320 mg, but no more than 480 mg a day.

Hydralazine hydrochloride, 50 mg to start, but never more than 250 mg a day.

Guanethidine sulfate, 12.5 mg a day to start, increasing to 100 mg a day, but no more than 300 mg.

Malignant Hypertension

The diagnosis of malignant hypertension depends on the rapid onset of developing symptoms, the diastolic blood pressure climbing above 130 or 150 mm Hg in a matter of weeks or even days. In blood pressure crises of hypertensive encephalopathy the rise of blood pressure is even more rapid. Other symptoms will appear, such as retinal involvement, hemorrhages, exudates, or papilledema, and, thereafter, evidence of renal impairment, loss of concentration of urine, proteinuria, elevated creatinine and BUN, intense headache, blurred vision, nausea and vomiting; and may lead to confusion, other neurologic symptoms, convulsions, and final coma. The accelerated evolution of the retinal changes is the best diagnostic criterion for malignant hypertension, with the consequent deterioration of cardiac and renal functions approaching insufficiency.

Malignant hypertension, and particularly the rapidly progressing hypertensive crisis, require emergency treatment with the patient hospitalized in an intensive care department, with specialized personnel. In severe cases give sodium nitroprusside or diazoxide, but avoid excessive drop of blood pressure. Patients less severely affected may be treated with reserpine, hydralazine, or methyldopa. Once the blood pressure is under control, follow the proper treatment for each individual patient. For more details, see the chapter on unconsciousness, under the heading "Stroke."

Sodium nitroprusside, vial containing 50 mg, to add to 500 ml of 5% glucose to provide 100 μg in each ml; give 0.5 to a maximum of 8 μg per minute in continuous intravenous drip; give higher dosages if needed and tolerated; watch for and avoid excessive drop in blood pressure.

Reserpine; give a daily dose of 0.1 mg, or continue the dosage established by previous treatment.

Vascular Renal Hypertension

Because surgery solves this problem in the majority of cases, efforts will be made toward an early, accurate diagnosis. Whenever the disease starts after age 50, the patient presents some evidence of arteriosclerosis, and on auscultation there are arterial bruits in the epigastric area or over the renal artery, with confirmation coming from radiologic or laboratory studies (intravenous urogram, renal scan, angiogram, increased renin activity in renal vein blood); and with the other usual symptoms of hypertension being present, there is strong evidence sustaining this diagnosis.

Discuss the desirability of a surgical procedure with an experienced urologist.

Arteriosclerosis

Hypertension may be a symptom of arteriosclerosis, but the diagnosis of this condition depends mostly on the onset of complications such as thrombosis, embolism, stenosis, aneurism, or evidence of organic brain syndrome (early forgetfulness, personality changes, confusion). An acceptable clue may be given by enlarged, tortuous, and somewhat hard peripheral arteries noted on the forehead, arms, or legs, or in X-ray films. Acroparesthesias are not rare, and plethysmographic changes may be noted. Causative factors of arteriosclerosis are diabetes, obesity, fat-rich diet, heavy smoking, and sedentarism, among others. These factors should be recognized and corrected as soon as possible to avoid the development of arteriosclerosis.

For treatment, carefully regulate the diet, with drastic reduction of saturated fats of animal origin, extra amount of fat-soluble vitamins, and perhaps some medication, as clofibrate, thyroid extract, estrogens, cholestyramine, and nicotinic acid. For more details, see the chapter on mental deterioration.

Clofibrate, 500 mg capsules; give one capsule four times a day, adjusting dosage according to response and tolerance.

Cholestyramine; use one package before each meal (three times a day).

Chronic Glomerulonephritis

Symptoms of chronic glomerulonephritis are vague and mild: febricula (not always present), indefinite malaise, scanty urine, and at times pain in the flanks. There may be the history of a previous acute glomerulonephritis following a streptococcal (or other type) infection. Rarely other symptoms will be present, such as headache, anorexia, retinal hemorrhages, modest dependent edema, and hypertension. But the main indications for diagnosis are found in the laboratory reports regarding the urine: hematuria, proteinuria, renal cells, and different kinds of casts. In the blood there is evidence of nitrogen retention, such as elevated BUN, creatinine, and so on.

Rest and diet are the essentials of treatment. The use of adequate antibiotics is advisable. Complications will be treated as they arise.

Pyelonephritis

Urinary tract infections are more frequent among women, and are increasingly so between ages 60 and 70. In acute pyelonephritis the symptomatology is that of a general infection, with a few symptoms pointing to urinary functions. In chronic pyelonephritis the most important symptoms are progressive hypertension and retention of nitrogenous products in the blood. There are cases presenting intermittent infectious bouts of fever, and urinary symptoms. Suggestive symptoms for diagnosis are bacteriuria, proteinuria, and casts formed with degenerated leukocytes and epithelial cells. The final diagnosis may be made by radiologic studies showing symmetric kidneys, cortical scarring, and blunted minor calyces, or biopsy.

Treat vigorously any urinary or other infection located elsewhere in the body. Recheck with some frequency for recurrences of the infection, which are quite frequent. In this instance, check for anatomical defects that may help to perpetuate infections. When hypertension and uremia are important factors, these conditions should be actively treated also.

Valvular Diseases

Most heart valve diseases do not present a substantial symptomatology with respect to blood pressure, except for mitral and aortic valve diseases. Not many patients with valvular disease reach advanced age; but these patients should be watched for thrombotic episodes, usually ending in a stroke. When there is also atrial fibrillation, the possibility of pulmonary edema is a constant threat.

Mitral insufficiency, in which most patients are female, presents a murmur heard during the whole systole, starting at the apex and spreading toward the axilla. Forceful beats are noted at this area on inspection, and a thrill may be palpated. Blood pressure is usually normal, but not too rarely there may be hypertension (also in mitral stenosis) whenever a good compensation by a large hypertophied left ventricle occurs.

Aortic insufficiency, in which most patients are male, presents a diastolic murmur heard at the upper right border of the heart, spreading to the right mid-border and the apex. Patients are pale and the pulse strong (water-hammer or Corrigan's pulse) and capillary pulsations are also noted. Moderately elevated systolic pressure is accompanied by a low diastolic. X-ray examination will disclose left ventricular hypertrophy.

It is always wise to request the help of a cardiologist and surgeon for evaluation of the need for valvular correction.

Climacterium

This word is ignored in some dictionaries, and minimized by authors who prefer that the term climacteric almost be synonymous with menopause. Menopause strictly means cessation of the menstrual flow; while in most languages, including English, climacterium refers to the physiologic changes that occur during the late years of life other than senility. The main symptomatology of the climacterium consists of vasomotor instability characterized by hypertension and flushes; other symptoms may be sweating, nervousness, chilling or itching sensations, asthenia and irritability, crying spells, palpitations, or headache. Women may present these symptoms more markedly than men, who very frequently do not complain of symptoms at all (there are women, also, who do not complain of symptoms of this type). The age for these symptoms is between 45 and 50 years for women; and about 60 years, for men. Naturally, all symptoms strictly climacteric in origin will improve and disappear at a time that varies according to the individual patient.

When there are no symptoms, or they are mild, there is no need for any treatment. In other instances, small, cyclical amounts of estrogens will be justified. For men, small amounts of androgens may be used.

> Conjugated estrogens, 0.625 mg, once a day, for 20 days a month, with 10-day pauses.

> Testosterone, 10 mg tablets, one or two a day, according to response and tolerance; it is best to give it three or four consecutive days every week, or in any other cyclic schedule.

Pheochromocytoma

Paroxysmal hypertensive crises are almost characteristic of pheochromocytoma, but elevated blood pressure may also be suspected. The typical attacks include intense headache, profuse perspiration, bothersome palpitations due to a forceful tachycardic pulse, vasomotor paleness or flushing, great irritability, dyspnea and possible anginal pains, and perhaps some neurological disturbances as well. Orthostatic fall of blood pressure is a frequent finding. Suspicion of pheochromocytoma because of the paroxysmal attacks is backed by finding elevated amounts of epinephrine and norepinephrine in blood and urine during the attack or immediately following it. The tumor is rarely palpable; more frequently it can be seen by radiologic studies.

Always consult a surgeon for evaluation of surgical removal of the tumor. Interim medical treatment may consist of phentolamine given by mouth. This drug is said to be no good for long-term treatment; when it fails, give phenoxybenzamine.

> Phentolamine, 50 mg tablets; give one every 4 hours, or even more frequently, according to response (avoid excessive fall of blood pressure!). Watch coronary patients very carefully.

> Phenoxybenzamine hydrochloride, 10 mg capsules, starting with one capsule a day and adjusting dosage individually by increments of 10 mg a day, every 4 or 5 days. Watch sclerotic patients carefully.

Diabetes Mellitus

Hypertension is a frequent symptom in diabetes, mentioned here to call attention to the fact that whenever a patient is discovered to have elevated blood pressure, a test for diabetes absolutely must be made. If diabetes is present, it has to be treated immediately. For more details, see other entries in this book.

Cushing's Syndrome

When the hypertensive patient also has excessive fat deposits on the face and around the shoulders, protruding abdomen and thin limbs, think of adrenocortical hyperfunction. Characteristic of the disease are the purplish striae and plethoric appearance of the skin. Regardless of this apparent strength, patients complain of asthenia, headache and backache, easy bruisability, impotence or amenorrhea, skin infections, and not rarely changes of mood (or true psychosis). Cortisol levels are elevated; and so are urinary 17-hydroxycorticosteroids. Also, special tests can be carried out for the disease (dexamethasone suppression, ACTH stimulation).

The only hope for a good treatment is an initial try with radiotherapy to the pituitary (mild cases), but usually the final attempt has to be surgical. Consult specialists for this evaluation.

Prostatic Adenoma

Patients with long-lasting prostatic adenoma may present some of the complications of the disease, and in this instance, hypertension may be found. Mostly, a complete clinical picture will be seen, that is, polyuria with urgency, sensation of a constantly filled bladder, hesitancy and straining when urinating, abnormal urinary stream, and nocturia; an enlarged prostate gland is noted on palpation; hematuria and symptoms of nitrogen retention may occur, as well.

Treat infections whenever present, and consult a urologist for evaluation of the need for surgical procedures.

Lead Intoxication and Colic

The classical "lead line" is rarely seen at the present time. Hypertension is not a frequent finding in lead poisoning, perhaps more easily noted during the crises of lead colic, with abdominal cramps and other neurological symptoms. Lead poisoning will be suspected whenever a possible contamination occurs. Other symptoms are: gastrointestinal symptoms, headache, leg cramps, pallor and malaise, asthenia, and even more severe central nervous system involvement. Hemograms may give the diagnosis, showing anemia and the typical stippled red blood cells. A well-known and prominent characteristic among the neurotoxic effects of lead poisoning is wrist-drop due to paralysis of the extensor muscles of the wrist.

Treat the condition symptomatically when necessary; and de-lead the patient by means of calcium disodium edetate and dimercaprol.

> Calcium disodium edetate, 15 to 25 mg for each kilo of body weight (for the elderly use the lower amount), repeated every 12 hours, for 5 days, by intravenous infusion; the series may be repeated after 2 days' rest, as needed.

> Dimercaprol, 3 to 4 mg for each kilo of body weight, intramuscularly, every 4 hours, for 2 days; decrease to 6 hours the third day, and then every 12 hours to a total of about 10 days of therapy.

Amputees

We wish to give only a brief reminder that some amputees may present some sort of reflex reaction leading to the presence of a hypertensive clinical picture.

The use of sedatives, like phenobarbital, or minor tranquilizers, like diazepam, will solve the problem in most cases.

DIASTOLIC HYPERTENSION

Diastolic hypertension refers to the elevation of the minimum diastolic pressure over the accepted 90 mm Hg, while the systolic pressure remains about at normal levels. Naturally, the pulse pressure is narrowed. This occurs most frequently in some cases of left ventricular failure, among patients with aortic stenosis, and in those with hyperthyroidism. Whenever there is diastolic hypertension, check for any of the above-mentioned causes.

Left Ventricular Failure

When physicans talk about heart failure, they are actually referring to failure of both right and left heart, though in most instances the main failure is that of the left ventricle. Symptoms of right ventricular failure are dependent edema with tender hepatomegaly and elevated venous pressure. Left ventricular failure causes, specifically, the following:

Exertional dyspnea and orthopnea
Paroxysmal nocturnal dyspnea
Cough and asthenia
Cardiac enlargement and gallop rhythm
Pulmonary venous congestion and râles

In a good number of cases left ventricular failure is accompanied by hypertension instead of the regular normal or low pressure. This may occur because a primary hypertension causes heart failure, and then other symptoms may also occur, such as anxiety.

Because heart failure with hypertension is usually due to hypertension, the treatment of the latter is the first concern. Therefore, treatment will start with rest, diet, and diuretics. Digitalis will take care of debilitated circulation. Frequently, it will be sound to give the diuretics first, and then resort to digitalis. If there is not a good response to diuretics and digitalis, vasodilators (sodium nitroprusside) will be tried. If there is an additional cause, treat it vigorously. For hypertension, the following schedule may be used:

Diastolic below 95 mm Hg: a diuretic, to be complemented or not with reserpine or methyldopa.

Diastolic up to 130 mm Hg: start the diuretic plus methyldopa; and complement with hydralazine or guanethidine.

Diastolic over 130 mm Hg: use the diuretic with guanethidine, and complement if needed with methyldopa.

In more severe or unresponsive cases, use the diuretic together with methyldopa and guanethidine; and complement if needed with hydralazine.

For cardiac failure itself, in addition to the diuretics, use digitalis; and for the elderly patient on rest, be careful to avoid decubitus ulcers and leg phlebitis. For this purpose use a water mattress, or change the patient's position frequently, and help with active or passive exercises.

Hydrochlorothiazide; give 25 to 50 mg every 12 hours.

Methyldopa; give 250 mg every 12 hours, increasing to as much as 500 mg ever 6 hours if needed and tolerated.

Guanethidine; give 10 mg to start (two or three times a day), and increase dosage if needed and tolerated (to 25 mg every 6 hours, or more).

Reserpine; give about 0.25 mg a day.

Hydralazine: give 25 mg every 12 hours; may increase dosage according to response and tolerance, to as much as 50 mg every 8 hours.

Digoxin, tablets containing 0.25 or 0.5 mg each; start with 2 mg in 24 hours (rarely more is needed—but remember that older people usually *need smaller* amounts of digitalis per day) in divided doses every 6 hours; beginning the second day the final maintenance dose will be given, namely. 0.25 or 0.5 mg a day. For other digitalizing schedules, consult a cardiologist.

Aortic Stenosis

Valvular diseases often cause dyspnea, at least as soon as cardiac failure begins; in fact, most symptoms are those of cardiac failure. In the case of aortic stenosis, exertional dyspnea occurs easily, and there is a systolic murmur at the second interspace on the right side, with concentric hypertrophy of the left ventricle. There may also be a thrill, on the same site. Radiologically, the elderly person will not only show left ventricle enlargement, but very frequently also calcifications in the aortic cusps. Many patients will present a combined form of aortic stenosis with aortic insufficiency, with obvious calcifications. Not rarely anginal pains will occur with exertional dyspnea and evidence of congestive heart failure, thus indicating a progressively severe case. The great majority of these patients will have elevated blood pressure.

There is no particular treatment for valvular disease, but the treatment is for heart failure, and angina pectoris. Nevertheless, even for patients of advanced age a consultation will be held with a cardiologist and a surgeon for evaluation of the advisability of providing a valvular prosthesis.

Hyperthyroidism

More frequent among women, hyperthyroidism may occur at any age. A fully developed clinical picture is easy to diagnose: general hyperirritability noted in all forms of motion, speech, walking, movements of the head and hands, and rapid sequence of thoughts; tachycardia and palpitations; perhaps atrial fibrillation with a normal or usually a mild elevation of the diastolic blood pressure; a more or less enlarged thyroid gland; tremor better noted on a paper placed on the extended hand; skin changes particularly noted in excessive perspiration, moist warmth, and hypersensitivity to heat; weight loss even though appetite and food ingestion are good; asthenia, dyspnea, and many other symptoms. Exophthalmos may be present. It is interesting to note that at least in warm countries diarrhea should be considered among the prevalent symptoms of hyperthyroidism. The laboratory will confirm the diagnosis, with elevated basal metabolism, and thyroid hormones, protein-bound iodine, T_4, T_3, and radioactive iodine uptake of the gland. Some elderly persons may show apathy instead of irritability.

Treatment will be initiated with antithyroid drugs, then resorting to radiotherapy, and, finally, surgery. Propylthiouracil is the drug of choice, alternatively with methimazole. Radioactive treatment (perhaps the choice for the elderly) has to be carried out by authorized personnel. Complications, including thyroid storm, are to be treated as they arise.

> Propylthiouracil, tablets containing 50 mg, to start with 300 to 500 mg in divided doses; readjust dose according to response and tolerance, the maintenance dose being about 50 to 100 mg a day; consider the first 2 months as a trial period.

Cardiac Tamponade

The triad of elevated diastolic blood pressure, feeble or distant heart sounds, and increased venous pressure, the last noted by bloating or exertional pains of the right upper abdomen, and enlarged neck veins, all these due to local venous engorgement, indicate an effusion into the pericardial sac. It may follow a wound or a bout of pericarditis with fever, dyspnea, and precordial oppression. X-ray findings will show an enlarged heart shadow.

Drain the effusion; surgery must be considered in case of recurrence.

HYPOTENSION

A systolic blood pressure below 90 mm Hg, usually accompanied by a diastolic pressure below 60 mm Hg, is considered indicative of hypotension, which may occur as a permanent condition, as a transient attack, or paroxysmally. Symptoms of hypotension are: asthenia, dizziness, cyanosis and coolness of extremities, bradycardia, and occipital headache. It does not constitute a disease by itself, but accompanies a number of medical conditions and is one of the principal factors in the development of shock. Hypotension does not need any special treatment, but the treatment of the causative disease, which should be carried out in all instances. If the state of shock is reached, it will be treated accordingly.

Orthostatic Hypotension

When the patient stands up, blood pressure falls. The big problem, particularly among the elderly, is that the patient may also fall because syncope is prone to occur; thus injuries are added to the other symptoms. In milder cases, there will be a minor dizziness with transient loss of vision. Causative or contributory factors or orthostatic hypotension are: any debilitating disease, anxiety, use of antihypertensive drugs, peripheral venous stasis, or a previous sympathectomy. In Shy-Drager's syndrome there are, in addition to the regular symptoms of postural hypotension, rigidity, tremor, dysarthria, diplegia, vertigo, incontinency, lack of inflexion in the voice, and other neurological symptoms.

Treat the causative factor, if known. Patients will avoid rapid change of position from supine to upright; reduce dosage of antihypertensive drugs, if they are being used; use an elastic stocking, if there is peripheral venous stasis; give a trial to ephedrine or fludrocortisone.

Ephedrine sulfate, 25 mg capsules or tablets; give one, three times a day, according to response and tolerance.

Fludrocortisone acetate, 0.1 mg, once a day.

Syncope; Shock; Coma

These conditions were discussed at length in the chapter on unconsciousness, a full section given to each. The reader is referred to that chapter for complete information.

Addison's Disease

Together with hypotension, or normal blood pressure in the lower limits, there are marked asthenia and hyperpigmentation of skin and mucosae, anorexia, diarrhea, nausea and vomiting, scanty body hair, irritability, easily produced syncopal attacks, small heart, enlarged lymphoid tissue, and occasional acute crises resembling acute abdomen. The laboratory will report low cortisol levels in blood and urine and also other low adrenal hormones, elevated potassium and blood urea nitrogen, and decreased natremia and glycemia.

Cortisone is the drug of choice for milder cases; desoxycorticosterone or fludrocortisone will be added in more severe ones. Small and frequent meals are to be rich in protein and carbohydrates. Protect the patient from stressful situations and infections of any kind. Check frequently for balance of electrolytes.

> Hydrocortisone, 10 mg a day, one dose on arising and a second at noontime (avoid administration close to sleep periods).

> Fludrocortisone, 0.05 to 0.1 mg in the morning, once a day or every other day (check blood pressure and ankle edema, for better dosage adjustment).

Hypopituitary Cachexia

Hypotension is the rule in this condition, together with a more or less marked loss of weight; intense asthenia; lack of resistance regarding stress, fasting, infections, and cold temperature; intolerance or actual loss of sexual activity, such as amenorrhea, dyspareunia, impotence; loss of hair and pale dry skin; and visual field defects (temporal fields). X-ray studies may reveal an abnormal sella turcica; bitemporal hemianopsia may be present; other findings may include hypoglycemia and a flat curve for glucose tolerance, and low blood levels for almost all the hormones produced by the pituitary gland. Do not mistake this disease for anorexia nervosa, in which there are evident psychopathic traits, no loss of hair and even apparent hirsutism, and most probably a normal blood pressure, or at least normal close to the lower limits. Most patients will not tolerate, and react poorly to, infections or any other stressful situation. Hemorrhage may cause an acute hypopituitary failure.

Substitution therapy should be the goal of treatment, but no complete pituitary preparations are yet available; therefore, the practical goal is to administer corticosteroids, thyroid, and sex hormones. But special care will be taken because corticosteroids may cause psychosis, and thyroid given without corticosteroids may cause an adrenal crisis. Hormonal replacement is to be continued throughout the patient's life.

> Hydrocortisone; give 10 mg two or three times a day (alternates are prednisolone or dexamethasone, in cases of edema). Proceed cautiously to avoid psychological reactions.

> Thyroid tablets; give 15 to 30 mg to start, gradually increasing to a maintenance dose of 60 to 120 mg, according to personal response and tolerance (avoid increases of more than 10 pulsations a minute, as a rough indication of tolerance), and do not ever give thyroid without corticoids.

> Sex hormones; give estrogens or testosterone in adequate doses, according to response and tolerance.

Liver Cirrhosis

Symptoms may start late in the course of the disease, at times with hematemesis; or with asthenia and weight loss; or anorexia, nausea, vomiting, or other gastrointestinal discomfort, including pain and diarrhea (rarely, constipation); or gonadal symptoms such as impotence, amenorrhea, fall of body hair, gynecomastia; and on physical examination, spider nevis, teleangiectases, palmar erythema, enlarged firm liver, mildly progressive jaundice, and, in the final stages, peripheral edema, ascites, pleural effusion, and other evidence of liver failure. When alcoholism is the basic cause, there are signs of peripheral neuropathy, particularly paresthesias, signs of pancreatitis, anemia glossitis, and parotid hypertrophy. Heralding oncoming coma there are assumed postures for intermittent lapses (asterixis), dysarthria, tremor, drowsiness, and delirium, all resolving into a late encephalopathy or coma. Enlarged veins will appear because of intrahepatic obstruction. Liver biopsy gives the diagnosis; but there are also elevated SGOT, LDH, bilirubin, alkaline phosphatase, and globulin.

There is not much to be done for the cirrhotic patient: general hygiene; strict abstinence from alcohol or any other toxic substance; a nutritious, moderately high-protein diet; vitamins supplementation; sodium restriction if there is a tendency toward fluid retention; and plenty of rest. Hemorrhages, ascites, encephalopathy, and comas require immediate hospitalization of the patient.

Acute Infections

In the acute stage of many infections, also in chronic infections, such as tuberculosis, there may be a more or less marked circulatory collapse with hypotension. This is not diagnostic in any event; so the evaluation of the condition rests upon other symptoms, which were reviewed in the immediately preceding chapter on fever. The reader is referred to that chapter for a better orientation.

Debilitating Diseases

It would be almost impossible to review here all debilitating diseases that may cause hypotension. Any debilitating disease may cause it, and it will be enough to mention the prevailing ones: cancer, anemia, and tuberculosis. In other words, when a patient shows a marked hypotension that cannot be ascribed to any of the foregoing entities, an effort will be made to rule out any of these common conditions.

> *Cancer:* check carefully for a location in the prostate gland, the lungs, or the gastrointestinal tract; but cancer may be found in any

other location as well. For more details see the chapter on tumors and ulcers.

Anemia: diagnosis is easy because of skin pallor and hemogram reports from the laboratory.

Tuberculosis: pulmonary location is usually revealed by evening febricula, cough, and expectoration; other locations may also present a similar febricula and a moderate symptomatology pertaining to the affected system or organ.

As can readily be imagined, diagnosis will not always be easy, depending on a large number of secondary factors, which have to be considered in each particular instance. For more details, the reader is referred to other sections of this book.

X. ARRHYTHMIAS

The accepted regular number of heart beats per minute is 75 to 80; below 60 beats a minute there is *bradycardia;* over 100, *tachycardia* (nevertheless, for a more scientific approach the limits are placed at 40 and 140). Also, the rhythm may be changed to constitute *respiratory arrhythmia, premature beats* or *extrasystoles, skipped beats, pulsus bigeminus, atrial fibrillation,* (formally called complete arrhythmia), *atrial flutter, ventricular fibrillation, pulsus alternans, embryocardia,* and the different *heart blocks* (sinoatrial, auriculoventricular, bundle branch, and Wolff-Parkinson-White block). Finally, there may be *cardiac arrest.*

Tachycardia

Tachycardia is characterized by a heart rhythm of over 100 beats a minute. It is one of the characteristic symptoms of the fever which accompanies most infectious diseases. It is also present in certain emotions, hyperthyroidism, all forms of stress, heart failure, hypotension, and a few cardiac diseases. The administration of epinephrine, atropine, and similar drugs also causes tachycardia. The clinical picture depends on the etiologic factor; otherwise, the only symptom is the greater speed of the pulse.

Treat the cause. Sedate the patient with phenobarbital, if so needed.

Paroxysmal Tachycardia

This occurs as paroxysms of sudden onset and a very rapid speed of the pulse, ordinarily between 170 and 200 a minute, or possibly 100 or 120 to over 240. Other symptoms are: a feeling of something like a shock in the chest, then a fluttering sensation, asthenia and nausea, and possibly angina-like discomfort or pain. There is always a risk of cardiac failure or shock.

The electrocardiogram gives a rapid but regular rhythm. In ventricular paroxysmal tachycardia there is not a regular EKG, but ST and T segments form as a wavy or undulating pattern. The EKG is essential for diagnosis.

For treatment, give a sedative (phenobarbital); perform any of the recommended maneuvers (carotid sinus compression with care in older patients who may respond with cardiac arrest!); or give an intramuscular injection of neostigmine (0.5 mg), or propranolol (1 or 2 mg by very slow intravenous administration), if symptoms are alarming (be careful particularly with propranolol). For ventricular tachycardia resort to cardioversion (very carefully for the elderly patient) or use quinidine, procainamide, lidocaine, or diphenylhydantoin. Prevention of paroxysmal tachycardia may be carried out with quinidine, propranolol, procainamide, or even full digitalization.

Bradycardia

There are no symptoms of bradycardia, except the slow pulse of less than 60 a minute; a rate below 40 pulsations a minute may lead to convulsions and a syncopal state. It has clinical significance only in cases of heart disease, meningeal reactions, intracranial pressure, or pain. There are individuals very sensitive to carotid sinus stimulation, who may present bradycardia, and even fainting, because of only a slight pressure on the neck by a tight collar.

Treat only the causative factor, if present. If the bradycardia becomes annoying, a small amount of atropine (0.3 mg, three times a day) may be enough.

Respiratory Arrhythmia

Also called sinus arrhythmia, this condition consists of a rhythm that is more rapid during inspiration and slower during the expiratory phase of respiration. It has little or no clinical significance.

There is no need for treatment; but small amounts of atropine or a sedative may terminate sinus arrhythmia.

Premature Beats

A condition also known as extrasystolia, the premature beat may be due to an atrial or a ventricular origin. Ventricular premature beats are more frequently noted; and both are among the most common causes of irregularity of heart rhythm. There is a meager symptomatology, mostly consisting of a feeling like a shock in the chest. On auscultation or on checking the pulse there is the anticipation of a beat that comes closer to the preceding one, with a longer pause following. The EKG shows several different patterns, from a cycle entirely normal except that it is closer to the preceding one and a little farther from the next, to juxtaposition or abnormalities of the regular waves, also coming ahead of time. There is a risk only in cases with coronary disease.

If digitalis toxicity is suspected, discontinue therapy for a while and check with a cardiologist. Diphenylhydantoin may be of help in many cases. Always check for myocardial infarction, and treat it if necessary.

Escape Beats

The extrasystole of escape beats, instead of coming ahead of time, as in the case of premature beats, comes later; that is, there is a long pause before the extra beat, which comes closer to the next one. It is better seen in the EKG, but may also be perceived by auscultation and checking the pulse. The symptoms are similar to those of the premature beats.

No treatment is usually needed; but if it is required, give atropine.

Pulsus Bigeminus

There are two beats that come close together and are separated by a longer interval from the next two beats; that is, a group beating in pairs. This is just a variety of the above-discussed premature beats, q.v. The only interest of pulsus bigeminus is that it frequently denotes digatalis toxicity, which has to be considered.

Atrial Fibrillation

This complete arrhythmia, each pulse being different from the preceding and the following ones, may present symptoms similar to those in paroxysmal tachycardia, namely, oppressive sensations in the chest, palpitations, and asthenia, which may lead to cardiac failure or shock if there is a poor cardiac reserve. Atrial fibrillation usually starts by paroxysms and at a later stage may become permanent. The only serious risk with fibrillation, when constant, is the formation of mural thrombi, with possible thrombosis. Fibrillation may be due to cardiac diseases, hyperthyroidism, injuries (including surgery), intoxications (mostly alcohol), vagal stimulation by abdominal distention, or unknown causes. The EKG is diagnostic. The condition is extremely frequent among the aged.

Quinidine (test tolerance!) and procainamide are generally considered the drugs of choice for the treatment of paroxysmal attacks. The treatment has to be continued a few weeks after the attack is over. In the case of an existing cardiac disease, digitalization seems to be preferred, before using quinidine or procainamide, for which reason digitalis should be preferred for the aged. Cardioversion is needed on some occasions, because of poor response to medication. In this instance, consult a cardiologist.

Quinidine sulfate, 100 or 200 mg in each tablet (there are also sustained-action tablets), to give 100 to 200 mg from one to four times a day (sustained-action tablets, once or only twice a day).

Procainamide, capsules containing 250 or 500 mg each, to give up to 2 or 3 g a day in divided doses.

Atrial Flutter

Symptoms may be similar to those of fibrillation, but when there is a regular atrioventricular response, the pulse appears to be regular. The diagnosis depends on EKG findings. The importance of flutter is that it almost always reflects an abnormal heart condition. Quinidine given for fibrillation may cause flutter.

Digitalis at a relatively high dosage is the drug of choice for paroxysmal flutter and for permanent flutter. It will restore the normal rhythm directly or after conversion to fibrillation. Propranolol is given when digitalis fails. Cardioversion is becoming a favored procedure for flutter, but because of the risks involved when treating the elderly, it is best to discuss the measure with a cardiologist.

Ventricular Fibrillation

Flutter or fibrillation of the ventricles also causes a complete arrhythmia, heart beats of different rhythm, which is usually rapidly followed by heart failure and prompt death. It may occur in a previously damaged myocardium, particularly in coronary insufficiency, and is precipitated frequently by the use of digitalis, quinidine, epinephrine, procainamide, emetime, or papaverine. There is an associated, and marked, hypotension, and on auscultation the heart sounds are hardly heard. The diagnosis is assumed by the clinical picture and confirmed electrocardiographically.

An immediate emergency treatment must be given to save the life of the patient, and in this case the risks of electrical defibrillation have to be taken. Until this can be accomplished, give external cardiac massage and oxygen or assisted respiration. In cases of repeated paroxysmal attacks, give a preventive treatment of quinidine or procainamide.

Pulsus Alternans

Pulsus alternans consists of alternating large and small pulsations, which are felt when checking from the radial artery if due to alternations of the left ventricle; also the condition may be detected by pressing a cuff around the arm at a pressure higher than the small beats but lower than the stronger ones (only these stronger beats will be perceived). If only the right ventricle is involved, the diagnosis depends on cardiac catheterization. It is due to previous cardiovascular diseases.

There is no specific treatment for pulsus alternans, but only for the causative cardiovascular disease, if it is known.

Embryocardia

In embryocardia the sounds of the heart resemble those heard during fetal life, that is, there is very little difference, if any, in the physical and acoustic qualities of the first and second sounds. It may be due to myocarditis, including the heart response to elevated fever in infectious diseases; and also in hypertension, renal diseases, or any other disease which may affect the myocardium.

The treatment is that of the causative disease.

Heart Block

The regular impulse conduction from atria to ventricles may be interrupted or blocked at any site in its way, thus constituting the different forms of heart block. For diagnosis, an EKG is mandatory.

Sinoatrial block may be due to excessive vagal tone, the use of digitalis or other drugs, arteriosclerosis, or rheumatic heart disease. Symptoms (dizziness or syncope) will occur only if the standstill period is long enough. In the "sick-sinus syndrome" bradycardia and tachycardia alternate. In sinoatrial block there are no audible sounds during the interval between beats. Treatment will be addressed to the causative factor; but in case of the sick-sinus syndrome, a pacemaker is usually needed; so consultation with specialists is mandatory.

Intraatrial block is mainly due to diseases of the auricular chamber. Usually no treatment is needed.

Auriculoventricular block reveals a myocardial disease or the use of drugs of the type of digitalis, quinidine, or procainamide. The block may be partial when only conduction is prolonged; second degree, when not all impulses reach the ventricle; and complete or third degree, when no atrial impulses reach the ventricle, which establishes a fixed rhythm of its own. In this situation syncope is likely to result from unusual effort, thus constituting the Stokes-Adams syndrome.

In all instances treat the causative disease. Intermittent blockings may, or may not, respond to ephedrine, isoproterenol, or epinephrine, the last to be given by intracardiac injection, when a cardiac standstill persists. Nevertheless, the implantation of a pacemaker should be discussed with a surgeon and a cardiologist in all cases, since this is the only good solution for the problem.

Bundle branch block gives no special symptoms and must be diagnosed by means of the EKG. The right bundle branch reveals cardiac disease, which has to be diagnosed and treated. The only treatment is to eliminate the causative disease.

Wolff-Parkinson-White Syndrome

This syndrome is characterized by a short P-R interval and a broad QRS complex. The chief purpose of the diagnosis is to be alerted to the possibility of fibrillation, flutter, or paroxysmal tachycardia, which frequently occur in these patients. These deviations may be prevented by the use of quinidine.

Cardiac Arrest

There is a sudden loss of consciousness, with apnea and absence of heart beat. With these symptoms there is no doubt of the cardiac arrest, and treatment must be started immediately, in less than 5 minutes, preferably less than 3.

The basic procedure is to use external cardiac massage plus assisted respiration (resuscitation procedures). While working, transfer the patient to the hospital to give countershock for defibrillation, or pass an electrical catheter pacemaker, or perform any of other lifesaving procedures under the direction of a specialist.

XI. EDEMA, CYANOSIS, PALENESS

EDEMA

Only tegumentary edema is considered in this review. Other forms of edema (pulmonary, and the like) have been considered in other sections, to which the reader is referred.

Heart Failure

Left ventricular failure will present the following symptoms: exertional dyspnea and orthopnea, paroxysmal nocturnal dyspnea, cough, asthenia, cardiac enlargement, gallop rhythm, pulmonary venous congestion, and râles heard on lung auscultation. When *right ventricular failure* occurs, there will be added, or there will appear in advance: elevated venous pressure, enlarged, tender liver, and dependent edema. Elevated blood pressure is a frequent finding in heart failure; but there may also be normal or low blood pressure.

For the treatment of heart failure with edema, diuretics and cardiotonics are advised: start with the diuretic (hydrochlorothiazide), and thereafter add the cardiotonic (digoxin).

Hydrochlorothiazide; give 25 mg (up to 50 mg) every 12 hours.

Digoxin: the first day give 0.5 mg every 6 hours (totaling 2 mg a day); continue with a maintenance dosage of 0.25 to 0.5 mg every 24 hours. Remember that the elderly usually need smaller amounts of digitalis; and that for different digitalizing schemes a cardiologist should be consulted.

Venous Obstruction

Any form of venous interruption of blood circulation will cause edema in the sites drained by that particular vein.

Phlebitis of limb (femoral vein) or superficial veins will present inflammation of the particular vein; or if the limb vein is somewhat deep, there will be turgor and cyanosis, the patient will complain of heaviness, and pain will be elicited on deep palpation or felt spontaneously; the febrile syndrome will also occur. For treatment, rest and anticoagulants will be considered the essentials, particularly rest.

Superior vena cava obstruction may start slowly or rapidly and present mediastinal symptoms (dry cough, anginal pain, paroxysmal dyspnea) plus the typical brawny edema with flushing of the head, involving the entire area of the arms and upper part of the trunk, neck, and face, where dilated veins are also seen. Most cases are due to malignancies growing in the mediastinum; and when emergency treatment is needed, it will consist of the intravenous administration of mechlorethamine to shrink the tumoral mass and ethacrinic acid to reduce edema; this will be followed immediately (24 hours) by irradiation of the mediastinum to shrink the tumor further (irradiation to be given alone in less severe cases).

Brachiocephalic vein obstruction will give a clinical picture similar to the above (superior vena cava) but affecting only one side of the neck and the corresponding arm. Obstruction of the *axillary vein* will give symptoms limited to the arm. A *cervical rib* will give symptoms similar to those of the axillary vein, but intermittent. Think of using anticoagulants and consult a surgeon.

Inferior vena cava obstruction will cause edema of both legs; if only one leg presents edema, it is usually due to the corresponding iliac vein.

Varicose veins may appear on any site of the body, but mostly on the legs. They appear as dilated, tortuous veins, with no other symptoms or at most some pain; but particularly in somewhat long-lasting cases there will be local edema with hyperpigmentation and possible ulceration. Usually, the diagnosis is obvious. Treatment may be conservative (elastic stockings) or surgical (excision).

Lymphatic Obstruction

Lymphedema may be a pitting edema at the start, but eventually turning brawny (hard, nonpitting), usually affecting the legs. It may reach such huge proportions as to deserve the name elephantiasis. Perhaps the most important cause of lymphedema is filariasis, but it may also be caused by fractures of the tibia, cancer, or irradiation. Also it may be due to repeated bouts of cellulitis, lymphangitis, or both; but these conditions are prone to occur in patients with lymphedema.

Use physical therapy (postural drainage, elastic stockings, and so on), or consult a surgeon.

Localized Infections

Local infections, in which the diagnosis is obvious the great majority of the time, may present more or less marked local edema. Such is the case with *furuncles* (the collection of pus appears surrounded by a mild edematous reaction), *carbuncle* (several furuncles draining together, usually with relatively marked surrounding edema), *anthrax* (marked local inflammation, ending in a black eschar and accompanied by notable edema and evidence of a generalized infection), *erysipelas* (with a central erythematous area, elevated border, and more or less marked edematous reaction), and *dacryocystitis* (at times evidenced only by the edematous reaction at the angle of the eye). All these infections are to be treated with local application of antibiotics, drainage whenever needed, and perhaps internal antibiotics as well.

General Infections

Trichinosis shows edema of the eyelids as an early symptom; and there are also, together with the febrile syndrome, urticaria, sweatings, subungual hemorrhages, muscle pains (especially the chest), mild gastrointestinal symptoms, and the hemogram with leukocytosis and eosinophilia; the history of having eaten raw pork helps the diagnosis. Treatment is carried out with corticoids and thiabendazole, with or without pyrvinium pamoate.

Filariasis causes marked edema, which frequently ends in enormous increases in size of legs and scrotum (elephantiasis); but not only is this adenitis and lymphangitis noted—other organs may also be involved; laboratory reports will reveal eosinophilia and the presence of microfilariae in the blood, and positive skin tests. Therapy gives poor results; diethylcarbamazine probably is the best drug for these patients.

Other diseases of an infective nature may develop edema, such as bacillary dysentery, ancylostomiasis, and so on. Repeated skin infections may cause edema.

Pressure Edema

This condition occurs mostly in the limbs and is due to ill-fitting orthopedic devices or badly applied bandages. The diagnosis is obvious, and the treatment only needs correction of the faulty procedure.

Postural Edema

Faulty positions are responsible for this sort of edema. They will occur under the following circumstances.

Prolonged bed rest because of long-lasting diseases or fractures requiring prolonged bed rest: dependent edema of the ankles will be noted as soon as these patients resume walking. No treatment is needed in the great majority of cases.

Prolonged immobility, as experienced by some prisoners during wartime, or people traveling for days in buses or trains: the best treatment is preventive (also curative), by exercising the legs at regular intervals.

High heels being worn for long periods: some women may develop edematous swelling around the ankles (pre- or retromalleolar), perhaps with some cellulitic involvement. The problem is solved by avoiding high heels.

Flat feet (not exactly postural edema, but closely related): a number of patients with flat feet will present ankle edema, which usually disappears when the anomaly is corrected by proper shoes.

Kidney Edema

Unlike cardiac edema, renal edema is not so much influenced by gravity; it is not exactly a dependent edema, mostly marked at the ankles, but may start on the eyelids and the face, or even may be generalized (anasarca). It gives a somewhat characteristic appearance to the renal patient, with a bloated pale face and swollen eyelids and conjunctivae, all more marked in the morning. It should not be confused with obstruction of the superior vena cava (there is also edema around the shoulders, the arms, and the neck), or myxedema (which will never present conjunctival edema). The causes of renal edema are the following:

Glomerulonephritis. In the acute form there are: history of a previous infection (usually streptococcal), headache, febricula, edema, anorexia, malaise, hypertension, retinal changes (hemorrhages), and laboratory evidence of renal impairment: nitrogen retention, hematuria, proteinuria, and casts. The chronic form, with its mild symptoms, may be followed by an acute stage, or the latter may appear after years of this damage, with a paucity of symptoms during latent periods; there is regular glomerulonephritic symptomatology when the corresponding clinical picture develops. Treat with antibiotics, and use a symptomatic approach during this acute exacerbation.

Nephrosclerosis. This may follow a well established clinical picture of essential hypertension, or a case of chronic glomerulonephritis. In both instances the symptomatology includes features of hypertension and renal insufficiency, with or without heart failure. To a pure hypertensive disease will be added a mild proteinuria, possible presence of casts, increased edema and hypertension, and more marked retinal changes; and a moderate or a malignant clinical course may follow. Treat hypertension and kidney insufficiency.

Nephrotic Syndrome

Edema is the dominant symptom in the nephrotic syndrome, with elevated proteinuria and hypoproteinemia. The accumulation of fluid is usually massive, including the serous cavities, notably ascites and pleural effusion. As a consequence there are shortness of breath, anorexia, and other symptoms due to mechanical impairment. Hypertension is frequently found. There is a *lipoid nephrosis* with an excessive amount of birefringent bodies in the urine, a relatively good renal function, and a good response to treatment with corticoids. *Membranous glomerulonephritis* is a progressive disease, prone to end in about 10 years, and not responsive to therapy. The *intercapillary glomerulosclerosis* of Kimmelstiel-Wilson, and perhaps other forms of renal impairment occurring following some infections or intoxications, and the renal impairment in SLE, can be included here, since the clinical picture and laboratory reports come very close to the pure nephrotic syndrome. In addition to the elevated proteinuria and decreased proteinemia, the laboratory will report hyperlipidemia, including elevated cholesterolemia, triglyceridemia, and lipoproteinemia, and more or less elevated nitrogen content of the blood and a mild anemia; in the urine there are also casts, cells, fat droplets, and other abnormalities of the sediment.

Corticoids used during the active stages and for a time during the remission of the disease are the best drugs to prescribe, in addition to adequate rest and a diet restricted in sodium, with a normal amount of proteins and calories. Treat the infective factor, if any. Hypertension, hyperpotassemia, and increased edema contraindicate the use of corticoids. When neither contraindicated nor effective, corticoids will be drastically reduced in dosage, and diuresis may respond to the change; if there is no response this way, re-start the administration of these drugs. Diuretics, or the simultaneous use of immunosuppressant drugs and diuretics, is also advised by some physicians.

> Prednisone; give large amounts, up to 80 or more mg a day in divided doses, for at least 3 or 4 weeks; if diuresis starts, reduce the dose at that time at a slow rate to adjust therapy to the minimum

active dosage, which will be continued for a long period of time (about 1 year), but intermittently, with the adequate amount given every other day.

Liver Edema

Cases with hepatic cirrhosis or cancer will very easily present ascites, and possibly other forms of edema. Only infrequently will ascites occur with choledocal obstruction or liver abscess, but this may happen.

Liver cirrhosis is asymptomatic for long periods; then it will present asthenia, weight loss, anorexia, nausea or other gastrointestinal symptoms, symptoms of decreased gonadal function, spider nevi, teleangiectasia, palmar erythema, enlarged firm liver, mildly progressive jaundice, and, finally, peripheral edema, ascites, pleural effusion, and other evidences of liver failure. Liver biopsy gives the diagnosis; check also for elevated SGOT, LDH, bilirubin, alkaline phosphatase, and globulin. Order a strictly hygienic life, and if there is ascites, hospitalize the patient for better care.

Cancer of the liver is noticed when a patient with a formerly assumed cirrhosis rapidly deteriorates. Liver biopsy and other means will make a final diagnosis. Treat symptomatically.

Choledocal obstruction has as its main symptom jaundice; liver abscess, the fever syndrome. Act accordingly.

Angioneurotic Edema

Though not a true edema, the giant urticarial lesions may appear as such. Itching may be the first symptom; but it is not rare that wheals open the clinical picture, perhaps with surrounding true edema when the size reaches huge proportions. There may be malaise and febricula; but the most important symptomatology comes from the diffuse swelling of tissues; both skin and mucosae, involving hands and feet, lips, eyelids, the genitalia, and, more importantly, nose, mouth, pharynx, and larynx. In this last instance there may be stridor and wheezing, similar to an asthmatic attack. Help from laboratory, radiologic, and other procedures is of little assistance. Try to find an active cause for the attack.

If there is respiratory involvement, give an injection of epinephrine; systemic *steroids are recommended*. A tracheostomy followed by administration of oxygen is needed, at times. Antihistaminics in a long-term treatment may offer some help, like corticosteroid therapy for more severe cases; but corticosteroids are to be avoided as much as possible because, if given, they are usually needed for the rest of the life of the patient.

Epinephrine, 1:1000 solution; inject subcutaneously 0.5 to 1 ml.

Cyproheptadine; give 4 mg every 4 or 6 hours.

Anemic Edema

A decreased number of red blood cells is a very frequent finding in medical practice. In most cases no other symptom is noted. Only when the anemic condition becomes marked will there be asthenia, dizziness, headache, spots before the eyes, irritability, febricula, loss of sexual desire, or amenorrhea; and in some special instances there will also be jaundice, splenomegaly, and heart failure with dependent edema. In other words, edema may occur with anemia, but it is always a very modest symptom. Nevertheless, an accurate diagnosis of the causative factor has to be made for all cases; so do a blood study.

> *Blood loss* may be external (obvious diagnosis) or internal (tachycardia, tachypnea, thirst, sweating, falling blood pressure, and final faintness or frank shock). Replace blood; close the bleeding point.

> *Iron deficiency* causes asthenia, pallor, spoon nails, papillary atrophy of the tongue, and other symptoms; there are hypochromia and microcytosis. Treat with ferrous sulfate.

> *Aplastic anemia* follows exposure to drugs or X-ray; there are pancytopenia and fatty bone marrow. Give testosterone or any other androgenic hormone.

> *Pernicious anemia* presents paresthesias and other neurogenic symptoms; there is pancytopenia, with hypersegmented neutrophils and typical oval macrocytes. Treat with cyanocobalamin.

> *Folic acid anemia* is frequent among alcoholics, but also under other circumstances; in the blood there are hypersegmented polymorphonuclears and in the marrow a megaloblastic maturation. Treat with folic acid.

> *Hemolytic anemias* usually present splenomegaly, increased number of reticulocytes, indirect bilirubin test elevated, and low or absent haptoglobulin; it may be due to the use of certain drugs, or neoplastic diseases. Coombs test is positive. Treat with corticoids, or consider splenectomy.

> *Secondary anemias* mostly present a symptomatology of the causative condition, which will be treated accordingly.

Cachexia

Any disease reaching the cachectic stage will provoke an anemic condition; but in all instances the symptoms of the primary disorder will be almost completely established and the diagnosis will be known for a long time before this situation occurs. Check more carefully for suppurative conditions, pituitary cachexia, prolonged malnutrition, and the like. Treat according to the cause.

Myxedema

When the thyroid function is so low as to allow the production of myxedema, the infiltration of skin and mucosae will occur so that the skin becomes hard, inelastic, dry, yellow, and puffy; and the tongue, large and thick. The nails become brittle, the hair is scanty (absence of the lateral ends of eyebrows), and other evidence will back the diagnosis of myxedema, such as slowness of all functions and mobility, a special type of hoarseness, impairment of cardiac function due to myxedematous infiltration, notable bradycardia, and decreased deep reflexes; and the laboratory will report low T_4 and radioiodine uptake, and a macrocytic anemia.

Thyroid extract or synthetic hormones will be used for treatment. In the case of myxedema/coma, give levothyroxine sodium by intravenous injection, together with hydrocortisone.

> Thyroglobulin (extract from hog thyroid); give 200 or more mg a day, adjusting the dosage to individual needs.

Hyperinsulinism

We merely wish to point out that long-lasting hyperinsulinic patients who become obese may also present some form of edema. This is of little concern for the final diagnosis, which depends on a careful evaluation of the clinical history, plus actual symptoms and laboratory tests. Treatment is surgical in most instances.

Hypo- and Avitaminoses

Deficiency in the intake of thiamine (vitamin B_1) and ascorbic acid (vitamin C) usually causes an edematous swelling of the skin.

Thiamine deficiency symptoms are: psychological changes, formication, paresthesias, and anorexia; and when the clinical picture of beri-beri develops, serous effusions, marked edema, polyneuritis with paralysis, and evidence of cardiac failure (dyspnea, tachycardia, and so forth). There is no thiamine in the urine. The best diagnostic orientation is given by the coincidence of large amounts of edema and polyneuritis. Treat with thiamine.

> Thiamine, to give no less than 30 mg a day; but it is better to adjust dosage to personal needs.

Ascorbic acid deficiency may cause a mild edema in many cases, though it is rarely mentioned in medical books. Actually, the main symptoms are the scurvy gums (swollen and bleeding), hemorrhages about the distal end of nails or other parts of the body, aches of muscles and joints, and also asthenia, irritability, weight loss, and a very low or total absence of ascorbic acid in the serum. Be sure not to call scurvy the hemorrhages often noted in the skin of elderly patients. Treat with ascorbic acid.

Ascorbic acid; give about 500 mg every day, adjusting dosage to personal needs.

Toxic Edema

Almost any drug and any allergen or toxin may produce reactive symptoms in certain subjects. The diagnosis depends on the clinical history of ingestion or exposure to the offending substance. The treatment will depend on the causative factor. Here we shall mention only the most frequent causes of such a toxic reaction.

Salicylates (including aspirin)
Quinine
Sodium
Potassium
Phenacetin (urticaria)
Carbon tetrachloride (late renal insufficiency)
Mustard gas
Formaldehyde (edema of the glottis after inhalation)
Hydrogen sulfide (pulmonary edema after inhalation)
Hypochlorites (edema of the upper respiratory tract)
Mercury (a late nephrotic syndrome)

Iodides
Bromides
Chronic alcoholism
Acids and alkalies (local swelling)
Chlorina (pulmonary edema)
Phenols (edema of the glottis, at times)
Potassium permanganate (laryngeal edema)
Rhus antigen
Parathion (pulmonary edema)
Pilocarpine (pulmonary edema)
Bee venom
Heavy metals

Localized Edema

Palpebral localization may indicate a local disease of the eye (orbital cellulitis, chronic dacryocystitis, sinusitis) or generalized infections, such as trichinosis or repeated erysipelas of the face; or other diseases, such as glomerulonephritis, myxedema, angioneurotic edema, or intoxication with sodium or arsenic, or only a personal predisposition to have bags under the eyes.

Mouth with edema should first suggest angioneurotic edema; myxedema gives a different appearance, with a thick, large tongue; and local infections will present evident symptoms (Vincent's angina, and noma).

Face with edema will point to glomerulonephritis, and then to myxedema, with an entirely different symptomatology; it also refers to allergies, and application of cosmetics.

Shoulders with edema will indicate an obstacle to blood circulation in the superior vena cava. Usually the neck and the face are also involved.

Limbs, when enlarged with edema, will mostly point to heart failure, but also renal edema and postural edema.

Penis: this organ, as well as the vulva, reacts easily with edema to cardiac failure and renal insufficiency. Filariasis usually affects the scrotum, but may involve the penis. Malignancies of the genitourinary tract may cause edema of the penis, as may local chronic diseases of an inflammatory type.

CYANOSIS

Cyanosis, a bluish darkening of the skin, indicates poor oxygenation of the blood. The cyanosis can be: *hypoxic,* or related to deficient provision of oxygen to the blood; *circulatory,* due to stagnation of the blood; *anemic,* accompanied by pallor, due to poor storage of oxygen in the blood; or *histotoxic,* due to tissue unable to use oxygen. Diagnostic procedures and treatment vary with each type of cyanosis.

Febrile Syndrome

The fundamental symptom is fever, which may present different curve patterns; but a change of color of the skin is present whenever the elevation of temperature is pronounced. Cyanosis may and does occur, but there is mostly flushing, and at times, pallor. There are also more or less marked tachycardia, polypnea, variable sweating, anorexia, possibly with nausea and vomiting, concentrated urine, and leukocytosis. Important accompanying symptoms are chills, pain, skin rashes, and symptoms from the different organs and systems. All febrile patients should have laboratory studies performed: a hemogram together with the adequate blood examinations required in each particular case, sedimentation rate, serology, culture, sputum examinations, cultures from different secretions or exudates, and urinalysis; and also the specialized techniques of electrocardiography, radiologic tests, radioisotope studies, or any other specialized procedure indicated.

Because most febrile attacks are infectious in nature, antibiotics and sulfa drugs are the most important medications in this therapy; but each particular febrile syndrome will be treated according to the causative factor.

Pulmonary Edema

This is an important diagnostic consideration in elderly patients who suffer from heart diseases, hypertension, pulmonary embolism, unusual physical activity, excursionists at high altitudes, inhalation of fumes or other toxic substances, and injuries to the head. The clinical picture may develop slowly or suddenly, with cough, wheezing, dyspnea, tachypnea and orthopnea, chest oppression, sweating, a frothy sputum leaking from the nose and mouth, and cyanosis that may occur with pallor. Auscultation reveals râles, first in bases and spreading to all pulmonary fields.

Give meperidine to allay anxiety and dyspnea; give oxygen or even assisted respiration to the patient resting in a sitting position; apply suction, if needed, or even perform a tracheostomy; give a diuretic intravenously; treat the etiologic factor aggressively. A phlebotomy, the application of a rotating tourniquet, or intermittent positive pressure breathing may be very helpful.

Meperidine, 50 mg, by intravenous injection.

Furosemide, from 20 to 40 mg (according to weight), by intravenous injection; may be repeated after 90 minutes.

Pulmonary Infarction

Symptoms are a sudden dyspnea, fever, substernal pain, anxiety, and maybe cyanosis, but the last is not a constant symptom. Cough with hemoptoic sputum during or following the foregoing symptoms is almost characteristic. Diagnosis is confirmed by the history of a previous thrombophlebitis and X-ray studies.

Emergency treatment together with surgical advice in evaluating need for embolectomy is wise. Start immediately with oxygen therapy, meperidine, levarterenol, and anticoagulants. For more details, see previous information.

Bronchial Cancer

In lung cancer there is a gradual onset with cough or hemoptysis, the overall clinical picture resembling pneumonia, pleurisy, atelectasis, or abscess. Complicating diseases may obscure the diagnosis of cancer. Cyanosis depends on the respiratory or circulatory impairment. The final diagnosis depends on X-ray findings of the characteristic shadows. Not rarely, a bronchogenic carcinoma is discovered because of its metastases. Also use cytologic study of the sputum, bronchoscopy, or any other means available.

Surgery is the only hope for cure. Chemotherapy and radiotherapy may be useful.

Chronic or Acute Pulmonary Diseases

Cyanosis is usually mild in *chronic* pulmonary diseases, such as tuberculosis, emphysema, bronchitis, or pleurisy. It may be more marked in pneumoconioses, in most of its varieties, and at times in pneumothorax.

More marked cyanosis may occur in some *acute* pulmonary diseases, such as pneumonia, bronchopneumonia, pneumothorax, pneumonic plague, acute asthmatic attacks, acute hemoptysis or atelectasis.

For information, see adequate entries in this book.

Laryngeal Obstruction

This usually occurs during meals, while chewing candies, or when using prosthetic appliances in the mouth. The patient suddenly chokes when a foreign body obstructs respiration. When it is impacted in the larynx, the outstanding symptoms are violent coughing and suffocation.

Emergency treatment is needed to dislodge the foreign body. Try doing so with your fingers in the patient's mouth, but with care not to push the object farther into the air passages; or wrap your arms around the patient's waist, making a fist with one hand and holding it firmly with the other to press violently toward the epigastrium as if intending to push the object out from below (the operation may be repeated several times). Otherwise, an emergency tracheostomy will be needed.

Mediastinal Diseases

Cyanosis is an important part of the "mediastinum syndrome," as follows:

Anterior mediastinum (also called superior mediastinum syndrome): cyanosis usually occurs with polycythemia; edema of the face, neck, and shoulders; pain in the thorax, the arm, or the phrenic nerve; decreased radial pulse; collateral blood circulation; and lethargy, which may be an initial symptom.

Middle mediastinum: cyanosis may occur late, when cor pulmonale develops; dyspnea is an important symptom, with dry cough; there are some pulmonary auscultatory symptoms.

Posterior mediastinum: instead of a pure cyanosis, there is usually congestion of one side of the face; dysphagia; cervico-brachial neuralgia or pain in the back; tachycardia, bradycardia, or asthmatic bouts; Horner's syndrome (palpebral ptosis, miosis, enophthalmos); and rarely ascites.

Diseases causing the anterior mediastinum syndrome are those affecting the superior vena cava, subclavian arteries, brachial plexus, and the phrenic nerve. The middle mediastinum syndrome occurs when trachea, bronchi, recurrent nerves, pulmonary vessels, and cardiac plexus are involved. Finally, the symptoms due to the posterior mediastinum are due to diseases involving the esophagus, sympathetic and parasympathetic fibers, and lymphatic channels. Most of the diseases involving this area are caused by masses growing inside the mediastinum, like adenitis and malignancies.

The treatment varies with the causative factor; and in most instances specialists should be consulted for a better evaluation of diagnosis and treatment.

Right Heart Failure

The main symptoms of right heart failure are elevated venous pressure, enlargement with tenderness of the liver, and dependent edema. To these symptoms those corresponding to left heart failure will sooner or later be added, namely, exertional dyspnea and orthopnea, peroxysmal nocturnal dyspnea, cough, asthenia, cardiac enlargement, gallop rhythm, pulmonary venous congestion, and râles heard on auscultation of the lungs. Normal or low blood pressure may be noted, but hypertension is a frequent finding. Cyanosis may be present, also.

Treat with diuretic and cardiotonic therapy, which can be found discussed in detail in other parts of this book.

Cor Pulmonale

The disease starts with chronic productive cough, exertional dyspnea, asthenia, and wheezing. The established disease will show a frank right heart failure, as described above. In short, cor pulmonale is simply a right heart failure in patients with pulmonary emphysema or chronic bronchitis. Cyanosis is marked in most cases; there will be distended neck veins; and the final diagnosis will be established with the aid of X-ray and electrocardiographic studies showing enlarged right ventricle and pulmonary conus and dilated artery (right axis deviation with peaked P waves).

Treat the pulmonary infection, usually with antibiotics (use the specific one). Put the patient on intermittent positive pressure breathing, and give bronchodilators. Use diuretics and digitalis for heart failure. For more details see other entries on heart failure. Note: In acute respiratory distress use corticoids and positive and expiratory pressure.

Valvular Diseases

Aged patients suffering from valvulopathies have to be closely watched for thrombotic episodes which may end in stroke, and atrial fibrillation which may end in pulmonary edema. Cyanosis does not constitute a constant finding in valvular diseases; but it may be noted in mitral stenosis and tricuspid insufficiency.

Mitral stenosis, in which most patients are women, has the following symptoms in moderate or severe cases: dyspnea and poor tolerance to exercise, flushed or cyanotic face, paroxysmal nocturnal dyspnea, intolerance to bed rest (patient prefers sitting position), developing pulmonary congestion, hemoptysis, atrial fibrillation (constant or transient) with the risk of stroke or pulmonary edema, and progressive heart failure. A presystolic murmur is heard at the apex.

Tricuspid insufficiency symptoms are those of right heart failure (q.v., above in this section). The insufficiency is diagnosed because of the murmur (holosystolic, long left sternal border), and the early occurrence of right heart failure.

Consult a cardiologist and a surgeon for evaluation of replacement surgery. Otherwise, treat heart insufficiency.

Pericardial Effusion

Pericardial effusion may run a clinical course reaching an alarming cardiac tamponade, with cyanosis that may become of some intensity, but always secondary to other more alarming symptoms. In the relatively slow course there are: pain or oppression in the precordial area; dyspnea, with cough (this is rarely absent), forcing the patient to lean forward for relief; at times a prominent dysphagia; and other symptoms due to the basic etiologic infection. At the stage of cardiac tamponade (which is also a primary consequence of injuries) there will be elevated diastolic blood pressure, feeble or distant heart sounds (the initial rub may persist), anorexia, bloating or exertional pains of the right upper abdomen, and enlarged neck veins.

Pericarditis itself is treated according to the etiological bacterial infection, such as tuberculosis or streptococcus or some other causes as heart failure, uremia, myxedema, or trauma. Only when symptoms of heart constriction become prominent, will paracentesis be performed for drainage of the pressing fluid. In an emergency, any physician can perform the surgical procedure; otherwise, it is better done at the hospital by trained personnel.

Acute Suppurative or Corrosive Gastritis

In both suppurative and corrosive gastritis cyanosis usually occurs to a marked degree. Suppurative gastritis presents a rather sudden onset with prominent symptoms: epigastric pain, bloated abdomen with tenderness and rigidity, very intense prostration, tachycardia, vomiting, dry tongue, and fever with chills. Corrosive gastritis follows the ingestion of an offending substance.

Suppurative gastritis may respond to a surgical approach under the protection of the specific antibiotic; so transfer the patient to the hospital under the care of a surgeon. In corrosive gastritis, neutralize the offending substance, check pain, relieve shock, and combat symptoms as they arise; it is much better if all this is done in the hospital.

Polycythemia

In all forms of polycythemia a more or less marked cyanosis appears among the most important symptoms. The increase in number of circulating red blood cells may be secondary to continuous residence at high altitudes, or any other form of hypoxia, as cardiovascular, pulmonary, or some similar diseases. Polycythemia vera is a chronic primary increase of erythrocytes due to unknown cause. Symptoms are almost the same in both instances, with cyanosis, possible bleeding, itching, paresthesias, and general malaise. When there is increased viscosity of the blood, there is a tendency to thrombosis. In secondary polycythemia there are also the symptoms of the causative disease. In polycythemia vera there may be hepatosplenomegaly and gout, and there is no decreased oxygen saturation of arterial blood; secondary polycythemia will show decreased oxygen saturation and will not present hepatosplenomegaly. Hemograms are essential for diagnosis, but good care has to be taken at times not to mistake polycythemia for leukemia (in myeloid leukemia the alkaline phosphatase value of leukocytes is low, while it is elevated in polycythemia vera).

To treat the causative factor in secondary polycythemia is to treat this disease. Polycythemia vera is better treated with radiophosphorus in older patients; but other chemotherapeutic agents may also be used. Venesection is a good approach for relief whenever practicable. Gout, if present, may be treated with allopurinol.

High Altitude

Patients living in cities at high altitude will present a compensatory increase in the number of erythrocytes. This is a physiologic response to the poorly oxygenated atmosphere, usually symptomless for the permanent resident, but which may cause altitude sickness for those who have traveled to a high altitude too rapidly or strenuously. Symptoms are cyanosis, dyspnea, tachycardia, headache, anorexia, mental disturbances (most frequently of the euphoric type), and even pulmonary edema ending with muscle twitching or cramps. Convulsions, and final unconsciousness and death may result.

Oxygen must be given to these patients. If they do not readjust rapidly to staying at high altitude, advise them either to return to lower places and attempt a gradual increase in altitude or to return to a lower altitude and stay there.

Intoxications

Toxic products capable of changing the physiologic properties of hemoglobin may cause cyanosis, which occurs with other symptoms of hypoxia, namely, dyspnea, headache, asthenia, mental troubles (of the euphoric type), and even convulsions. Other symptoms due to different individual toxic irritants may also be present. There may be a history of exposure to the offending substance.

> *Sulfa drugs:* cyanosis will be the result of production of methemoglobinemia; other symptoms are of the gastrointestinal type, skin rashes, headache, peripheral neuritis, renal reactions, and allergic symptoms. Some patients will show cyanosis preferentially on the lips and nails, and men on the glans penis.

> *Barbiturates:* added symptoms are sleepiness, depressed respirations, ptosis of eyelids, lowered blood pressure, soft and possibly irregular pulse, twitching of muscles, and neurological symptoms.

> *Aniline analgesics,* such as acetanilide or acetophenetidin, if abused, will also cause dyspnea, asthenia, vertigo, anginal pains, rashes, weak and irregular pulse, and final profound depression with respiratory failure.

> *Nitrites:* there is not exactly a cyanosis, but a marked flushing of the face together with violent headache, dizziness, dilated pupils, muscle relaxation, and other symptoms.

> *Quinine:* there may be a rapid rejection of the drug, with tinnitus, deafness, skin reactions (cyanosis, rash, purpura, urticaria), diarrhea, and hypotension.

> *Arsenicals:* there are intense gastrointestinal symptoms, thirst, depression, neurological impairment, and garlic odor to the breath.

Diagnosis is obvious in most cases, but it may be helped by identification of the offending substance or the altered hemoglobin in the blood.

In all instances the basic treatment is, first, liberation from exposure to the toxic substance, then efforts to neutralize its effects, and, finally, efforts to cope with the symptoms. In the case of sulfa drugs, force fluid ingestion of up to 4 or more liters a day, provided there is normal kidney function; and if there is anuria, try dialysis or a diuretic. For barbiturates, if damage is from moderate to severe, assist respiration through a patent airway; give stimulants, and other supportive measures. Severe cyanosis with aniline analgesics is treated with methylene blue (1 or 2 mg for each kilo of body weight, intravenously) and blood transfusions; assist respiration, if necessary. Nitrites require assisted respiration with pure oxygen and administration of methylene blue (warn of coloring of urine blue). Quinine intoxication usually requires treatment for shock. Arsenical intoxication may require the use of BAL (dimercaprol) in 10% oil solution, preceded by an antihistaminic to avoid unpleasant reactions, the dose of BAL depending on the intensity of the poisoning.

Traumatic Cyanosis

Following generalized injuries, as in car accidents, even in the absence of organ damage, a very marked cyanosis may occur. In the majority of cases it is of secondary interest and needs no treatment.

Acute Adrenal Insufficiency

When a clinical picture occurs similar to an acute abdomen accompanied by cyanosis, hypotension, dehydration, pain and tenderness at the costovertebral angle, headache, asthenia, fever, shock, lowered blood sodium and cortisol, and elevated potassium, the diagnosis of acute adrenal insufficiency is justified. It will follow an acute infection, withdrawal from cortisone therapy, unusual stress (trauma, surgery), or any other similar strain.

Shock will be treated vigorously on an emergency basis with oxygen, intravenous fluids and plasma, vasopressors, and cortical hormones, hydrocortisone preferably. Watch for hypokalemia (flaccid paralysis), which may follow cortical therapy.

> Hydrocortisone, to start with 100 mg by intravenous drip; repeating every 6 hours the first day, every 8 hours the second day; and to follow with gradual reduction of dosage.

Raynaud's Disease and Phenomenon

Intermittent, paroxysmal attacks of pallor, cyanosis, or both, occurring in the distal ends of the fingers or, rarely, the thumbs, are followed by recovery characterized by redness, throbbing, and paresthesias. As the condition worsens, there is atrophy leading to gangrenous reactions of the affected digits. Raynaud's phenomenon is present in systemic lupus erythematosus, thromboangiitis obliterans, arteriosclerosis, tuberculosis, leukemia, polycythemia, cervical rib, scalenus anticus syndrome, and scleroderma. Raynaud's disease is more frequent among women; Raynaud's phenomenon is more frequently unilateral, involving one or two fingers.

Since attacks are precipitated by cold or emotions, these causes will be avoided as much as possible. Also, because smoking deteriorates these patients, it will be strictly prohibited. Regional sympathectomy may be considered; so consult a surgeon. The use of reserpine or nicotinic acid has been recommended.

Reserpine; give 0.25 mg (up to 0.5 mg), by mouth every day.

Nicotinic acid, tablets containing 50 or 100 mg each; give 50 or 100 mg, two or three times a day.

PALENESS

Paleness has nothing to do with the scarce pigmentation of tissues; a dark skin may be pale, while a very white skin may be ruddy. Of course, hypopigmented tissues are also called pale. According to this evaluation, pallor will be due to anemia, in the first place, and also to conditions involving vasoconstriction. When due to hypopigmentation, it may be familial, racial, or the product of lack of sunlight.

Anemia

All forms of anemia will cause a more or less marked pallor. Other symptoms will be: asthenia, cephalalgia, dizziness, spots before the eyes, and, most important, the corresponding changes in the hemogram.

Iron deficiency: the basic symptoms of anemia are accompanied by hypochromia, microcytosis, low serum iron, absent bone marrow hemosiderin, and increased total iron-binding capacity. Treat with ferrous sulfate (200 mg, two or three times a day).

Posthemorrhagic anemia follows a clinical picture of internal hemorrhage if there is not an obvious external hemorrhage. For more details see the chapter on unconsciousness. Emergency transfusions are usually needed, after measures to stop bleeding.

Pernicious anemia: to the basic anemic symptoms are added neurological troubles, paresthesias from peripheral neuritis, and a sore, smooth tongue. The hemogram presents oval macrocytes, hypersegmented neutrophils, pancytopenia, and also a mégaloblastic bone marrow. A reliable diagnostic test is a good response to injected cyanocobalamin, which is the drug of choice for treatment. Start with 100 μg one to three times a week until complete recovery is achieved, then followed by 100 μg once a month for life.

Folic acid deficiency presents the same clinical picture as pernicious anemia, but usually linked to malnutrition. Check for blood levels of vitamin B_{12} and folic acid. This anemia will not respond to cyanocobalamin administration, but to folic acid. Give 1 mg of folic acid every day for treatment.

Aplastic anemia: among the symptoms there will be a bleeding tendency (purpura), tachycardia, and recurrent infections with hyperpyrexia; but always suspect exposure to X-ray radiation or to a toxic drug; the idiopathic forms are more important in the earlier years. There will be pancytopenia, fatty bone marrow, and a tendency to macrocytic red cells. There is hemosiderin in the bone marrow. Treatment requires the elimination of the etiologic factor, transfusions of packed red cells, and testosterone in large amounts by injection. Surgery may be required, as splenectomy or a bone marrow transplant.

Hemolytic anemia: except for those due to hemolytic agents, parasitism, bacterial toxins, chemicals, autoantibodies, transfusions with incompatible blood, leukemia, Hodgkin's disease, systemic lupus erythematosus, carcinomas, and other systemic diseases, hemolytic anemias are usually of a hereditary type and are not to be considered here. In these patients the anemic syndrome is accompanied by splenomegaly and possibly jaundice, occasionally ending in shock. The anemia is normocytic, and there is evidence of active hemopoiesis. Check and treat the causative factor; give transfusions and corticosteroids, and consider splenectomy when the treatment fails.

Other secondary anemias: the anemic syndrome occurs with symptoms of *cirrhosis, cancer, uremia,* or *infections* (beta-hemolytic streptococci, clostridia, meningococci, plasmodia, bartonellae, escherichiae, or tuberculosis). There are *intoxications* (nitrites, penicillin, acetanilide, phenylhydrazine, benzene, potassium chlorate, spider venoms, or snake venoms), or diseases *invasive of the bone marrow* (metastasic carcinoma, multiple myeloma, and others). The symptoms of the causative disease will determine the etiologic diagnosis. Needless to say, the treatment depends on the cause.

Bleeding Diseases

These diseases will cause symptoms of internal bleeding, external hemorrhages are obvious, and the associated symptoms of iron deficiency are plain. For more information see the chapter on unconsciousness, for the different types of bleeding. Treatment consists of transfusions and stopping the bleeding.

Hypertension

It is not exceptional that some patients with hypertension, particularly when due to renal diseases of the type of glomerulonephritis, may show paleness of the face, perhaps in some relationship to the edematous infiltration of the tissues. This is mentioned here only to alert the physician to this possibility; it will not be an essential feature of the diagnosis. For more details, see other entries.

Transient Paleness

A transient paleness linked to the causative factor may occur in the following cases.

Cold weather will cause paleness before it provokes symptoms of abnormal behavior, asthenia, and a course leading to stupor and coma. Cover the patient with blankets allowing gradual rewarming, with good care to maintain a patent airway at all times.

Myocardial infarction may be accompanied by paleness, but this is only a secondary symptom in the constellation of anguishing and constricting chest pain occurring with hypotension, arrhythmia, and other evidence of cardiac failure and final shock. For more details see other entries.

Shock and *syncope* may also cause paleness. For complete information see the corresponding sections in the chapter on unconsciousness.

Use of epinephrine: following an injection of epinephrine, among the possible symptoms that might arise, local or generalized paleness is paramount. To reverse the action of epinephrine, phentolamine, propranolol, or phenoxybenzamine may be used (phentolamine: give 5 mg, or less, intravenously; propranolol: also by slow intravenous injection, 1 mg, which is better used under electrocardiographic control).

XII. WEIGHT CHANGE

Normal weight depends on height and sex; but according to the usual tables given by health departments or insurance companies the range within each group varies considerably, and more so when different social groups are considered. In general, it should be said that weight toward the lower side is more desirable for elderly people. Here is an acceptable table of weights for older persons, according to height; figures are approximate.

				Weight			
Height		*Men*			*Women*		
1 m 52 (5′0″)	—			50 kg	(110 lb)	± 5 kg
1 57 (5′2″)	57 kg	(125 lb)	± 5.5 kg	52.5	(115)	
1 62 (5′4″)	60	(133)		56	(123)	± 5.5
1 67 (5′6″)	63.5	(140)	± 6	59	(130)	
1 72 (5′8″)	68	(150)		62	(137)	± 6
1 78 (5′10″)	71	(155)	± 7	66	(145)	± 6.4
1 83 (6′0″)	75	(166)		—		

A workable rule for estimating weight from any table entry (entries could be memorized) is too add or subtract for each 2 centimeters of difference in height 1 kg for women and 1.5 kg for men; for instance, a man who weighs 70 kg and is 1.67 m tall, will be about 6 kg above his desired weight because there is a difference of 10 cm from 1.57 to his height of 1.67, and $10 \div 2 = 5 \times 1.5 = 7.5$ kg, which should be added to 57, the weight for 1.57, thus giving 64.5 kg.

WEIGHT GAIN (OBESITY)

Estimation of excessive fat storage can be made from the absolute body weight (above 20% of the average weight for a particular individual) or measuring skin-fold thickness over the triceps muscle, not to be over 20 mm for females or a little less than 30 mm for men after 60 years of age. But in the great majority of cases, excessive or deficient weight can be assessed at first sight.

Overeating

Ingesting 500 calories more per day than the needed amount means a weight increase of about 0.5 kg a week. This is the most common way of gaining weight or reaching the condition of true obesity. The main symptom is compulsive eating. Other symptoms will come from physical difficulties in carrying the excessive weight. From the metabolic point of view, there are no important changes. Naturally, to be sure of the correct diagnosis other causes must be correctly eliminated.

The only treatment is to reduce the amount of ingested calories, which reduction must be reevaluated at short intervals because the organism tries to readjust to the amount of food eaten. In no instance should the rate of losing weight be greater than 2 to 4 kilos a month.

Cushing's Disease and Syndrome

The obesity is of the buffalo type, that is, involving the upper abdomen, thorax, shoulders, and face. A characteristic is the presence of purple striae on the skin; and there are also hirsutism, easy bruisability, thin extremities, asthenia contrasting with the strong and plethoric appearance, and various psychotic symptoms. Most patients are hypertensive, show a diabetes-like glucose tolerance, have osteoporosis, and produce large amounts of cortisol and other corticoids. A pneumoperitoneum may reveal enlarged or tumoral adrenals. Special tests may be carried out for a more accurate estimation of the condition—the dexamethasone suppression test, ACTH stimulation test, and others.

The only hope for cure is the surgical approach, or in some cases, radiotherapy to the pituitary gland. A specialist should be consulted for evaluation. Testosterone may be of help in special cases. Following surgery a permanent treatment with hydrocortisone will be prescribed.

Hypogenitalism

During the physiologic hypogonadism of the climacterium a tendency to gain weight is common for both women and men, starting at about 50 years or 70 years, respectively. Other symptoms are those corresponding to the climacterium, namely, hot flushes, or personality changes. The diagnosis is made by exclusion of other causative factors for obesity.

A little help with diet and gonadal hormones can be given; if the latter are used, always administer them with interruptions of several days.

Hypothyroidism

Moderate hypothyroid states may lead to some gain in weight, but other symptoms are of a far greater clinical interest. These are: dry and cold skin, thick tongue, bradycardia, cold intolerance, great asthenia, changes of the voice, notable slowness of mental and physical functions, and the low findings for thyroid hormones.

Only in cases of true hypothyroidism will some amounts of thyroid hormones be given to the patient. In each instance, the adequate dosage must be adjusted individually. An increase of 10 pulsations above the normal rate for that person is a warning of developing intolerance to the particular dose used.

Diabetes Mellitus

In the insulinoplethoric type of adult onset diabetes, there is a marked tendency to obesity. Consequently, whenever a gain in weight is accompanied by increased thirst and urination, itching of the skin, evidence of peripheral neuropathy, and changes of visual acuity, or even is without any accompanying symptoms, it will be wise to check for glucose tolerance and for hyperglycemia and glycosuria. These findings will prove the occurrence of diabetes, which is not a rare disease among the elderly.

In a large number of cases diet alone will suffice to control the situation. The main objective among these obese diabetics is to reduce weight; so fewer calories will be allowed in the diet, also curtailed in saturated fats and in refined and simple sugars. A second step, if diet alone does not suffice, is to add insulin or an oral hypoglycemic drug. For more details, see other entries in this book.

Hypoglycemia

The constant tendency to hypoglycemia of the hyperinsulinic patient increases appetite and, consequently, causes a gain in weight. This will occur in patients with a pancreatic tumor or simple cell hyperplasia, or those with other diseases that may also help the production of hypoglycemia, such as Addison's disease, hepatic insufficiency, or hypopituitarism. Symptoms may be scanty, only hunger and perhaps flushing and sweating; or the clinical picture may be more important, with chilliness, numbness, dizziness, headache, tachycardia, palpitations, hypertension, behavioral changes (may mimic drunkness), and final coma.

One or two lumps of sugar will control the situation and is a confirmatory test for diagnosis. A practical dietary schedule consists of frequent small feedings taken ahead of the regular crises. But the best therapy is the surgical removal of the tumor or tumors, or of a part of the hypertrophied pancreas.

Lipodystrophia Progressiva

This is a rare disease; it usually starts early in life, but patients, mainly females, may reach advanced age. The fully developed clinical picture shows a body apparently formed from two different portions, a superior very thin one, and an inferior very fat one, united at about the iliac fossae in front and the upper side of the buttocks on the back. Most cases will present the tendency to gain weight just at the lower parts of the body, while the upper part does not vary too much in thinness. The diagnosis is easy just from inspection; the problem is that a reducing diet will not change the lower fatness but will increase thinness at the upper levels.

To obtain some results, at least in a few cases, a try will be given to a moderately hypocaloric diet helped with small amounts of corticoids, carefully watching for tolerance and response.

Central Nervous System Lesions

If no explanation is found for a case of obesity, before accepting it as due to overeating, check carefully for brain tumors, mainly of the base and cerebellum; encephalitis, particularly of the chronic type, and meningitis; bone growths within the skull, as in the Stewart-Morell syndrome, or following a trauma to the head. In these cases obesity is only a secondary symptom. The treatment will depend on the causative lesion.

WEIGHT LOSS (LEANNESS)

Similarly to obesity, consider that leanness occurs when the weight is 20% below the ideal. In many instances, even a weight 15% below the normal range will give the impression of leanness.

Underfeeding Leanness

Underfed persons will lose weight, even though the human organism normally tries to protect itself from damaging situations. For psychopathic personalities, see anorexia nervosa in the next entry. Also, those misled by bad counseling about desirable body shape might diet and lose weight to an unhealthy degree.

The rational treatment is reassurance and overfeeding.

Anorexia Nervosa

Most patients are young females, but this condition may also be seen at more advanced ages. There is a morbid, psychological refusal to eat, which starts gradually; as deterioration is produced, there is a loss of weight, with evidence of dehydration, hypothermia, intolerance to cold, lanugo-like growth of hair on the body, and a final truly cachectic condition. In pituitary cachexia there are loss of hair, extreme asthenia, and hypotension, and estimates of most hormonal findings are on the low side. These findings are normal or only moderately low in anorexia nervosa.

The treatment is better carried out in the hospital; otherwise, failures are the rule. Psychotherapy is to be continued for a long time. Perhaps a try could be given to corticoid therapy, which might increase the need to eat, but with extreme care because of psychological implications.

Gastrointestinal Disease

Weight loss is one of the symptoms of a large number of gastrointestinal diseases, but only a secondary symptom, of not much diagnostic importance. Consider the following diseases as possible cause of weight loss:

Esophageal diseases that make swallowing difficult.

Pyloric stenosis, with vomiting and foul eructations.

Gastric diseases, including gastritis, peptic ulcer and cancer.

Enteritis and colitis, mostly with diarrhea.

Parasitic infections, especially teniasis; and diseases of the liver or the pancreas.

Each of these diseases requires special diagnostic procedures and treatment. For more information, see relevant entries.

Infectious Diseases

Acute or chronic infectious disease will cause weight loss because of diminished food intake or excessive losses, pyrexia, diarrhea, or a combination of each. Consider, for instance, cholera, a disease that in only a few days may take a considerable number of kilos out of the body. An early diagnosis of tuberculosis, if not revealed by a constant cough or an unexpected hemoptysis, may be disclosed by a persistent weight loss. Take a temperature curve in every case of weight loss of unknown etiology; it may be an infective process, which will be revealed because of febricula or a frank fever. The reader is referred to the chapter on fever, where more information on this subject will be found. Any infectious disease is a potential cause of weight loss.

Hyperthyroidism

Think of this condition whenever a patient is losing weight in spite of a good appetite and good food intake, and at the same time presents a rapid rate of both mental and physical activities. The pulse is rapid, and fine tremors are present, better seen from a paper placed on the extended hand. The skin is sweating; there is diarrhea; and there are asthenia, irritability, palpitations, and other symptoms of an elevated basal metabolism, and an increased amount of thyroid hormones in the blood, particularly T_3 and T_4. These findings and some special tests will confirm the diagnosis of hyperthyroidism.

Treatment should start with antithyroid drugs (propylthiouracil). The second choice will be radioactive iodine, and the last resource, subtotal thyroidectomy. Radioactive therapy and surgical removal are to be performed by expert personnel.

> Propylthiouracil; give 100 or 200 mg every 6 or 8 hours, until control of symptoms and improved laboratory findings are achieved; then adjust dosage to the minimum effective daily amount.

Hypopituitarism

Symptoms depend on the severity of pituitary dysfunction and vary from mild to an extreme cachectic condition. There is a more or less marked loss of weight together with hair loss. It is important to differentiate it from anorexia nervosa, which may present a striking clinical resemblance to hypopituitarism. Symptoms are: a very intense asthenia, the skin dry and hypopigmented with a special pallor, hypotension, intolerance to fasting and cold, and if there is a pituitary tumor, an enlarged sella turcica, as seen by X-ray, and decreased visual fields. In fluoroscopy the heart is seen to be small. Laboratory reports will disclose low amounts of all hormones, particularly ACTH, TSH, LH, FSH, T_4, ketosteroids, and corticoids.

Supplements to the corticoids, sex hormones, and thyroid hormones are needed for the rest of the life of the patient once hypopituitarism is established, unless some recovery occurs by posthemorrhagic necrosis, or reactive hypopituitarism.

> Hydrocortisone, to give 20 to 30 mg a day, in divided doses.

Testosterone or estrogens (for men or women), in moderate amounts, preferably with days of omission.

Thyroid extracts; give an adequate amount to each individual patient, according to tolerance.

Arteriosclerosis

In advanced cases of arteriosclerosis or in cases affecting the mesenteric arteries, there may be weight loss. In the first instance symptoms are most impressive because there is the clinical picture of cachexia with evidence of a complete bodily deterioration. These patients usually present a progressive increase of symptoms, including the natural arterial occlusive complexes and not rarely the apparition of successive little strokes. Other symptoms and signs of sclerotic deterioration will occur. In sclerosis of the mesenteric arteries, together with the weight loss there are abdominal pain and diarrhea. Plain X-ray films, arteriography, plethysmography, and other procedures may help in diagnosing arteriosclerosis, though this is not an easy task. Hypercholesterolemia with or without hypertriglyceridemia may be illustrative.

Elderly persons with a tendency to arteriosclerosis, as hereditary, longlasting blood increase of cholesterol and triglycerides, will do better trying to prevent the advance of the disease with adequate diet, low amounts of saturated fats, and the treatment of any possible causative condition, such as diabetes and obesity. Clofibrate and cholestyramine may also help. For occluded vessels only surgery offers relief.

Nervous System

There are a number of psychological derangements that decrease appetite and cause weight loss. The symptoms are those of the primary disease, and the thinness is only secondary. These diseases are only mentioned by name: depression, anxiety, schizoid reaction or a fully developed schizophrenia, neurasthenia, lesions similar to those that cause obesity, and the troublesome clinical picture of anorexia nervosa, which has been discussed.

Lipodystrophia Progressiva

This disease was discussed in the section of this chapter devoted to obesity. Because of its peculiar clinical picture—obesity of the inferior half of the body together with thinness of the superior half—it is recalled here. Nevertheless, only in the fully developed cases will there be a severe weight loss leading to disappearance of the fat deposit as described by Bichat, in the malar area, which mostly only occurs in very severe cases of thinness. There are many patients who are thin in the upper part of the body and frankly obese in the inferior part; but the same response to hypocaloric diets will occur in all these patients, that is, they will lose fat from the upper areas of the body, and none from the lower parts; conversely, if given a hypercaloric diet, they will gain weight by fattening the lower part of the body.

The treatment is difficult. A try could be given to a moderately hypocaloric diet helped with small amounts of corticoids; but care will be observed for tolerance and response.

Cachexia (Cancer)

When this stage is reached, the diagnosis of cancer is already established, and the hope for some results from surgery, radiotherapy, or chemotherapy practically lost.

Constitutional Thinness

There are cases, usually running in families, of persons who are constitutionally thin. No matter how accurate an examination is performed in search of a causative factor for weight loss, none is found. These people are naturally thin, and they do not complain of symptoms. Most of them are relatively tall. Very rarely there will be some asthenia, digestive troubles, or hypotension.

No treatment is usually needed, but a try with a hypercaloric diet will be offered, particularly to those who complain of asthenia.

XIII. TUMORS AND ULCERS

TUMORS

Not rarely patients complain of a ''lump'' or a ''mass'' they noticed developing somewhere in the body. It may happen in the skin, a mucosa, the bones, or any of the systems, and its size may be from the size of a pea to that of a grapefruit or larger.

Eyelids

Enlargement of all or part of one or both eyelids may occur in cases of *blepharitis,* which is merely an inflammaton of the palpebral border, which appears red and thicker than normal, with minute scales and agglutination of the eyelashes. This condition is due to many of the infective diseases of the eye, such as conjunctivitis, dacryocystitis, sty, and chalazion, or possibly due to refractive errors, or infectious diseases. Treat the basic cause and use local ointments.

In the case of a sty there is a growth localized in one of the glands with symptoms of local collection of pus, as a small, round, and tender induration. In chalazion there is also a small, round mass, farther from the border of the eyelid than the sty. Both may need drainage or excision; but the sty may respond to antibiotic therapy.

In *xanthomatosis* there is a yellowish noninflammatory growth around the eyelid. These masses are easily excised or cauterized with trichloroacetic acid, 30 to 50% solution.

Parotid Area

Mumps is not expected in old age, but an exceptional case may occur. Symptoms will be parotid gland swelling with moderate fever, and discomfort while chewing. Gland involvement will be less severe as age advances; treatment is only symptomatic.

In *Stensen's duct obstruction* there is also a painful swelling of the parotid, which increases in size during mealtimes and decreases in the intervals; if it is infected, there will be fever, more intense pain, and marked swelling, with edema of the skin and final abscess formation. A calculus may be disclosed by sialographic studies; it will be dislodged surgically, the abscess drained, and antibiotic therapy used for the infection.

Postoperative parotitis may present symptoms similar to duct obstruction, starting as a unilateral swelling with pain, trismus, and fever; in a mild form the onset is slowly progressive, symptoms are moderate, and the second gland becomes involved while the process in the first is subsiding; in a fulminating type there are chills and the symptoms are of rapid onset and severe character, with large edematous reaction of the affected side and the possibility of death within 48 or 72 hours. Use an aggressive antibiotic treatment together with the needed surgical procedures for evacuation of pus.

Mixed tumors present a hard, irregular mass after a very slow growth that may take years to develop. There will be no nerve involvement, even though these tumors, when left alone, may reach enormous proportions. They require surgery.

Parotid carcinoma is more frequently found before 60 years of age, but cases may occur thereafter; the growth is relatively slow, but not as slow as in mixed tumors, the consistency is similar, but there will be facial nerve involvement, and there may also be adherences to the skin and involvement of regional lymph glands. Early surgical excision is the best hope for cure.

Submaxillary Area

Submaxillary adenitis usually grows rapidly from moderately hard and isolated lymph nodes to form a more dense aggregate, which is a tender, palpable mass when the patient comes to the physician. It is secondary to some mouth involvement such as gum infection, or tooth abscess. Treatment is directed to the causative factor.

Actinomycosis may present a very hard mass, like a stone, with multiple draining sinuses leaking a secretion that contains the characteristic sulfur granules. Of course, the actinomycotic lesion may start in other places, but this is the usual site. The drug of choice is penicillin, but surgical procedures (drainage, resection) are helpful at times.

Cellulitis of the floor of the mouth causes a brawny swelling of the submaxillary area, with fever and chills, local pain, evidence of toxicity, and the characteristic thickening of the floor of the mouth, which may end in the formation of an abscess. Adequate treatment requires large doses of antibiotics, better if the specific one is given; but since surgical drainage is also required in most instances, the help of a surgeon is required.

Osteomyelitis of the jaw may show a mass on the bone, which mass extends upward and downward and will usually end in an abscess. The diagnosis is made by X-ray, and the treatment is with adequate antibiotics and surgery.

Wharton's duct obstruction will provoke a swelling of the submaxillary gland, which very frequently occurs in a matter of minutes, mostly without pain. It will only occur if there is an infection. Increase in size will occur when sour food is eaten. The diagnosis is easy in most instances, by digital examination and X-ray studies. Treatment is surgical.

Mixed tumors are not rare in this area, since one in every 10 of these tumors will originate here. Symptoms are similar to those occurring in the parotid gland (see the corresponding entry, above), but centering in the submaxillary gland. Surgery will solve the problem for diagnosis (biopsy) and treatment (excision).

Carcinoma, most frequently metastatic, will appear as a gradual growth which eventually becomes extremely hard and fixed. Check carefully any lesion, either tumoral or ulcerative, in the lips, tongue, gums, or any other part of the mucosa of the mouth. After complete excision, recheck for a few years, since recurrence is not rare.

Frontal Area of the Neck

Adenitis: an enlarged nodule noted in the submental area is usually a lymph node inflamed because of an infection of the lower lip, the tongue, or the floor of the mouth; but it may also indicate a malignancy, if the original lesion appears to be a chronic one, which is of primary importance to the elderly, even when the primary lesion is not evident. The treatment is that of the primary lesion, unless the nodule is abscessed and needs drainage.

Fistulae are mostly seen in the lateral area of the neck; but also appear on the frontal area in cases of tuberculosis, actinomycosis, or osteomyelitis.

Diagnosis may depend on laboratory or radiologic studies, and treatment will be followed according to the original disease.

Parathyroid tumors are mostly noted at the back of the upper or lower poles of the thyroid gland, but they may appear anywhere in the vicinity of this gland (some may grow even in the mediastinum). Parathyroid tumors are not easily palpated or differentiated from thyroid nodules. Their existence may be assumed by abnormal calcium and phosphorus metabolism and bone symptoms, or renal calculi. Surgical excision is usually needed.

Thyroid Tumor

A general engorgement or frankly developed mass in the frontal area of the neck, either in the midline, unilateral, or bilateral, which follows the movements of the trachea, generally corresponds to a goiter, which is the name given to the enlarged thyroid gland.

Simple goiter and *nodular goiter* consist of a generally enlarged gland, or a gland presenting irregular nodulations. There is no associated thyroid symptomatology. The treatment is surgical; but a try may be given to bismuth therapy, which may be effective in reducing hypertrophied thyroids—if they are not excessively large.

> Bismuth subsalicylate, each ml containing 130 mg; give 1 ml once a week, for 8 or 10 weeks, intramuscularly.

Exophthalmic goiter (over which a bruit may be heard) is diffuse and not very large, but the associated symptoms dominate the clinical picture. They are: tachycardia, tremor (better seen from a paper placed on the extended hand), irritability and nervousness (more rarely psychopathic symptoms may be present), an attitude of tension in physical and mental functions, and moist and thin skin, at times with excessive sweating; the patient appears warm to the touch and has diminished tolerance to heat, good or increased appetite which may accompany weight loss, a tendency to diarrhea as an important complaint (at least in warmer countries), bright and staring eyes, frequently with exophthalmos and lid lag, and other minor symptoms that are not always present, as leg edema, cardiac fibrillation, and splenomegaly. The diagnosis is backed by laboratory findings: elevated levels of thyroid hormones in the blood, particularly T_4, and increased uptakes of the thyroid gland for radioiodine and radio-T_3; the uptake limited to the hypertrophied nodule in cases of nodular goiter. Other findings are frequent, but less informative, such as hypocholesterolemia, hyperglycemia, elevated serum calcium and phosphate, and leukocytosis.

Medical suppression-depression of the hyperfunctional gland is to be tried first, by means of propylthiouracil or a similar antithyroid drug. The second choice will be the administration of radioiodine therapy. Finally, surgery will be done, but always keeping in mind that this procedure is risky among older patients, particularly those debilitated by aging or chronic diseases.

> Propylthiouracil, tablets containing 50 mg, from 300 to 500 mg a day in divided doses to start; maintenance dose usually from 50 to 100 mg a day, according to response and tolerance.

Thyroiditis may be Hashimoto's lymphadenoid goiter, the suppurative type, subacute thyroiditis, or Riedel's woody thyroiditis.

In Hashimoto's lymphadenoid goiter there is a slow, progressive enlargement of the gland with very few, if any, associated symptoms; but it may run toward myxedema or thyrotoxicosis in late stages. Treat with thyroid extracts to maximal tolerance, and give corticoids if indicated.

Suppurative thyroiditis is not frequent; it will cause pain, tenderness, redness, and other evidence of local infection, even to fluctuation. Give antibiotics and drain if necessary.

Subacute thyroiditis is painful, radiating to the ears, and causes dysphagia. Treat with corticoids, salicylates, thyroid extracts, or propylthiouracil.

Riedel's woody thyroiditis presents a very hard gland, adherent and causing great discomfort (dysphagia, dyspnea, and so on). Surgery is often needed.

Thyroid Cancer

Unfortunately, elderly patients with no previous history of goiter are subject to fatal *anaplastic cancer* of the thyroid, which appears suddenly and grows, rapidly invading the gland and the neck (affected side), provoking pressure and pain. Also, for these patients *follicular cancer* presents a dangerous prognosis, although the variety may be encapsulated or invasive; presenting symptoms are similar to a benign adenoma (no lymph node metastasis for encapsulated ones, and systemic or lymph node metastasis for the invasive type, affecting bones and lungs). *Papillary cancer* is less dangerous, even after metastasizing to lymph nodes; there is a hard infiltration of a lobe of the thyroid, not rarely with lymph node infiltration (which may be the first sign of the disease). *Medullary cancer* grows slowly, infiltrates surrounding tissues, and presents hard lymph nodes when metastasizing.

Biopsy by needle aspiration seems to be a good diagnostic procedure, particularly if done by an expert. Only 10% of suspected cases will give positive results, and operation will be avoided in a substantial number of patients. The final diagnosis will often depend on the findings following thyroidectomy. An important note of precaution: Watch for the possible development of cancer in those patients exposed to radiation in former years (X-ray, radioactive iodine), though it is probable that danger disappears after 20 years (some extend the possibility to 40 years).

There is almost no hope for the patient with anaplastic cancer, which will be treated with radiation therapy (patients will succumb to metastases). The follicular cancer usually responds well to total lobectomy, unless there is capsular invasion and involvement of lymph nodes (a thorough search for invaded lymph nodes should precede surgery). Papillary cancer will be evaluated by an expert surgeon, to decide the extent of excision to be carried out. Medullary cancer will usually be treated by total thyroidectomy. Suppressive doses of dessicated thyroid are of little use in advanced age.

Sides and Back of the Neck

Signal or *sentinel node* is a relatively hard and nontender adenopathy noted upon the left clavicle, beside the sternocleidomastoid muscle. It signals a malignancy from an intra-abdominal organ, the stomach, most often.

Pancoast's tumor is a carcinoma of the apex of the lungs, which grows very slowly, extending into the supraclavicular area, with pain that may spread to the arm, and other symptoms of Horner's syndrome (ptosis of the upper eyelid, miosis, enophthalmos, narrowing of the palpebral fissure). Treatment is as for bronchogenic carcinoma.

Hematoma usually occurs around the sternocleidomastoid muscle, growing suddenly and rapidly, not painful (but causing discomfort), and fluctuating after a few days. Avoid surgery.

Esophageal diverticulum is relatively frequent among older patients; it is a mass latero-posterior to the thyroid cartilage with a characteristic change in size from day to day (or hour to hour!), increasing after food intake. Choking and regurgitation are also characteristic symptoms. Radiologic studies will give a final diagnosis. Call a specialist for evaluation of the need for surgery.

Lateral aberrant thyroid is a very rare occurrence, its importance lying in the fact that it is a thyroid cancer in almost all cases. Otherwise, it is more frequent among youngsters than among the elderly.

Carotid body tumor is not a frequent finding, but the mass may reach a large size, can be moved only transversally (not vertically), is deeply located, and may give pressure symptoms. Surgery is the only solution.

Lipoma is not rare in the posterior area of the neck, appearing as a soft, flat, mostly irregular and lobulated mass of variable size. Disregard the small ones; only extirpate large ones causing discomfort.

Carbuncle most frequently arises on the nape of the neck; it is an inflammatory reaction, with swelling and presenting multiple openings secreting pus. Drain it, and use antibiotics generally and locally; check for diabetes.

Lymph Nodes

Enlarged lymph nodes may appear individually, independent of the others, or they may coalesce; they may be soft or hard, tender or not; and the size varies considerably. The finding of adenopathy may have but little clinical significance, but it will always help in the diagnosis.

Tuberculosis: small nodules may be noted in the neck and perhaps in other areas, in patients with some evening fever, cough, weakness, and night sweats.

Infectious mononucleosis symptoms are mild chills and fever, following a catarrhal upper respiratory syndrome, frequently together with an erythematous rash and always with the diagnostic adenopathy behind the ears and on the back of the neck. It is very rare among the elderly.

Plague symptoms are: sudden hyperpyrexia, marked malaise and prostration, muscular pains, and enlarged lymph nodes in axillae and groins.

Tularemia: lymph nodes enlarge and drain during the disease. There are, also, recurrent chills, acute onset of fever, local reaction at the site of the inoculation, and profuse sweating.

Brucellosis: an undulant type of fever in patients who sweat, present enlarged lymph nodes in the neck and axillae, feel extremely weak, and have pains in the head and joints, may call for the diagnosis of this disease.

Syphilis: following the chancre of inoculation there will be mild fever, generalized adenopathy, sore throat, malaise, and many different dermic symptoms, such as generalized erythema, papulosquamous lesions on the palms, soles, and mucous membranes, pustules, and nodules. This can happen with non-sexually-active older persons.

Lymphogranuloma venereum: draining inguinal buboes, soft and with a tendency to coalesce, with several openings and a later marked scarring, follow the initial lesion on the genital area and the rapidly fading vesicles or ulcers.

Sarcoidosis may show multiple enlarged lymph nodes located on different parts of the body, with fever, articular pain, weight loss, skin lesions of erythema nodosum, papules, and plaques; that is, a very variable clinical picture characterizes sarcoidosis.

Leukemia: there may be a sudden onset of fever, or the start may be slower, with acute sore throat, articular pains mimicking rheumatic fever, petechiae, ecchymoses, and other bleeding due to thrombocytopenia, all coming together with generalized adenopathies, hepatomegaly, and splenomegaly. It is frequent in advanced age.

Vincent's angina starts suddenly with fever and inflammation, bleeding, and pain in the mouth, which shows profuse salivation and extreme fetor. Regional adenopathy is marked.

Hodgkin's Disease

This disease, which is rare among older patients, may occur with fever, adenopathy, pruritus, and sweating. The nodes are firm and painless, usually of different sizes within the same group, and may adhere to deeper structures, but the skin stays free above them. Cervical nodes are first to appear; other enlarged nodes develop in the mediastinum, at times obstructing respiration. When a patient presents fever, adenopathies, pruritus, and sweating, get a biopsy of a lymph node, which will give the final diagnosis. An important step in the investigation is the establishment of the stage of the disease: *stage I,* or single adenopathy; *stage II,* with two or more discrete lymph nodes limited to one side above the diaphragm; *stage III,* as above, but on both sides, between the spleen and Waldeyer's ring; and *stage IV,* with extensive involvement outside the lymph nodes, in the bones, lungs, liver, and skin.

Treatment, better given by a specialist, will consist of irradiation over a large field, of 3000 to 4000 Rad, in 4 weeks, of isolated regional groups of lymph nodes, for stages I, II, and III. Stages III and IV require immunosuppressive drugs, such as nitrogen mustard, chlorambucil, and vinblastine in resistant cases.

> Nitrogen mustard (mechlorethamine): dissolve 0.4 mg per kilo in sterile water and give it in a 5-minute injection of physiologic saline infusion, in the evening, after a light lunch not followed by supper. Repeat every 2 months. Sedatives and antiemetics will help against unpleasant side effects.

> Chlorambucil may follow instead of the prospective doses of nitrogen mustard: 0.2 mg for each kilo of body weight per dose, after meals, 2 to 4 times a day according to hematologic response, for 3 to 6 weeks.

Combined therapy, which gives maximum advantage with minimum risk, uses nitrogen mustard, vincristine, procarbazine, and prednisone, or any similar combination:

Weeks 1–2:	Procarbazine, 150 to 200 mg daily. Prednisone, 60 mg a day. Days 1 and 8, nitrogen mustard, 7 to 10 mg, i.v.; vincristine, 2 to 4 mg, i.v.
Weeks 3–4:	Rest.
Weeks 5–6:	As weeks 1–2, without prednisone.
Weeks 7–8:	Rest.
Weeks 9–10:	As weeks 5–6.
Weeks 11–12:	Rest.
Weeks 13–14:	As weeks 1–2.

Sebaceous Cyst

A wen is a globular mass of variable size (pea to apple), in the subcutaneous tissue and slightly protruding from the skin. In the puncta where the cyst is attached to the epidermis, there is at times a plug of sebaceous material, and this site produces a dimpling in the skin when pushed (lipomas produce multiple dimplings when similarly moved). Sebaceous cysts are found wherever there are sebaceous glands, but very frequently in the neck, the scalp, the back, the scrotum, the vulva, and so on. Sebaceous cysts do not cause symptoms other than bulging from the skin; but the big problem in older patients is their increased frequency and their possible transformation into malignant growths.

Surgical removal of the entire sack is the treatment, unless electrocoagulation is preferred. In any of these instances the procedure is better carried out by a specialist because there is always the risk of incomplete removal.

Keratosis

Also called keratosis senilis because of its prevalence at older ages, it consists of horny growths forming slightly elevated flat dry papules, sharply outlined and of a yellowish, gray, or grayish-black color. The surface appears rough to the touch; and the lesions grow, usually, on skin exposed to sunlight. The problem with keratosis is its transformation into malignant growths; in this instance the lesions increase in size more rapidly, and the boundaries are hyperemic (because of increased vascularity).

The potentially malignant lesion (rapid growth and hyperemic surroundings) must be totally excised, including a small margin of the normal skin. Other lesions may be treated with keratolytic substances or by electrodesiccation. It is better to ask a specialist to treat these lesions; but in case of need an ointment with salicylic acid may be used.

Salicylic acid, 10% ointment in petrolatum base, to apply on the lesions.

Leprosy (Hansen's Disease)

The clinical picture of leprosy is extremely slow in its course. It usually starts with multiple nodules, mainly in the face and the dorsum of hands and feet, growing on an exanthematic area of variable color (from clear to a darker hue). This is the nodular form of leprosy, which may reach tremendous deformities of the affected tissues (facies leontina, elephantiasis of hands or feet). Initially, the nodules are pink or somewhat cyanotic; at advanced stages they become dark brown. Nodular outbreaks may occur at times. The outcome of the nodules is resolution, leaving a superficial pigmented scar, or ulceration, leading to extensive mutilations. There is a different clinical picture of leprosy, the maculo-anesthetic leprosy, in which the skin shows more or less regularly limited rounded patches of a color from pink to dark brown, or even completely white (achromic), which spots are totally anesthetic. These two clinical pictures may mix in the same patient. Other symptoms are: nerve thickening with resultant polyneuritis, trophic ulcers, and bone resorption (shortening of digits).

Two different forms of leprosy may occur: the tuberculoid type, with macules and marked nerve involvement; and the lepromatous type, with a predominance of nodular lesions. The diagnosis is made by detection of mycobacteria in scrapings from the nasal septum or the affected skin. Also, biopsy of a nerve may be diagnostic.

Deformities will not respond to drug therapy, even in case of practical cure of the disease. Treatment has to be given for years, since the lepromatous type takes from 3 to 8 years for an adequate regression. Patients under treatment need not to be isolated. The "lepra reaction" to medication has to be avoided by cautious increase of dosages, according to effects and tolerance, and the use of corticoids.

> Dapsone, tablets containing 50 mg each, to start with 25 mg twice a week, increasing very cautiously to a maximum of 600 mg a week. Check for "lepra reaction" or anemia, fever, jaundice, or granulocytopenia. This drug is said to cause cancer.

Fibroma

Fibromas grow from the deep layers of the skin at any site in the body, and are also found in the stomach, the intestines, the uterus, the breast, and other locations. These are benign tumors; but it must be remembered that when exposed to continuous irritation or trauma, they may turn malignant, for which reason all those fibromata growing where exposed to permanent irritation (such as that caused by a collar, a shoe, or a belt) should be removed. These tumors are of slow growth, move freely under the skin, are more or less regular in shape, and are hard to the touch. The most important variety for the general practitioner is the *neurofibroma*, Von Recklinghausen's disease, noted along nerve paths, mostly beneath the skin; but there are cases in which the tumors arise from the skin in the form of tumors of variable size (in this instance mostly in large numbers, almost covering the whole body surface), and accompanied by patches of pigmentation of the skin, of a brownish color.

Older people may have the disease present, either brought from youth or becoming apparent at this time of life. In some cases neurological symptoms may occur, particularly paresthesias or pain. Removal of fibromas will be done only when discomfort is caused by them.

Lipoma

Clinically, they are similar to fibromas, but of a softer consistency, perhaps giving the tactile sensation of fluid, generally lobulated, and may reach great proportions. Locations preferred are the back, the shoulders, the upper arm, and the buttocks. They are relatively freely movable beneath the skin, and when moved they cause multiple dimpling of the skin, not a single dimple like sebaceous cysts. The only treatment is surgical excision, a must for abdominal lipomas which may reach enormous proportions.

Carcinoma

The departure point for diagnosis may be either a tumor or an ulcer, usually starting as a polypoid formation projecting above the skin level, but also as an ulceration invading the tissues more or less deeply. The two main forms are the basal cell carcinoma, or epithelioma, and the epidermoid carcinoma.

Basal cell epithelioma is the most frequent form of cancer, to which both men and women are equally subject, but which will appear more frequently among persons exposed to sunlight and wind, sunbathers, those dedicated to outdoor sports, fishermen, farmers and construction workers, hunters, and also those exposed to irradiation, chronic nonmalignant ulcers and scars, and certain drugs, as arsenic, nitrites, or coal-tar products. Fortunately, this form of cancer is of slow growth and of relatively low malignancy, giving high rates of cure, made better by early diagnosis. It starts as a papule that grows slowly and finally ulcerates at the center, presenting a grayish color and with a teleangiectatic translucent border. The diagnosis can be made by inspection, but it is better to perform a biopsy. Excision is the cure.

Epidermoid carcinoma starts as a keratotic papule, which may also be ecchymotic, and after a time suddenly increases its rate of growth, becoming fungoid, with a central ulcer on an indurated base and bordered by a hard edge. Unfortunately, this tumor is more malignant than the former, particularly when located on mucocutaneous junctions around the mouth, the nose, the eyes, and the vulva. Again, the diagnosis may depend on a biopsy, and the excision has to be performed as early as possible.

Melanoma

This highly malignant tumor is usually diagnosed in the skin or in the retina. The lower extremity gives a larger rate of incidence, head and neck coming next. Hyperpigmented patches in the eye, the soles, and palms, beneath the nails, and in the genitalia are to be strongly suspected. Other patches with increased vascularity on the borders are also suspicious, as those growing satellite moles, increasing in size, changing in color, or ulcerating. Adenopathy is the rule with melanomas. Biopsy requires an extensive resection; and an early radical excision is the only hope for cure.

Fibrosarcoma

This is the typical case in which a patient visits the physician to complain of a "lump" or "mass" growing anywhere in the body. It starts as a nodule that is firm, smooth, and painless; it may increase in size, ulcerate, and bleed, and develop with a foul odor. The diagnosis depends on a biopsy; and the only effective treatment is surgical ablation, wide and deep.

Tumors in the Eye

Most eye tumors grow in the conjunctiva. A brief review is offered here.

Melanoma of the malignant type starts at the limbus with rapid growth and not rarely with little pigmentation, but always diffusely infiltrating. The only hope for cure is the enucleation of the eye.

Epitheliomas also grow at the limbus, but the tumor is slow-growing, red, and small, generally with a good blood supply, which is a good diagnostic clue. Surgery is the only treatment; the size will depend on the type.

Pinguecula is a small and yellowish nodule, like embedded drops of fat. It has to be excised.

Pterygium grows similarly to pinguecula, but is fleshy and vascular, and presents a triangular shape, slowly invading the cornea. A very careful excision is to be performed by a specialist.

Tumors in the Mouth and Pharynx

Most malignant growths will be found in the lips and tongue, being a very frequent occurrence among older people, particularly smokers and alcoholics.

Cancer in the mouth is best diagnosed by exfoliative cytology of *all* local lesions, since there are no characteristic symptoms for any variety of cancer, which may start as a small leukoplakia-like patch, an erythema, an aphtha, a swelling, an ulcer, or simply local pain. Treatment will be carried out by a specialist, since it consists of a combination of surgery and radiation, and subsequent prosthesis is often needed.

Benign tumors are *fibromas* (slow-growing, freely movable, more or less regular in shape, somewhat hard to the touch), which should be excised because of the continuous irritation of mastication; *epulis,* presenting as pedunculated tumors arising from the periodontal membrane in the interdental spaces, are to be removed with or without the adjacent teeth, according to attachment of the tumor; also *papillomas* and *hemangiomas* must be removed.

Leukoplakia is, as implied in the name, a white plaque, noted on the tongue, which actually presents little, if any, elevation from the mucous level. It is considered to be a precancerous lesion, which should be excised.

Tumors in the Larynx

The common symptom for almost all forms of tumoral lesions of the larynx is a change of voice, particularly noted as hoarseness.

Papillomas will cause aphonia and possibly dyspnea; diagnosis is made by laryngoscopy, and treatment by excision by ultrasound therapy.

Polyps of the vocal cords usually appear after violent vocal strain, which is followed by persistent hoarseness. The polyp has to be excised.

Polyposis of the vocal cords usually occurs in the heavy smoker who uses the voice excessively. The voice drops in pitch and volume, and becomes monotonous. Treatment includes stripping of the cords and avoidance of smoking.

Carcinomas are to be suspected in all older patients who, without any apparent cause, start to speak with hoarseness. It is very important to make an early diagnosis by laryngoscopy with or without biopsy for a more conservative treatment with radiotherapy or laryngofissure, before the resection of the entire larynx becomes necessary.

Tumors in the Abdomen

Inguinal hernia is easily recognizable when fully established because the mass projects from the inguinal area into the scrotum, the spermatic cord cannot be palpated, and the tumoral tension increases with the act of coughing; furthermore, the tumor can be reduced with the patient on the bed. Initial hernias are only felt when a finger is placed into the inguinal canal and the patient is asked to cough. There is a pressure against the finger, as the inguinal mass tries to project from the inside. Surgery is the only repair for hernia; in the meantime, a well-adapted truss should be worn at all times while out of bed.

Epigastric hernia is neither frequent nor rare among elderly people; it appears as a nodular mass in the epigastric area, and is treated surgically.

Umbilical hernia is relatively frequent among older women, noted because of the protrusion of the umbilical area. It also is treated surgically.

Gastric cancer must be diagnosed before it becomes palpable, at which time it is too late for any efficient therapy. At this stage, it may not only be felt but also seen as a large epigastric mass; at times a lateral approach is needed to feel the enlarged stomach. A good radiographic study is the only means for an accurate early diagnosis, when surgery is the only hope for cure.

Acute gastric dilation may come after surgery, prolonged immobilization, or myocardial infarction, and starts with a marked abdominal distention, epigastric pain, profuse and persistent vomiting of fluid stained with bile, tympanism to percussion, dyspnea, thirst, and other evidence of dehydration. There are no borborygmi heard as in the case of mechanical obstruction of the higher portions of the small bowel, which also shows a smaller distention. X-ray films will help the diagnosis. Immediately start a Levin tube for constant mild suction, which is curative in most instances in less than 48 hours. Restore electrolyte balance.

Intestinal obstruction also presents abdominal distention, with crampy pain, fecal vomiting, and interruption of the passing of gas and feces. The best procedure for diagnosis of the type of obstruction—be it, strangulation, complete, mechanical, or partial obstruction, or closed loop obstruction—is a good X-ray film. Surgery is to be performed only when the patient is in good condition, after relieving distention with continuous gastric suction, and improving dehydration with correction of the water and electrolyte balance.

Perigastritis presents a painful hard mass in the epigastrium or a little to the right; pain is continuous or may be alleviated by a change of position, and there is usually a previous diagnosis of peptic ulcer. Febricula may also occur. In some special cases the patient wastes and becomes cachectic, and gives the erroneous impression of cancer. The diagnosis is achieved by X-ray studies; and treatment consists of allaying pain (codeine or meperidine) and controlling the source of the infection (start with gentamycin or kanamycin if necessary, before the specific antibiotic is known.)

Intestinal cancer, when palpable, seems to be a movable large mass at the umbilical area, the flank, or the hypogastrium; a typical symptomatology consists of constipation alternating with mucous, bloody, or simple diarrhea; obstruction may supervene. When there is any suspicion, do radiologic and endoscopic studies, on which the possibility of an early diagnosis is based, leading also to a possible cure by surgery or a hopeful treatment with radio- or chemotherapy.

Cancer of the colon starts with a change in bowel habits, mucus or blood with feces, and intermittent cramps. This is true with malignancies of the terminal colon, which may be touched by rectal examination or seen by proctosigmoidoscopy. A cancer of iliocecal location is almost painless, but is easily detected on local palpation because the mass is usually large; it may also cause symptoms of occlusion. Again, the only hope is early surgery.

Other masses in the right iliac fossa to be considered must include, first, the relatively frequent hard tumoral mass from *pseudotumoral appendicitis,* noted in older patients; also consider all forms of *appendicitis,* accompanied by the typical clinical picture; *terminal ileitis* also presents an inflamatory mass, with cramps and several loose stools, which are not bloody.

Fecal impaction easily occurs among the senile, and with the increasing longevity of these patients it will not be rare to see more and more cases. For days, there will be no formal defecation, but only a watery fecal material passed; mucus or blood may be added, not always accompanied by pain. On abdominal palpation fecalomas are noted in varied position; but the main diagnostic indication is the firm, rubbery, and putty-like mass impacted in the rectum and noted on digital examination. The treatment is digital dislodging (perhaps the easiest way); but a sigmoidoscopy, cleansing enemas, and high colonic irrigations are indicated. If the digital dislodging causes pain, give some sort of anesthesia.

Liver

Practically all cases of tumoral liver can be presented under the common heading of *hepatomegaly* because even when there are nodular formations, the whole clinical picture refers to an enlarged liver. That is, if when exploring a patient, we find the total hepatic area to be increased, or the border is found at a lower position, we may refer to an enlarged liver; and we may consider for diagnosis all cases of diffuse or only regional liver enlargement as hepatomegaly.

Hepatomegaly in *acute infections* is only a part of the febrile syndrome plus the particular symptoms of the causative infection: typhoid fever, malaria, syphilis, brucellosis, dysentery, kala-azar, Chagas' disease, spirochetosis icterohemorrhagica, and others.

Hepatic abscess is much less frequent than it was years ago, but still is relatively prevalent at older ages; it starts with fever, and pain in the hepatic area, which is also tender to the touch; rarely, fluctuation is felt; there may also be jaundice; X-ray films may show the corresponding diaphragmatic elevation (right side abscess), or the liver scanning, the presence of intrahepatic abscesses. Treat aggressively with antibiotics of the kanamycin or gentamycin type (better the specific antibiotic!), and resort to surgical drainage if there is no control of the infection in a reasonable time. Think of hepatic abscess if there is a previous appendicitis, portal phlebitis, or dysentery.

Parasitary hepatomegaly is usually noted in tropical countries or people coming from these countries. Keep in mind malaria, dysentery, hydatid cysts, or Chagas' disease.

Heart failure (right ventricle involvement) is perhaps the main cause of tender hepatomegaly among the elderly, which is one of the outstanding symptoms of the complete syndrome. Not rarely, it is accompanied by a mild jaundice and other dyspeptic symptoms. For a more complete review, see other, more detailed entries in this book. Note: Not too rarely this tender hepatomegaly will be the first symptom of heart failure.

Liver cirrhosis always provokes hepatomegaly, more marked in biliary cirrhosis than in nodular cirrhosis. Other symptoms are: jaundice (earlier in biliary cirrhosis), dyspeptic symptoms, local pain in the hepatic area, itching (more frequent in biliary cirrhosis), diarrhea (more frequent in nodular cirrhosis), and in both types a late occurrence of ascites and edema. In nodular cirrhosis there may appear the well known spider nevi, palmar erythema, and teleangiectasia. Biopsy may give particular signs, but in general differentiation of one from the other type may sometimes be very difficult, and is a matter that should be left for the specialist. Add to these complexes a special bronzing of the skin and evidence of diabetes when bronze or bronzed diabetes (hemochromatosis) develops.

If there is obstruction causing biliary cirrhosis, the obstruction will be relieved surgically; otherwise, the treatment will be supportive and symptomatic. For nodular cirrhosis, avoid the ingestion of toxic substances (alcohol, in the first place), give an adequate diet, advise rest, and treat ascites and edema with sodium restriction and diuretics if so needed. Also, symptoms and complications will be treated as they arise, particularly anemia, hemorrhages, and encephalopathy. Hemochromatosis is treated with intermittent phlebotomies and the use of chelating agents, such as deferoxamine (500 mg ampoules, to give two to start, followed by one every 6 to 8 hours, intramuscularly, not to exceed 4 or 6 g in 24 hours, watching for cataract formation, and not to be given to patients with renal insufficiency).

Hepatitis may cause hepatomegaly in some, but not all, cases; but the diagnosis will depend more on the infectious syndrome and the laboratory findings (elevated SGOT, SGPT, LDH).

Fatty liver is a uniformly enlarged organ, diagnosed by percutaneous biopsy, due to diseases that symptomatologically dominate the clinical picture: alcoholism, diabetes mellitus, obesity, starvation, poisoning with carbon tetrachloride or yellow phosphorus, gout, and some chronic infections. The treatment is that addressed to the causative factor.

Neoplasias of the liver may be primary (hepatoma) or metastatic. In both instances the enlarged liver is also tender, and the diagnosis depends mostly on percutaneous biopsy. Treatment is only palliative and symptomatic.

Diseases of the gall bladder may or may not cause hepatomegaly, but not rarely will present an enlarged mass consistent with the liver, usually with pain and tenderness, not rarely jaundice and perhaps fever. The diagnosis is usually made radiologically; the treatment will be addressed to each particular disease.

Spleen

Splenomegaly is usually diagnosed by percussion or palpation, more rarely by simple inspection. When there is the possibility of palpating the organ, other signs helpful for diagnosis are elicited, such as consistency, shape, and so forth.

Many *infectious diseases* will cause a marked splenomegaly, which in some instances is a good diagnostic help. Nevertheless, the enlarged spleen is a relatively minor sign amid the specific symptomatology for any particular disease: typhoid fever, malaria, bacteremia, brucellosis, spirochetosis icterohemorrhagica, tuberculosis, and trypanosomiasis, and less frequently in other infectious diseases.

Splenohepatomegaly is a very important finding in many cases of nodular cirrhosis, including the alcoholic type; it is also of interest in biliary cirrhosis, hemochromatosis, splenic anemia with liver cirrhosis, polycythemia vera, and even a few cases of neoplasias of the liver. In all these cases the specific symptomatology rather than the splenomegaly will orient the diagnosis. Also, in some infectious diseases this combination is suggestive in the diagnosis, as in typhoid fever, malaria, brucellosis, spirochetosis icterohemorrhagica, and a few others. But, again, the diagnosis depends on the complete infectious clinical picture.

Leukemia in all its forms will cause a more or less marked splenomegaly, of little diagnostic interest in many cases, except for *myelocytic leukemia,* in which the splenomegaly reveals a large, hard, nontender, notched spleen, occurring with vague symptoms of asthenia, mild adenopathy, and characteristic findings in the hemogram (marked leukocytosis including young granulocytes). Treatment is usually rewarding in the sense of symptomatic improvement, but not as a lifesaving procedure. Busulfan is the drug of choice, but the scheduling of administration will be left to a specialist. In *lymphocytic leukemia* symptoms are similar, and the diagnosis usually made from the hemogram; but these patients may show a hemorrhagic tendency and more marked adenopathy. For this form of leukemia chlorambucil is the drug of choice, but its use is better left to a specialist.

Hodgkin's disease may cause splenohepatomegaly, but only late in the disease, when it is fully developed and the diagnosis already made. Only rarely will the splenomegaly occur early.

Hemolytic jaundice is a congenital disease not rarely evidenced in old age by an enlarged spleen, with jaundice, anemia, abdominal discomfort, and other vague symptoms, all backed by laboratory findings of hyperchromic, mild anemia with small spherocytes, and a negative Coombs test. Aplastic crises with headache, abdominal pain, fever, and pancytopenia may occur. Splenectomy will be evaluated; for the aplastic crises, use transfusions.

Polycythemia vera presents a characteristic splenomegaly with hepatomegaly (which will differentiate this disease from other secondary polycythemias), vague generalized symptoms, itching, paresthesias, a bleeding tendency, and a dusky red color to the skin. Thrombosis causing cerebral or coronary symptoms, peptic ulcer, and other complications may arise. The hemogram will reveal an increased red cell count, with elevated figures for hematocrit and hemoglobin. For treatment consider phlebotomy (when the hematocrit is over 55%), but for older patients the use of radioisotopes seems to be preferable (to be given by specialists).

Infarction of the spleen may cause minimal pain and minimal splenomegaly, or may cause an acute abdomen with local and generalized peritonitic symptoms. The diagnosis is difficult; the treatment, surgical.

Spleen abscess usually follows an infection in the peritoneum or elsewhere in the body; a more or less intense febrile syndrome, or the accentuation of a previous one, will occur together with a more or less marked splenomegaly and local pain. Treatment will include antibiotics (preferably the specific one, but at least those against intestinal flora), with or without surgical drainage.

Primary splenic neutropenia is very rare among the elderly; the spleen is large, several fingers below the costal margin, and there are marked leukopenia and recurrent infections. Surgery is to be considered.

Felty's syndrome is just a rheumatoid arthritis with splenomegaly and leukopenia. Treatment is as for rheumatoid arthritis.

Kidney

A *movable kidney* may be felt (mostly at the right side), but it is a normal size and no other symptoms are usually noted (some may present intermittent hydronephrosis).

Hydronephrosis will show a large, renitent kidney, with some pain on palpation, and fever if there is pyonephrosis. Radiologic studies will help in diagnosis. Send the patient to a urologist for treatment.

Polycystic kidneys are usually diagnosed in earlier years, showing large kidneys, pain noted in the flanks, hematuria, possibility of urinary infections, and eventually hypertension and other symptoms of uremia. The diagnosis is made by an intravenous pyelogram. The treatment consists of prevention of infections, management of hypertension whenever present, and care for the uremic syndrome. Consider a kidney transplant or dialysis after renal insufficiency starts.

Pyelonephritis may present enlarged kidneys, but the diagnosis will not depend on this not-too-frequent finding.

Carcinoma of the kidney is more frequently found among males, the enlarged kidney being a symptom secondary to hematuria, local pain, and fever. Polycythemia and hypertension are occasionally noted. The best diagnostic procedure is pyelography; the best curative procedure, surgery performed in due time.

Breast

The breasts of all female patients must be carefully examined in each periodic visit to the physician, particularly during and after the climacteric years. Also, males should be examined at this age because gynecomastia is not too rare, especially when certain medications are given, estrogens in particular.

Carcinoma of the breast is to be feared whenever a mass is noted in the breast, until it is proved to be benign in nature. For a long time the only symptom is the presence of a painless mass (except for "inflammatory carcinoma"), from firm to hard and with ill-defined borders, when touched;

also, it may start as an erosion of the nipple with swollen surroundings that are not changed at times. Mammography will confirm the diagnosis; but this procedure may also detect cancer before any symptom is present. Skin with an orange-like pitted retraction or nipple retraction, mainly noted when the mass is pushed together, with breast enlargement, redness and edema of the skin, pain, fixation of the mass, and adenopathy will appear in more advanced cases. In final stages there are skin ulcers, edema of the arm, extensive adenopathy, and metastases to bones, lung, liver, brain, and other sites. The final diagnosis is given by regional biopsy. The stages are considered as follows: stage I, when there is only a mass in the breast; stage II, when enlarged nodes are found in the corresponding axilla; stage III, when the tumor infiltrates neighboring skin or bones, and the axillary nodes are fixed; and stage IV, when there are metastases.

Treatment will be evaluated for each individual patient, depending on extent and age. It will be a radical mastectomy, or a simple mastectomy with radiation. Hormonal therapy will start with estrogens and be followed with androgens according to the response. Chemotherapy (fluorouracil or thiotepa) will be used as a last resort.

Diethylstilbestrol; give 10 to 15 mg every day.

Testosterone propionate; inject intramuscularly 100 mg, three times a week.

The *inflammatory breast carcinoma* presents symptoms like the above, but the growth is very rapid, there is local pain, and the covering skin is red and warm. The disease is always fatal, and any form of treatment usually disappointing.

Fibroadenoma of the breast is also a very frequent disease, more frequently found during earlier years, appearing as a capsulated mass, nonadherent to neighboring tissues, elastic, without nipple retraction and adenopathies, and painless. Surgical removal is the logical approach.

Cystic mastitis remnants will rarely be seen after the climacteric. Cysts are nonadherent, painless, and usually (but not necessarily) multiple and bilateral. Surgery is the most widely recommended approach, though it has to be evaluated at a time when these cysts have a spontaneous tendency to disappear.

Intraductal papilloma, which is rare, may be felt on palpation, but it can be so small as to be impossible to palpate. The main symptom, then, is a bloody discharge from the nipple, which will be examined at short intervals, for diagnostic purposes. Surgery is the treatment of choice.

Cystosarcoma phylloides grows very rapidly and usually reaches a great size. It must be carefully and totally removed; otherwise, it may recur.

Tuberculosis of the breast is very rare these days, but may occur, affecting the upper outer quadrant following an injury to a patient carrying the infection. It starts as an inflammatory, painful nodulation; the skin soon becomes inflamed, and some of the symptoms of cancer (orange-like skin, retraction of the nipple, and so on) may also occur. Finally, suppuration and fluctuation will take place. It is best to perform an early biopsy. Treat tuberculosis.

Breast abscess very rarely will occur without lactation. The abscess symptoms will give the diagnosis. Treat with antibiotics and drainage.

Gynecomastia will occur not rarely among older patients, either unilateral or bilateral. It is a tender nodule located at the site of the normal gland. These patients may be running a previous liver cirrhosis, may have a testicular tumor, may be hyperthyroid, or may use estrogens, reserpine, or methyldopa. In case of diagnostic doubt, ask for a biopsy. Most cases will resolve spontaneously, for which reason surgery will be delayed for at least 2 years.

Prostate

Prostatic tumors are only detected by rectal examination, a procedure to carry out with all patients complaining of pollakiuria, dysuria or urinary retention, nocturia, abnormal urinary stream (decreased and hesitant), tenesmus, hypogastric pain, hematuria, or other, less frequent symptoms (nocturnal erections, cystitis, impotence). Naturally, in the case of urinary retention a hypogastric tumor due to the dilated bladder will be noted (usually hard and round).

Benign hypertrophy is extremely frequent. All the symptoms listed above are present in the great majority of cases. The adenoma may be of small, medium, or large size. Those of larger size may add symptoms of renal insufficiency; and more frequently than with the smaller sizes, symptoms of infection may also occur. The disappearance of the central crease of the gland will be noted by rectal examination, and then the enlargement of the lobes, which will be felt as hard (not stony) and smooth. Prostatic symptoms may worsen owing to tranquilizers and drugs used for hypertension. Also, retention may be due to ingestion of alcohol, exposure to cold, immobilization, and perhaps attempts to retain urine for prolonged periods. The main clues to differentiate it from cancer are the disappearance of the median lobe or crease, the rubbery—not stone—consistency of the gland, and the smoothness of its surface. Since the best therapeutic approach is surgical, a urologist will be consulted for final evaluation of the process.

Prostatic cancer, unfortunately, is still one of the most frequent diseases of elderly patients. The clinical picture is exactly like benign hypertrophy, perhaps without any symptoms during the earlier stages. Main differential signs are: a less bulky tumor, of stony-hard consistency, and the nodular, irregular surface; the gland is fixed to surrounding structures, and the serum acid phosphatase is elevated. An early diagnosis may help the performance of a curative radical prostatectomy. Otherwise, estrogen treatment with bilateral orchidectomy is the best procedure. Call a urologist for evaluation.

Prostatitis presents an enlarged and painful prostate gland. It will follow a previous infection, most probably affecting the urinary system. The treatment will be directed to the specific infection.

Fibromyoma of the Uterus

Most cases occur during the years of gonadal activity, but because they remain for a while or are due to estrogen therapy, others will be diagnosed during or after the climacterium. The enlargement will suggest a pregnant uterus, but it will be noted to be irregular on palpation. At this time of life, the only symptoms due to these fibromyomata are those due to pressure over the organs in the neighborhood.

Because many of these tumors will resolve by themselves at this time of life, a gynecologist will be called for evaluation of procedures to follow.

Bladder

Retention of urine in the bladder is characterized by an incomplete urinary voiding with subsequent enlargement of the organ, which is palpated in the hypogastrium as a round, smooth mass, central or lateral, more or less painful to pressure. In the chronic process with incomplete voiding there is a slow increase in bladder volume, with not too marked symptoms until those corresponding to renal insufficiency begin to appear. The acute retention is accompanied by pain and fruitless efforts to void. The following instances involve urinary retention.

Prostatic retention is the most commonly diagnosed such condition, usually starting as an incomplete retention with slow increases in volume of the bladder occurring in a patient with a prostatic tumor (see above, in this section). At times an acute retention will be the first symptom of prostatic tumor. Infection is not rare in these cases. Help the patient to void, and then treat the basic prostatic problem. First try a sedative and heat applied to the hypogastrium; then catheterize the patient.

Urethral retention may be due to impacted calculi, impacted foreign bodies, or urethritis (acute or chronic). The diagnosis of the previous urethral disease will aid in recognition of urinary retention. Patients should be hospitalized, since surgical procedures are generally needed. Treat the basic problem.

Tumors of the bladder are usually preceded by hematuria before urinary retention will occur. The carcinomatous infiltration will also cause pollakiuria, rigidity of the bladder walls, and finally pain and cachexia. In all instances of hematuria, particularly if persistent, the help of a urologist will be sought because the only diagnostic procedure is cystoscopy. The treatment is also for the urologist to decide.

Spastic neck of the bladder is a reaction that may occur in older patients who do not have prostatic hypertrophy but may react this way even to the occurrence of a more or less complete retention of urine. Perhaps, this is a form of the neurogenic bladder, q.v. in the next entry.

Neurogenic bladder results from injury to this organ or diseases of the nervous system or nervous supply. One of the important symptoms of this disease is urinary retention, either complete or with urinary overflow. Upper cord lesions may cause retention because of spasticity of the neck of the bladder, while in acute spinal injuries or injuries to the lower part of the cord, the bladder will become flaccid. Comatose patients will present urinary retention. The diagnosis depends on serial urographic studies, but the help of both a urologist and a neurologist will be required. They will evaluate both diagnosis and treatment. In cases of acute injury with urinary retention, start catheterization immediately to avoid distention. In all instances prevent infection.

Testicles

Cancer of the testicles is more frequent at younger ages, but it may appear at any time in life. The testicle is enlarged and painless; even the normal testicular pain elicited on pressure is not felt, but a dragging inguinal pain may bother the patient. The tumor very rarely will adhere to the scrotum, gynecomastia may develop, and in transillumination the tumor will not be seen. Hormonal findings may deviate from normal, according to the type of tumor. Pulmonary metastases occurs relatively early in most cases. Surgery, radiotherapy or the use of antitumoral drugs will be evaluated according to each case.

Hydrocele is a frequent disease, with an enlarged scrotum due to fluid accumulation in the tunica vaginalis; the testicle is pushed up and backward, but the gland may be found below the liquid if it mainly involves the epididymus. On palpation, fluctuation is perceived, and it appears very clear in transillumination. It has to be differentiated from testicular tumors, which do not transilluminate, and hernia which transmits abdominal pressure on coughing. In *hematocele* the symptoms are the same, but without a tumor visible in transillumination. Treatment is surgical.

Elephantiasis of the scrotum, due to filariasis or to edema from kidney tumor, can reach enormous proportions.

Epididymitis presents an inflammatory mass on the supero-posterior area of the testicle. It may be secondary to tuberculosis present elsewhere in the body, in this instance with little or no pain, and hard nodulations that alternate with caseous areas, which may fistulize. Treat the tuberculosis. If it is due to other infective agents, treat the causative factor.

Orchitis is inflammatory and painful swelling of the testicles, usually accompanied by fever and other symptoms of the causative infection (typhoid fever, pneumonia, brucellosis, and the remote possibility of mumps among older persons). Also, injuries to the testicle may cause orchitic symptoms.

Vulva

Cancer of the vulva arises from previous leukoplakia or kraurosis, in a large number of patients. The tumor is neglected because of the prevalence of itching from other causes in many instances, until it becomes locally more distinctive. Radical surgery will be considered for most patients; so consult a gynecologist.

Bartholinitis causes a periodic or more or less continuous painful swelling of either or both sides of the introitus, noted as an inflammatory tumoral mass in the inferior portion of the affected labium, which may end in abscess formation. Treat with the corresponding antibiotic, and drain whenever needed.

Penis

Venereal diseases will rarely occur, but may present the inflamed and indurated coinlike mass of the chancre found in syphilis.

Cancer of the penis occurs in the prepuce, more rarely in the penis, and is more of an ulceration than a tumor, at least at the beginning. Request a biopsy. Surgery is the only hope for cure.

"Fracture" of the shaft of the penis may follow intercourse or an external traumatism; a tense, painful mass results, with some distortion of the organ, and in some cases urinary retention. First try rest and cold applications, and use a catheter if there is retention of urine. Consult a urologist if the hematoma does not reabsorb in a reasonable time.

Plastic induration of the penis consists of a hard fibrous mass noted by palpation; the organ is curved toward that side, particularly during erection. There is no agreement yet on how to treat this disease: surgically (removal of the induration), by radiotherapy (frequent reactions), by local injection of corticoids into the fibrous mass, by administration of vitamin E, and so forth.

Infective lesions of the penis, such as phimosis, balanoposthitis, chancre, and so on, will cause swelling of the glans or the whole organ, with redness and congestion. In syphilis, the chancre will be noted as a coinlike induration, hard enough to make a whole body of the painless, punched-out ulcer.

Condyloma acuminatum is a wartlike tumoral mass, generally multiple, growing as a crown around the balano-prepucial sulcus, which may be diagnosed by simple inspection. These lesions may also be found around the vulva and the anus. Treatment is by surgical removal or local antiseptic applications, such as podophyllin.

Podophyllum resin, 20 to 25% in tincture of benzoin. Extreme care should be taken to avoid contact with uninvolved skin (wipe off immediately, if this occurs!). Allow the medication to remain in contact with the lesions for at least 8 to a maximum of 24 hours, then wash out with soap and water. Do not apply or allow to remain beneath the prepuce.

Intracranial Tumors

An efficient procedure for diagnosing intracranial tumors consists of the adequate grouping of proofs derived from symptoms of intracranial hypertension, neurologic symptoms from the location of the tumor, and the specialized techniques for detection of these masses within the skull.

The general symptomatology is as follows. Elderly persons may start the clinical picture with evidence of some form of mental deterioration, to which are added headache, vomiting (projectile, in many instances), bradypnea, bradycardia, and, with time, papilledema, meningismus, and a moderate febricula. The triad headache, projectile vomiting, and papilledema are strongly suggestive of tumoral intracranial hypertension. The spinal fluid will show increased pressure.

Focal symptoms are as follows:

Parietal lobe: contralateral hemiplegia, with motor or sensory seizures; if the left side is involved, there is also aphasia.

Temporal lobe: frequent psychomotor seizures, usually with aphasia or visual defects.

Frontal lobe: paramount mental deterioration; not rarely with convulsive seizures, aphasia, or anosmia.

Occipital lobe: mainly visual symptoms, such as hemianopsia, hallucinations, and papilledema.

Cerebellar: predominance of disturbances of coordination and equilibrium.

Thalamus: ipsilateral pains of the head, trunk, and extremities; hemianesthesia with hyperreactive sensations; and perhaps motor changes, as well.

Corpus striatum: athetosic or choreic symptoms, and intestinal hypertonus.

Corpus callosum: slowly developing hemi- or quadriplegia, or paresis, possible contracture of the left hand, mental symptoms, and ataxia.

Pontocerebellar angle: deafness, either sudden or progressive, always an important symptom; vertigo; facial paresis; lack of corneal reflex. The diagnosis should be made from the first two symptoms, deafness and vertigo.

Diagnostic aids may be very effective in achieving prompt and accurate knowledge of the cause of the syndrome being studied. A computerized scanning of the brain will give very good information about shape, size, and location of a tumoral mass. The spinal tap, electroencephalography, radiologic studies, echoencephalograms, angiography, and other tests will round out the diagnostic procedure.

For symptoms due to intracranial edema, and only in a transitory way before surgery, mannitol may be administered. Surgery is the main procedure for a complete cure; if it is not feasible, chemotherapeutic agents will be advised.

Mannitol, 10% solution, to be given intravenously.

ULCERS

A loss of the covering layers of skin or mucous surfaces constitutes an ulcer. These ulcerations are easily noted by patients themselves, who visit the physician because of them. They also fear cancer because of ulcerations; but, again, not all ulcers are cancerous. There are many of traumatic origin, and others are infective, or, more rarely, of a nervous etiology.

Carcinoma

Polypoid formation may be the initial symptom of cancer, but very frequently the patient will show a more or less ample crater of an ulceration invading more or less deeply into the tissues. If it is a grayish ulcer, it may be a basal cell epithelioma; if the ulcer is on an indurated base with a relatively hard border, an epidermoid carcinoma.

Basal cell epitheliomas are very frequent among the elderly, particularly those who are exposed to sunlight and wind, and also those exposed to irradiation, chronic nonmalignant ulcers or scars, or certain drugs. The initial papule ulcerates and shows a grayish color and a teleangiectatic translucent border. The diagnosis may be made by simple inspection, but it is better to perform a biopsy. Excision is the best curative procedure. For more details, see in the above section on "Tumors."

Epidermoid carcinomas start as keratotic papules, but soon turn into a rapidly growing ulceration, fungoid in type, with a central ulcer on an indurated based surrounded by a hard border. They may grow at mucocutaneous junctions around the mouth, the nose, the eyes, and the vulva. Diagnosis depends on biopsy; and an early removal is mandatory if cure is to be achieved.

Decubitus Ulcer

At pressure points, namely, sacrum area, hips, occiput, ankles, elbows, heels, and ears, decubitus ulcers will start as red, tender erythemas, in patients confined to bed for long periods. At a second stage the affected area turns cyanotic and indurated. Finally, it will vesiculate, or it will go directly into ulceration because of tissue necrosis, which is the terminal stage, not rarely invading tissues to the bone. The diagnosis is easy because the patient is usually a thin, debilitated, aged, bedridden subject. The occurrence will be more likely if the patient is paralyzed.

Prevention is the best treatment, since in a great number of cases decubitus ulcers announce carelessness on the part of the nursing personnel; patients will be turned at least once every hour, and helping devices will be used whenever necessary. Developed ulcers will need the same procedures as for prevention, plus local care and surgery if sufficiently extensive and deep.

Gout

Only in late stages of chronic gout, one or more of the affected joints will ulcerate, and there will be, perhaps, a secretion rich in urates. Because this situation will occur after several more or less typical gouty attacks have occurred, the diagnosis will be easily established. For confirmation, request measurement of uric acid levels, which will be above 8 mg%. For more information see other entries in this book.

Leprosy

Mainly the nodules in nodular or lepromatous leprosy will ulcerate to cause extensive mutilations. From these ulcers the mycobacteria are relatively easily isolated. The diagnosis depends entirely on the evaluation of the former symptoms of nodular infiltration of the skin of the face, and the dorsum of hands and feet. In the tuberculoid type, there will be little ulceration of tissues; but the macular spots are anesthetic. Bacteria can be recovered for diagnosis from the nasal septum. For treatment, start with dapsone, or any other sulfone drug. For more information see the corresponding entry in the above section on "Tumors."

Ulcers on the Ankles

Any ulcerative disease can express its symptomatology at the ankles; but the two most frequent causes will be discussed here, namely, varicose ulcers and ulcers due to arterial occlusion.

Varicose ulcers are not rare among older people, either those presenting large varicose veins or those with almost invisible varicosities. These ulcers are noted at the lower half or lower third of the leg, and show a reddish hamlike color, with irregular vertical borders. They are very similiar to syphilitic ulcers, but do not present the indurated base. There is usually one ulcer on the affected ankle, but multiple ulcers are not rare, the size ranging from a few millimeters to a few centimeters. A good diagnostic sign will be the presence of extensive dilation and tortuosity of the corresponding veins, which may be accompanied by weakness and fatigability of the muscles of the leg, cramps, ankle edema that may disappear during bed rest, and other vague uncomfortable sensations.

A conservative treatment will always be tried first, unless lesions are too extensive or threatening. Start with bed rest (the leg higher than the thigh and the thigh higher than the heart), keeping the ulcer moist and clean with a saline warm dressing; and as a second step, use an Unna's paste boot or a zinc gelatin bandage. If there is infection, use antibiotics. Evaluation of surgery will be done in consultation with a specialist.

Arterial occlusion will cause gangrene if suddenly established, but more of an ulceration if progress is slow. This is not a rare occurrence among diabetics, or those with neurologic problems, particularly those with senile changes. When the arterial occlusion causes gangrene, this is preceded by a more or less extended phase of true ulceration. This ulceration may be at the ankles, but more frequently will be noted at the distal portion of the limbs. Oscillometry will show a frankly diminished oscillometric pattern for the extremity. Treatment is better followed with a specialist, since the surgical procedures will vary according to the particular lesions involved. The first attention will be given to those with acute occlusion, by means of epidural injection of procaine or papaverine, and the use of anticoagulants.

Procaine, 1.5% solution; inject about 25 ml epidurally.

Heparin, 10,000 units by injection (either route), adjusting dosage according to clotting time, to between 20 and 30 minutes.

Warfarin, to be started at the same time as heparin (the latter to be discontinued as soon as warfarin begins to work), 10 to 20 mg, dosage to be adjusted according to prothrombin time (between 15 to 30% of normal).

Tuberculosis

These ulcers are of an irregular size and shape, and the borders are detached from the deeper layers, where granulated ulcerations are found and surrounded by a violet halo. There may be pain, caseous material, and fistulization. Diagnosis is made by detection of the *Mycobacterium;* and perhaps by finding the lesions around the mouth or the anus in patients with chronic tuberculosis.

Treatment is that of tuberculosis and local cleansing.

Actinomycosis

These are very deep ulcers, even reaching bones or other organs, mainly with typical fistulae (discharging from several sinuses a yellowish pus containing the causal *Actinomyces*). The lesions are mainly noted in the cervicofacial area, at times following a tooth extraction or revealing bone rarefaction. As already indicated, the diagnosis is made by finding the *Actinomyces* in the pus from the ulcers.

The treatment of choice is penicillin, first by injection for 1 or 1½ months, followed by the oral route, until several months after all lesions are completely healed. Sulfonamides may add some help.

> Penicillin; give 12 to 20 million units a day by injection, during 1 or 1½ months (less if possible); to change to penicillin V potassium, 1.6 million units (1 g) every day.

Ulcers of the Tongue

Traumatic ulcers are noted in relation to a tooth, usually badly infected, and may have an indurated base. Others are due to prosthetic devices, and they may even be produced by chronic cough. In most instances the diagnosis is evident. The treatment consists of cleansing the site and avoiding further irritation.

Cancer is relatively frequent in older patients, most frequently among men. It may appear at any site, mostly on the borders, the dorsum, or the frenulum of the tongue and not rarely in relation to a previous lesion of leukoplakia. It may be suspected when the patient is unable to protrude the tongue from the mouth. In these cases the only hope of cure is surgery, if in time.

Tuberculous ulcers are similar to those found on the skin, with irregular size and shape, detached borders, granulomatous ulcerations, and the coexistence of a previous known tuberculous lesion. Keep the site clean, and treat the tuberculosis.

Syphilis will cause primary and then secondary lesions. The chancre will occur most frequently in the tip of the tongue, most likely as an indolent erosion; in the secondary lesions try to obtain a pertinent serodiagnosis, particularly if multiple lesions are found. Treat with penicillin or other specific antibiotic.

Glanders

Glanders is not a frequent disease, affecting mostly those involved with horses or other equines, and usually developing a painful ulcer at the site of infection and other ulcers first in the nose but also in the pharynx and the larynx. The disease may start abruptly with elevated temperature and chills, headache, and prostration. Lymphangitis and adenitis are the rule with these ulcers. Rhinitis, when it occurs, gives a typical course to the disease; the mucosa swells and ulcerates, the secretion turns purulent and sanguinolent, and respiration becomes difficult. There may also be a chronic form, but in the chronic cases the ulcers look like abscesses close to an articulation. The diagnosis is made by identification of the causative germ, preferably before the ulcers open.

This is a very severe disease, and the treatment must start as early as possible. Use the specific antibiotic, or a combination of two antibiotics.

Sufadiazine, 500 mg tablets; take 4 to 12 tablets a day in divided doses until complete clearance of symptoms.

Chlortetracycline; 250 mg tablets, take four a day between meals; if the case is too severe, favor injection.

Chloramphenicol, 250 mg tablets; take four a day between meals; or take it by injection if the case is too severe.

Streptomycin, 500 mg by intramuscular injection, repeated every 6 hours. All the antibiotics are to be used until complete clearance of all symptomatology.

Vulvar Ulcers

Herpes genitalis starts with vesicles but ends with ulceration. There are fever, chills, and other symptoms. This is associated with herpes virus 2, which is carcinogenic. Check for serum antibodies. Cleanse the area. Try to differentiate herpes simplex and zoster. For more details see "Ulcers of the Penis," the next entry.

Syphilis, very rare in old age, may present the initial chancre as a punched-out ulcer, coinlike, indurated, hard to the touch, painless, with adenitis (no pain, not purulent), and the characterisitic serodiagnosis. Treatment is carried out with penicillin or any suitable antibiotic. For other stages, the diagnosis is more difficult, mostly depending on serology.

Acute vulvar ulcer is in a way somewhat similar to aphthous stomatitis, which may simulate other diseases, but has a tendency to spontaneous resolution and frequent recurrences. Keep the area clean.

Chancroid finally forms a soft painful ulcer from the initial macule or vesicopustule. The base is necrotic, and the lesion erythematous and accompanied by painful adenitis with matted nodes. Usually there are fever and chills; and the culture gives the final diagnosis (the causative *Hemophilus*). The treatment consists of local cleansing (soap and water), aspiration of buboes, and administration of tetracycline or sulfisoxazole.

Tetracycline; give 500 mg, four times a day, by mouth, for 2 weeks.

Ulcers of the Penis

Cancer of the penis begins as an ulcer rather than a tumor; it seems to be similar to a chancre, but with irregular borders; it bleeds easily, and the corresponding adenopathy is late in occurring. If in doubt, perform a biopsy, and treat with surgery.

Balanitis will present an ulcerated mucosa, inflamed, red, and with a purulent discharge. This may occur in cases of obesity, diabetes, or simply old age; it must be differentiated from other more serious infectious diseases. In all instances a culture and perhaps a serodiagnostic test will be made. The treatment will consist of local cleansing and the adequate antibiotic.

Syphilis, again, is rare in old age. It will present the chancre as a punch-out, coinlike indurated ulcer, hard to the touch, with no pain in the corresponding adenitis, and with the characteristic serology. The ulcers corresponding to other stages are so varied that it is much better to depend on the serology. Treat with penicillin or any other suitable antibiotic.

Herpes will start with vesicles, but will end in ulceration. The diagnosis will be that of herpes genitalis (due to herpes virus 2) or simplex or zoster. In the first case herpes antivirus will be checked for diagnosis. Generally the beginning of herpes simplex is itching and burning, while that of herpes zoster is pain and a radicular distribution of vesicles.

Gangrene

This is the death of tissues, usually due to loss of vascular supply of nutrients followed by bacterial infection and final putrefaction, restricted to more or less ample areas, and usually manifested as dry gangrene (less infected, or not at all) or moist gangrene with a varied symptomatology.

Senile gangrene is due to arteriosclerosis after 70 years of age. It appears in the legs, is preceded by symptoms of sclerosis (intermittent claudication), and particularly pain in bed, and is relieved by sitting with the legs hanging down. Try surgery, improve blood supply, or give symptomatic treatment.

Diabetic gangrene is similar to senile gangrene, but occurs in a diabetic.

Thromboangiitis obliterans rarely will appear in later years.

Drug gangrene is due to ergotism, epinephrine, or local application of caustics.

Physical agents (cold, heat, electricity, radiation, and so on) may cause gangrene.

Other causes may be nervous diseases, Raynaud's disease, trauma, infection, and all possible causes of gangrene that usually require surgical treatment, or at least the advice of a specialist.

XIV. SKIN PROBLEMS

The aged patient presents multiple problems related to the skin, some of them discussed in the foregoing paragraphs and others left for grouping here as follows: (1) itching, (2) pain, (3) vesicles, (4) lymph nodes, (5) jaundice, (6) maculae papules, (7) pigmentations, (8) erythema, and (9) bleeding. There are final sections devoted to reactions to drugs and location of symptoms.

ITCHING

The first problem to consider when an elderly person complains of itching is diabetes, but also senile itching may be a very important symptom. Other diseases to consider here are kraurosis, radiodermatitis, gout, jaundice, uremia, Hodgkin's disease, leukemia, neurodermatitis, and other toxic and allergic causes of itching.

Diabetes Mellitus

Pruritus is one of the first symptoms of diabetes among the elderly. Unfortunately, itching is a very frequent complaint in this age group; consequently, efforts will be made to determine the true nature of the symptoms by searching for other common initial symptoms occurring at this time. In the first place, consider asthenia or easy fatigability—which may be due to different causes! Also, any of the frequent complications of the disease may accompany or precede itching; retinopathy, neuropathy, nephropathy, or a less characteristic arteriosclerotic complex. If blood circulation to the lower extremities is impaired, there will be local coldness, drying, scaling, and cracking of the skin. Do not wait for coma (ketoacidotic or hyperosmolar nonketonic), polydypsia with polyuria, or polyphagia with weight loss, to make the diagnosis. Suspicion of diabetes will be aroused by any person over 60 or 70 years of age complaining of pruritus, particularly if accompanied by asthenia, blurred vision, retinitis or initial cararact, paresthesias, previous attacks of hypoglycemia (confusion, sweating, dizziness, hunger), or any early manifestations of usual complications (arteriosclerosis obliterans—with or without gangrene; retinopathy—microaneurisms, exudates, hemorrhage, cataract, glaucoma; sensory neuropathies with lightning pains or numbness, neurogenic diarrhea, foot lesions, nephropathy, and infections, of the skin or systemic). Do not forget that a large number of older diabetics are obese (66%), and a large number are hypertensive (50%).

Pruritus may also be induced by drugs, of which a large number may cause itching, so that the diagnosis may depend upon knowledge of drug administration; by liver diseases, usually accompanied by jaundice, spider angiomas, and the corresponding elevation of bilirubin or other liver tests; by cancer, also accompanied by weight loss and local signs, and detected by X-ray examination and biopsy; by anemia, usually revealed by pallor, weakness, blood counts, and possibly lymphadenopathy or splenomegaly; by skin disease, with rash, such as rosacea (center of face), eczema, pemphigus, or diseases with parasites, such as lice, crabs, or scabies; and by other diseases, such as Hodgkin's disease, polycythemia, myxedema, nephropathies, gout, and reticulosis, among others. Finally, care will be taken to differentiate it from psychogenic pruritus, usually with other symptoms of a stress situation, as in forced retirement; and above all the very frequent senile pruritis must be ruled out, with drying of the skin, exacerbated during fall and winter, and showing xerosis of the lower legs (reticulation, rhomboidal, phomboidal scaling).

Laboratory diagnosis depends on the finding of glycemic levels over 120 mg%, fasting, or over 215 mg%, 2-hour postprandial (245 mg% after 70 years of age).

Usual complications are the ketoacidotic, marked asthenia, confusion, polydypsia, and ketoaciduria, which end in diabetic coma; decreased blood flow to leg and foot, with coolness, cramps, pain (at rest), claudication, and lack of pulsations, with possible ulceration and gangrene; retinopathy, as microaneurisms, hemorrhages, exudates, newly formed vessels, and final blindness if allowed to progress; blurred vision, also due to cataracts or glaucoma; coronary artery insufficiency, angina, or infarction; and glomerulosclerosis with edema, hypertension, elevated blood urea and creatinine, which may lead to uremia; then sclerosis of brain vessels with mental deterioration and a possible final stroke; neuropathy of any type, sensory (lower leg symptoms), motor (paresias or paralysis) or visceral (diarrhea or postural hypotension); infections of the lungs, the genitourinary system, and mainly the skin; and also other complications of the mouth, the eye (other than the retina), the pancreas, the gall bladder, bones, or joints, all easily related to the diabetic cause.

Treatment starts with diet alone, or insulin is added if a satisfactory control is not achieved, namely, fasting blood sugar below 130% or below 150 mg%, 2-hour postprandial. Give no less than 150 g of carbohydrate and 80 g of protein. Weekly adjustments will add lente or NPH insulin if there is no control: 20 units before breakfast if glycosuria is + + + +; or 10 units, if only + +. Tolbutamide (1500 mg a day), acetohexamide (500, rarely 750 mg twice a day), tolazamide, or chlorpropamide are the recommended oral antidiabetics; including phenformia (50 mg b.i.d. of the long-acting preparation) for the obese diabetic patient.

Senile Itching

This is one of the most troublesome symptoms that may affect elderly people. It must be stated that it is not truly due to senility but to lesions of vascular, uremic, or hepatic origin, without which the itching will very rarely be present. Also, it may be provoked by excessive dryness of the skin due to overuse of soaps and bathing, and, at the present time, by the use of heating during the wintertime without the necessary humidification of the air. When the older patient complains of itching, try to diagnose the cause, if possible, because its treatment may improve the condition.

Try to treat the causative factor, if known; and avoid the use of unnecessary measures that may irritate the skin. Wet the skin with water, and apply petrolatum thereafter to keep the moisture in place. Rarely, the skin will be too moist, and then the use of drying agents will be recommended. Do not allow the patient to bathe too often; advise just the necessary cleansing of the body, better with the use of bath oils. Only in very difficult cases may the use of corticosteroids be recommended, particularly in restricted areas of lesions that cause itching. Also, antihistaminics will be used in some selected cases that could be allergic in origin.

Petrolatum, ointment; apply locally.

Bath oil, any one of the well-known brands, such as Alfa-Keri, Lubath, Nivea, and others.

Cyproheptadine, 4 mg tablets; take one, three or four times a day.

Kraurosis of the Vulva

Itching from a lesion of leukoplakia is characterized as kraurosis of the vulva, with atrophic changes, smoothness, the labia also atrophic, all appearing whitish or slightly pigmented. It will not be mistaken for diabetes, particularly when both conditions exist in one patient. Itching is the most characteristic symptom.

Large doses of vitamin A have been advised, and have been beneficial to many patients. Some advise using it together with dilute amounts of hydrochloric acid. Also estrogen therapy has been of some use. But care should be taken not to confound these areas with malignancies which require surgery.

Radiodermatitis

Radiodermatitis occurs as a reaction to excessive amounts of radiation, generally following radiotherapy for malignant diseases. The first effect noted is an itching erythema localized at the site of the radiation and accompanied by falling-out of hair. According to the dose received, other general effects may also occur, such as depression of the blood-forming organs or even their total destruction, dysfunction of the gonads if still relatively active, and other inflammatory or ulcerative lesions in any of the organs in the vicinity of the action of the active rays.

There is no known treatment; only symptomatic help will be given to these patients. Give transfusions of whole blood if needed, or even of marrow cells. Electrolytes and antibiotics will be used in all instances when needed.

Gout

Not rarely pruritus will be felt in gout, particularly during recovery from acute attacks. Also, in chronic or atypical forms of gout some sort of itching may be noted. Nevertheless, the acute attack is characterized by pain, redness, heat, and swelling in the affected joint, most frequently at the base of the great toe. It comes with general complaints of fever, chills, and tachycardia.

Colchicine is the drug of choice, the response being so effective that when it fails, the diagnosis may be doubted. For more details, see other, more detailed entries in this book.

Uremia

In chronic uremia the diagnosis is already made; but either as a warning or simply as a finding, pruritus may be extremely intense, revealing the intensity of the intoxication. These cachectic stages are relatively frequent among older patients, especially when there are also arteriosclerotic changes involved. A very interesting feature of the pruritus is its increase following almost any form of internal medication, which the physician must always have in mind. With these patients, check the mental condition first, and their stability of character. Neuromuscular changes are frequent, as well as gastrointestinal manifestations and hypertension in advanced cases. The laboratory diagnosis will depend on the finding of elevated nitrogenous components, anemia, and acidosis; and a urine of fixed density, casts, and proteinuria. Uremia is generally a late stage of glomerulonephritis, with predominance of proteinuria, hematuria, and urine casts; or nephrosclerosis, with hypertension with renal insufficiency, chronic pyelonephritis, and persistent bacteriuria.

Each causative disease should be treated. Give a diet of no more than 1 g of protein for each 2 kilos of body weight, with essential amino acids and sufficient vitamins and calories. Fluids, sodium, potassium, calcium, and phosphate will depend on individual findings. If dialysis seems to be needed, discuss the problem with a specialist.

Hodgkin's Disease

This disease, very rare among elderly persons, may start with pruritus, enlarged lymph nodes (a frequent initial symptom), and sweating. The enlarged adenopathies are firm and painless, reach different sizes, and may adhere to deeper structures but not to the skin. Mediastinal lymph nodes can obstruct respiration. Fever is low or absent among the elderly. In the case of a patient with pruritus, adenopathies, and sweating, ask for a biopsy of a lymph node. The state of the disease is estimated as follows: stage I, with a single adenopathy; stage II, with two or more discrete nodules on one side above the diaphragm; stage III, as above, but on both sides; and stage IV, extensive involvement outside the lymph node area.

Enlist a specialist to check the treatment. Irradiate a large field, 3000 or 4000 Rad in 4 weeks, on isolated regional groups, for stages I, II, and III. For stages III and IV it is better to give immunosuppressive agents, (nitrogen mustard, chlorambucil, and vinblastine). Maximum advantage with minimum risk will be obtained by combined therapy with procarbazine, prednisone, nitrogen mustard, and vincristine (or a similar combination):

Weeks 1–2:   Procarbazine, 150 to 200 mg daily.
Prednisone, 60 mg daily.
Nitrogen mustard, intravenous injection of 7 to 10 mg, only on days 1 and 8.
Vincristine, intravenous injection of 2 to 4 mg, only on days 1 and 8.
Weeks 3–4:   Rest.
Weeks 5–6:   As weeks 1–2, but without prednisone.
Weeks 7–8:   Rest.
Weeks 9–10:   As weeks 5–6.
Weeks 11–12:   Rest.
Weeks 13–14:   Repeat completely the first 2 weeks of treatment.

Leukemia

In practically all forms of leukemia a relatively intense pruritus may occur, perhaps before other symptoms. That is, a combination of pruritus with fever may be suggestive. Soon, there may be added sore throat, enlargement of the lymph nodes in several regions of the body including splenomegaly and hepatomegaly, and bleeding in the form of petechiae or ecchymoses with thrombocytopenia and the particular hemogram for each variety of leukemia, namely, acute myelocytic, acute lymphocytic, and so on.

Ask a specialist to handle the treatment, since each variety responds better to a particular drug schedule, such as a start with Cytoxan, Oncovin, Ara-C, and prednisone for acute myelocytic leukemia; or vincristine and prednisone, for acute lymphocytic leukemia.

Neurodermatitis

Pruritus starts the symptomatology on a normal skin, which secondarily becomes lichenoid because of the continuous scratching (diamond-shaped lesions bordered by normal tiny dermic creases). The most common sites for these lesions are the arms and legs, but also the neck, the face, the anus, and the pudenda.

Psychotherapy is very important. Minor tranquilizers may also be of minor help. The best topical treatment is the application of corticosteroids.

Diazepam, 2 mg tablets; give half or one tablet every 8 hours.

Dexamethasone cream, to apply locally.

Cyproheptadine, 4 mg tablets; take half or one tablet every 8 hours.

Parasitism

Check in all cases for parasites, and act accordingly.

PAIN

There are a large number of diseases, either dermatological or general, that may cause skin pain. A complete list is practically impossible. The following list may be supplemented by examining the corresponding chapter on "Pain" earlier in this book. Also, see our book on *Pain: From Symptom to Treatment.*

Acne

This is a disease of youth, when the activity of gonadal hormones starts; it is rarely seen in the elderly, whose pilosebaceous follicles show very little energy; but it may be seen, particularly following gonadal therapy, when that is used. Pain, moderate but increased with pressure, starts the symptoms. Lesions are superficial and begin as a comedo, which develops into a papule, then a pustule, and finally a scar. Acne centers on the face and head, and the upper parts of the chest and back.

These painful lesions only require warm compresses; only when there is a frank collection of pus will an incision with a small scalpel be warranted. To avoid new lesions, tetracycline or clindamycin have been recommended.

Folliculitis

The clinical course is similar to that of acne with the main difference being a deeper setting in this instance. Pain is more intense, and inflammation more prominent. The lesion is a small nodule surrounding a hair, and may end in pustulation.

Cleanse with sodium bicarbonate solution, and continue wet compresses for at least 15 minutes. Use local antibiotic ointments or creams, such as neomycin or any other similiar drug. Systemic antibiotic therapy will be used if the above measures fail.

Sodium bicarbonate, 3% solution (8 teaspoonfuls to 1 liter of tap water).

Neomycin, 1% ointment or cream; apply locally every 6 to 8 hours.

Furuncle

Occasionally, aged patients will present furuncles rather than acne or folliculitis. The infection is greater in furunculosis, invading the perifollicular area. There is a very painful elevated pustule with necrosis of its central portion. Pain is more intense in the fingers, nose, and ears. Furuncles also center in the axillae, breasts, and buttocks, but may be found anywhere in the body.

Treatment is as for acne, indicated above.

Carbuncle

Several furuncles develop in the same area and are confluent. Pain and inflammation are considerable. Cellulitis extends to the surrounding area, and the tumor makes a frank elevation above the skin level. Systemic manifestations (fever, malaise) are the rule. The presence of several openings draining pus is diagnostic.

Use the adequate antibiotic systemically; otherwise, choose the proper broad-spectrum antibiotic. Moist heat may help to allay pain and localize the process. Mature lesions may be incised superficially, and the area protected with antibiotic ointments or creams (preferably, the specific one), covered with bandages. At times, analgesics are needed.

Pustules

These are small purulent lesions centering superficially in the skin, which may be due to different clinical entities, being the late stage of acne, folliculitis, furuncle, carbuncle, chicken pox, smallpox, herpes, and the like. The most important is the so-called malignant pustule, or anthrax, ordinarily originating on the hand, arm, face, or neck. Anthrax presents little or no pain, but the enlarged lymph nodes are frequently painful. The dark pustule surrounded by a red halo and showing vesicles is characteristic.

Treat as carbuncle, described above.

Pemphigus

Characteristic for diagnostic purposes is the appearance of large vesicles or bullae directly arising from a normal skin or mucosa (no erythematous halo around the vesicle). As soon as the bulla breaks, there is a painful erosion in the skin. Diagnosis is suggested when the epidermis can be easily detached from the dermis by lateral pressure (Nikolsky's sign); but in cases of difficult diagnosis a biopsy of the skin is mandatory (acantholysis detected by the Tzanck test). Anti-intercellular antibodies have been detected.

The patient should be hospitalized, for better care. Intravenous infusions (blood, feeding) may be needed. Bed rest is imperative. Local skin lesions will be treated with wet dressings; soothing mouthwashes should be given before eating; and the basic treatment will include very large doses of corticoids, better directed by a specialist, who will also evaluate the need for immunosuppressive therapy.

Sodium bicarbonate, 3% solution (8 teaspoonfuls in 1 liter of tap water).

Neomycin, 1% solution; use as such.

Tetracaine, 2% solution; instill a few drops.

Prednisone, up to 150 mg, by injection, the first day; to be continued by oral administration, decreasing the dosage rapidly to maintenance levels.

Impetigo

In the first stage of impetigo the vesicles are swollen, and the erosive surface is frankly purulent. As soon as the vesicle breaks, the lesion becomes painful. It is easily autoinoculated.

Keep the area clean, and keep it wet with compresses, for at least 15 minutes, every 12 hours. Larger lesions must be opened, and the necrotic tissue trimmed away; then cover the lesion with antibiotic ointments or creams.

Sodium bicarbonate, 3% solution (add 8 teaspoonfuls to 1 liter of tap water).

Neomycin, 1% ointment or cream; apply every 6 to 8 hours.

Ecthyma

There is a painful, shallow ulcer covered with a crust, surrounded by an erythematous halo, with a history of a previous impetigo, or a previous trauma. The lower parts of the legs are most frequently afflicted.
Treat as impetigo.

Cellulitis

Be on the alert when an elderly person develops fever, chills, and local change in any area of the skin, which becomes swollen, red, warm, painful, and tender. There is usually a previous local infection, and it is not rare that cellulitis reappears at the same site. Deep cellulitis is more difficult to detect (local discomfort, pain and tenderness, and generalized symptoms). Anaerobic infections are shown by crepitation of trapped gases when the skin is pressed, and the secretion has a bad odor. Leukocytosis and elevated erythrosedimentation rate are reported. Whenever possible, try to obtain a culture and determine the sensitivity of the offending germs to antibiotics.
Rest and elevation of the affected part (usually a leg), local heat, analgesics, and antipyretics are good treatment. The basic treatment is the use of the specific antibiotic, or start with a penicillase-resistant penicillin. Use gas gangrene antitoxin, if it is found applicable.

Nafcillin, 500 mg to 1 g, by intravenous injection, every 4 to 6 hours; may change to oral administration, 1 g every 4 to 6 hours, after improvement is noted. Continue for some 4 days after complete disappearance of local and general symptomatology.

Oxacillin, to be given as indicated above for nafcillin.

Cephalothin, 500 mg to 1 g; by intramuscular or intravenous injection, every 4 to 6 hours (do not give over 6 g a day by i.v.).

Gas gangrene antitoxin, 50,000 units, by intravenous injection, every 4 to 6 hours, in addition to high doses of penicillin and adequate surgery, when anaerobes are present.

Erysipelas

There is fever, moderate, but practically always with chills. A bright red spot starting near the nose or mouth, or from a fissure anywhere on the body, is almost diagnostic. Relatively soon, it spreads, forming a red and swollen area with a sharply demarcated and slightly elevated border. Vesicles or bullae may or may not be present. The causative germ is a beta-hemolytic streptococcus. Constant findings are elevated erythrosedimentation rate and a marked leukocytosis.

Nontreated erysipelas is lethal to the older patient, but the use of a specific antibiotic is almost sure to be curative. Penicillin is the first choice, but erythromycin, cephalosporin, and so on, may be used. Local treatment will be of help, with bed rest, hot packs, and acetylsalicylic acid.

> Crystalline penicillin G, 300,000 to 600,000 units or more, if needed, by intramuscular or intravenous injection, every 3 to 6 hours. The antibiotic is to be given for at least 2 to 4 days after disappearance of local and systemic symptoms.

Abscesses

Abscesses are deep infections leading to purulent painful tumors that usually terminate in fluctuation, which is the warning sign. They mostly follow local infections (injections, osteomyelitis, and so on) or visceral infections (prostate, kidney, and so forth). In each particular instance the local symptomatology depends on the site of the infection, which is added to a general infective syndrome, usually with fever, tachycardia, and malaise. Brief information will be given here.

Intracranial abscesses will provoke headache, convulsions, and increased intracranial pressure with vomiting and papilledema. They usually depend on previous known infections.

Dentoalveolar abscesses are secondary to a previous suppurative pulpitis; they provoke local inflammation of the gums and edema of the face.

Peritonsillar and *retropharyngeal abscesses* cause severe sore throat with swelling and tenderness of the pharynx, and finally pus formation.

Spinal epidural abscess causes severe pain in the back as the first symptom. It is aggravated by motion of the spine and accompanied by neurological reactions, as paresis or paralysis or paresthesias.

Hepatic abscess is amebic in origin with pain on the right side of the epigastrium, exaggerated by motion and radiating to the lower chest or right shoulder. There is a similar syndrome provoked by *subdiaphragmatic abscess,* but the elevation of the right hemidiaphragm disclosed by X-ray will establish the diagnosis.

Perirenal abscesses start abruptly with fever, chills, prostration, pain in the corresponding costovertebral angle, nausea, and vomiting, and tenderness on palpation. The roentgenographic examination will give the diagnosis.

In a large number of cases abscesses may be treated as carbuncle; but also in many instances they require a specialized treatment, particularly with surgery (at least, for drainage), and mainly large doses of specific or broad-spectrum antibiotics.

Hidradenitis Suppurativa

Because of the decay of sweat glands this is not as frequent a disease in the elderly as in younger people, but it still may occur as a firm and painful tumor in the axilla, showing the infection of a sweat gland; it may be present in the nipple or the anogenital area as well. The distinction has to be made from furuncle, which is more painful and less firm than hidradenitis.

In the axilla, pain is always annoying, requiring compresses at the beginning; but when there is a collection of pus, only an incision with a small scalpel will control it. In severe cases, the affected glands must eventually be removed surgically. While the lesions are painful, an analgesic may be helpful. Antibiotic therapy, if specific against a sensitive germ, might be curative.

Herpes Simplex

Most cases will occur as a mild disease, showing only the vesicular lesions. Others will occur following an acute illness and present fever and chills. The clinical picture will show a cluster of small vesicles appearing on the face or on any other part of the body, most frequently around the mouth or the genitals; the base is erythematous; the attack may be accompanied by pain, burning, or itching, and regional adenitis may be present with variable tenderness of the enlarged glands. After a few days, the vesicles dry and form a crust, but in moist areas they may be secondarily infected. It is not rare that after a time a second attack of herpes simplex appears at the same site as the first. Clinically, some resemblance to herpes simplex might be shown by herpes zoster, impetigo, varicella, drug eruptions, lymphogranuloma venereum, chancroid, and even syphilis. Diagnosis is confirmed by culture of the virus, increased serum antibodies, and biopsy (all this mainly needed for vaginal herpes).

Avoid the possible precipitating factors, such as fever, nervous tension, sunburn, or indigestion, for prevention of recurrent attacks. Do not forget that *corticosteroids are positively contraindicated in herpes simplex*. There are contradictory reports (but any of these remedies should be tried) on the favorable effects of local application of ether for cutaneous lesions, or idoxuridine (IDU) for use in superficial herpetic keratitis. Methylene blue solution applied and followed by white light exposure has been recommended for herpetic ulcerations in the mouth. Usually, drying agents are recommended, such as camphor spirit, bismuth formic iodide, 70% alcohol, or epinephrine solutions. Since moisture worsens the lesions, when they appear in wet areas dust them with the bismuth powder or use a lotion.

Anesthetic ether; apply a soaked gauze or cotton sponge for a few minutes.

Aqueous methylene blue, 0.1%, applied to ulcers, followed immediately by direct exposure of the area to sunlight or white light for 10 minutes.

Idoxuridine, 0.1% solution, one drop to the affected eye once an hour during the day and every 2 hours during sleep time.

Bismuth formic iodide, powder; apply locally twice a day.

Corn starch, 12 g, and zinc oxide, 12 g.

Glycerin, 6 cc.

Lime water, 60 ml.

Epinephrine, 1:100 solution; apply locally twice a day.

Herpes Zoster

People over 50 years of age are the usual victims of the disease, and they are the ones who particularly suffer from the residual pain following fever and chills. The vesicular rash of herpes zoster starts similarly to that of herpes simplex: tense vesicles on an erythematous base, the base perhaps less inflamed. The differences are in the distribution, always along the path of a nerve for herpes zoster. Pain most frequently precedes the eruption and persists during the course of the disease, and very frequently increases, even after disappearance of the lesions. Incidence is more marked in the cranial nerve area or in the intercostal nerves, but any nerve may be involved, almost always only on one side of the body—although herpes zoster, rarely, may be generalized. At times gastrointestinal disturbances may occur.

Bed rest is indicated for most patients; and even hospitalization, in severe cases. Oral analgesics will be given in cases that either respond well or do not show great intensity of symptoms. In herpes zoster *in contrast to herpes simplex,* corticoids are helpful, as the basic treatment. Local care should be carried out as for herpes simplex (see above). An ophthalmologist should be consulted when the ophthalmic nerve is involved. Residual neuralgia (which occurs in 10% of elderly patients) may respond to the local injection of corticoids or a local anesthetic.

Prednisolone, 10 mg, every 6 hours for the first 4 days; then reduce the dosage gradually, and terminate its administration at an even more gradual pace.

Triamcinolone acetonide, 40 mg by intragluteal injection, to start therapy, but not to be repeated; or:

Triamcinolone acetonide, 40 mg, suspension: infiltrate the affected area.

Lidocaine, 2% solution; infiltrate 1 to 5 ml into the affected area; this procedure may be repeated if needed.

Other forms of herpes zoster may show certain other characteristics, but are easily diagnosed and treated in many cases. But in cases of *otic herpes zoster* there may be a sudden onset of pain, a sensation of fullness in the ear, tinnitus, and slight deafness. Eventually, the characteristic vesicles appear, together with swelling of the area and a corresponding lymphadenopathy. Pain may reach an excruciating degree in cases of herpes zoster of the geniculate ganglion (7th and 8th cranial nerves may be involved). Analgesics should be given for relief; acetylsalicylic acid, codeine, a mixture of acetylsalicylic acid and codeine, meperidine, propoxyphene hydrochloride, and corticoids.

Corticoids may be useful both for pain and for the duration of the disease, which is lessened in many cases, particularly if they are given at an early date. Also, vitamin B_{12} can help.

Prednisone, 10 mg, by mouth, every 6 hours, at the start; to be decreased after 2 or 3 days, and after 7 to 10 days of therapy, to continue decreasing the dosage even more, but very gradually.

Cyanocobalamin, 1000 mg daily, by intramuscular injection, to continue for 1 or 2 weeks following disappearance of the lesions.

Intertrigo

These are inflamed opposing skin surfaces that become painful when rubbed one side against the other (beneath the breasts and in the axillae, the groins, the anal region, and even between the interdigital spaces).

The only way to avoid discomfort is to prevent rubbing of the opposed skin surfaces in the acute stage. Wet dressings may help.

Sodium chloride, 1% solution (2 teaspoonfuls in a liter of water).

Sodium bicarbonate, 3% solution (8 teaspoonfuls in a liter of water).

Potassium permanganate, 100 mg, tablet, to be dissolved in 1 liter of water (warn against discoloration of the skin and staining of clothes).

Contact Dermatitis

Allergic patients may develop the disease when they come in contact with the allergenic substances. When it reaches the state of red swelling and bullae formation, there is pain in addition to itching. Tests can help the diagnosis of this sensitivity.

In chronic cases, advise a thorough cleansing of the area, using the above solutions, and keeping the lesion protected with drying powders. The use of local treatment is advisable, even for mild cases as the only treatment; wet compresses will be applied to the lesions. Use the following:

Talcum powder.

Sodium bicarbonate, 3% solution (8 teaspoonfuls in 1 liter of water).

Patients with severe acute contact dermatitis will receive corticoids.

Prednisone, 40 mg, to start, by mouth, in three divided doses (20, 10, 10) the first day; decrease by 5 mg, each following day; discontinue gradually over 6 days.

Erythema Nodosum

This may be an independent clinical entity, ordinarily associated with systemic symptomatology; but it also may appear with other diseases, as streptococcal infections, rheumatic fever, endocarditis, or tuberculosis. There are tender, red nodules, often in the anterior aspect of the tibia; rarely, in the arms or other parts of the body. After a time, the red color changes to bluish and brown. Patients should be hospitalized; if a known infection is present, it should be treated adequately; and if lesions need local help, use wet dressings. Pain felt in lesions may be helped with analgesics.

Sodium bicarbonate, 3% solution (8 teaspoonfuls in 1 liter of water).

Erythema Multiforme

Symmetrical lesions are characteristic in the distal limbs, showing concentric rings; in severe cases they are combined with bullae on the mucosae. The Stevens-Johnson syndrome, a severe form of erythema multiforme invading all visible mucosae, is a relatively frequent finding.

When there is an underlying disease—infection, rheumatism, lupus, ulcerative colitis—treat it vigorously also. Bed rest is imperative if there is fever. The initial painful lesions will be treated with wet dressings.

Sodium chloride, 1% solution (2 teaspoonfuls in 1 liter of water).

Sodium bicarbonate, 3% solution (8 teaspoonfuls in 1 liter of water).

Neomycin, 0.1% solution, to use as such.

But it mostly seems advisable to use antibiotic therapy, with a tetracycline, or sulfapyridine; and corticoids in more resistant cases.

Tetracycline, 250 mg, tablets, one every 6 hours, for 12 days.

Sulfapyridine, 500 mg, every 6 hours, also for 12 days.

Prednisone, 10 mg, every 12 hours, the first 2 or 3 days; then 5 mg, every 12 hours, for another 2 or 3 days; finally, decrease gradually to total stoppage in 3 days.

Ulcers

An entire chapter in this book is devoted to ulcers, which may be consulted. Only a very brief review is given here.

When the skin loses its superficial layers and becomes ulcerated, pain is one of the most important associated symptoms. Ulcers may be due to trauma, infective diseases, circulatory insufficiency, nervous ailments, or cancer. Perhaps the most frequent form is the varicose ulcer in the legs, associated with evident varices and always pigmented. The diagnosis depends on the associated symptoms and signs.

Initial ulcers may be improved by use of topical antibiotic preparations, preferably in powder form, under adhesive absorbent bandages, which will allay pain. Also provide a water or an air mattress. If needed, analgesics might be given.

Codeine, 60 mg, by mouth, every 4 to 6 hours.

Propoxyphene hydrochloride, 65 mg, by mouth, every 4 hours.

Chronic ulcers will be better evaluated by a surgeon, since cancer may be a possibility. Should a cancerous ulcer provoke pain, opiates of the type of morphine will be given.

Morphine sulfate, 15 mg, by subcutaneous injection, as needed and tolerated.

Methadone, 10 mg, by subcutaneous injection, as needed and tolerated.

Gangrene

This necrosis of tissues nourished by an obstructed artery, which also was reviewed earlier, occurs most frequently in the distal parts of the limbs. The first symptoms are decrease in the variations in local temperature and in local warmth; and also some paresthesias. Fully developed, it is severely painful in both of the two types: dry gangrene, which shows a dark, almost black mummified area; and moist gangrene, infected by putrefying bacteria, and showing sloughing of tissues and foul odor. Its causes may be arteriosclerosis (senile gangrene), diabetes, thromboangiitis obliterans, emboli, arteritis, ergotism, freezing, heating, electricity and other traumas, nervous disease, and Raynaud's disease.

Treatment is surgical; the patient has to be sent immediately to a specialist. In the meantime, to allay pain, which may reach great proportions, opiates must be given.

> Morphine sulfate, 15 mg, by subcutaneous injection, as needed and tolerated.

> Methadone, 10 mg, by subcutaneous injection, as needed and tolerated.

> Meperidine, 100 mg, by subcutaneous injection, every 4 hours, or as needed and tolerated.

Trauma

Any injury will provoke pain in the skin: contusions, abrasions, lacerations, and wounds. The diagnosis is obvious in each instance.

When some sort of surgical repair must be made, the patient will be referred to a specialist. Local anesthesia will suffice in most instances; and rarely analgesics are to be given thereafter.

> Procaine, 1% solution, 1 to 3 ml, to infiltrate the wounded area.

> Codeine, 30 or 60 mg, by mouth, every 4 to 6 hours.

VESICLES

A vesicle or vesicula is a small epidermic bladder or sac containing a liquid, usually serous and transparent, which may become purulent or hemorrhagic; it is variable in size but not too large because in the latter case it constitutes a bulla. The general physician, who has to deal with some diseases that present vesicles, will keep in mind that: vesiculation follows a clinical picture of a general disease; if there is a general syndrome together with it, the syndrome presents some changes when the vesiculation takes place; the vesicle appears directly on the skin, or follows a previous macula or papule; the vesicle has a halo of erythema, or has no halo at all; the vesicle has an umbilication or other signs of trabeculation; and the vesicle breaks, leaving a bleeding spot, or slowly forming a crust. In this section, a few of the practical problems dealing with vesicles will be briefly reviewed.

Herpes Simplex

Mild cases of herpes simplex will characterize the clinical picture of the disease; but among the elderly, the disease will not rarely be accompanied by fever and even chills. A large number of febrile diseases will present herpes simplex. Clusters of small vesicles on an erythematous base appear anywhere on the body (around the mouth or the genitals, more frequently) with pain, burning, or itching. Regional tender adenitis may occur. In a few days the vesicles dry and form a crust, except in moist areas where they may become infected. Second attacks are not rare, in the same site as before. Be sure of the diagnosis (particularly in cases of vaginal herpes) by biopsy, culture of the virus, or increased serum antibodies, since *corticoids are formally contraindicated* in herpes simplex.

Try, in spite of contradictory reports, the local application of ether on the cutaneous lesions, or of idoxuridine (IDU) for superficial herpetic keratitis. Also, try methylene blue solution followed by white light exposure for herpetic ulcerations of the mouth, and drying agents, particularly when the lesions appear in wet areas.

> Anesthetic ether; apply a soaked gauze or cotton sponge for a few minutes.

> Idoxuridine, 0.1% solution, one drop to the affected eye, once an hour during the day and every 2 hours during sleep time.

> Methylene blue, 0.1% aqueous solution, applied to ulcerations and followed by direct exposure to sunlight or white light for 10 minutes.

> Bismuth formic iodide, powder; apply locally twice a day.

> Epinephrine, 1:100 solution; apply locally twice a day.

Herpes Zoster

Unfortunately, this is a frequent and at times severe disease affecting elderly persons. The *ophthalmic herpes zoster* is perhaps among the prevalent forms, lesions found over the cutaneous distribution of the nasociliary and other branches of the ophthalmic nerve, that is, around one eye from the forehead to the nose on one side of the face. There are also edema, inflamed tissues, and even corneal ulcerations, which usually terminate in opacities. In this form as in all other forms of zoster, pain may initiate the symptoms, at times reaching the intensity of agony. In other forms of zoster the lesions may be similar to varicella, but are limited to only one side of the body, corresponding to the cutaneous distribution of one nerve. The disease may start as an ordinary infection with fever, chills, and malaise. Also, in the case of *otic zoster* there will be a sudden pain with fullness of the ear, tinnitus, slight deafness, and even vertigo or nystagmus. There may be facial paralysis; and the vesicles are seen on the auricles and the canal.

No specific therapy is available, but pain can be relieved, and the disease shortened, by the adequate use of corticoids. It is extremely important to differentiate herpes zoster from herpes simplex, particularly when located in the ocular area because corticoids are positively contraindicated in herpes simplex. Other analgesics can be tried. Persisting neuralgia after disappearance of skin lesions might respond to infiltration of the affected area with triamcinolone acetonide (see above) and lidocaine solution.

> Prednisone; start with 40 to 50 mg a day, in divided doses; decrease slowly to smaller amounts as soon as improvement is noted; and after 7 or 10 days of therapy, discontinuance will be started, also at a slow pace.

> Triamcinolone acetonide, 40 mg suspension for intramuscular injection in the gluteal areas as the starting medication, to afford rapid relief; then, continue as stated above.

> Acetylsalicylic acid, 600 mg, in tablets, every 4 hours, preferably with meals.

> Codeine, 60 mg, by mouth, every 4 to 6 hours.

> Meperidine, 100 mg, by mouth, every 4 or 6 hours.

> Lidocaine, 2% solution, 1 to 5 ml, for each specific painful area.

> Procaine, 0.5% solution; inject a total of 200 ml in some 50 to 100 different points; the procedure may be repeated once a week, for a few weeks.

Variola

Rarely will this disease be seen today, but until its total disappearance, we shall be aware of severe headache, among the initial and outstanding symptoms of variola, together with pains in the muscles and back. If pain is accompanied by an abrupt elevation of temperature, with chills and marked malaise, then the patient comes from the very few places where smallpox is still reported, the physician must suspect that disease. Good evidence will be a fall in temperature about the third day and the appearance of a rash of light-red macules on the mouth, forehead, and temples, which rapidly spread to the head, neck, limbs, and trunk, and possibly to the muscosal surfaces, axillae, palms, and soles. The macular character rapidly, and all at the same time, changes into papules, *umbilicated vesicles,* and then pustules. This central depression does not occur in varicella, which might have been one of the diagnostic considerations. With the developing rash, the other symptoms worsen, especially the headache. Initially the blood count shows leukopenia, changing to leukocytosis, as the pustular character of the rash progresses. Viral inclusion bodies occur in the blood and tissues, including Guarnieri's bodies in the rabbit's eye after inoculation.

Rigid isolation and report are mandatory, with forced bed rest and symptomatic treatment for pain, itching, undernutrition, and dehydration. Pain may respond to acetylsalicylic acid alone or combined with another analgesic.

Septicemia (Bacteremia)

In a few cases patients with septicemia will present vesicles, or other similar symptoms. Bacteria invading the circulating blood may provoke fever, commonly of the hectic (septic) type, mostly with chills, at least at the onset, and headache, as well as frequent skin rashes. Bacteremia ordinarily spreads from a known infected area, and is suspected when from such an infection there is no improvement in due time, or if, instead, there is an exacerbation of septic symptoms. Of course, the site of origin may be unknown (cryptogenic bacteremia). Most commonly bacteremia follows: erysipelas, having the characteristic well-delineated red area with swollen borders, located mainly around the mouth or the eyes, but also on limbs or trunk; or tonsillitis, otitis, urinary sepsis, or dental abscess. In turn, bacteremia may produce new focal sites of infection, particularly in the heart (check continuously for early detection of endocarditis), central nervous system (mainly meningitis), vascular system (thrombophlebitis), lungs (abscess, pneumonia, infarct), or skeletal system (osteomyelitis). Blood cultures will establish the diagnosis, in most instances.

The basic treatment depends on the offending infective organism and its sensitivity to antibiotics, which will be administered accordingly.

Pneumonia

Pneumonia is a disease ordinarily of sudden onset, characterized by sharp pain in the diseased side of the thorax, accompanied by elevation of temperature, chills, headache, and cough, with or without expectoration. This is one of the characteristic diseases with herpes, of only a few vesicles, ordinarily in the peribuccal area, mostly the upper lip. The production of a pinkish sputum rapidly turning to a rusty hue is one of the characteristic features of pneumonia. Dyspnea with tachypnea and a special expiratory grunt are very frequently found. Early, fine râles are heard on auscultation, and finally all the well-known signs and symptoms of the disease are well developed. There are forms of pneumonia among the elderly that present very little symptomatology, but in all cases, the roentgenological examination gives the diagnosis.

The acute disease with marked symptomatology will most proably be a *pneumococcal* infection. In *hemolytic streptococcal pneumonia* the pharynx is swollen and inflamed, the tonsils are covered with exudate, and, not rarely, there is a pleural effusion. *Staphylococcal pneumonia* ordinarily occurs as a complication of other staphylococcal infections, either postoperatively, following attacks of influenza, or as a form of hospital (or any other concentration of people) infection by resistant strains. *Klebsiella pneumoniae* is suspected when consolidation rapidly spreads from lobe to lobe. In *tularemia pneumonia* there is a history of some contact with wild animals, particularly rabbits. The onset of *viral or mycoplasmal pneumonia* infection is slow and shows few symptoms. *Aspiration pneumonia* follows the introduction of foreign matter (food) into the respiratory system.

For *pneumococcal pneumonia* give penicillin, cephalothin, or cephaloridine.

For *Klebsiella pneumoniae* give kanamycin, gentamycin, or chloramphenicol.

For *Hemophilus influenzae* use ampicillin or chloramphenicol.

For *streptococcal pneumonia* start with penicillin or erythromycin.

For *staphylococcal pneumonia* use oxacillin, nafcillin, or cephalothin.

For *viral pneumonia* use a tetracycline.

For *aspiration pneumonia* use ampicillin and a corticoid.

More details will be found in the corresponding entry in the chapter devoted to "Pain."

Encephalitis

In cases of encephalitis, there are many persons who develop crops of herpetic vesicles. These generally appear on the face, but may be seen elsewhere also. Together with the typical clinical picture of herpes simplex there are also fever, chills, and a respiratory syndrome which may mimic influenza; but soon neurological symptoms appear, such as tremors, muscle spasms, changes in reflexes and behavior, insomnia or somnolence, diplopia (in most cases a very important symptom), sialorrhea, or paresis. The encephalitic syndrome may be viral in origin or secondary to known diseases also of an infectious nature. Thus, there are California encephalitis, the Eastern or the Western equine encephalitis, the St. Louis encephalitis, and finally Venezuelan encephalitis, as well as encephalitis due to typhoid fever, pneumonia, influenza, abscesses, and others. The diagnosis is made by examination of the spinal fluid, determination of its cellular and chemical characteristics, and the isolation of the causative virus or other germ.

The patients must be isolated, in bed, and good hospital care observed from the beginning, particularly with respect to nutrition (intravenous or nasogastric), oxygen, control of convulsions, maintenance of an airway, and intracranial pressure. See some other treatment details in the following entry, on "Meningitis."

Meningitis

Crops of herpetic vesicles, usually abundant, may be noted in a large number of cases of meningitis, extended over the face and elsewhere. If it occurs with rigidity of the neck, contracture of other muscles, opisthotonos, strabismus, abdominal rigidity, irritability of all the senses, delirium, intense headache or nasal itching (a very suggestive sign, when present) bradycardia, and fever with chills, the possibility of meningitis comes to mind. Signs that should be elicited for confirmation are Kernig's (painful extension of a flexed leg), Brudzinski's (flexion of one leg when the other is forcefully flexed against the abdomen; also, flexion of the legs when the neck is flexed by force), Babinski's (plantar reflex reversed), and increased pressure of the spinal fluid, which also shows increased cells, protein, and a characteristic decrease of glucose content. The causative factor must be determined. Check the fluid for culture and sensitivity to antibiotics.

As in the above entry, keep the patient in bed with good hospital care, monitoring all vital signs, maintaining correct nutrition (intravenous or nasogastric if needed), with maintenance of a free airway and oxygenation, and control of convulsions and intracranial hypertension. If hypovolemic shock threatens, give isotonic electrolytic solution plus isoproterenol, add corticoids if there is delayed response. Cerebral hypertension due to edema will respond to mannitol; intravascular clotting, to heparin; and, most important, the causative factor should respond to antiobiotherapy—start with penicillin, and change to the specific antibiotic as soon as it is known.

Saline solution, isotonic, for intravenous use, 2 to 3 liters a day.

Isoproterenol, 0.2 mg in each ml; add 2 to 4 mg to each liter.

Prednisolone, 5 to 10 mg or more a day.

Mannitol, intravenously, 2 g per kilo of body weight every 24 hours.

Heparin, the amount needed to keep coagulation between 20 and 30 minutes.

Penicillin G, 20 million units a day, intravenously.

Malaria

The sequence *chill–fever–sweating* is characteristic of malaria. When the chill is intense, there are general shivering, chattering teeth, and difficulty in talking. Many patients will also present crops of herpes simplex vesicles around the mouth. The temperature reaches 40°C or more, and is usually accompanied by headache. Each attack lasts for the same period of time and is repeated at predictable intervals, according to the type of parasite involved: *Plasmodium vivax,* 5 to 8 hours, occurring every other day; *Plasmodium falciparum,* 20 to 36 hours, every fourth day; *Plasmodium malariae,* also every fourth day. The diagnosis depends on the identification of the parasite in blood smears. Control of paroxysms with the adequate antimalarial drug is also diagnostic. Attacks may last for more or less time, repeat at shorter intervals, be more or less violent, or be entirely irregular. Splenomegaly after the second or third paroxysm is a very important diagnostic sign. Untreated cases, because of a delayed diagnosis, may result in severe complications.

Plasmodium vivax and *P. malariae* infections are treated with primaquine, quinine, or amodiaquine: alternates are chloroquine, quinacrine, pyrimethamine, or chlorguanide. *P. falciparum* infection frequently responds with a complete cure to chloroquine, amodiaquine, or quinine, as well as to alternates such as quinacrine, or chlorguanide. In cases of *P. falciparum* resistant to the above medications, a combination of primaquine and quinine or pyrimethamine can be used. It is best to have any antiplasmodial drug in its highest concentration at the time of release of the merozoits into the bloodstream (chill).

Primaquine phosphate, 26 mg (15 mg base), by mouth every 8 hours, for 14 days.

Quinine sulfate, 600 mg, by mouth, every 8 hours, for 14 days. Watch for cinchonisn (tinnitus, deafness, vertigo, visual disturbances, headache, or hemoglobinuria).

Chloroquine phosphate, 1 g, first oral dose; then 500 mg, every 6 hours, for the rest of the day; thereafter, 500 mg a day, for 2 days.

Amodiaquine hydrochloride, 600 mg, oral dose, the first day; thereafter, 400 mg a day, for 2 more days.

Quinacrine hydrochloride, 200 mg, oral dose, every 5 hours to a total of five doses; thereafter 100 mg every 8 hours, for 6 days (in case of *P. vivax* and *P. malariae*) or up to 10 days (*P. falciparum*).

Pyrimethamine, 50 mg, oral dose, for the first day; thereafter, 25 mg a day, for 2 additional days (for 10 days in case of *P. falciparum* infection).

Chlorguanide hydrochloride, 300 mg, oral dose, every 12 hours, for 10 days (only once a day in cases of *P. falciparum*).

Influenza

In influenza there is a rapid onset of the disease, with fever, chills, muscle aches, a coryza-like syndrome with nasal stuffiness, cough, sore throat, and chest pains. Many patients will show crops of vesicles, particularly around the mouth. Malaise may reach true prostration, and many other people will deteriorate very rapidly. Weakness may develop during the course of the disease, and may persist for several weeks. Laboratory findings of leukopenia and isolation of the causative virus would probably be a help in the diagnosis. Many times there will be serious doubt as to whether a patient has a severe cold or influenza in a mild form. Usually the symptoms are more severe in influenza, present or residual weakness is greater, and the prevalence of similar cases favors the diagnosis. In bronchitis and pneumonia there are definite pulmonary symptoms, and the blood count shows no leukopenia but leukocytosis. Bronchitis and pneumonia are frequently a complication of influenza, and will be suspected when fever does not subside in 4 or 5 days or reappears after a frank remission. This is a dreadful complication for elderly patients who frequently succumb to it rather than to the influenza.

Immunization against influenza should be done in weakened patients and persons over 65 years of age, just ahead of the usual epidemic season, in November.

The treatment is purely symptomatic. Bed rest is ordered until 1 or 2 days following return of the temperature to normal. Antipyretic and analgesic drugs should be prescribed, either alone or with codeine, if coughing is troublesome. When other respiratory symptoms are bothersome, such as nasal stuffiness or sore throat, adequate medication should be recommended: nasal decongestants, sprays, or gargles. Complications—particularly staphylococcal pneumonia—should be treated as required, if possible, with the specific antibiotic.

Miliaria

These are very small maculo-papules that rapidly turn into superficial, red, and thin-walled vesicles which only in severe cases will present fever and other signs of heat prostration. The lesions appear only in overheated areas of the skin, particularly those exposed to bright, hot sunshine; they usually cause burning or itching. The disease occurs mostly in hot weather.

Use cooling, antipruritic lotions, drying lotions, antipruritic powders, and the needed treatment when there are secondary infections.

Anthrax

The most important of pustules may be those known as malignant pustule, or anthrax. It develops with a relatively large papule that presents a purple or black center, which vesiculates and is surrounded by an erythematous skin with smaller vesicles. The center ulcerates and turns into a necrotic eschar. There are the corresponding adenitis and a syndrome of acute febrile illness;

all symptoms worsen, and shock may occur at the sloughing of the eschar. The causative germ can be recovered.

Give a tetracycline if the case is not too severe, or large doses of penicillin if needed.

Tetracycline, 500 mg every 6 hours, by mouth.

Penicillin, by intravenous injection, 10 million units every day.

LYMPH NODES

Adenopathies may be found in any region of the body with lymph nodes. The enlarged lymph nodes may be independent or coalescing, hard or soft, tender or painless, adherent or nonadherent to surrounding tissues, and the size may vary considerably. At times, the presence of adenopathies may help in diagnosing a disease, but in many instances they have very little clinical significance.

Hodgkin's Disease

This disease, relatively rare among elderly people, was dealt with at the beginning of this chapter. The important diagnostic clues are adenopathy, fever, pruritis, and sweating. Large nodes may be seen first, which are firm and painless, adherent to deeper tissues but not to the skin, and of different sizes. The number and the location of the enlarged nodes give the classification of the four stages of the disease.

The disease can be treated with maximum advantage and minimum risk with combined therapy using procarbazine, nitrogen mustard, vincristine, and prednisone, or any similar combination.

Plague

In bubonic plague the start is rapid, but headache may be mild. There will be evident adenopathies, elevated temperature with chills, tachycardia, hypertension, irritability, restlessness, incoordination, delirium, hepatomegaly, and confusion. In pneumonic plague the symptomatology becomes extremely severe, and coughing, blood tinged sputum, and other signs of a progressing pneumonia appear. Other forms of plague are septicemic, meningeal, or pharyngeal plague. Confirm the diagnosis at the earliest possible moment, to start therapy, with specimens from aspirated nodes, blood, and sputum, and also complement fixation and agglutination tests, similarly checking all known contacts.

Use streptomycin as the antibiotic of choice, but if necessary use tetracyclines or chloramphenicol as a substitute. Maintain regular hospital care.

Carbuncle

It has been stated above, in this chapter, that a carbuncle is the coincidence of several confluent furuncles. At the same time, the corresponding lymph nodes are enlarged, and systemic manifestations are the rule, with fever, malaise, and the presence of several openings draining pus.

Start immediately with a broad-spectrum antibiotic, to use the specific one as soon as it is determined.

Lymphogranuloma Venereum

This disease rarely will be found at advanced ages, but may occur with sexually active patients. The diagnosis is made by draining inguinal buboes, which are soft and have a tendency to coalesce, have several openings draining pus, and later will present a marked scarring. It starts with an initial lesion on the genital area (vesicles or ulcers which fade rapidly) and a general disease syndrome with fever, headache, conjunctivitis, and joint pains; a positive Frei test and complement fixation will give the final diagnosis.

Tetracyclines are the specific antibiotic. Help locally with warm compresses, aspiration of secretions, dilation of strictures, and relief of pain.

Tetracycline, 500 to 1000 mg, every 6 hours, for 10 to 20 days.

Sarcoidosis

Diagnosis is made by the finding of multiple enlarged lymph nodes located on different parts of the body, which appear together with fever, joint pains, weight loss, skin lesions of the type of erythema nodosum, papules, and plaques. This is a variegated clinical picture, the diagnosis of which requires biopsy from the superficial lesions and a positive Kveim test.

Corticoids may serve to arrest the developing progressive lesions; and some cases will also respond to hydroxychloroquine for disfiguring skin lesions and hypercalcemia, but it is not to be given for more than 6 months, because of ocular damage. Relapses are the rule.

Prednisolone, start with 40 mg a day, and decrease the dosage after 2 weeks to a maintenance dose of 15 to 20 mg for 6 months; then discontinue it gradually.

Hydroxychloroquine, 200 mg tablets; give two to four a day.

Tuberculosis

Together with the regular symptomatology there may be small lymph glands felt in the neck and perhaps other areas of the body. The better diagnostic signs will be fever, cough, weakness, and night sweats.

The treatment will be carried out with two or more of the well-known antitubercular drugs.

Tularemia

Lymph nodes enlarge and drain during the course of a disease that presents recurrent chills following an acute onset of fever. There is also profuse sweating, and a local reaction at the site of the inoculation. Different clinical pictures may be present, such as pneumonia, usually with the regular symptomatology, but at times with only a few râles with marked decrease of breath sounds or a typhoid- or meningitis-like syndrome.

Streptomycin is the antibiotic of choice, to be given alone or, if there is not an evident improvement, together with a tetracycline or chloramphenicol. Keep the patient at rest, and give good hospital care.

> Streptomycin, 500 mg, every 6 hours, by intramuscular injection, until in 4 to 6 days the temperature falls to normal.

Brucellosis

This type of undulant fever usually presents enlarged adenopathies in the neck and the axillae, and the patients sweat profusely, feel extremely weak, and have pains in the head and joints. The diagnosis depends on the finding of one of the causative brucellas, or the increase of the agglutination titer over 1:100 during the course of the disease.

Tetracyclines are the specific antibiotic, to be given together with corticoids to the severely ill patient (corticoids not for more than 3 or 4 consecutive days!). Take good care of other symptoms.

Syphilis

As with lymphogranuloma venereum, some still-sexually-active aged patients may present the disease. The chancre of inoculation is followed by generalized adenopathy, fever, sore throat, malaise, and dermic manifestations. The laboratory examination will help with different blood or microscopic tests for syphilis.

Penicillin is the treatment of choice.

Leukemia

Here we merely remind the reader that there may be a sudden onset of fever, acute sore throat, articular pain, petechiae, ecchymoses, and other forms of bleeding due to thrombocytopenia, together with generalized adenopathies, hepatomegaly, and splenomegaly. Good hematologic studies will be decisive in diagnosing each variety of leukemia, thus helping in the choice of adequate treatment.

Vincent's Angina

Regional adenopathy is a prominent symptom when the disease starts suddenly with fever and local changes in the mouth: inflammation, bleeding, pain, profuse salivation, and extreme fetor. It starts as an acute tonsillitis and ends in necrotizing ulcerations. The laboratory will find one of the two main causative factors. (*Fusobacterium* or *Borrelia*).

Prefer peroxide and Fowler's solution locally as a mouthwash. Consult a specialist.

Peroxide, 10 cc in 20 cc water. Rinse mouth every 2 hours.

Follow with Fowler's solution of arsenic, 4 cc to 200 cc of water as a mouthwash every 4 hours. *Do not swallow*. Discontinue in 5 days.

JAUNDICE

There is evident clinical jaundice, with yellowish discoloration of conjunctivae, mucosae, and skin, when the bilirubinemia is over 3%; and a chemical hyperbilirubinemia without evident jaundice when the blood bilirubin is between 1.5 and 3%.

Cholangitis

Patients will show jaundice, fever, and a sharp pain in the epigastrium towards the upper right quadrant, with muscle guarding and tenderness on pressure (particularly if the patient makes an inspiratory movement). This syndrome may be due to inflammation of the bile ducts (cholangitis) or of the gall bladder (cholecystitis). The diagnosis is made radiologically.

Use broad-spectrum antibiotics, and consult a specialist.

Cancer

In dealing with older patients, cancer must be considered if jaundice develops together with a palpable gall bladder and other signs of deterioration. This may be a cancer of the head of the pancreas. Also, the cancer may involve the gall bladder or the bile duct. A good radiologic study will help. In all these cases consult a specialist.

Hepatitis

When a patient presents jaundice after starting with fever and upper respiratory and gastrointestinal symptoms, or urticarial rash and joint pains, look for the presence of hyperbilirubinemia and hepatic damage with elevated SGOT (over 40 u), SGPT, (over 45 u), and LDH (over 200 mu). If the Australian antigen is present, it will be a case of serum B hepatitis.

Only in cases of coma or fulminant hepatitis will corticoids be given.

Yellow Fever

If jaundice, hematemesis, and albuminuria appear in a feverish, severely ill patient, the diagnosis probably is yellow fever. There will also be chills, congested face, severe prostration, pains, and perhaps capillary bleeding. The virus can be isolated and serologic conversion confirmed. These patients live in or come from countries with yellow fever.

Treatment is only symptomatic.

Spirochetosis Icterohemorrhagica

Jaundice and hemorrhages characterize this disease, which starts abruptly with high fever, chills, pain in the abdomen and muscles, intense cephalalgia, red conjunctivae, capillary bleedings, and purpura; and after about 5 days the liver enlarges and jaundice appears. During the first 10 days the leptospirae may be found in the blood, and thereafter in the urine.

Treat with tetracyclines or with penicillin.

Meningitis

Rarely jaundice may be seen in these patients, but it may occur, and the physician must be ready to make the corresponding diagnosis.

Pancreatitis

The presence of jaundice is of little diagnostic help in cases of pancreatitis, though it occurs frequently. There is a sudden onset of epigastric pain, more marked on the left side; fever with tachycardia and marked hypotension, possibly to the extent of shock, pallor, abdominal distention and other gastrointestinal symptoms, and marked prostration. On physical examination there will be tenderness on pressure over the epigastrium and possibly a mass. Leukocytosis, elevated serum amylase (over 600 Somogyi units), and X-ray studies will help the diagnosis.

Give antibiotics against the intestinal flora, or the specific one as soon as known. Treat symptoms carefully in the hospital.

MACULAE-PAPULES

A short review of many diseases that present macules or papules will be presented here.

Smallpox

The initial rash of smallpox appears more frequently on the face and surrounding areas, but during the stage of macules and papules the diagnosis rarely will be made. These lesions turn into vesicles, which are umbilicated and appear of the same maturity. Treatment is symptomatic.

Relapsing Fever

This disease presents a sudden onset of fever, chills, and joint and muscle pains, headache, and an early erythema on trunk and limbs, eventually turning into red maculae, which may also be petechial. The total clinical picture subsides, to recur after 2 weeks. The laboratory will disclose the causative *Borrelia,* and patients should be treated with a tetracycline, penicillin, or chloramphenicol.

Salmonellosis

Maculae of a rose color that fade under pressure are noted on the trunk and abdomen during the course of a disease which grows worse and worse as time passes. The laboratory will differentiate between the different types of typhoid and para-typhoid fevers. The treatment is with ampicillin or chloramphenicol.

Rickettsioses

Different clinical pictures may occur, which may be diagnosed by laboratory procedures by means of the Weil-Felix reaction and the finding of specific antibodies. In most instances the rash helps to make the diagnosis, as follows.

Epidemic (classic) typhus shows the rash first on trunk and axillae, and then spreading to the rest of the body, occasionally becoming confluent or purpuric; there is no invasion of face, palms, and soles.

Endemic (murine) typhus presents a rash that is slightly petechial.

Trench fever starts the rash on chest and abdomen.

Rickettsialpox rash appears all over the body.

Rocky Mountain spotted fever rash appears on wrists and ankles, spreading toward the center of the body; it may be petechial.

Q fever presents no rash; only a few patients may show jaundice.

Tetracyclines or chloramphenicol are the best choice for treatment.

Bacteremia

Many patients with bacteremia will present a rash with papules, vesicles, or pustules, usually with purpura and petechiae, and many also show meta-static abscesses or localized infections, as pericarditis, endocarditis, arthritis, or meningitis. The fever is of the septic type, accompanied by chills. The diagnosis will be established through repeated blood cultures, particularly in the presence of a widely spread infectious process.

All these patients should be treated in the hospital, caring especially for electrolyte balance, general nutrition, and clearing of the infection whenever possible. The use of penicillin plus gentamycin will start the treatment for gram-negative species; use oxacillin or methicillin if infection is staphylococcal.

Penicillin G; give 20 million units a day by slow intravenous injection.

Gentamycin, 3 to 6 mg per kilo of body weight in 24 hours, in divided doses every 6 hours, intramuscularly.

Methicillin, 2000 units every 6 hours, in an intravenous drip lasting 30 minutes.

Tularemia

An inflamed papule on a finger, arm, eye, or mouth appears at the site of inoculation at the same time that fever with chills suddenly occurs, with prostration, headache, and gastrointestinal distress. Then the papule pustulates, ulcerates, and produces a scanty secretion, and local adenopathy will be noted with profuse suppuration. At this time a pneumonia may develop, the spleen enlarges, and other complications may occur. Isolate the causative germ from any one of the secretions. If contact with wild rodents is known, the diagnosis will be helped.

Treat with a combination of streptomycin plus tetracycline.

Cat's Scratch Fever

There is a papule with a central vesicle which may ulcerate, or the ulceraton may start as an injury, where a person was scratched by a cat a few days before. Also, there is a suppurative local adenopathy, and a febrile syndrome. A positive skin test may be made with antigen prepared from the pus.

Tetracyclines are recommended to shorten the disease, but their usefulness is uncertain. Also, some patients may improve after aspiration of the pus from enlarged nodes, or after excision.

Rat Bite Fever

In the streptobacillary infections a morbilliform rash is more frequent; in sodoku, it is a roseola-like urticarial rash. There is a remittent type of fever, usually with chills, and in some cases articular pains. In sodoku the lymph nodes are enlarged and will harbor the causative germ, which in streptobacillary infection will be obtained from blood or joint fluid.

Treatment with penicillin is effective. Alternates will be tetracycline for streptobacillary infections, and streptomycin for sodoku.

Yellow Fever

A macular eruption occurs in some patients with yellow fever, but the suspicion of the disease will start when there are a high fever, jaundice, and albuminuria in a patient with flushed face, tachycardia, headache, and other generalized pains. The patient should live or come from a country with endemic yellow fever.

Only a good symptomatic care can be given to these patients.

Dengue

There is a rapid onset of fever, chills, aches all over the body (breakbone fever), and a scarlatiniform or a maculo-papular rash that starts at the fall of the fever, and disappears promptly, followed by desquamation. Diagnose the disease by finding the germ in the blood during the acute stage. Treat symptoms.

PIGMENTATION

Chronic Adrenal Insufficiency

This diagnosis is not too frequently made with the elderly patient. Of course, in those cases in which the gland has been removed, the diagnosis will have been established before symptoms, including hyperpigmentation. In other instances, there is a tendency to a better tolerance of the disease when it starts during or after the sixth decade. If the diagnosis is deferred until hyperpigmentation, this will show first an increase of the intensity and number of moles, together with a darkening of knuckles, the genital areas, and most especially the gums. When these symptoms are noted, it will be good practice to test adrenal function. It will be unwise to delay the diagnosis until the whole body is hyperpigmented, with a fall of hair (particularly at the axillae), weakness, fatigability, anorexia, or other gastrointestinal distress, hypotension, and a rather small heart. Check for urinary excretion of keto- and hydroxycortocosteroids and the amount of corticol in the blood:

also it will help to know the level of ACTH and of sodium and potassium. Special tests can also be performed.

Most cases will respond well to cortisone or hydrocortisone, plus desoxycorticosterone or fludrocortisone. If the latter are added, beware of potassium depletion; but in all instances some sodium supplements are to be given.

> Cortisone; give 10 mg every 8 hours.

> Desoxycorticosterone; start intramuscular injections to supply 1 to 4 mg a day; after good response is obtained, it will suffice to inject the corresponding trimethylacetate only once a month in a dosage of about 50 mg.

> Sodium, a supplement of about 10 to 15 g a day.

Hemochromatosis

More frequently diagnosed among older people, the disease is often recognized because an already known diabetic patient develops hepatomegaly, and some evidence of splenomegaly may also appear, with heart enlargement, perhaps with symptoms of insufficiency, and most important the skin pigmentation. The latter has been described as a bronze color (bronzed diabetes), but it may vary from slate gray to brown—very easily confounded with the pigmentation of adrenal insufficiency (in which there is no hepatomegaly). Elevated iron in blood and in hepatic biopsies are characteristic.

Treat with phlebotomies, extracting about 500 ml every month, until the excessive iron storage has been depleted. Try deferoxamine in all cases, a chelating agent that has given good results in many patients. Treat other symptoms.

> Deferoxamine, ampoules containing 500 mg each; give 1 g at the start and two additional 500-mg doses every 4 hours; and thereafter 500 mg every 12 hours, all injected intramuscularly. Watch very carefully for cataracts and for renal insufficiency.

Porphyria

There are several clinical pictures of porphyria, not all reaching old age. The most important in older patients, the so-called porphyria cutanea tarda, is more frequent in men who are alcoholic. Hyperpigmentation of skin and even teeth occurs, particularly on the exposed areas, and other dermic symptoms may be hypertrichosis, pellagra-like erythema, easily produced congelations, and scleroderma, all reflecting an increased photosensitivity. Other symptoms of porphyria are dependent on the gastrointestinal system, neurological, or ocular. If there are more symptoms due to liver damage, it is better to think of a symptomatic form of porphyria. The urinary uroporphyrins are increased, giving the urine a red color. Since the urinary excretion of porphyrins is increased, these can be measured by laboratory means, thus confirming the diagnosis.

Recently, the administration of chloroquine has been advised as very effective. This should be tried. Otherwise, resort to phlebotomy, 500 ml every 2 weeks, until restoration of porphyrins to relatively normal levels.

Chloroquine, 125 and 250 mg tablets, take 250 mg a day during course of 5 to 7 days.

Pellagra

This disease, with its name derived from the Italian word for "skin" and its first accurate medical description from Asturias (Spain), can be diagnosed at any age. The discoloration appears on the dorsum of the hands, but in any other site also subject to the effects of physical agents or sunlight, such as the neck, the face, ankles, and feet (particularly when barefooted); and finally the skin turns dry, cracked, bright, and darkly hyperpigmented. The other prevalent symptoms are diarrhea and mental disorders, thus completing the three D's of diagnosis: dermopathy, diarrhea, and dementia. The etiologic factor links with deficient nutrition.

Niacinamide is the basic treatment; 500 mg daily, to be given by mouth, if possible, or by injection if there is a lack of cooperation, or there are well developed mental symptoms calling for higher doses. Other vitamins of the B group should also be given.

Xanthomatosis

The different xanthomatoses are forms of hyperlipemia or better hyperlipoproteinemia manifested by abnormal fat deposition in the skin, the tendons, and the eye, and even atherosclerosis. In addition to the latter symptoms, there are also xanthelasma (yellow patches of a soft nature developed around the eyelids), xanthoma tendinosum (similar, but harder, yellow patches developing in the tendon sheaths), arcus senilis (noted as a whitish ring around the cornea), and, finally, any change noted in the blood supply due to interference by atheromatous plaques.

Low-fat diets are essential in the treatment of these conditions, with unsaturated fats or the use of clofibrate, according to the case.

Clofibrate, 500 mg capsules; take four a day.

Acanthosis Nigricans

More of a warning than a disease itself, acanthosis nigricans develops in most instances of abdominal cancer, at times as a very early stage of development. It presents papillary growth of a very dark hue, almost black, thick and wrinkled, of a velvet-like appearance. This is noted mainly in the axillae, the neck and lower areas of the abdomen or groins. In all these instances, check for the abdominal cancer.

Liver Spots

Not rarely liver diseases will present some dermic symptoms, which will help in diagnosing the condition, even though they may not be constant. Remember the spider nevi, the telangiectasias, the palmar erythema, the chloasma-like discoloration, and hyperpigmentations similar to those noted in hemochromatosis though less marked.

Syphilis

Melanodermias, leukodermas, and other dyschromias may appear in or complicate all cutaneous forms of syphilis, which are manifold.

Leprosy

Persons who have had close relationships during youth with patients in infected places are usually the subjects of the disease, which makes it a rare occurrence in old age. Nevertheless, a long-delayed incubation period or infection due to tattooing or other similar procedures makes older patients possible subjects. Relatively large areas, up to 10 cm in diameter, become discolored from pink to red, or from violet to dark brown. Most of them are round, with clearly defined borders, noted on the extensor surface of the limbs or the back of the trunk. Some patches may have irregular borders, with a white-yellow center and a dark red border. Most of these spots are anesthetic. Later thickening of the lesions, the development of trophic ulcers, and bone resorption, causing a great distortion of limbs, will be almost diagnostic. There are two types of leprosy, the malignant lepromatous type, with nodular lesions rich in bacilli and with a negative lepromin test; and the progressive tubercular type, with few or absent nodular lesions, severe nerve involvement, fewer bacilli in the lesions, and a positive lepromin test.

Dapsone, amithiozone, or rifampin is used.

> Dapsone, 100 mg tablets; start with 25 mg twice a week, increasing gradually to a maximum of 300 mg twice a week, watching very carefully for intolerance. Recently this compound has been reported to be carcinogenic.

Vitiligo

This complete lack of pigmentation on relatively symmetrical areas of the skin, knuckles, elbows, or forehead, is surrounded by a border of somewhat increased pigmentation, as if the pigment were pushed away. This may occur at any age, in about 1% of the general population. The general problem of the disease is just the disfigurement it causes; but back in 1954 this was presented for the first time as the diabetes-vitiligo polysyndrome, stating that it was not a coincidence of two different syndromes but a consequence of one cause, in this case with the characteristic of almost a very mild diabetes. Thereafter, in England it was found that over 3% of all diabetics do present vitiligo; and more recently cases of glandular insufficiency with vitiligo were presented in the United States.

Toxic Pigmentation

We shall simply mention that dyschromias may be due to arsenic, silver salts, gold salts, picric acid, or hydroquinons.

Physical Agents

Also, dyschromias may be due to sunlight, radium, radiotherapy, ultraviolet light, and infrared rays.

ERYTHEMA

A very large number of diseases present erythematous reactions of the skin, but only a few will be mentioned here.

Scarlet Fever

This disease has been reviewed in some detail in other entries, but it is appropriate to say here that it may also be seen in relatively elderly individuals following an infection with hemolytic streptococci, particularly pharyngitis. A diffuse pink or red skin flush starts on the abdomen, flanks, lateral parts of the chest, and skin folds, here as darker lines, and with a characteristic pallor around the mouth, though the tongue is red with protruding papillae. The rash blanches on pressure and desquamates after the disease is over. Always watch carefully for nephritis, endocarditis, or septicemia. Check related persons for streptococcal infections.

The specific antibiotic should be given; but the starting treatment will use penicillin G benzathine, 1.2 million units, intramuscularly.

Relapsing Fever

This disease may start with an erythematous rash on trunk and limbs, which finally turns into red spots that may become petechial. It has a sudden onset: fever, chills, tachycardia, headache, body pains, gastrointestinal symptoms, and at times some upset of the respiratory system. Hepato- and splenomegaly, mental changes, and other complications may complete the picture. In about 3 to 10 days the fever decreases, and in 2 weeks there is a relapse of the whole syndrome; which may occur up to 10 times if the disease is untreated. The diagnosis is made by finding the corresponding *Borrelia* in the peripheral blood.

Tetracycline or penicillin is the best treatment, but given only at the start of an attack or during the afebrile period.

Rickettsial Diseases

These patients will present an influenza-like syndrome with cough and pains, with gradual appearance of more severe symptoms, such as elevated fever with chills, disabling prostration, headaches, and the positivity of the Weil-Felix reaction or the specific antibodies. In most instances, a rash appearing about 2 days after the initial symptoms will give the diagnosis. In epidemic classic typhus it starts on trunk and axillae, spreads to the rest of the body, and may become confluent or purpuric; in endemic murine typhus it is slightly petechial; in trench fever it starts on the chest and abdomen; in rickettsialpox it is generalized (all over the body); in Rocky Mountain spotted fever it begins on wrists and ankles, spreading toward the center of the body; and in Q fever there is not a true rash, but some jaundice.

Tetracyclines or chloramphenicol are the antibiotics of choice.

Secondary Syphilis

Beware of the bizarre and variegated symptomatology of secondary syphilis. It appears 6 or 8 weeks after inoculation (chancre), with slight fever, adenopathies, and other manifestations; most of the lesions are moist and rich in treponemas. Depend on laboratory tests to confirm the suspicion of the disease.

Penicillin, or erythromycin or a tetracycline, will be the remedy of choice.

Salmonellosis

Rose spots noted on the trunk, which fade under pressure, may help the diagnosis, when the clinical picture shows a worsening of all symptoms. Under the circumstances, do blood cultures during the first week, the Widal test during the second, and check for the germ in the stools after the third.

Ampicillin or chloramphenicol is the best treatment.

Cellulitis

The disease starts with fever and chills, malaise, and the characteristic erythema, warm, painful and swollen, with the borders poorly defined (not as in erysipelas, that is, sharply demarcated, with some elevation). In the case of cellulitis due to anaerobic germs, there is also crepitation noted to the touch.

Try to use the specific antibiotic, in all instances. In the meantime, use oxacillin, nafcillin, or erythromycin if the others are not tolerated. Surgery and the regular local care are used.

Oxacillin, 1000 mg every 6 hours, by mouth (or injection).

Erythromycin, 500 mg, as above.

Polyvalent gas antitoxin, to be given in all anaerobic cases, 50,000 units every 4 to 6 hours, by intravenous injection.

Erysipelas

Symptoms are similar to those of cellulitis, but the elevated borders here are sharply defined, red, warm, painful, and swollen. In severe erysipelas there are vesicles formed. The disease starts with a very bright red spot around the mouth, the trunk, or the extremities.

Local care, plus penicillin or erythromycin, gives good results.

Yellow Fever

Several times we have stated that whenever a patient lives in or comes from an infected country, yellow fever has to be suspected as soon as that feverish patient appears very ill and presents jaundice and black vomit, because of hematemesis, and shows albuminuria. The reason we mention this disease now is that not rarely it begins with an erythematous face. Laboratory tests will help the diagnosis (done in specialized centers).

Symptomatic care is the only help that can be given.

Dengue

Breakbone fever usually presents a sudden onset with elevated temperature, chills, prostration, depression, occasional sore throat, headache, and intense aches all over the body. There is also a skin rash, which will suggest the diagnosis when it occurs with fever and intense body pains. There is usually, after a few prodromal days, a defervescence with sweating, when the rash appears. Note that the rash may assume different dermatological characteristics.

Treatment is symptomatic.

Dermatomyositis

An erythematous rash during the prodromal stage occurs in most patients, with edema or not, appearing on extensor surfaces of the limbs, the face, or the eyes. The muscles beneath the rash are swollen and painful. There are other symptoms of toxemia and involvement of other systems. In older patients, check very carefully for the existence of malignancies.

Lymphangitis and Lymphadenitis

Lymphangitis usually occurs together with lymphadenitis. The first is due to a local infection and starts with fever, chills, general aches, and streaks of redness running from the site of infection to the corresponding lymph nodes. In thrombophlebitis there are similar streaks of redness, but without any noticeable adenitis. In cases of lymphadenitis, it may start with the corresponding lymphangitis, or may occur without it.

In all these instances check for the causative microorganism and give the specific antibiotic. Meanwhile, start with oxacillin or with erythromycin.

BLEEDING

Coagulation Defects

Except for senile purpura and thrombocytopenic purpura, most of the coagulation defects are very rarely seen in elderly persons. Nevertheless, a few of these defects will be considered.

Senile purpura seems not to be any particular disease of older people but the occurrence during this stage of life of disseminated intravascular coagulation or thrombocytopenic purpura. It may also be a deficiency of vitamin K or the existence of other endogenous substances preventing normal coagulation of the blood. In *disseminated intravascular coagulation* there is profuse bleeding, usually accompanied by collapse; bleeding from the nose, the mouth, or the anal area may reach large proportions, and there will be numerous petechiae and ecchymoses in the skin. The laboratory will report an almost total hemostatic failure, with no clot formation but a normal bleeding time, a low platelet count, and increased prothrombin and partial thromboplastin time. Heparin is effective, but check for a possible underlying cause, which should be treated as well. In cases of *deficiency of vitamin K* there is no bleeding history, but a history of poor feeding, malabsorption, prolonged antibiotherapy, or excessive use of anticoagulants; there are ecchymoses and other bleedings (but not joint bleeding). The laboratory reports will disclose a decrease of factors, IIa (normal factor V), VII, and X. Vitamin K in any of its forms is the best treatment. The *circulating anticoagulants* syndrome is noted for its prolonged coagulation time, provoking ecchymoses, hemarthroses, and gastrointestinal bleeding (including tongue and pharynx) and may appear in previously healthy older people. The coagulation time is largely over 30 minutes, and partial thromboplastin time is also prolonged; but prothrombin time is normal, as are bleeding time and platelet count. Very large doses of factor VIII (AHF or Hyland Antihemophilic Factor) are needed. For thrombocytopenic purpura, see next paragraph.

Thrombocytopenic purpura may occur at any age, and is a disease of very poor prognosis. There is always a low platelet count, a poor clot retraction, prolonged bleeding time, and a clinical picture with easy bleeding from all sites but without splenomegaly. Splenectomy is advised as the treatment of choice for these patients.

Hemorrhagic telangiectasis is a hereditary disease that has its peak incidence at about the sixth decade. Of course, there are other similar cases in the family, with telangiectasias appearing on the face, lips, tongue, mouth, nose, and hands (particularly the tips of the fingers and the toes). Anemia is the consequence of these bleedings, since these lesions are opened by minimal trauma. There is no treatment, but transfusions and iron may help in cases of uncontrollable bleeding.

Meningitis

Skin hemorrhages are a relatively frequent finding in all cases of meningitis: petechiae in mucous membranes, or an occasional hemorrhagic rash. In less than 4 days these hemorrhages disappear. The rest of the disease and its treatment will follow the regular known steps.

Rickettsial Diseases

The characteristic rash of rickettsial diseases may become purpuric in many instances; otherwise, there will be the regular pattern in each case, as seen in other entries in this book.

Dengue

In Asiatic countries, less frequently in other areas, there will be a petechial rash and other internal hemorrhages in addition to the regular clinical picture of the disease: sudden onset, elevated temperature, chills, headache, and very intense aches all over the body. There is leukopenia, and the causative virus can be recovered. There is no known treatment.

Dysentery

Both the amebic and the bacillary dysentery will present bloody stools, which testify to the intestinal hemorrhages. Other symptoms are: fever, copiousness of stools, abdominal crampy pains, and some evidence of dehydration. In bacillary dysentery try to avoid antibiotics, but give ampicillin (or a tetracycline) in case of need; in amebic dysentery use emetine followed by a tetracycline and finally diiodohydroxyquin.

Bacteremia

In many cases of bacteremia, petechial or purpuric lesion may occur. It will occur with the septic, spiking fever with chills and with other symptoms that indicate the origin of the infection, such as pericarditis, endocarditis, meningitis, arthritis, and others. The progression of the disease may provoke a massive hemorrhage, hypotension, renal failure, shock, and final death. Repeat blood cultures frequently until the causative germ is found. Maintain perfect nursing care, and give the specific antibiotic after previously starting with penicillin plus gentamycin if a gram-negative sepsis is assumed; or oxacillin for staphylococcus.

Endocarditis Lenta

Hemorrhages are an outstanding part of the clinical course of the disease, occurring from bruises and appearing in the mucosae, the skin, the retina, and epistaxis, and beneath the nails. The rest of the symptomatology will show a gradual onset of temperature with chills or chilly sensation, indefinite aches, night sweats, malaise, and evidence of some possible embolism (visual disturbance, hemiplegia, abdominal or respiratory pains). Not rarely heart murmurs will be heard, and blood cultures will be positive during the first week.

Prevent this infection in patients with heart disease who have to be operated on in the urogenital system or the mouth. Start the treatment with kanamycin, if possible. Most gram-negative infections will respond well to gentamycin or kanamycin.

Malaria

Hemoglobinuria (black water fever) may complicate long-lasting falciparum infection or other forms incorrectly treated. The clinical picture in these cases will be fever, hemoglobinuria, anemia, and jaundice. The rest of the picture will be consistent with the common type of the infection.

Spirochetosis Icterohemorrhagica

Together with the icteric symptom there will be hemorrhages characterized by capillary bleedings and purpura in the skin. The disease starts abruptly with elevated fever, chills, markedly red conjunctivae, severe headache and other pains in the abdomen and muscles, vomiting, and hepatomegaly with jaundice appearing the fifth day. Some cases may show symptoms of nephritis or meningeal irritation. The leptospirae are seen in the blood (first 10 days of disease) or in the urine (after 10 days).

Treat with tetracycline or penicillin, as soon as possible; and keep a constant watch for renal failure.

Plague

Plague may display a clinical picture called the black plague, presenting a rapid hematogenous spreading noted by purpuric spots. The rest of the clinical picture does not differ from the regular pattern, and the diagnosis is made as usual by blood cultures or the aspirate of buboes.

The patient is hospitalized as soon as possible, with the best possible nursing care and treatment, starting immediately with streptomycin plus tetracycline.

Polyarteritis Nodosa

The general symptomatology of polyarteritis nodosa includes fever; pains in the abdomen, loins, and muscles; arthritis; hypertension (half the patients); and involvement of multiple organs and systems, including the blood vessels. Usually, cases will show dermic manifestations of purpura, but also erythema, urticaria, subcutaneous nodules, and edema; and some may start with bloody stools. Diagnosis is made by the wide combination of symptoms, and confirmed by biopsy findings.

If there is a general reaction to a particular drug, it should be stopped immediately. The rest of the treatment will be supportive, but corticoids occasionally give some help.

Erythema Multiforme

The characteristic dermatologic lesions, which occasionally may become hemorrhagic, are symmetrically distributed on distal parts of the limbs or on the mucous membranes, and are of an annular, target-type pattern with concentric rings, with erythematous macules, papules, wheals, or bullae. There are fever, malaise, and articular pains, not rarely following herpes simplex eruption, most frequently during the spring or fall. Recurrences are not uncommon. The Stevens-Johnson syndrome presents more prevalent hemorrhages and is a more severe disease.

In the severe cases, corticoid therapy is justified.

REACTIONS TO DRUGS

Here the reader will find a list of the drugs that have more frequently been found to provoke reactions, noted by dermic symptoms.

ACTH
Aminopyrine
Anovulatory drugs
Antipyrine

Allopurinol
Androgens
Antimalarial drugs
Arsenicals

Barbiturates
Birth control drugs
Bromosulphthalein

Bromides

Busulfan

Carisoprodol
Chlordiazepoxide
Chlorpropamide
Coumarin

Chloramphenicol
Chloroquine
Corticoids
Cyproheptadine

Dextran
Diphenylhydantoin

Dextropropoxyphene

Enzymes and extracts
Erythromycin

Ephedrine

Gold
Guanethidine

Griseofulvin

Halogens
Hydantoin

Heparin

Insulin
Isoniazid

Iodides

Lithium

Meprobamate
Methyldopa

Mercury

Neomycin

Novobiocin

Opium

Paraaminosalicylic acid
Phenolphthalein
Phenylbutazone

Penicillin
Phenothiazine
Procaine

Quinacrine

Quinidine

Reserpine

Salicylates
Streptomycin

Serums
Sulfa drugs

Tetracycline
Thiouracil

Thiazide
Tolbutamide

LOCATION OF SYMPTOMS

In the great majority of instances, the location of dermic symptoms is of little diagnostic help. Nevertheless, some indications may be gained by considering location, as follows:

Head

The initial rashes of smallpox and dengue appear most frequently on the face and surrounding areas. Other erythematous initial rashes may also appear in this vicinity, as Boston exanthem.

Eyes

Some sort of conjunctivitis, reactional to the causative factor, is seen in the following instances:

Common cold: mild disease, with upper respiratory symptoms.

Scarlet fever: usually together with a relatively severe angina.

Erysipelas: the main lesion appearing as redness of skin delimited by an elevated border.

Influenza: a severe "common cold" together with pains all over the body.

Typhus and other rickettsial diseases: conjunctivitis and dermic rash (see above, for distribution of these rashes).

Smallpox: evidence of a very severe disease, followed by the appearance of maculae.

Spirochetosis icterohemorrhagica: with jaundice and bleeding.

Meningococcemia: with stiff neck and other neurologic syndromes.

Tularemia: with enlarged, draining lymph nodes and papules that ulcerate.

Trichinosis: with edema of the eyelids, and local hemorrhages.

Diphtheria: with pseudomembranous angina.

Neck

Adenopathy occurs in infectious mononucleosis.

Chest

Several rashes start on the chest.

Path of a Nerve

Vesicles appearing over the cutaneous distribution of a nerve (ophthalmic, geniculate ganglion, intercostal) are indicative of herpes zoster.

Trunk

Think of relapsing fever, typhoid fever, typhus, and dengue.

Limbs

In secondary syphilis lesions may appear on palms and soles; also in erythema multiforme. The rash may appear on wrists and ankles in Rocky Mountain spotted fever.

XV. SURGERY FOR THE ELDERLY

TO PROLONG LIFE OR PROLONG AGONY

It is not easy to decide in favor of or against a drastic procedure when the life of the very old patient is in deadly danger. In other words, will the medical decision prolong life and thus merely prolong agony? In this book, the reader has very frequently seen the suggestion to call an experienced surgeon for advice, because when dealing with older people all problems increase in geometrical proportion to age.

On the othe hand, successful surgery should solve these problems, not merely attack them without regard to future events. The surgeon has to be conservative, because his skill is judged on his ability to save lives. This often means the performance of almost impossible feats of mind and hands, but surgeons want to serve the patient, not astound the spectators.

For this reason, whenever the family physician sends the aged patient to a surgeon for a solution to his problems, the first advice returned to the physician is "the less surgery, the better," and this is almost always right.

In consequence, the seven following questions have to be carefully answered, if there is genuine desire to serve the patient:

What are the chances of survival with or without an operation?
What are the risks of surgery or of non-surgery?
What are the advantages and disadvantages of operating?
What are the desires of the patient himself?
What is the attitude of the family regarding the problem?
What does a future in a nursing home mean?
What can be done in this particular case?

Risks

This comes very close to the above criteria. If the risk of the disease is a small risk, leave it alone; if the risk is great, act. If the risk is neither great nor small, and there is a little chance for medical treatment, treat medically until the last moment because there is always risk in any surgery done on the older patient.

Resulting Comfort

The risk of the result of the operation and the risks of leaving the patient with the punishment of suffering are to be measured. The only advantageous situation will occur when the operative risk can compare favorably with the risks of doing nothing to help. No matter that the operation poses a severe limitation of activities or imposes a number of operations to follow; it will always be beneficial if the suffering from the disease is avoided by this means.

The Attitude of the Patient

A negative attitude in a patient is a black cloud on the horizon. On the contrary, if the attitude is positive, even miracles can be expected. The reason for this is clear: either consciously or unconsciously he will disobey and contradict, or will obey and accept all that the surgeon tries to do to help. It is true that there are persons who die because they will.

The Attitude of the Family

Families play a very important role in all these decisions. In the first place, there is some relationship, pleasant or unpleasant, between patient and relatives. Even in the best-regulated families a moment will arrive when the elder feels like an alien at home. Or the elderly person can be so troublesome and unpleasant that even the most loving relatives cannot cope with him. Patients will try to hide symptoms or to gain advantage with ailments. Getting family members to be frank with one another is most advantageous, for it is not a matter of their not doing what they cannot afford. We must believe that our society will pay for those who need the help—but we must not attempt to achieve results that cannot possibly be sustained.

Nursing Home

Most families will not be able to do what they are expected to do following surgery. At times the care of the patient requires long hours of attention, which will not always be available. Then the patient, and at times a lovely family, will resent the situation. Of course, the problem is greater with the nursing homes, which do not always give what they offer and what, by minimum standards, they should give. We are tempted to write a long chapter on this subject, but for understandable reasons we hold our peace.

What to Do

Repeatedly we have advised consultation of a specialist—a surgeon, ophthalmologist, urologist, or the like—whenever the decision of whether to operate must be made. This is the best procedure, the most humane, and also the least risky, now that the practice of suing the doctor has reared its ugly head.

Diabetes mellitus poses very difficult surgical problems. On the other hand, the diabetic patient is prone to need surgery. What should be done? When the disease affecting a diabetic patient follows a bad course, it is better to take the risk and operate. Take, for instance, acute cholecystitis.

Myocardial infarction requires delay until 3 months after the attack to make surgery less of a risk.

Peptic ulcer will be treated medically, but in cases of hemorrhage or perforation the surgeon will probably prefer to do operations of a similar technique (vagotomy, simple plication, pyloroplasty). If after about 4 weeks of a well-followed medical treatment there is no improvement, a suspicion of malignancy will arise, and perhaps more complex operations should be carried out. At times the procedure has to be decided upon after opening the abdomen.

Prostatic problems are usually treated by means of transurethral resection, preceded by catheterization and fluid therapy if there is renal insufficiency. It seems that these operations are well tolerated.

Cancer of the bladder is generally treated by fulguration of the tumor as seems advisable after periodic cystoscopy.

Appendicitis will be accepted by most surgeons as a cause for immediate operation, because of the disease itself, or because not rarely it is the clinical picture of right colon cancer.

Diverticulitis does not require operative procedures in most instances, except when there is a notable hemorrhage, or urinary tract symptoms are also prominent, there is an abscess not improved by medical treatment, there is fistulization (to the small intestine) and/or peritonitis, there is an important suspicion of cancer, or recurrent symptoms do not improve as they should with medical treatment. Most surgeons accept a safe one-stage resection.

Hernia will safely be operated on when needed, by herniorrhaphy with local anesthesia, but in all instances care will be taken for the diagnosis of a concomitant malignancy. Hiatal hernia rarely needs surgery, except in emergencies.

Gastrointestinal cancer requires a laparotomy, and the procedure is decided on on the spot. This holds true for gastric cancer. For cancer of the colon, surgery is also accepted by most surgeons because of the high rate of cure.

Intestinal obstruction will require early surgical exploration when no improvement is obtained by intubation.

Intestinal infarction is very frequent among the aged and usually responds to surgery.

Gallstones should not wait until emergency cholecystectomy is required, but an elective operation should be performed, or even a relatively minor cholecystostomy under local anesthesia. Surgeons usually advise operating for gallstones when they are symptomatic, when there is diabetes mellitus, when there is obstructive jaundice, and in frequent episodes of pancreatitis.

Abdominal aneurisms usually require surgery when they are large enough in diameter (over 7 cm), when there is hypertension, or when there is a progressive enlargement of the sac or local calcification. It is unwise to wait until rupture occurs because very few patients will be saved then.

Index of Drugs